Wolf-Heidegger's

Atlas of Human Anatomy

Volume 1

Petra Köpf-Maier, Berlin

Wolf-Heidegger's

Atlas of Human Anatomy

Volume 1

Systemic Anatomy, Body Wall, Upper and Lower Limbs

6th, completely revised
and enlarged edition, 2005

643 figures of which 510 are in color

KARGER

Editor

Univ.-Prof. Dr. med. Petra Köpf-Maier
Professor of Anatomy
Charité – Universitätsmedizin Berlin
Campus Benjamin Franklin
Institute of Anatomy
Königin-Luise-Strasse 15
D-14195 Berlin (Germany)

This Atlas is published in two volumes:
Volume 1: Systemic Anatomy, Body Wall, Upper and Lower Limbs
Volume 2: Head and Neck, Thorax, Abdomen, Pelvis, CNS, Eye, Ear

Until 1989 the Atlas was published as
'Atlas of Systematic Human Anatomy', vol. I–III
1st edition 1954
2nd edition 1960
3rd edition 1972
Spanish translation: Salvat Editores S.A., Barcelona
Portuguese translation: Editora Guanabara Koogan S.A., Rio de Janeiro

Since 1990 the Atlas is published as
'Wolf-Heidegger's Atlas of Human Anatomy'
4th edition 1990
Indonesian translation: EGC Medical Publisher, Jakarta
Japanese translation: Nishimura Co., Ltd., Tokyo
Portuguese translation: Editora Guanabara Koogan S.A., Rio de Janeiro

5th edition 2000
Chinese translation: Xi'an World Publishing, Xi'an
Italian translation: Edi-Ermes s.r.l., Milano
Japanese translation: Medical Sciences International, Ltd., Tokyo
Polish translation: Wydawnictwo Lekarskie PZWL, Warsaw
Portuguese translation: Editora Guanabara Koogan S.A., Rio de Janeiro
Spanish translation: Marban Libros, Madrid
Turkish translation: Günes Bookshops & Publishing Ltd. Co., Ankara

The original Latin nomenclature version with German and English captions is also available under the titles: 'Wolf-Heideggers Atlas der Anatomie des Menschen' / 'Wolf-Heidegger's Atlas of Human Anatomy'
Bd./Vol. 1: Allgemeine Anatomie, Rumpfwand, obere und untere Extremität/Systemic Anatomy, Body Wall, Upper and Lower Limbs: ISBN 3-8055-7662-5
Bd./Vol. 2: Kopf und Hals, Brust, Bauch, Becken, ZNS, Auge, Ohr/Head and Neck, Thorax, Abdomen, Pelvis, CNS, Eye, Ear: ISBN 3-8055-7663-3
Complete set: ISBN 3-8055-7664-1

Library of Congress Cataloging-in-Publication Data

Wolf-Heidegger's atlas of human anatomy – 6th, completely rev. and enlarged [English] ed. / [editor] Petra Köpf-Maier
p. cm.
'The original Latin nomenclature version with German and English captions is also available under the titles: 'Wolf-Heideggers Atlas der Anatomie des Menschen'/ 'Wolf-Heidegger's atlas of human anatomy'' – T.p. verso.
Includes bibliographical references and index.
Contents: v. 1. Systemic anatomy, body wall, upper and lower limbs – v. 2. Head and neck, thorax, abdomen, pelvis, CNS, eye, ear.
ISBN 3-8055-7667-6 (v. 1: alk. paper) – ISBN 3-8055-7668-4 (v. 2: alk. paper)
1. Human anatomy-Atlases. I. Title: Atlas of Human anatomy. II. Wolf-Heidegger, G. (Gerhard) III. Köpf-Maier, P. (Petra)
[DNLM: 1. Anatomy-Atlases. QS 17 W859 2005]
QM25.W633 2005
611'.0022'2–dc22 2004057765

KARGER
Basel • Freiburg • Paris • London • New York • Bangalore • Bangkok • Singapore • Tokyo • Sydney

Printed in Switzerland on acid-free paper by Reinhardt Druck, Basel
ISBN 3-8055-7667-6

The editor dedicates
this book to her grandson

Leander Leonin

Homage to Those Who Bequeathed Their Bodies to Science

'Hic locus est ubi mors gaudet succurrere vitae'

'This is the place where death delights in helping life'
(Inscription above the Anatomical Theatre of Bologna)

The present atlas of human anatomy shall not begin without paying due homage and returning thanks to those who freely bequeath their bodies to anatomy. Such donations testify to an admirable, unselfish, and idealistic sense of sacrifice, and nothing can compensate for the invaluable service rendered to science and to society. Anatomy and medicine owe these individuals a tremendous debt of gratitude. By bequeathing their bodies, they enable medical students to learn through real observation and direct 'grasping', and even now, at the beginning of the twenty-first century, there is no substitute for this. Thus, even beyond death, these altruistic people help the living – medical students, physicians, and patients alike. This is how the above inscription should be interpreted, and students should make every endeavour to be worthy of these voluntary and generous body donations by respecting and honoring the dead as well as by working hard and learning eagerly.

Contents

Contents of Volume 2:
Head and Neck, Thorax, Abdomen, Pelvis, CNS, Eye, Ear

Preface to the 6th Edition

With his *Atlas of Systematic Human Anatomy,* Professor Dr. Gerhard Wolf-Heidegger edited a standard work among the anatomy atlases between 1950 and 1971. This is now its 6th edition.

In the preceding 5th edition, published in 2000, the editor had already thoroughly modified the Atlas:

- Most of the black-and-white anatomical drawings were colored didactically;
- Numerous new, generally topographically orientated illustrations were added;
- All technically outdated X-ray plates were replaced by new ones;
- Many new X-ray plates and radiological sections, i.e. computed tomograms (CTs) and magnetic resonance images (MRIs) as well as ultrasonograms were included, and
- CTs and MRIs were consistently matched with anatomical sections for comparison.

This clinically and radiologically oriented new concept of the earlier, more systematic, editions of the Atlas, and in particular the combination of anatomical sections, CTs, MRIs and ultrasonograms for comparison, was received very favorably by many readers, users and reviewers of the 5th edition.

This course has been held in the 6th edition and more clinical aspects have been integrated, with the long-term objective of turning the Atlas into a clinically focused work. This also conforms with the new programs leading to the MD degree, which have been implemented in Germany as of the 2003/4 winter term, stipulating that preclinical studies must integrate much more clinical topics.

Concretely, this clinically oriented remodeling of the present 6th edition consists of the following innovations:

- Numerous **clinically relevant illustrations** have been added, such as the motor segments of the spine, the venous circulation in the lower limbs, the arrangement of the cervical fascia, and the projection of the heart and cardiac valves onto the surface of the thorax, or the portocaval anastomoses. The resulting clinical situations, such as disc herniation, formation of varices, spread of inflammation in the neck, location of the cardiac auscultation points, or the bypass circulation of a stenosed hepatic portal vein, are shown in order to illustrate how clinical phenomena may easily and correctly be inferred from anatomical and topographical situations.
- Typical **manifestations of paralysis** of the main arm and leg nerves are illustrated as well. A perturbed function of nerves cannot be understood without knowing their normal function – or to put it differently – clinical symptoms of nerve paralysis can be explained easily and correctly based on the normal anatomical function of nerves. In the present context, this means that there is no clinical understanding without well-founded anatomical knowledge.
- In volume 2, the **section of interest to dental students** has been considerably enlarged. New illustrations of the temporomandibular joint, the structure of teeth, the topographical relation of the upper teeth to the maxillary sinus, the toothless aged skull, the trabeculae and trajectories in the upper and lower jaws as well as the typical fracture lines of the facial skeleton and skull base have been added.
- The common **eponymous synonyms** of anatomical designations used in the Atlas have been integrated into the labeling of the figures and the subject index. An eponym is a term that is composed of a proper name – often that of the person who first described a given structure. Eponyms are generally short expressive designations that are usually less complicated than the corresponding anatomical term, and are thus generally preferred to the anatomical term in current clinical use. They should thus be learned and known as well.
- In addition to these innovations, the 6th edition of Wolf-Heidegger's Atlas now employs the **'Terminologia Anatomica'**, the approved anatomical nomenclature adopted and published a few years ago. Moreover, as far as possible, the synonyms mentioned in the Terminologia Anatomica have also been included in the labeling of the figures and the subject index.

Without the enthusiastic collaboration of experienced graphic artists knowledgeable in anatomy, it would not have been possible to include so many new anatomical illustrations in the 6th edition of Wolf-Heidegger's Atlas. First and foremost, the editor would like to acknowledge Mrs. Gertrud Heymann-Monhof, who had already designed many of the anatomical illustrations of the 5th edition. She has also prepared most of the new illustrations of the 6th edition with her confirmed artistic power and deep understanding of the world of anatomical structures (*vol. 1:* figs. 4a,b, 5c, 6a–c, 24, 45, 49a–c, 70a,b, 71a,b, 102, 103a–e, 148, 149, 178a–d, 179a–d, 180a–d, 181a–c, 262a–d, 298a,b, 299a–d, 300a–d, 301a–d, 302a–d; *vol. 2:* figs. 8a,b, 14, 16, 27c, 30c, 31a–d, 32c,d, 39b, 40, 41a–d, 52a,b, 53a–c, 116, 117a,b, 158a,b, 159a–c, 222, 223, 233a–d, 237a–c, 272, 273, 274, 275, 317, 345, 346, 348, 349, 350a,b, 351b, 352b, 362a,b, 363a,b). Mr. Hendrik Jonas, who had already collaborated on the 5th edition as well, has drawn figures 141a,b, 142a–c, 259a,b of *volume 1* and figures 49a,b, 51a–c, 54a–c, 56d, 68e of *volume 2* in a style admirably suited for Wolf-Heidegger's Atlas.

I would also like to cordially thank Professor Dr. Martin Herrmann, Ulm, as well as Privatdozent Dr. Reimer Andresen, Güstrow, for our many discussions concerning the new concept of the present Atlas and the provision of new radiographs. Many thanks also to Professor Dr. Gottfried Bogusch, Institute of Anatomy of the Charité, Berlin, for granting access to the Anatomical Collection of this institute. This has considerably facilitated the preparation of new illustrations of the head and, especially, the teeth. I would also like to extend my thanks to Dr. Frank Neumann, dental surgeon in Berlin-Reinickendorf, for the generous provision of numerous radiographs for the design of page 55 in the second volume. Dr. Andreas Winkelmann, Berlin, has given me his support for the inclusion of eponyms and the preparation of the lists of eponyms. I thank him very much for his expert collaboration.

My special thanks go to Dr. h.c. Thomas Karger, the Publisher, who has actively engaged in the project of Wolf-Heidegger's Atlas during the past years until today. He has consented high financial investments and has always lent an understanding ear to my concerns and wishes while preparing the 5th and 6th editions. Mr. Hermann Vonlanthen has initiated and supervised the implementation of all the technical measures for producing the 6th edition and transferring the data to a new software. Mr. Beat Pfäffli designed the layout of the new illustrations, carried out the text corrections and coordinated all the work connected with the Atlas: his expertise and untiring enthusiasm have significantly contributed to the realization of the present 6th edition of Wolf-Heidegger's Atlas.

Mrs. Monika Risch has assisted me very efficiently during the preparation of the present new edition and has thus enabled me to work on this Atlas; I would like to thank her very much.

I also thank the readers, users and reviewers of the 5th edition of Wolf-Heidegger's Atlas for their numerous letters and oral comments. They contained many valuable remarks and suggestions for improvements, which I have taken into account and integrated into the present 6th edition whenever possible. In this connection, I would like to express my thanks to my colleague Professor Dr. Renate Graf from our institute, who made many valuable suggestions for improvements and additions, especially in the field of head and neck anatomy; I have largely used them for the present 6th edition. This has permitted the chapters on the head and neck, of special interest to dental students, to be augmented in a clinically relevant manner.

I do ask the readers and users of the present 6th edition of Wolf-Heidegger's Atlas to let me know their criticisms, suggestions for improvements or modifications because only a lively dialogue between the author and the readers and users of a textbook or an atlas, resp., will enable this work to be improved over the years and tailored to the needs of its readers and users.

Berlin, Autumn 2004 Petra Köpf-Maier

Preface to the 5th Edition

Macroscopic anatomy is a fundamental branch of medicine without which clinical facts cannot be understood.

Throughout history, the importance of anatomy for medicine – and thus for medical studies – has fluctuated considerably. Five hundred years ago, at the end of the Renaissance, Leonardo da Vinci and Andreas Vesal laid the foundation stones of modern anatomy and modern medicine. In those days, anatomy – then exclusively macroscopic – was the only fundamental speciality medical students were confronted with during their studies, along with the clinical subjects internal medicine, surgery and botany (in the meaning of use of herbal drugs).

The first half of the twentieth century saw the development of microscopic anatomy besides macroscopic anatomy; physiology became an independent speciality and physiological chemistry and biochemistry made huge progress. Research in these fields provided new knowledge on functional and molecular interactions in the mammalian organism which fundamentally altered our understanding of diseases and opened new perspectives in clinical diagnosis and therapy. As a consequence of these developments, macroscopic anatomy was somehow relegated to the background during the 1960s and 1970s, and seemed to have retained its essential importance only for surgical specialities.

Apart from these developments, new diagnostic imaging technologies have become clinically established in the second half of the twentieth century: computed tomography, magnetic resonance imaging and ultrasonography. These imaging techniques opened up new visions of the morphology of the living organism, enabled a very detailed identification of structures and thus laid the foundation stone of rapid and unexpected progress in clinical diagnosis. However, the interpretation of normal and pathologically altered structures in two-dimensional images of the human body with all these techniques demands extremely precise anatomical knowledge. In recent years, this has led to the revival and to a considerable increase in the significance of macroscopic anatomy both for clinical medicine and the education of medical students.

Successful clinical work without well-founded knowledge in topographical and sectional anatomy is thus no longer possible. This is the reason why the editor urges present and future medical students to study macroscopic anatomy intensively.

As a matter of fact, it is the establishment of the new imaging techniques in clinical medicine that prompted this new revised version of Professor Wolf-Heidegger's Atlas of Human Anatomy, which had been continued by H. Frick, B. Kummer, and R. Putz in its 4th edition, and the supplementation of its 5th edition with numerous anatomical sections, computed and magnetic resonance imaging tomograms and ultrasonograms. Such a new design of an atlas of the anatomy of the whole human body is only possible with the collaboration of many enthusiastic forces. Thus I am deeply indebted to Dr. R. Andresen and Priv.-Doz. Dr. D. Banzer (Berlin) for most of the new radiographs as well as the computed and magnetic resonance tomograms included in this atlas. Prof. Dr. G. Bogusch (Berlin), Prof. Dr. E. Fleck (Berlin), Dr. M. Jäckel (Göttingen), Dr. H. Kellner (Munich), Priv.-Doz. Dr. T. Riebel (Berlin), Priv.-Doz. Dr. C. Sohn (Heidelberg), Dr. D. Zeidler (Berlin) and Prof. Dr. W.G. Zoller (Munich) contributed some further radiographs, tomograms and ultrasonograms for which I would like to thank them.

I am moreover deeply indebted to Prof. Dr. M. Herrmann (Ulm) who provided the anatomical sections for most of the computed and magnetic resonance tomograms of the present atlas and thus considerably enriched it. The sections on which these illustrations are based were prepared and photographed by Mr. E. Voigt (Ulm), whom I would like to thank as well.

I also express my thanks to Mrs. G. Heymann-Monhof, Mr. H. Jonas, Mrs. H. Heinen, Mrs. I. Tripke, Mrs. C. Naujok and Mr. F. Geisler who prepared about 230 new anatomical drawings for the present edition.

My special thanks go to Dr. h.c. Th. Karger for his constructive collaboration during the past years. Dr. Karger always lent an understanding ear to my concepts, which were often difficult and expensive to realize, and was a partner whose expert advice and understanding always helped me in my work with the atlas. Many thanks in particular to Mr. B. Pfäffli as well as to all the personnel of S. Karger Publishers and Neue Schwitter AG who helped in the production of Wolf-Heidegger's atlas.

Mrs. M. Risch, my secretary, has been a great and dependable help over the past years, which has eased my work in many respects. I would like to thank her as well.

This new edition of Wolf-Heidegger's *Atlas of Systematic Human Anatomy* has been supplemented by numerous new anatomical drawings, radiographs, tomograms, ultrasonograms and anatomical sections. As the editor, I am confident that this new edition will indeed 'help one to see' – one of the most difficult things, according to the quote from Goethe, which Wolf-Heidegger chose as the motto for the first edition of his atlas – and that it will give medical students better access to anatomy and clinical medicine:

> 'What is the hardest of aught? What seemeth the simplest to you:
> With your eyes to see that which is in front of your eyes.'
>
> Johann Wolfgang von Goethe,
> Distichon 155 of the 'Xenien' (translated by M. Pfister, Berlin)

Berlin, Spring 1999

Petra Köpf-Maier

Information for Users

1. Anatomical Nomenclature

In the present atlas, all anatomical structures are consistently designated according to the 1998 Issue of the Terminologia Anatomica (TA), the currently approved international nomenclature. For reasons of consistency, terms like 'urogenital diaphragm' have also been deleted although the editor and many other anatomists do not fully understand the reasons for their elimination from the TA.

If the TA mentions two or three synonyms for a structure, they appear in the subject index with a cross-reference to the main entry (preferred term). Space allowing, these synonyms are also mentioned in the figures following an equal sign (=) and the preferred term.

2. Spelling

The German spelling conforms to the 'old' German spelling rules, as used in Switzerland, that is spelling with 'ss' instead of a sharp 's'.

3. Eponyms

An eponym is a term frequently used in the clinical routine that includes a proper name – often that of the person who first described the structure. Eponyms are expressive and less complicated than the anatomically correct terms and are thus preferred in clinical use. Current eponyms appear as follows in the present atlas:

- The name of the person after whom the eponym was named is printed in parentheses and capital letters behind the respective anatomical term in the figure.
- Tables that match the eponyms and the anatomical terms and vice versa have been inserted before the subject index. The first table also includes the main biographical data of the persons after whom the eponyms were named.
- The corresponding cross-references have been included in the subject index.

4. Abbreviations

The following current abbreviations are used throughout:

Singular			Plural		
A.	=	*Arteria*	*Aa.*	=	*Arteriae*
Lig.	=	*Ligamentum*	*Ligg.*	=	*Ligamenta*
M.	=	*Musculus*	*Mm.*	=	*Musculi*
N.	=	*Nervus*	*Nn.*	=	*Nervi*
Proc.	=	*Processus*	*Procc.*	=	*Processus*
R.	=	*Ramus*	*Rr.*	=	*Rami*
V.	=	*Vena*	*Vv.*	=	*Venae*

Moreover, to save space, the following abbreviations had to be used in some instances:

cut.	=	*Cutaneus*
F.	=	*Fonticulus*
Ggl.	=	*Ganglion*
Gll.	=	*Glandulae*
lymph.	=	*Lymphoideus*
Pl.	=	*Plexus*
Var.	=	*Variation*

5. Brackets and Parentheses

The synonyms of the TA are placed in square brackets [ ] if they do not appear with an equal sign (=) behind the main entry. These equivalent terms also appear in the index; an arrow refers to the main entry.

Parentheses ( ) are used to note terms also shown in parentheses in the TA, moreover for designing varieties, complementary information and explanations. The relative size of the figure, expressed as a percentage of the original size, is also shown in parentheses in the legends.

Terms commonly used moreover, but not mentioned in the official TA, are indicated in pointed parentheses ⟨ ⟩.

6. Formation of Genitives

Unless they are official designations of the TA, complicated Latin genitives have been avoided since these days only few students have a sufficient command of Latin. Instead of the complete genitive, we have generally first indicated the generic term (bone, artery or nerve) and then, on the following line, without a comma, the specific term:

Examples:	*Os occipitale* *Pars basilaris*	or	*Glandula thyroidea* *Lobus sinister*

7. Dashes

A dash *following* (left column) or *preceding* (right column) an entry indicates that one or several specific entries for the same body part will follow. The generic term is shown above it – usually without a pointer:

Examples:	*Corpus fibulae*	or	*Plexus brachialis*
	Facies lateralis –		*Pars infraclavicularis*
	Margo anterior –		*– Fasciculus lateralis*
	Facies medialis –		*– Fasciculus medialis*
	Margo interosseus –		*– Fasciculus posterior*

8. Dots and Pointers

If dots on a pointer identify two or more anatomical structures or if several dots appear on the pointer, the various designations are separated by a comma; their order follows that of the arrangement of the anatomical structures in the figure. In both columns, the labellings are arranged according to the following general principle: left first, then right; in the case of branched pointers, above first, then below.

9. Notation of Sizes

Unless otherwise indicated in the legends, the anatomical drawings in the present atlas always represent the situation in adults; the percentages given in parentheses in the legends denote the relative size of the specimen. With a view to the considerable biological variations in body size, the percentages were rounded off and should only be considered as indicative.

10. MRI Tomograms

Enhancement of the tissue-specific relaxation parameters T_1 and T_2 in MRI tomograms is noted in the legends as T_1 or T_2 weighting. T_1- and T_2-weighted tomograms represent the various structures of the human body in different brightnesses and different contrasts. Thus, in T_1-weighted tomograms, liquid-filled spaces appear black, muscles dark and the bone marrow white. In T_2-weighted tomograms, liquid-filled spaces appear white, bones dark and muscles light gray.

11. Tomograms and Anatomical Sections

In current clinical practice, transverse (axial) computed and magnetic resonance imaging tomograms of the human body are always viewed from caudal, that is from below and looking up. This is the reason why, in the present atlas, the anatomical sections – with the few exceptions noted in the legends – are also viewed from caudal, that is from the patient's feet. While this view of the tomograms and sections is doubtless difficult for beginners, it does correspond to the physician's perspective when he approaches the supine patient from the foot end of his bed. The accompanying figure illustrates this view from caudal (bottom) to cranial (top) and makes clear that in this perspective the organs located on the patient's right (R) side appear on the left in the figure and the organs located on the left (L) side appear on the right side of the figure.

R

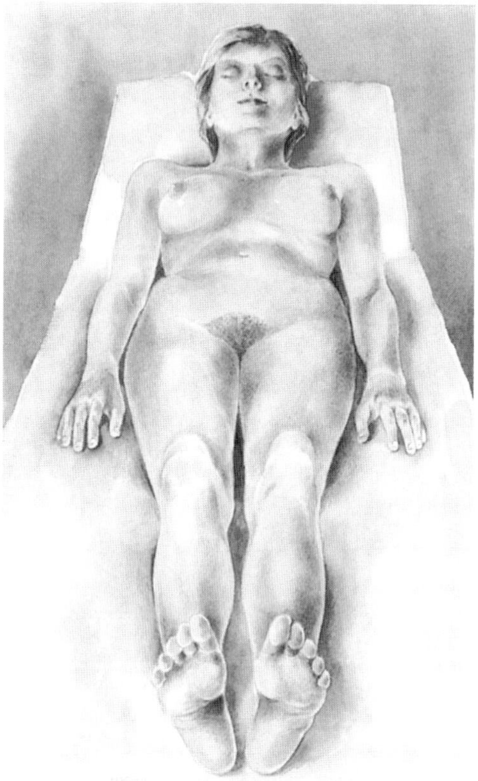

L

(Painted by G. Heymann-Monhof, Berlin)

Systemic Anatomy

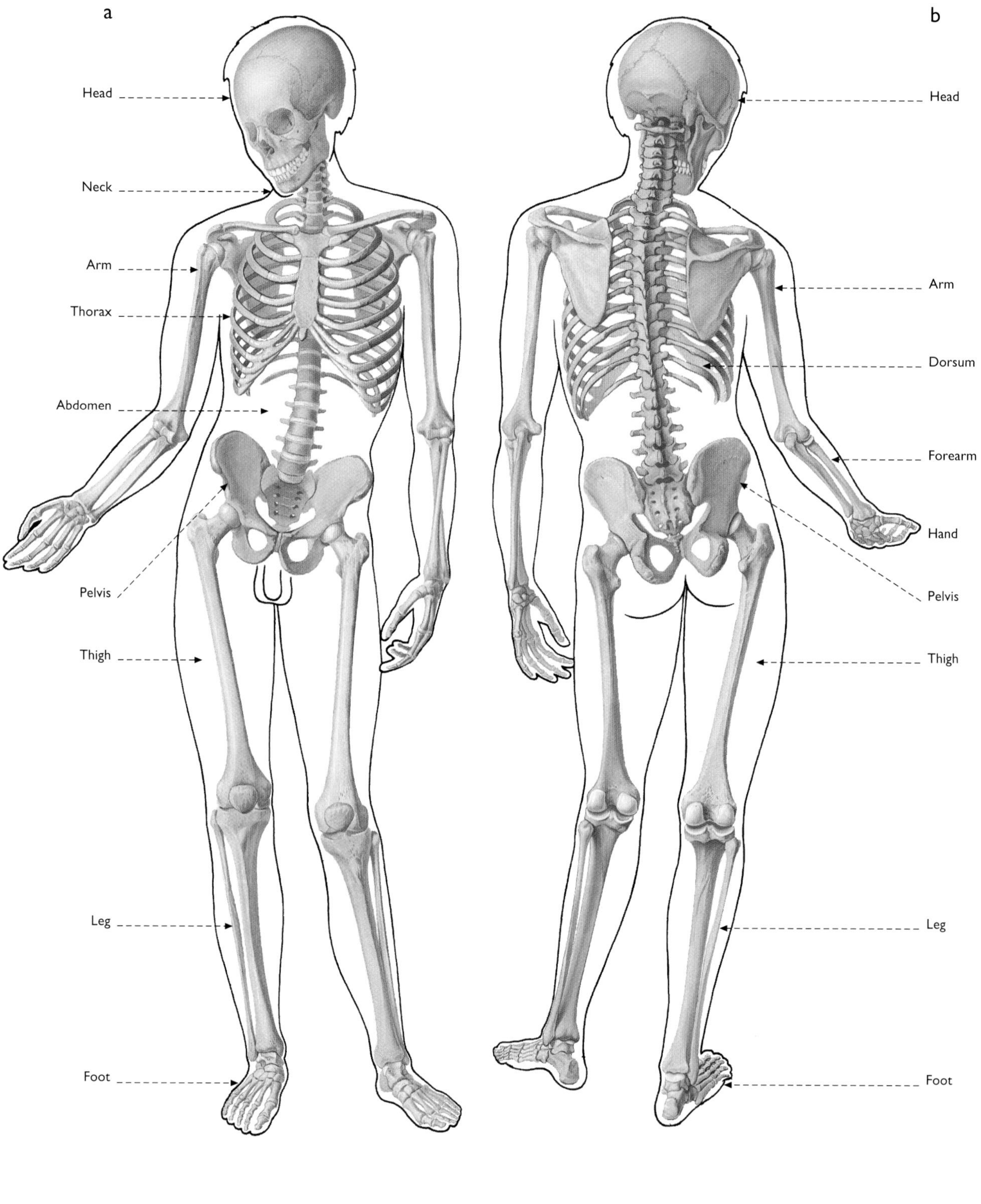
a
Head
Neck
Arm
Thorax
Abdomen
Pelvis
Thigh
Leg
Foot
b
Head
Arm
Dorsum
Forearm
Hand
Pelvis
Thigh
Leg
Foot

2 Skeleton and parts of the human body (10%)

Male skeleton

a Ventral aspect

b Dorsal aspect

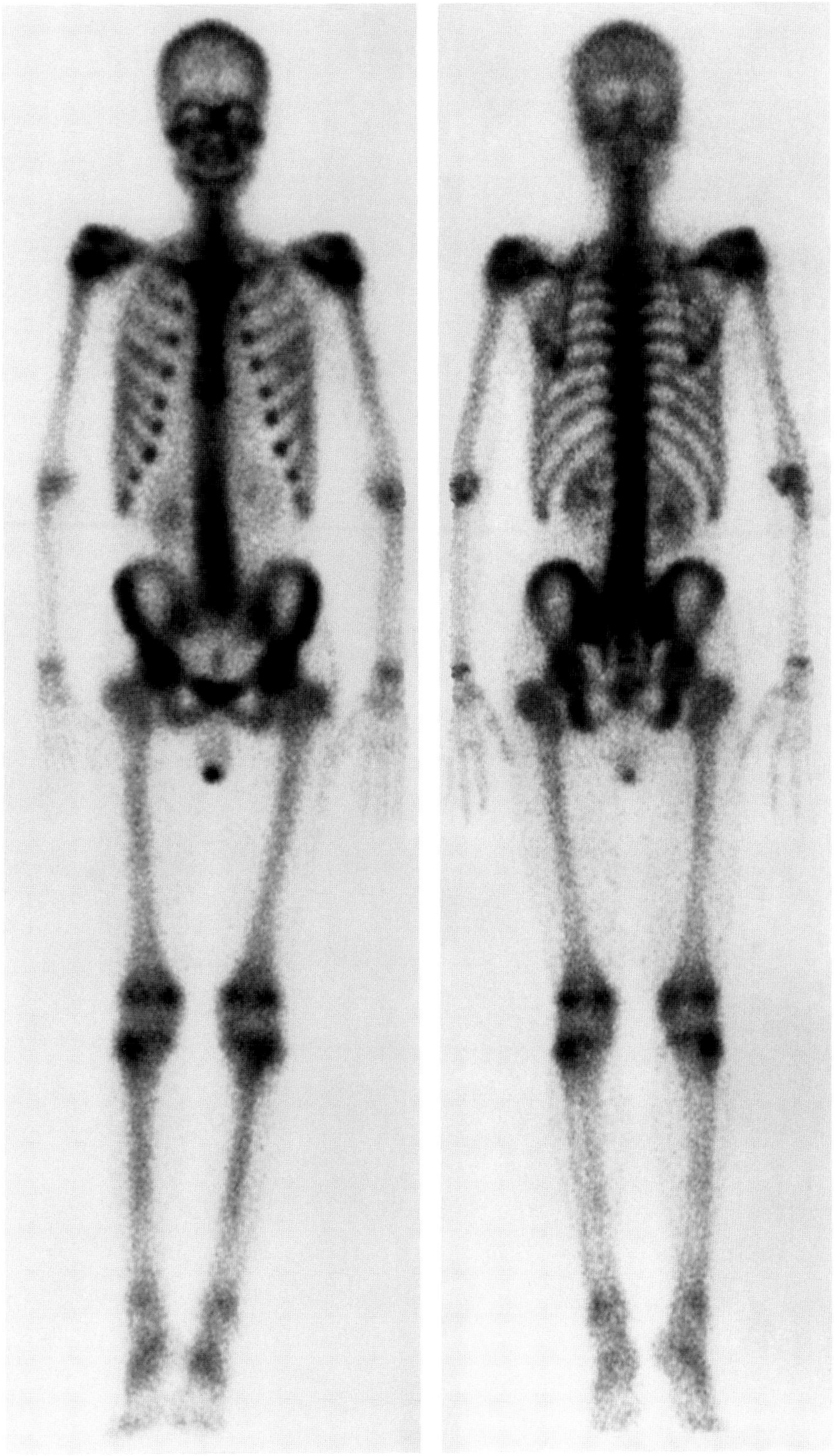

3 Skeleton of the human body (10%)

Male skeleton, scan of bones using ^{99m}Tc

a Ventral aspect

b Dorsal aspect

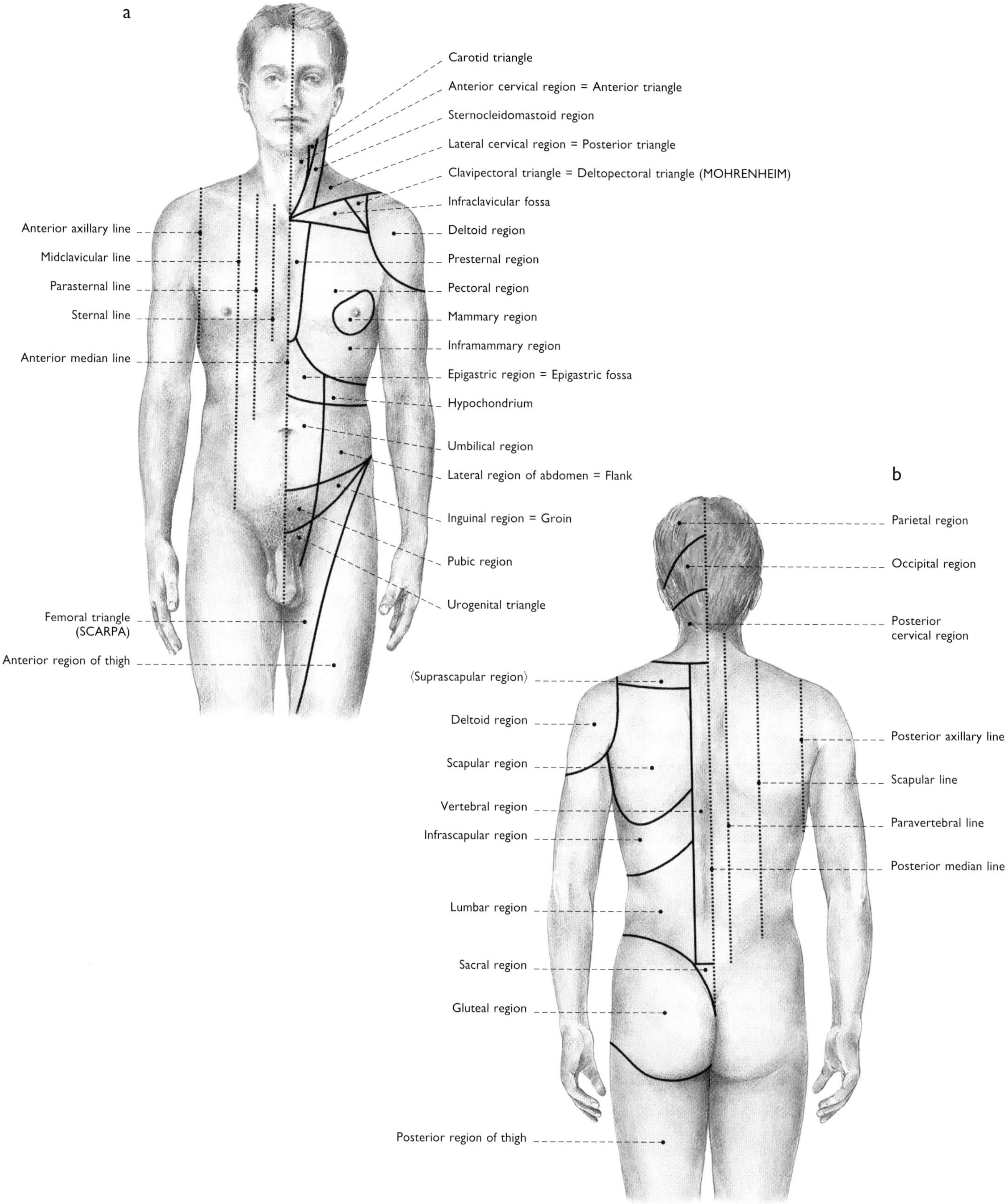
a
Carotid triangle
Anterior cervical region = Anterior triangle
Sternocleidomastoid region
Lateral cervical region = Posterior triangle
Clavipectoral triangle = Deltopectoral triangle (MOHRENHEIM)
Infraclavicular fossa
Anterior axillary line
Deltoid region
Midclavicular line
Presternal region
Parasternal line
Pectoral region
Sternal line
Mammary region
Inframammary region
Anterior median line
Epigastric region = Epigastric fossa
Hypochondrium
Umbilical region
Lateral region of abdomen = Flank
Inguinal region = Groin
Pubic region
Urogenital triangle
Femoral triangle (SCARPA)
Anterior region of thigh
b
Parietal region
Occipital region
Posterior cervical region
⟨Suprascapular region⟩
Deltoid region
Posterior axillary line
Scapular region
Scapular line
Vertebral region
Paravertebral line
Infrascapular region
Posterior median line
Lumbar region
Sacral region
Gluteal region
Posterior region of thigh

4 Regions and lines of the human body

a Ventral aspect
b Dorsal aspect

1 Coronal (= frontal) planes
2 Horizontal (= transverse = axial) planes
3 Sagittal, paramedian planes
4 Median plane (= plane of right and left symmetry)
5 Sagittal axes
6 Transverse axes
7 Longitudinal (= vertical) axes

a

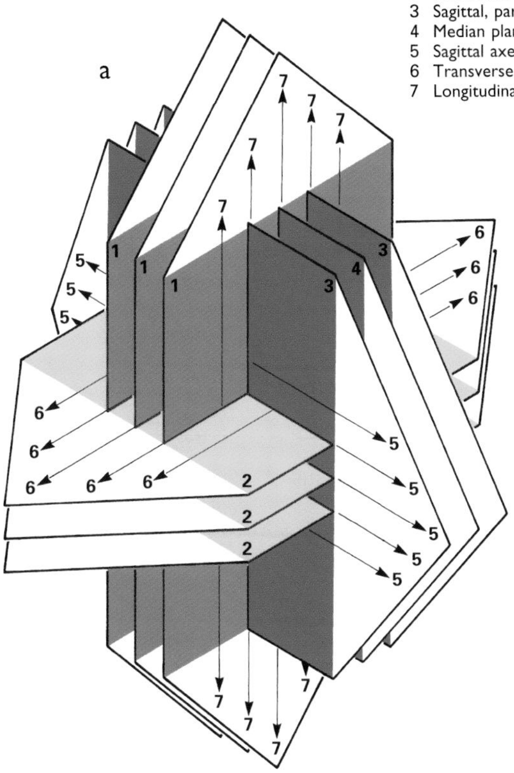

b

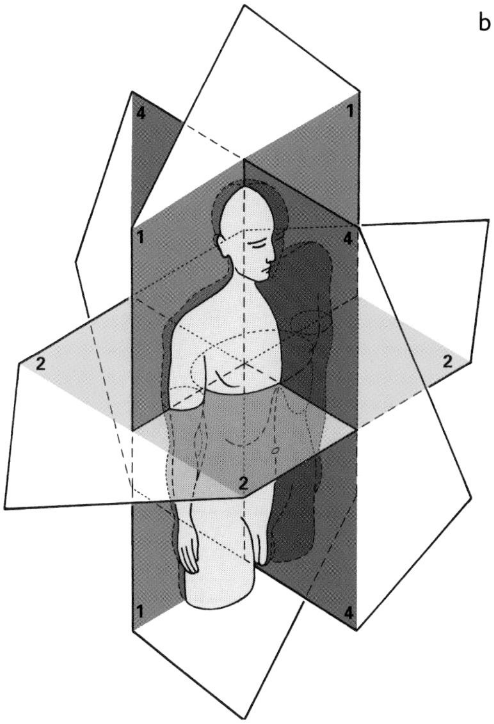

c

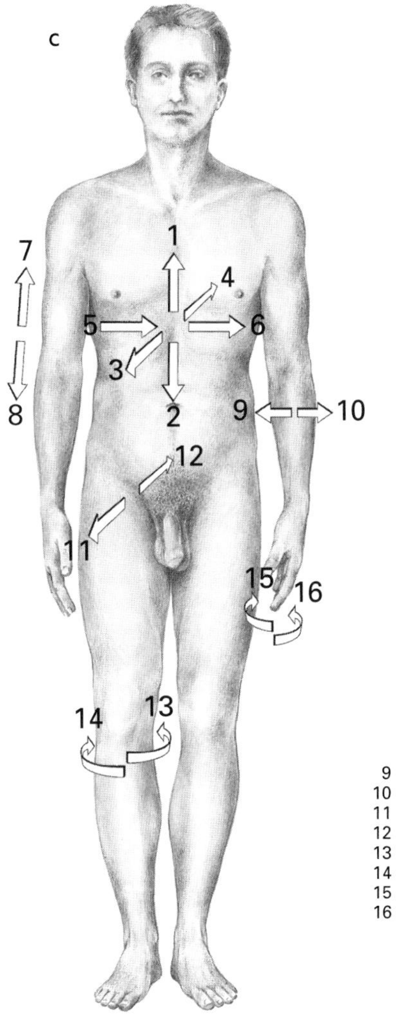

1 Cranial, superior
2 Caudal, inferior
3 Ventral, anterior
4 Dorsal, posterior
5 Medial
6 Lateral
7 Proximal
8 Distal

9 Adduction
10 Abduction
11 Flexion
12 Extension
13 Medial (= internal) rotation
14 Lateral (= external) rotation
15 Pronation
16 Supination

5 Planes and axes

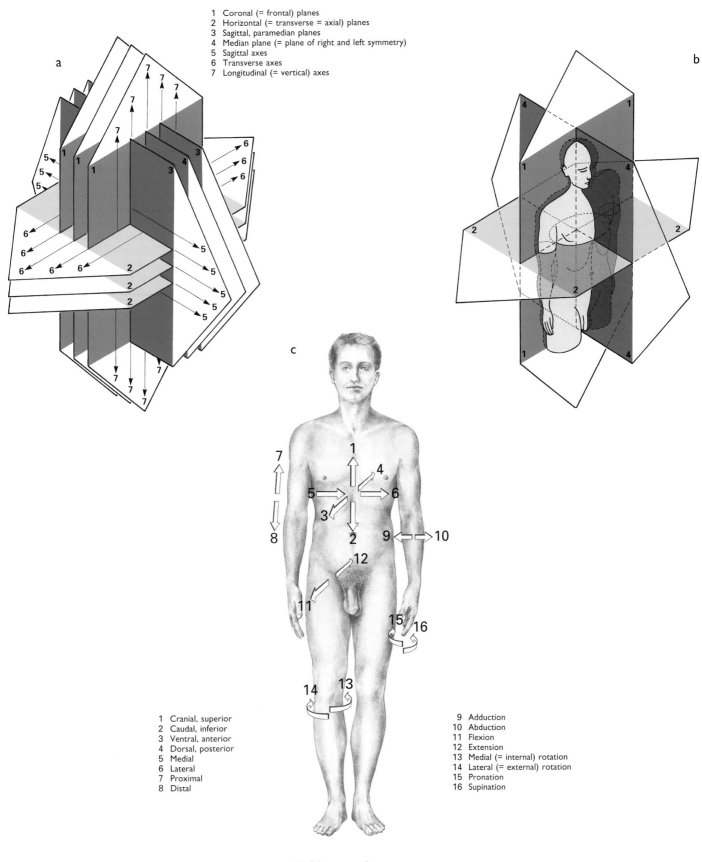

a Planes and axes
b Planes
c Spatial orientations and directions of motion

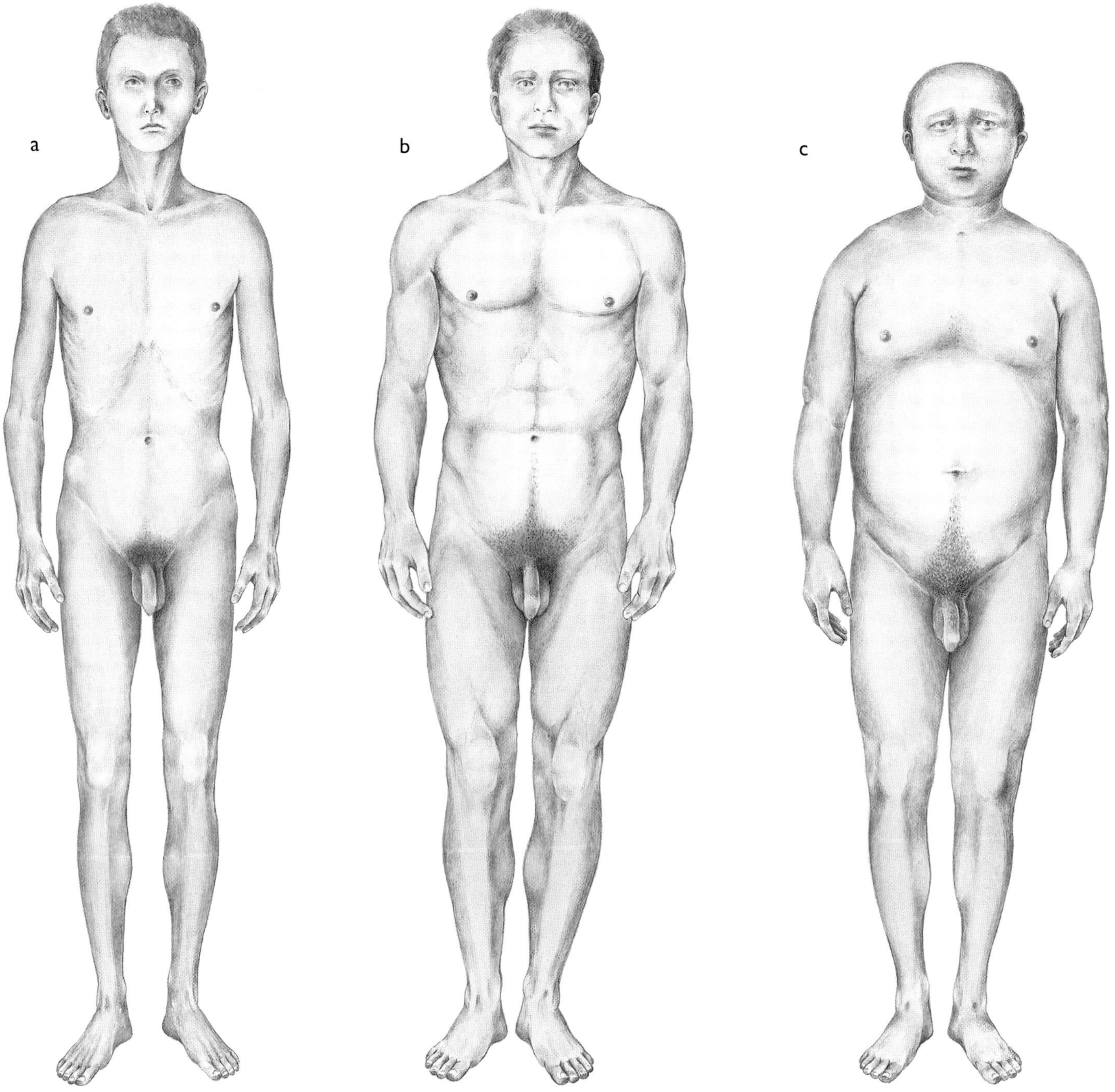

6 Body types

Ventral aspect
- a Leptosomatic person
- b Athletic person
- c Eurysomatic, pyknic person

a

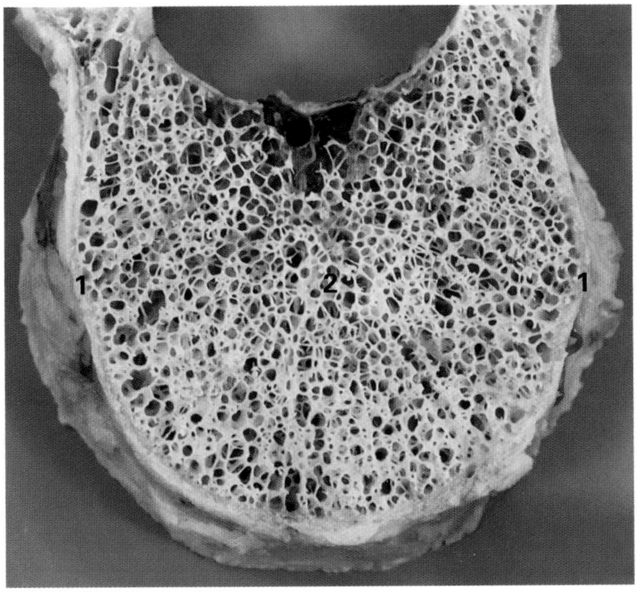

b

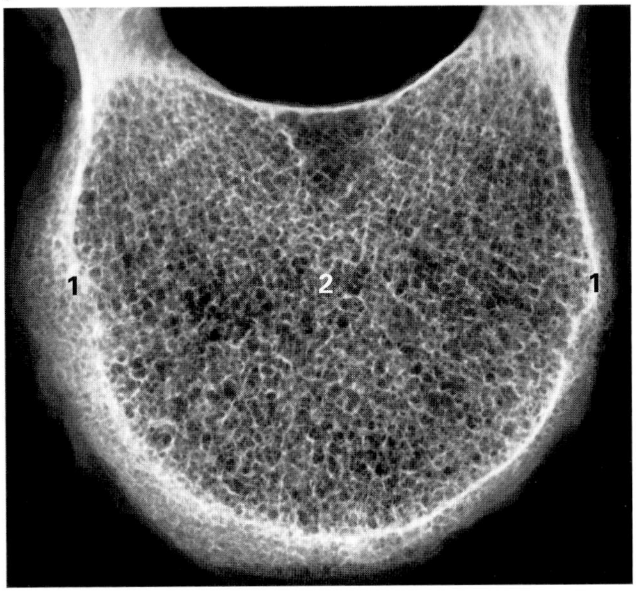

1 Compact bone
2 Spongy bone = Trabecular bone

c

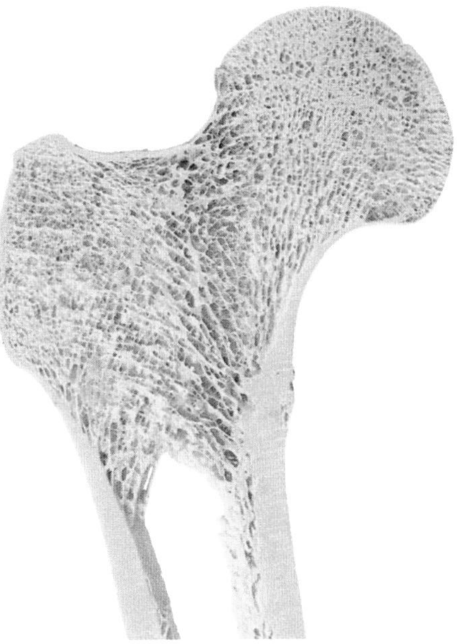

d

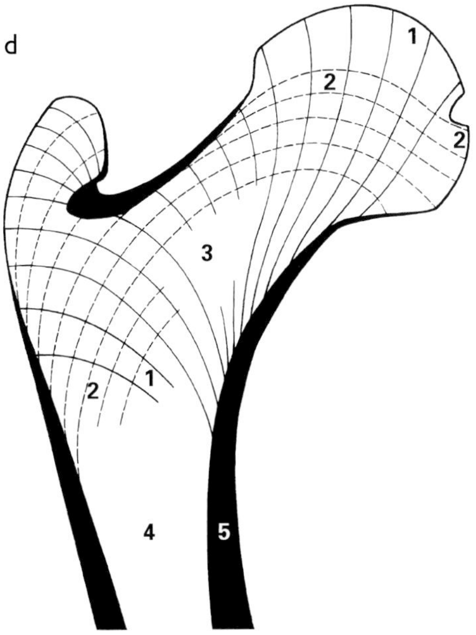

1 Compressive stress trajectories (solid lines)
2 Tensile stress trajectories (dashed lines)
3 WARD's triangle
4 Medullary cavity
5 Compact bone of shaft

7 Compact and spongy bones

a, b Vertebral body (200%)
- a Anatomical cross-section
- b Corresponding radiograph

c, d Trabecular architecture, proximal end of the femur (80%)
- c Coronal section
- d Stress trajectories

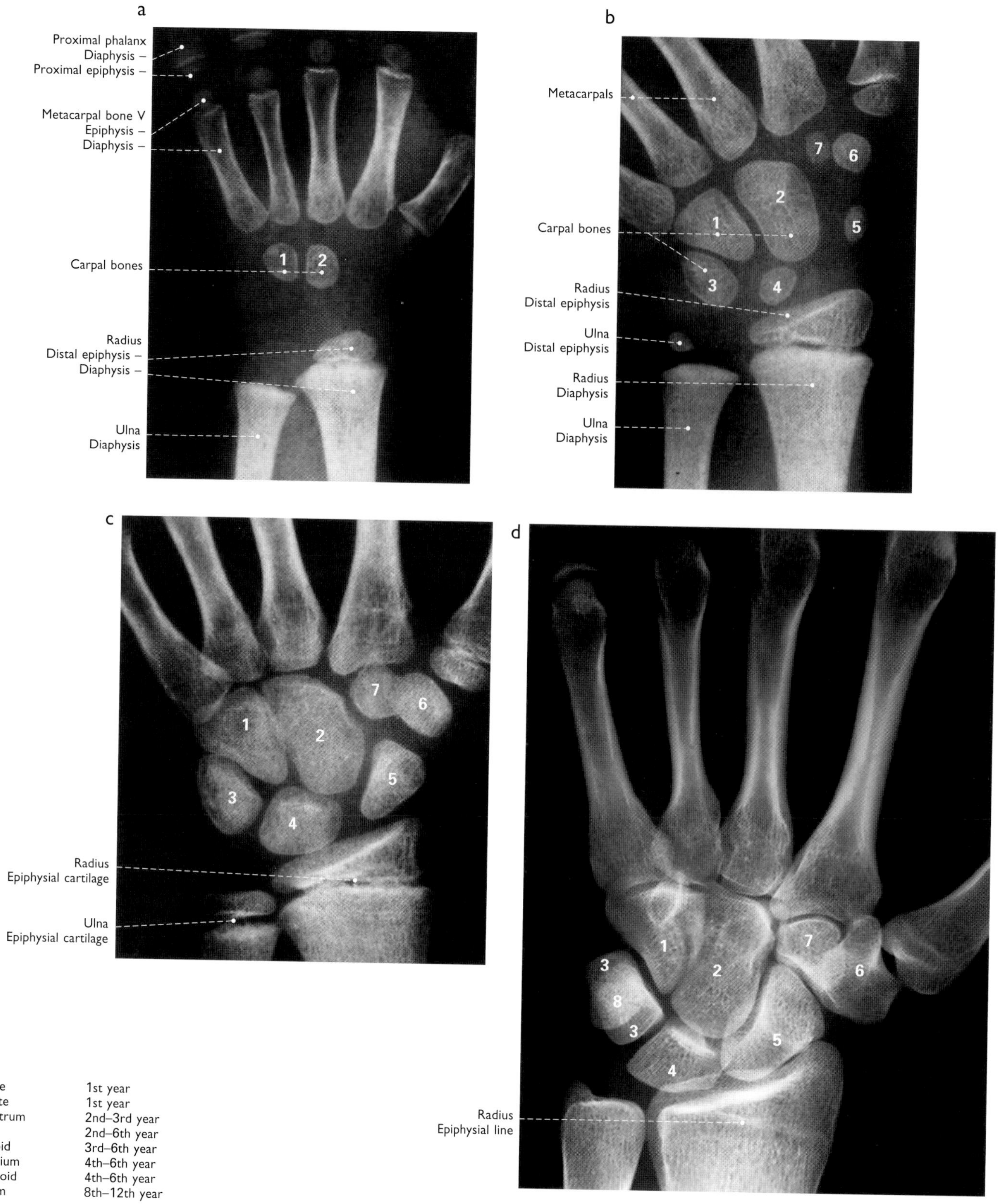
a
Proximal phalanx
Diaphysis –
Proximal epiphysis –
Metacarpal bone V
Epiphysis –
Diaphysis –
Carpal bones
1
2
Radius
Distal epiphysis –
Diaphysis –
Ulna
Diaphysis
b
Metacarpals
Carpal bones
Radius
Distal epiphysis
Ulna
Distal epiphysis
Radius
Diaphysis
Ulna
Diaphysis
1
2
3
4
5
6
7
c
Radius
Epiphysial cartilage
Ulna
Epiphysial cartilage
1
2
3
4
5
6
7
d
Radius
Epiphysial line
1
2
3
3
4
5
6
7
8
1 Hamate 1st year
2 Capitate 1st year
3 Triquetrum 2nd–3rd year
4 Lunate 2nd–6th year
5 Scaphoid 3rd–6th year
6 Trapezium 4th–6th year
7 Trapezoid 4th–6th year
8 Pisiform 8th–12th year

8 Development of bones

Dorsopalmar radiographs of the hand (100%)

a 1st year of life
b 2nd year of life
c 12th year of life
d 26th year of life

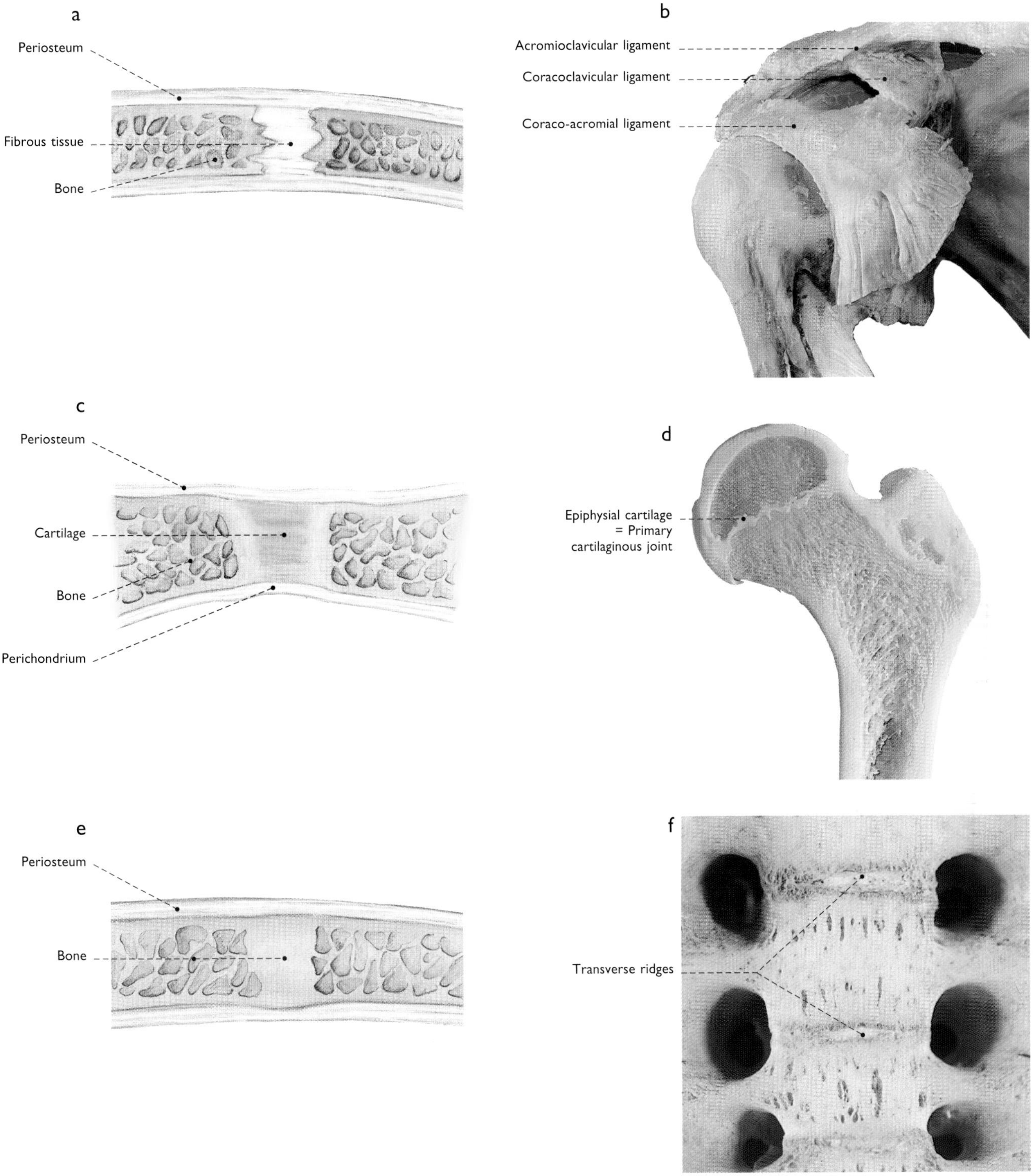
a
Periosteum
Fibrous tissue
Bone
b
Acromioclavicular ligament
Coracoclavicular ligament
Coraco-acromial ligament
c
Periosteum
Cartilage
Bone
Perichondrium
d
Epiphysial cartilage
= Primary
cartilaginous joint
e
Periosteum
Bone
f
Transverse ridges

9 Joints

a Fibrous joint (syndesmosis)
b Example, ligaments of the pectoral (= shoulder) girdle (75%), ventral aspect
c Cartilaginous joint (synchondrosis)
d Example, epiphysial cartilage in the proximal part of the femur of a 12-year-old child (75%), coronal section
e Bony union (osseous joint, synostosis)
f Example, sacrum (200%), ventral aspect

a

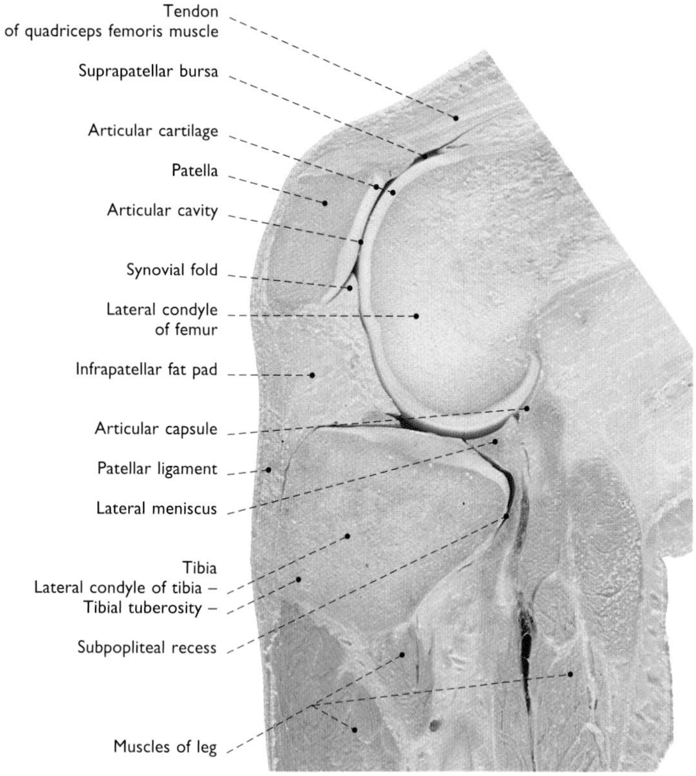
Tendon
of quadriceps femoris muscle
Suprapatellar bursa
Articular cartilage
Patella
Articular cavity
Synovial fold
Lateral condyle
of femur
Infrapatellar fat pad
Articular capsule
Patellar ligament
Lateral meniscus
Tibia
Lateral condyle of tibia –
Tibial tuberosity –
Subpopliteal recess
Muscles of leg

b

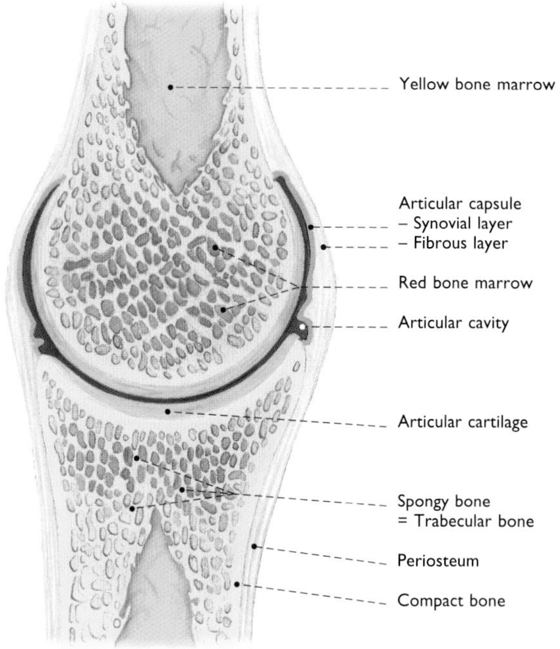
Yellow bone marrow
Articular capsule
– Synovial layer
– Fibrous layer
Red bone marrow
Articular cavity
Articular cartilage
Spongy bone
= Trabecular bone
Periosteum
Compact bone

c

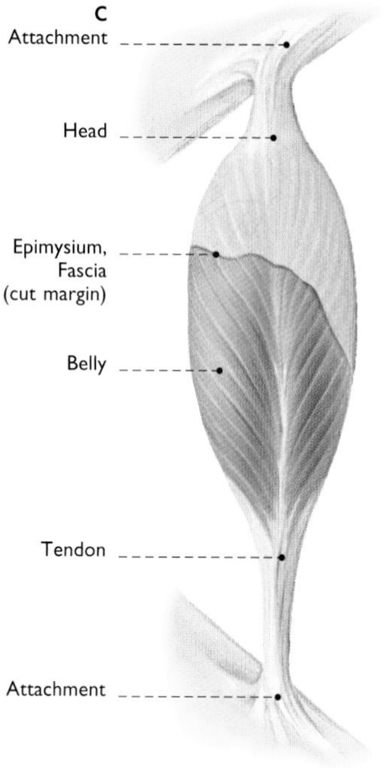
Attachment
Head
Epimysium,
Fascia
(cut margin)
Belly
Tendon
Attachment

d

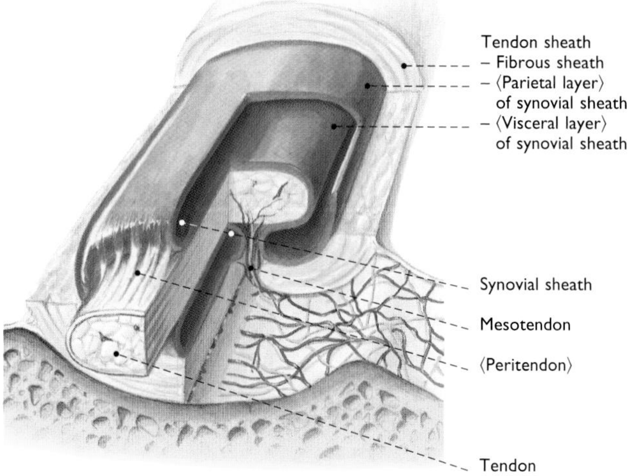
Tendon sheath
– Fibrous sheath
– ⟨Parietal layer⟩
of synovial sheath
– ⟨Visceral layer⟩
of synovial sheath
Synovial sheath
Mesotendon
⟨Peritendon⟩
Tendon

10 Synovial joint = diarthrosis, muscle and tendon

a Flexed right knee joint, sagittal section (60%), medial aspect of the lateral part
b Schematized section through a synovial joint
c Parts of a muscle
d Tendon sheath, schematic representation

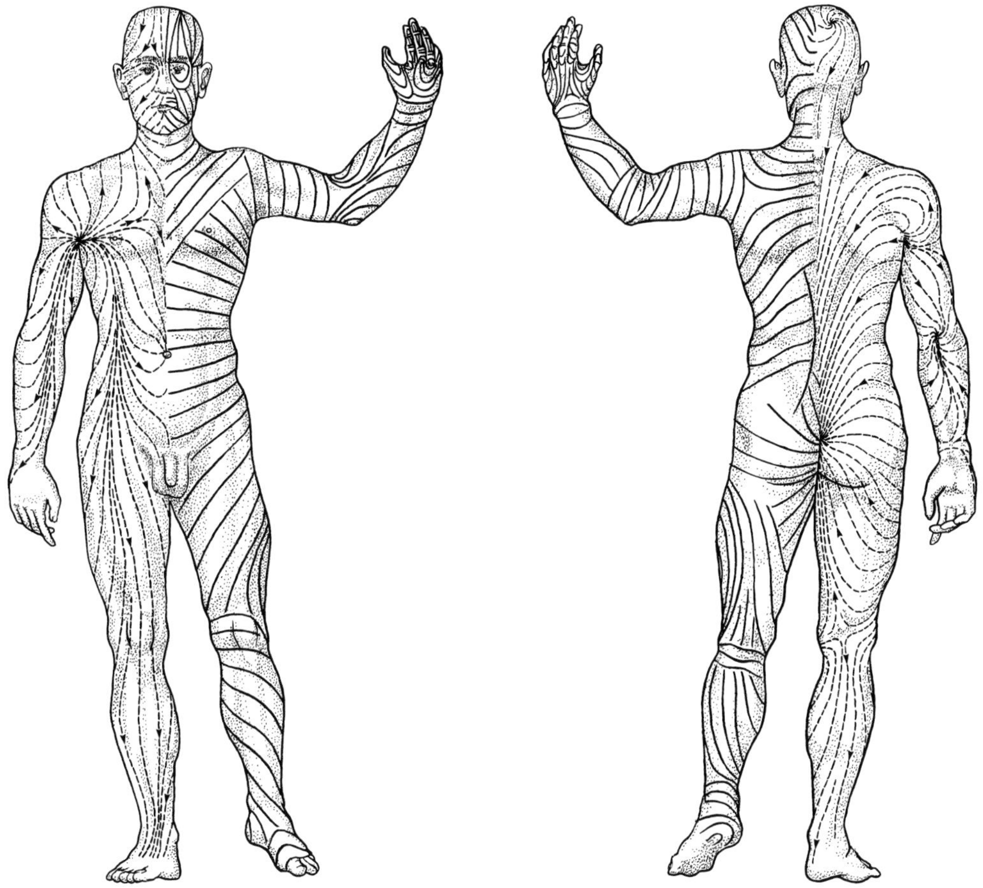
a
b

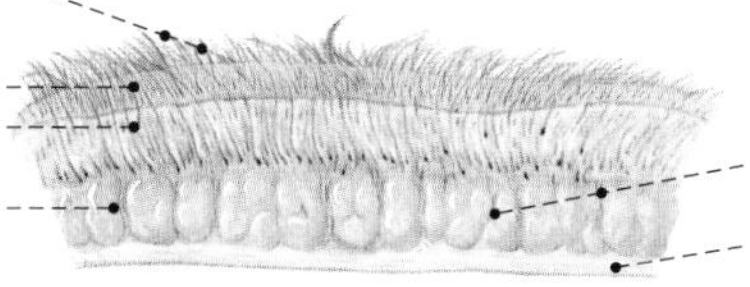
c
Hairs
Skin = Cutis
Epidermis
Dermis = Corium
Subcutaneous tissue
Retinacula of skin
Epicranial aponeurosis

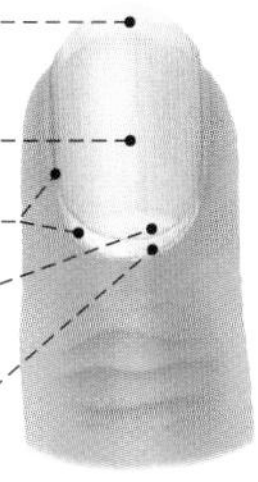
d
Free border of nail
Body of nail
Nail wall
Lunule
Eponychium

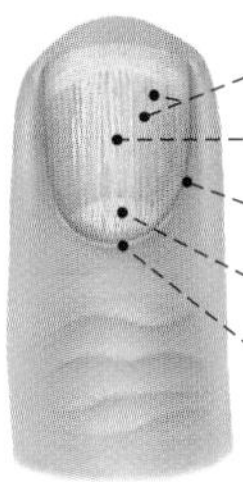
e
⟨Crests of nail bed⟩
Nail matrix
⟨Furrow⟩ of nail matrix
Lunule
Nail wall
(with the edge
of eponychium)

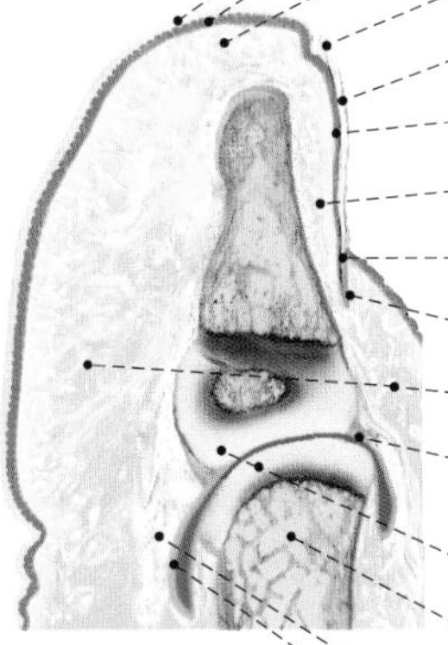
f
Epidermis
– Stratum corneum
– Stratum germinativum
Dermis = Corium
Free body of nail
Body of nail
Nail matrix
Hyponychium
Eponychium
Nail wall
Subcutaneous tissue
Synovial layer,
Synovial fold
Articular cartilage
Middle phalanx
Articular capsule
– Fibrous layer
– Synovial layer

11 Skin and fingernail

a, b Hair streams (flumina pilorum) on the right, tension lines (cleavage lines, LANGER's lines) on the left side of the body
- a Ventral aspect
- b Dorsal aspect
- c Skin of the head (400%), cross section

d, e Fingernail, dorsal aspect
- d Distal phalanx with nail (80%)
- e Distal phalanx without body of nail (80%)
- f Distal phalanx (200%), longitudinal section

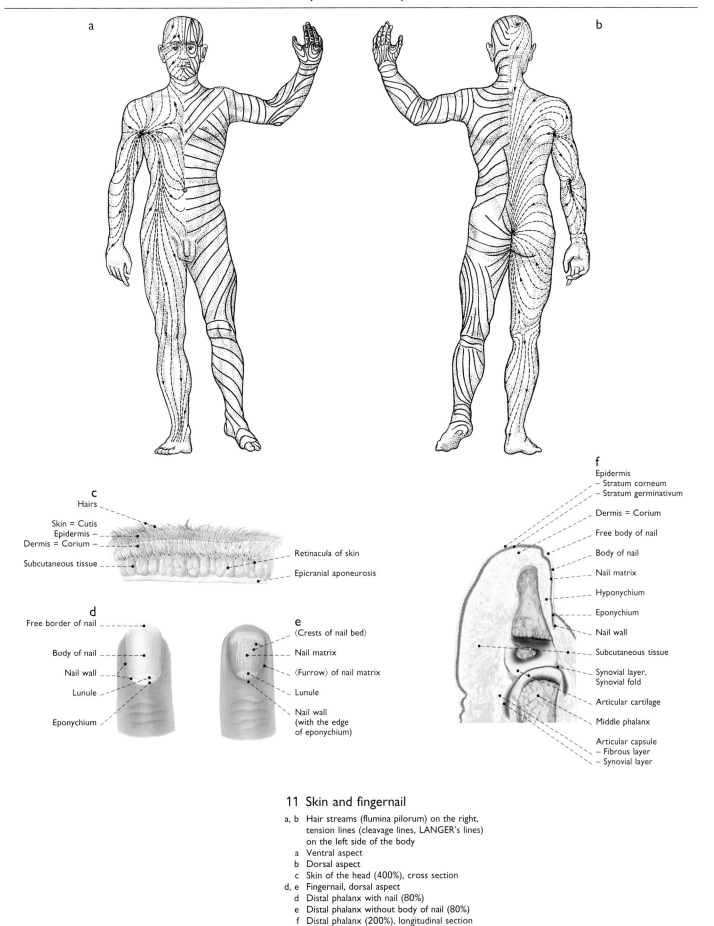

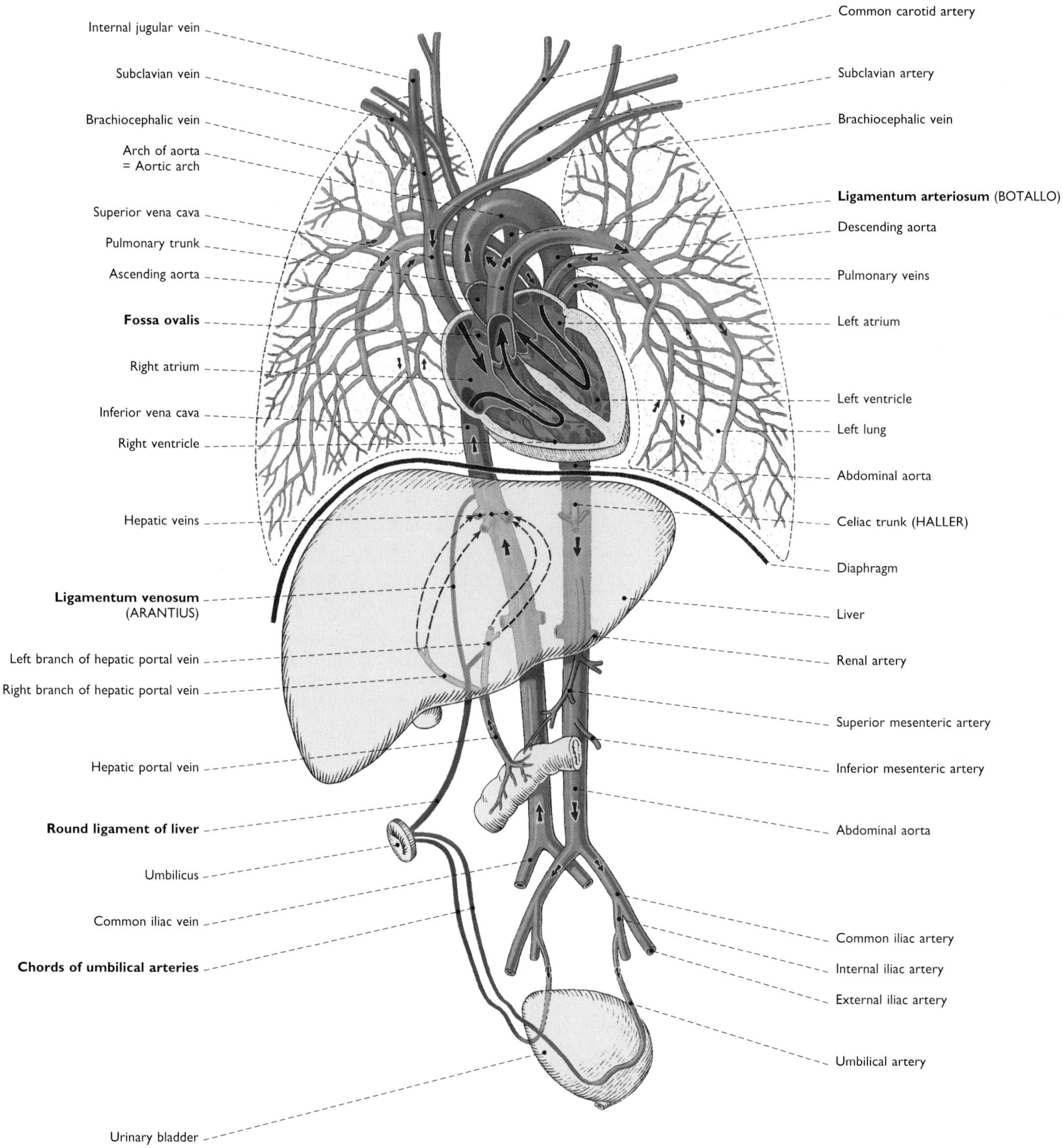
Internal jugular vein
Subclavian vein
Brachiocephalic vein
Arch of aorta
= Aortic arch
Superior vena cava
Pulmonary trunk
Ascending aorta
Fossa ovalis
Right atrium
Inferior vena cava
Right ventricle
Hepatic veins
Ligamentum venosum
(ARANTIUS)
Left branch of hepatic portal vein
Right branch of hepatic portal vein
Hepatic portal vein
Round ligament of liver
Umbilicus
Common iliac vein
Chords of umbilical arteries
Urinary bladder
Common carotid artery
Subclavian artery
Brachiocephalic vein
Ligamentum arteriosum (BOTALLO)
Descending aorta
Pulmonary veins
Left atrium
Left ventricle
Left lung
Abdominal aorta
Celiac trunk (HALLER)
Diaphragm
Liver
Renal artery
Superior mesenteric artery
Inferior mesenteric artery
Abdominal aorta
Common iliac artery
Internal iliac artery
External iliac artery
Umbilical artery

Arterial (oxygenated) blood **red**,
venous (deoxygenated) blood **blue**,
obliterated embryonic vessels **brown**

12 Adult cardiovascular system
Ventral aspect

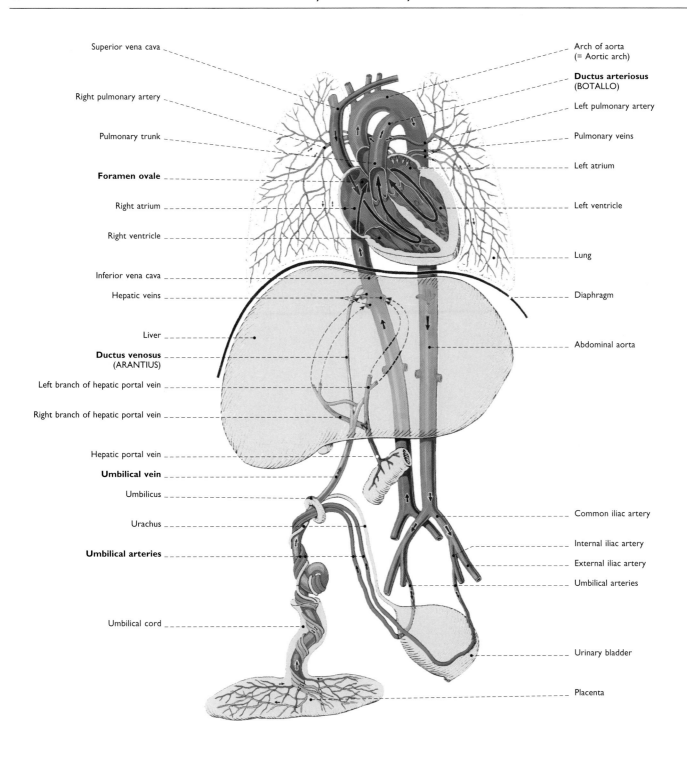

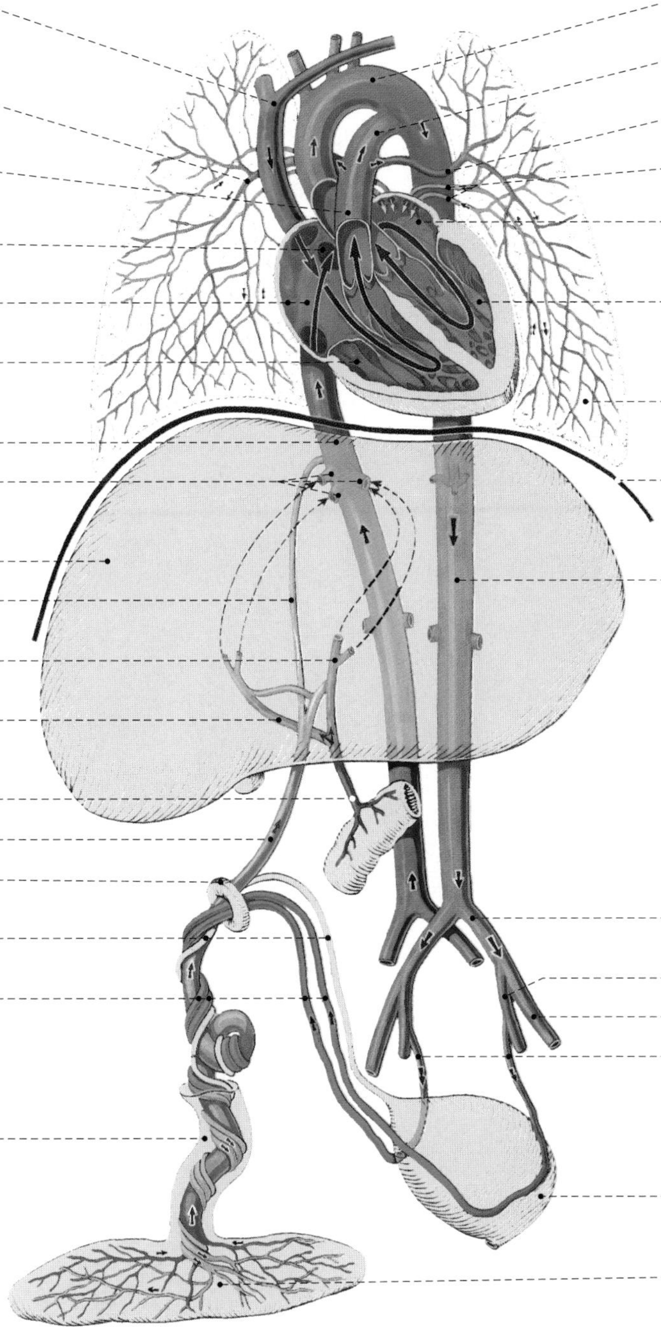
Superior vena cava
Right pulmonary artery
Pulmonary trunk
Foramen ovale
Right atrium
Right ventricle
Inferior vena cava
Hepatic veins
Liver
Ductus venosus
(ARANTIUS)
Left branch of hepatic portal vein
Right branch of hepatic portal vein
Hepatic portal vein
Umbilical vein
Umbilicus
Urachus
Umbilical arteries
Umbilical cord
Arch of aorta
(= Aortic arch)
Ductus arteriosus
(BOTALLO)
Left pulmonary artery
Pulmonary veins
Left atrium
Left ventricle
Lung
Diaphragm
Abdominal aorta
Common iliac artery
Internal iliac artery
External iliac artery
Umbilical arteries
Urinary bladder
Placenta

Arterial (oxygenated) blood **red**,
venous (deoxygenated) blood **blue**,
mixed blood **violet**

13 Fetal cardiovascular system

Ventral aspect

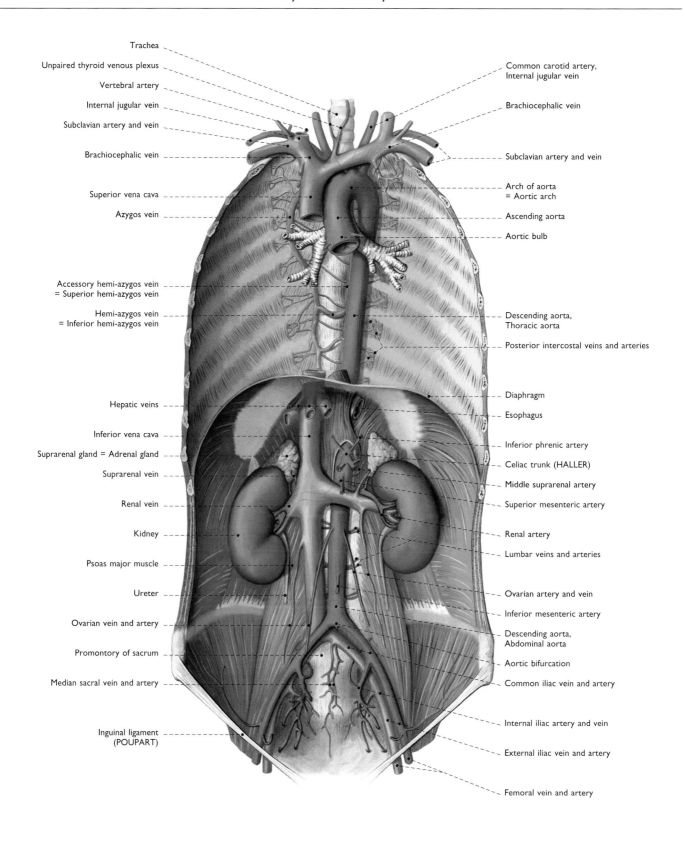

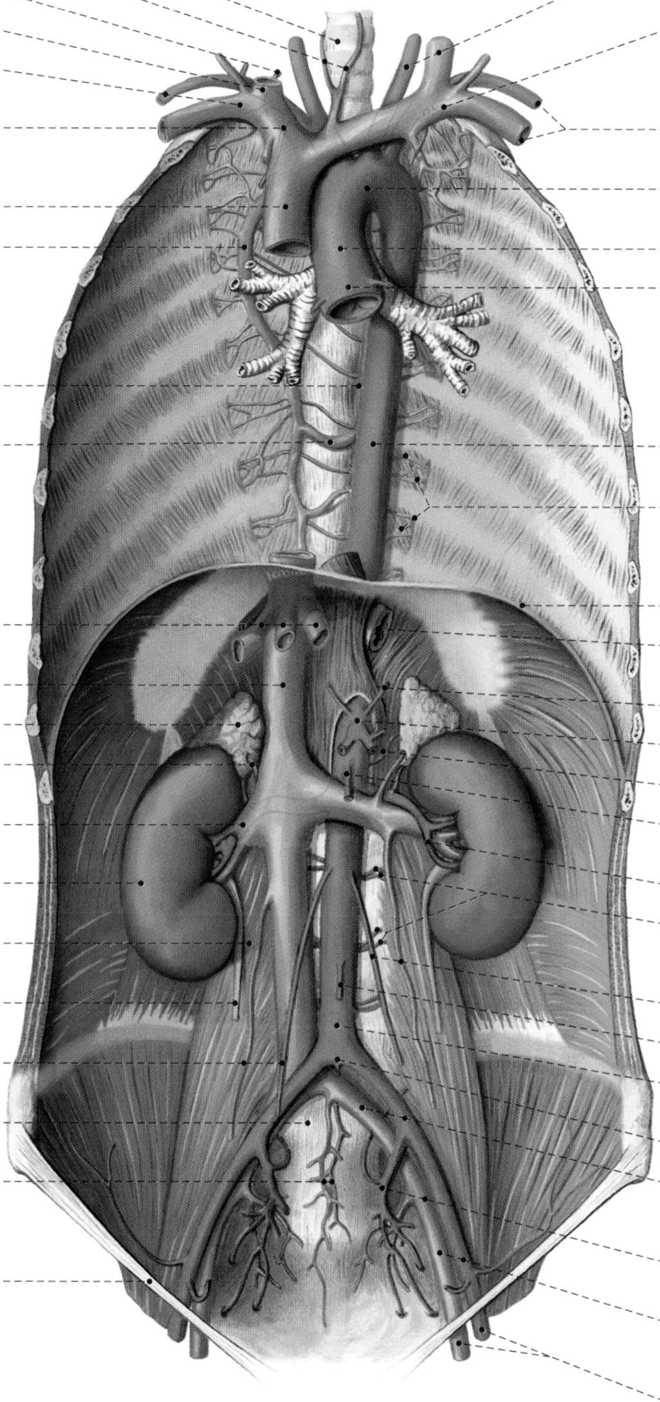
Trachea
Unpaired thyroid venous plexus
Vertebral artery
Internal jugular vein
Subclavian artery and vein
Brachiocephalic vein
Superior vena cava
Azygos vein
Accessory hemi-azygos vein
= Superior hemi-azygos vein
Hemi-azygos vein
= Inferior hemi-azygos vein
Hepatic veins
Inferior vena cava
Suprarenal gland = Adrenal gland
Suprarenal vein
Renal vein
Kidney
Psoas major muscle
Ureter
Ovarian vein and artery
Promontory of sacrum
Median sacral vein and artery
Inguinal ligament
(POUPART)
Common carotid artery,
Internal jugular vein
Brachiocephalic vein
Subclavian artery and vein
Arch of aorta
= Aortic arch
Ascending aorta
Aortic bulb
Descending aorta,
Thoracic aorta
Posterior intercostal veins and arteries
Diaphragm
Esophagus
Inferior phrenic artery
Celiac trunk (HALLER)
Middle suprarenal artery
Superior mesenteric artery
Renal artery
Lumbar veins and arteries
Ovarian artery and vein
Inferior mesenteric artery
Descending aorta,
Abdominal aorta
Aortic bifurcation
Common iliac vein and artery
Internal iliac artery and vein
External iliac vein and artery
Femoral vein and artery

14 Blood vessels of the trunk (30%)

Ventral aspect

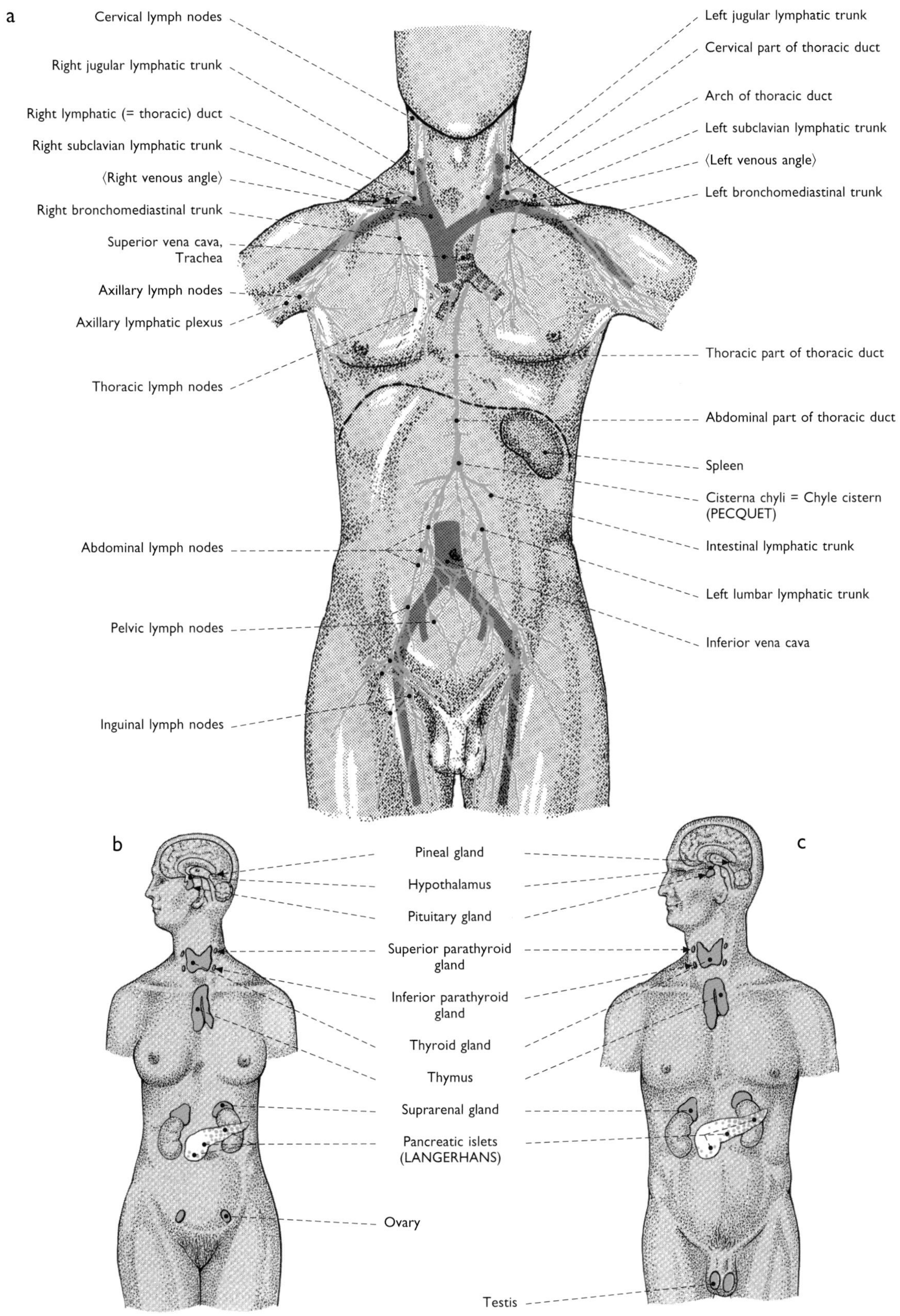
a
Cervical lymph nodes
Right jugular lymphatic trunk
Right lymphatic (= thoracic) duct
Right subclavian lymphatic trunk
⟨Right venous angle⟩
Right bronchomediastinal trunk
Superior vena cava, Trachea
Axillary lymph nodes
Axillary lymphatic plexus
Thoracic lymph nodes
Abdominal lymph nodes
Pelvic lymph nodes
Inguinal lymph nodes
Left jugular lymphatic trunk
Cervical part of thoracic duct
Arch of thoracic duct
Left subclavian lymphatic trunk
⟨Left venous angle⟩
Left bronchomediastinal trunk
Thoracic part of thoracic duct
Abdominal part of thoracic duct
Spleen
Cisterna chyli = Chyle cistern (PECQUET)
Intestinal lymphatic trunk
Left lumbar lymphatic trunk
Inferior vena cava
b
c
Pineal gland
Hypothalamus
Pituitary gland
Superior parathyroid gland
Inferior parathyroid gland
Thyroid gland
Thymus
Suprarenal gland
Pancreatic islets (LANGERHANS)
Ovary
Testis

15 Lymphoid system and endocrine glands

Ventral aspect

a Lymphatic trunks and ducts, lymphoid organs

b Female endocrine glands

c Male endocrine glands

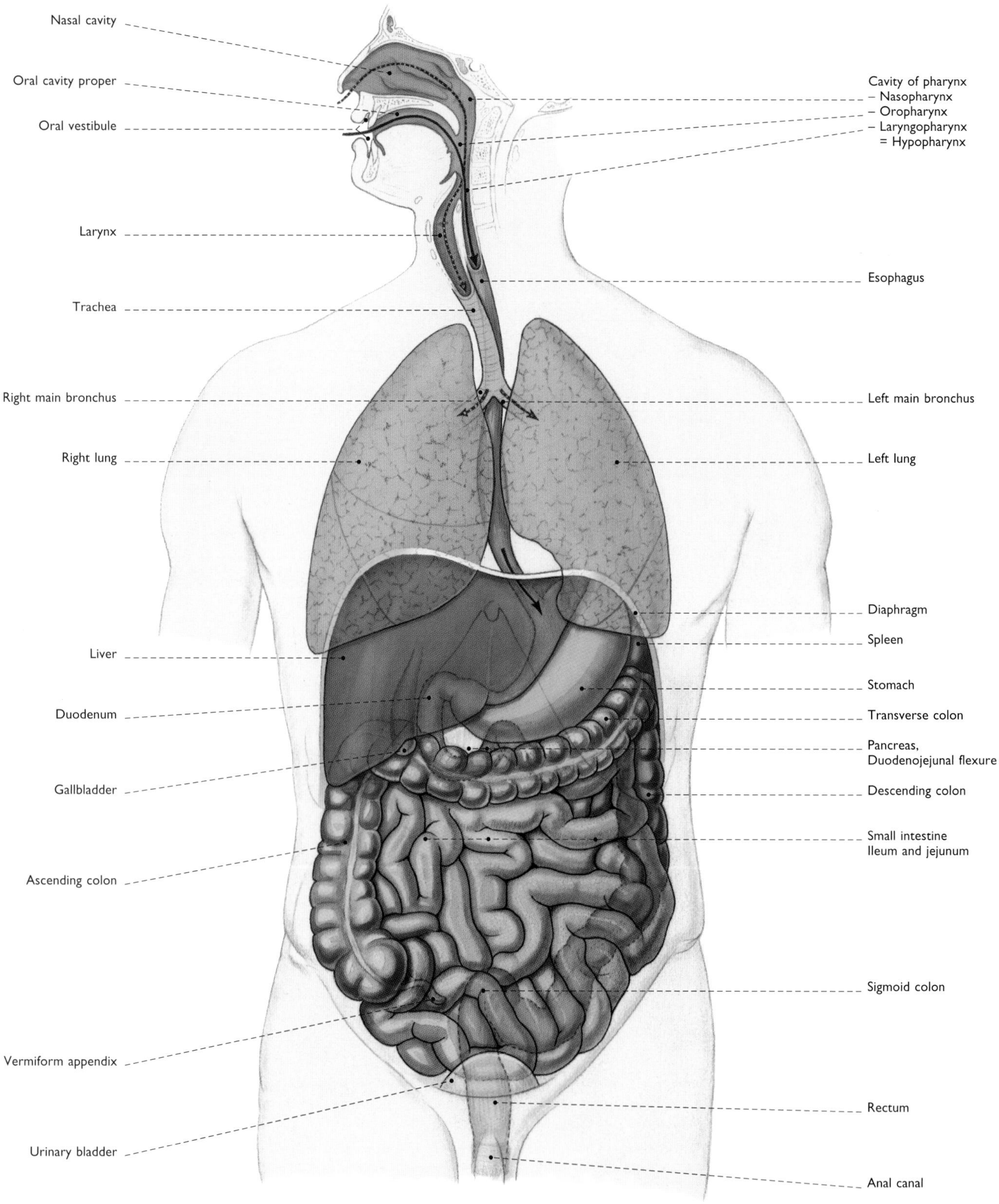
Nasal cavity
Oral cavity proper
Oral vestibule
Larynx
Trachea
Right main bronchus
Right lung
Liver
Duodenum
Gallbladder
Ascending colon
Vermiform appendix
Urinary bladder
Cavity of pharynx
– Nasopharynx
– Oropharynx
– Laryngopharynx
= Hypopharynx
Esophagus
Left main bronchus
Left lung
Diaphragm
Spleen
Stomach
Transverse colon
Pancreas,
Duodenojejunal flexure
Descending colon
Small intestine
Ileum and jejunum
Sigmoid colon
Rectum
Anal canal

16 Alimentary and respiratory systems (25%)

Ventral aspect

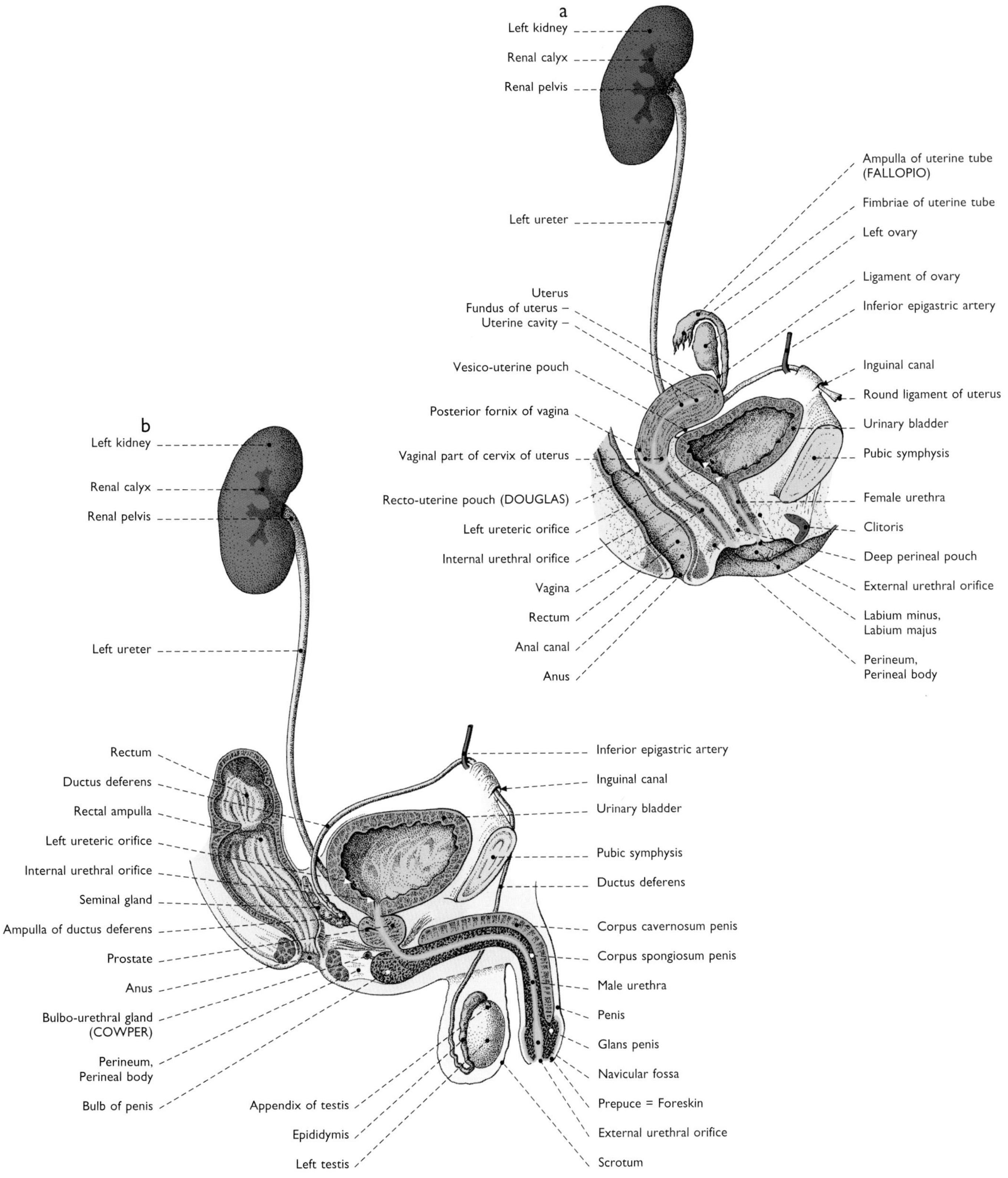
a
Left kidney
Renal calyx
Renal pelvis
Left ureter
Uterus
Fundus of uterus –
Uterine cavity –
Vesico-uterine pouch
Posterior fornix of vagina
Vaginal part of cervix of uterus
Recto-uterine pouch (DOUGLAS)
Left ureteric orifice
Internal urethral orifice
Vagina
Rectum
Anal canal
Anus
Ampulla of uterine tube (FALLOPIO)
Fimbriae of uterine tube
Left ovary
Ligament of ovary
Inferior epigastric artery
Inguinal canal
Round ligament of uterus
Urinary bladder
Pubic symphysis
Female urethra
Clitoris
Deep perineal pouch
External urethral orifice
Labium minus, Labium majus
Perineum, Perineal body
b
Left kidney
Renal calyx
Renal pelvis
Left ureter
Rectum
Ductus deferens
Rectal ampulla
Left ureteric orifice
Internal urethral orifice
Seminal gland
Ampulla of ductus deferens
Prostate
Anus
Bulbo-urethral gland (COWPER)
Perineum, Perineal body
Bulb of penis
Appendix of testis
Epididymis
Left testis
Inferior epigastric artery
Inguinal canal
Urinary bladder
Pubic symphysis
Ductus deferens
Corpus cavernosum penis
Corpus spongiosum penis
Male urethra
Penis
Glans penis
Navicular fossa
Prepuce = Foreskin
External urethral orifice
Scrotum

17 Urinary and genital systems (40%)

Schematized median section, medial aspect of the left half

a Female
b Male

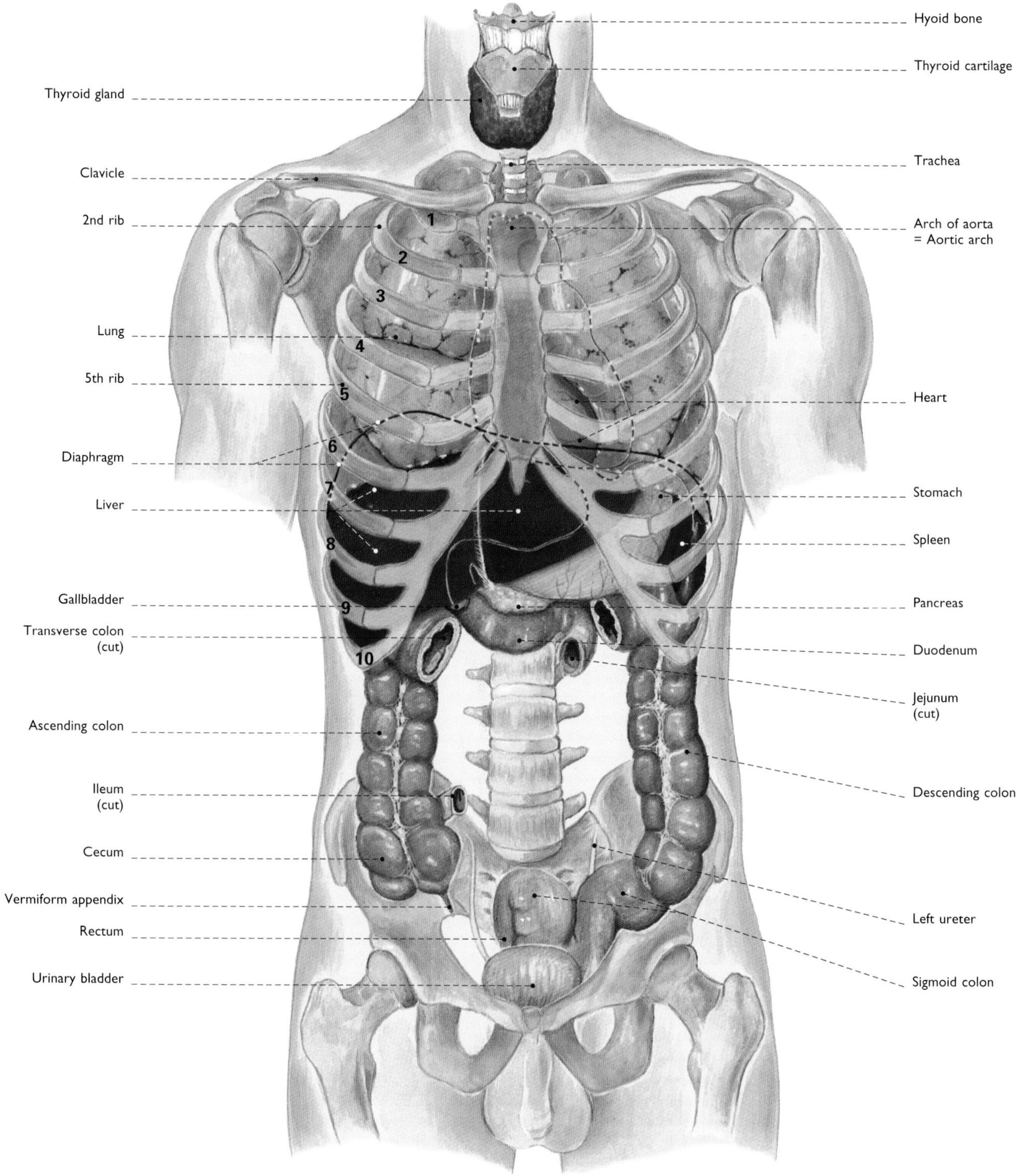
Hyoid bone
Thyroid cartilage
Thyroid gland
Trachea
Clavicle
2nd rib
Arch of aorta
= Aortic arch
1
2
3
Lung
4
5th rib
5
Heart
6
Diaphragm
7
Stomach
Liver
8
Spleen
Gallbladder
9
Pancreas
Transverse colon
(cut)
10
Duodenum
Jejunum
(cut)
Ascending colon
Descending colon
Ileum
(cut)
Cecum
Vermiform appendix
Left ureter
Rectum
Sigmoid colon
Urinary bladder

18 Surface projections of thoracic and abdominal viscera (25%)

Jejunum, ileum, and transverse colon were removed. Ventral aspect

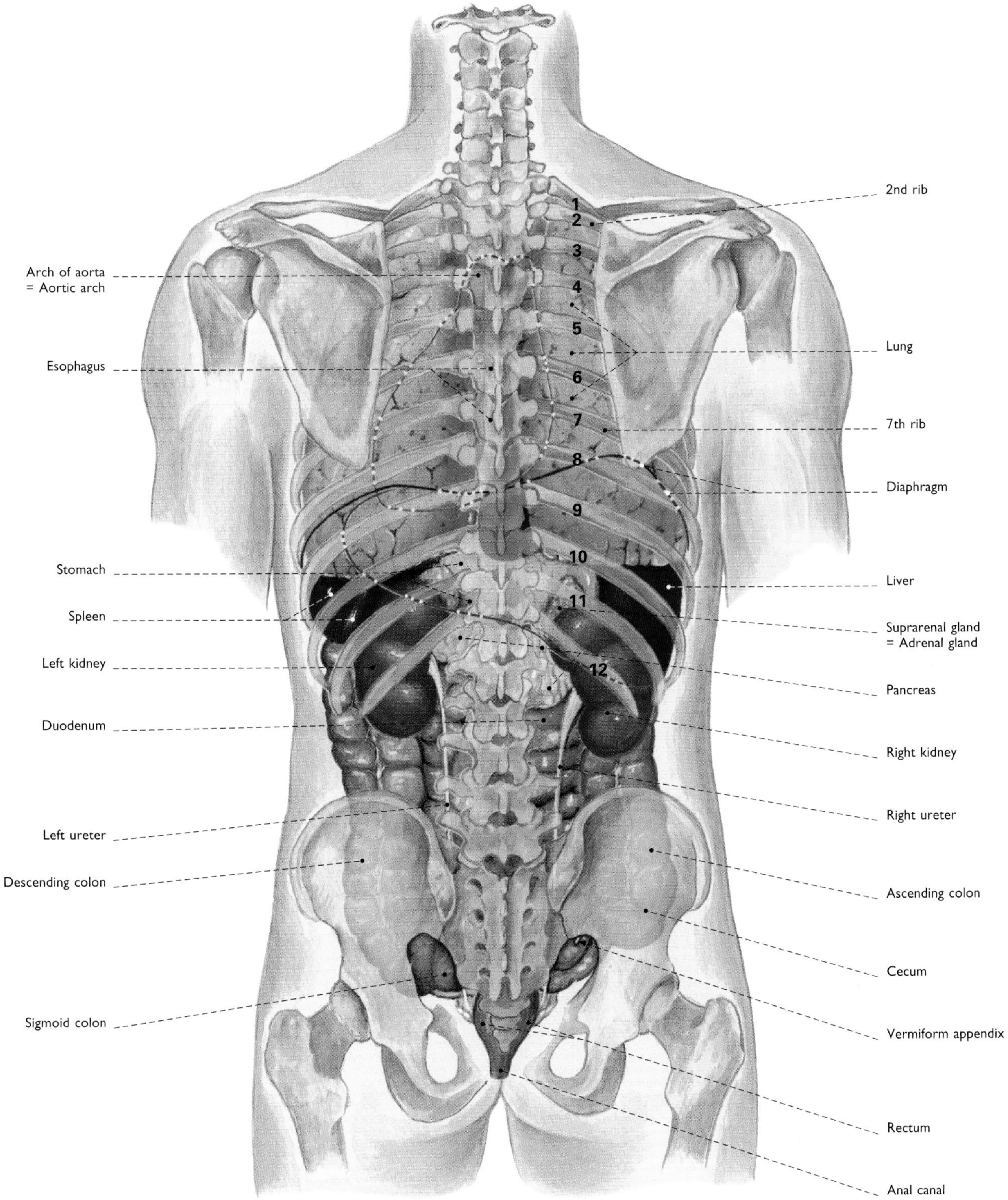
2nd rib
1
2
3
4
5
6
7
8
9
10
11
12
Arch of aorta
= Aortic arch
Lung
Esophagus
7th rib
Diaphragm
Stomach
Liver
Spleen
Suprarenal gland
= Adrenal gland
Left kidney
Pancreas
Duodenum
Right kidney
Right ureter
Left ureter
Descending colon
Ascending colon
Cecum
Sigmoid colon
Vermiform appendix
Rectum
Anal canal

19 Surface projections of thoracic and abdominal viscera (25%)

Dorsal aspect

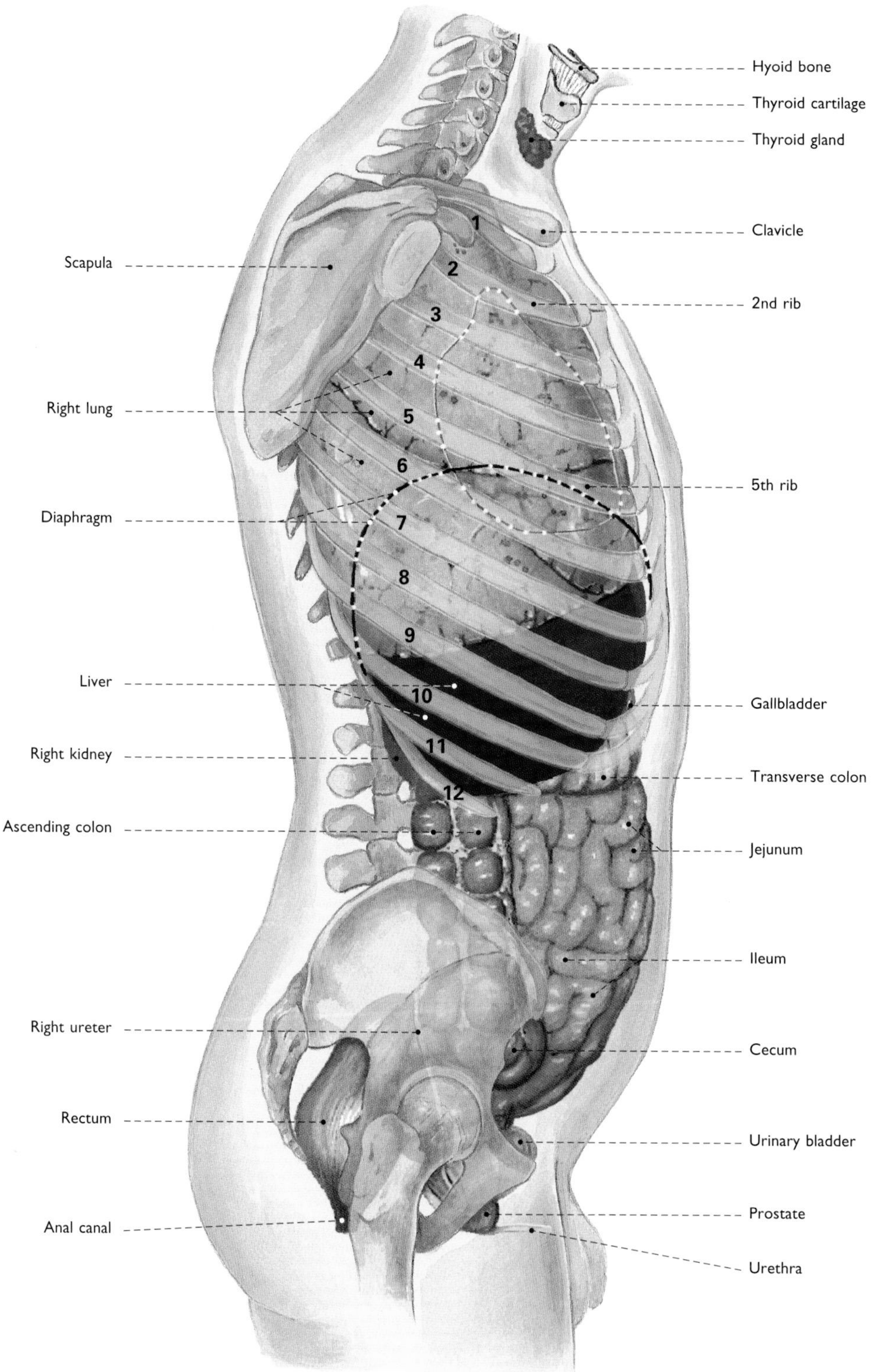
Hyoid bone
Thyroid cartilage
Thyroid gland
Clavicle
Scapula
2nd rib
Right lung
5th rib
Diaphragm
Liver
Gallbladder
Right kidney
Transverse colon
Ascending colon
Jejunum
Ileum
Right ureter
Cecum
Rectum
Urinary bladder
Anal canal
Prostate
Urethra
1
2
3
4
5
6
7
8
9
10
11
12

20 Surface projections of thoracic and abdominal viscera (25%)

Right lateral aspect

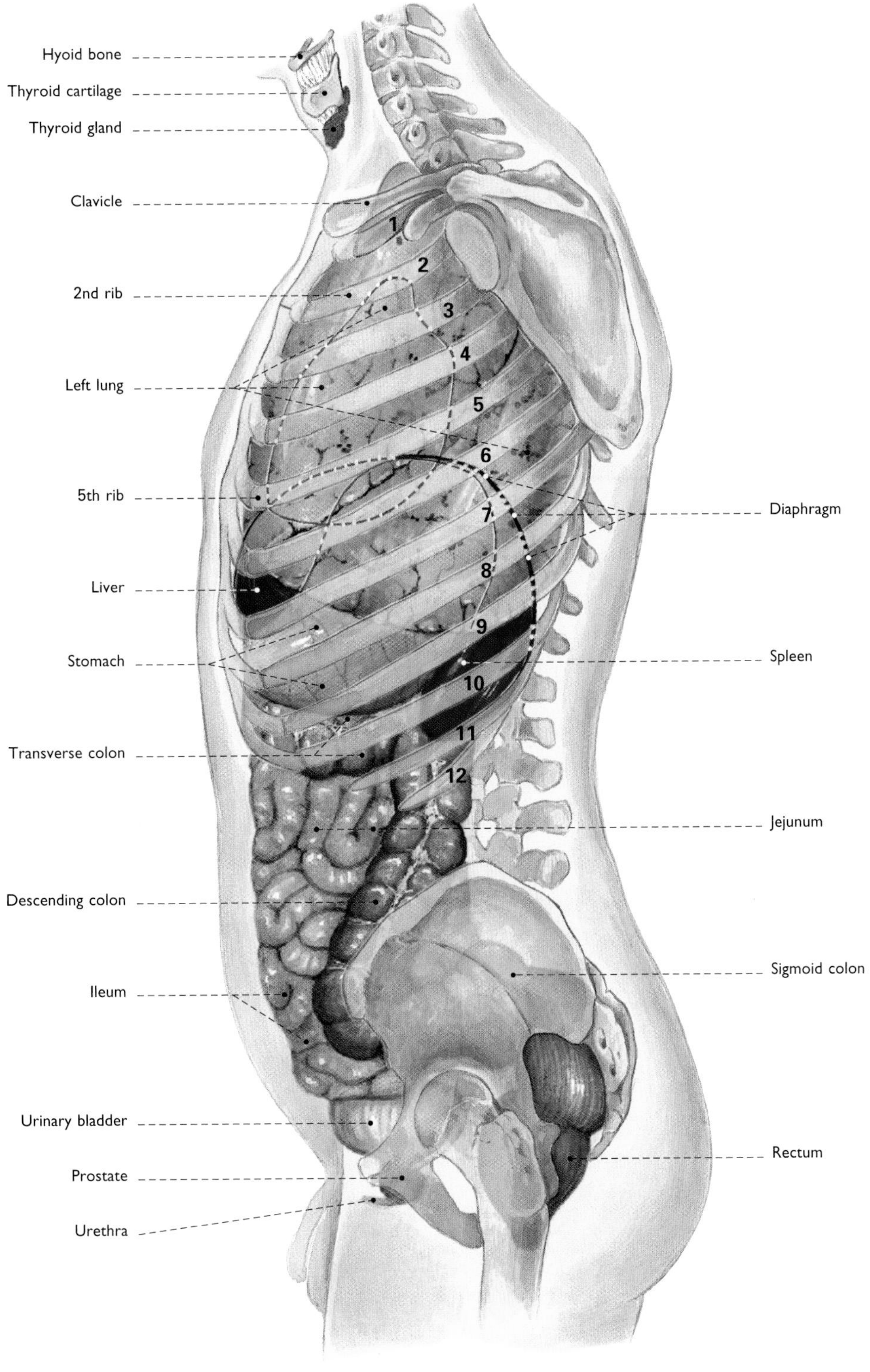
Hyoid bone
Thyroid cartilage
Thyroid gland
Clavicle
2nd rib
Left lung
5th rib
Liver
Stomach
Transverse colon
Descending colon
Ileum
Urinary bladder
Prostate
Urethra
Diaphragm
Spleen
Jejunum
Sigmoid colon
Rectum
1
2
3
4
5
6
7
8
9
10
11
12

21 Surface projections of thoracic and abdominal viscera (25%)

Left lateral aspect

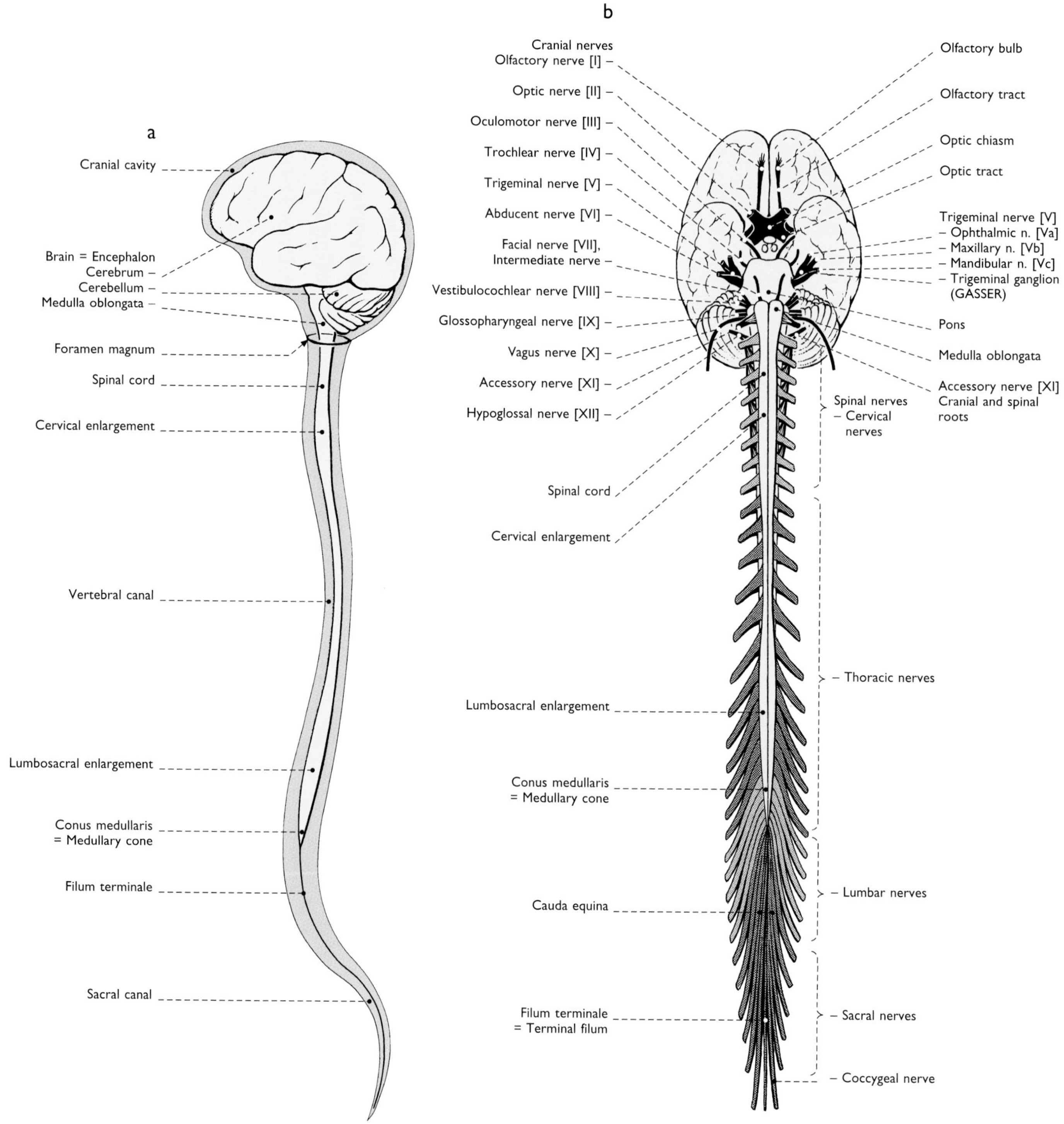
a
Cranial cavity
Brain = Encephalon
Cerebrum
Cerebellum
Medulla oblongata
Foramen magnum
Spinal cord
Cervical enlargement
Vertebral canal
Lumbosacral enlargement
Conus medullaris = Medullary cone
Filum terminale
Sacral canal
b
Cranial nerves
Olfactory nerve [I]
Optic nerve [II]
Oculomotor nerve [III]
Trochlear nerve [IV]
Trigeminal nerve [V]
Abducent nerve [VI]
Facial nerve [VII], Intermediate nerve
Vestibulocochlear nerve [VIII]
Glossopharyngeal nerve [IX]
Vagus nerve [X]
Accessory nerve [XI]
Hypoglossal nerve [XII]
Spinal cord
Cervical enlargement
Lumbosacral enlargement
Conus medullaris = Medullary cone
Cauda equina
Filum terminale = Terminal filum
Olfactory bulb
Olfactory tract
Optic chiasm
Optic tract
Trigeminal nerve [V]
– Ophthalmic n. [Va]
– Maxillary n. [Vb]
– Mandibular n. [Vc]
– Trigeminal ganglion (GASSER)
Pons
Medulla oblongata
Accessory nerve [XI] Cranial and spinal roots
Spinal nerves
– Cervical nerves
– Thoracic nerves
– Lumbar nerves
– Sacral nerves
– Coccygeal nerve

22 Central and peripheral nervous systems

a Central nervous system, left lateral aspect
b Cranial and spinal nerves, ventral aspect

a

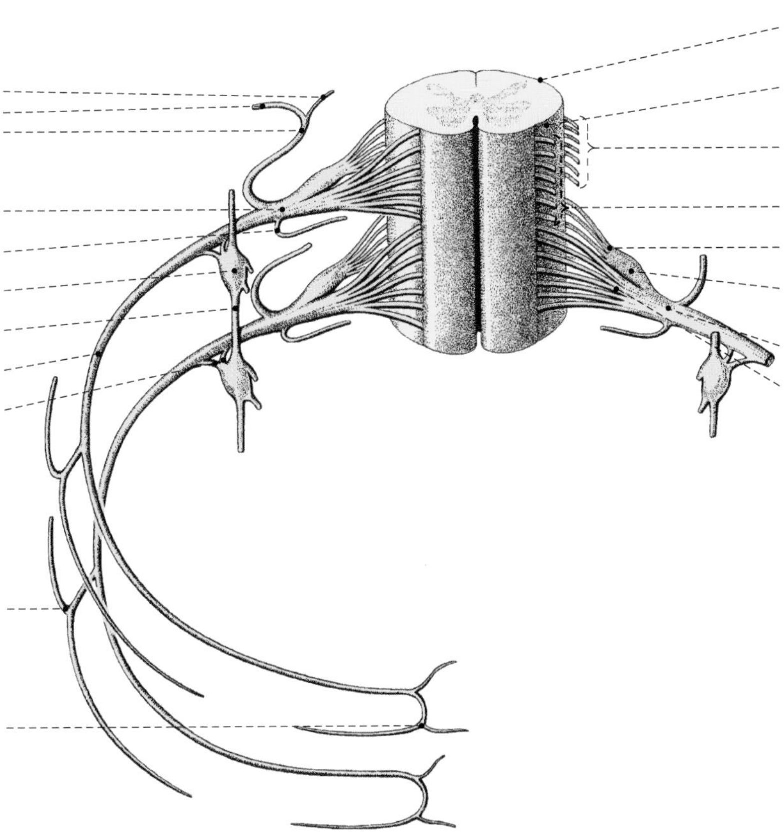
Medial branch
Lateral branch
Posterior (= dorsal) ramus of spinal nerve
Trunk of spinal nerve
Meningeal (= recurrent) branch of spinal nerve
Ganglion of sympathetic trunk
Interganglionic branch
Anterior (= ventral) ramus of spinal nerve
Gray and white rami communicantes of spinal nerve
Lateral pectoral cutaneous branch
Anterior pectoral cutaneous branch
Posterolateral sulcus of spinal cord
Anterolateral sulcus of spinal cord
Posterior rootlets
Anterior rootlets
Posterior (= sensory) root
Spinal ganglion = Dorsal root ganglion
Trunk of spinal nerve
Anterior (= motor) root of spinal nerve

b

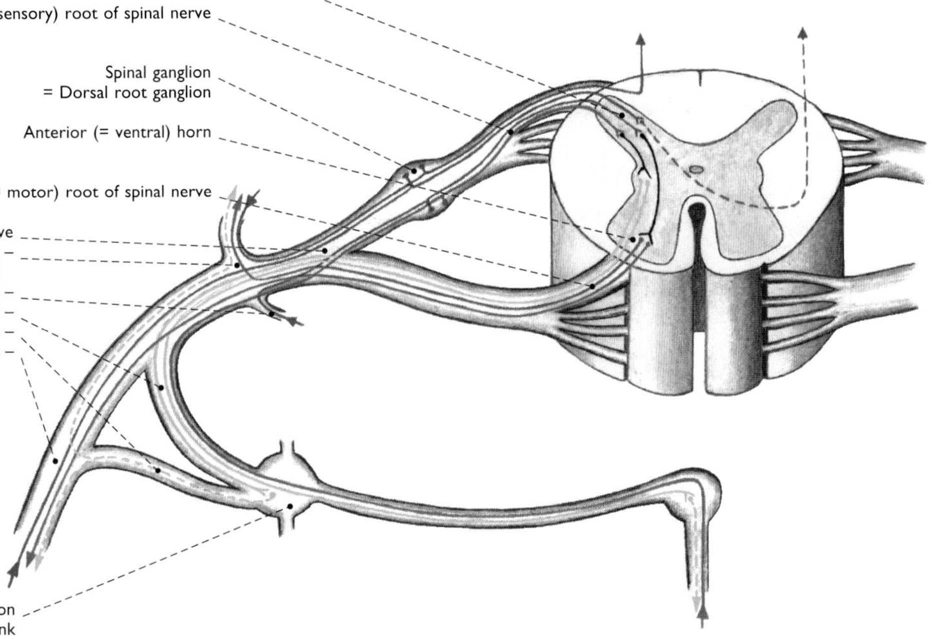
Posterior (= dorsal) horn
Posterior (= sensory) root of spinal nerve
Spinal ganglion = Dorsal root ganglion
Anterior (= ventral) horn
Anterior (= motor) root of spinal nerve
Spinal nerve
Posterior (= dorsal) ramus
Meningeal (= recurrent) branch
White ramus communicans
Gray ramus communicans
Anterior (= ventral) ramus
Ganglion of sympathetic trunk
Somatic efferent nerve fiber
Somatic afferent nerve fiber
Visceral efferent nerve fiber
Visceral afferent nerve fiber
Interneuron
The interrupted lines indicate postganglionic visceral or secondary somato-afferent fibers, respectively.

23 Spinal cord and spinal nerves

Ventral aspect

a Distribution and

b Construction

of typical spinal nerves (thoracic nerves)

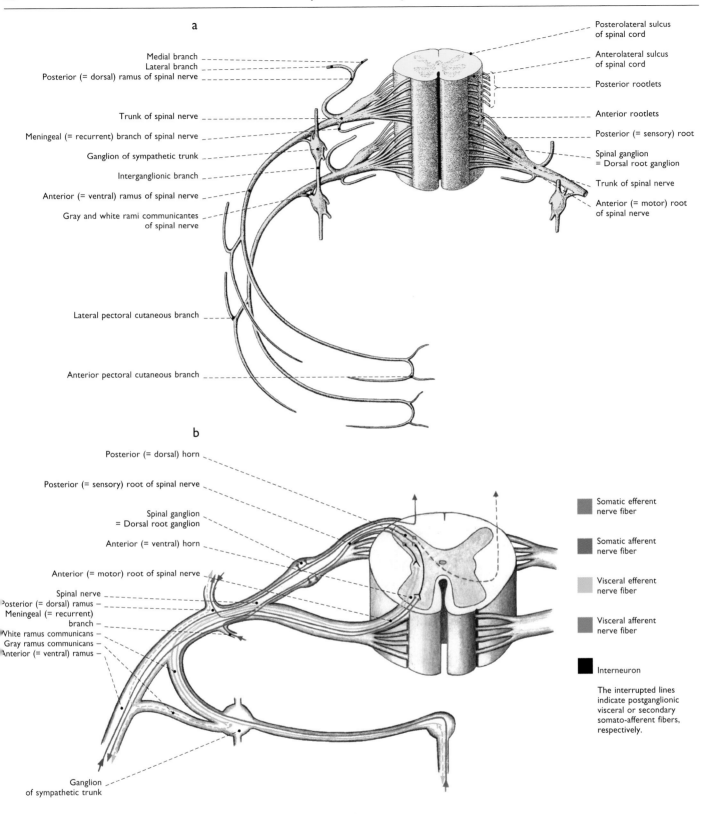

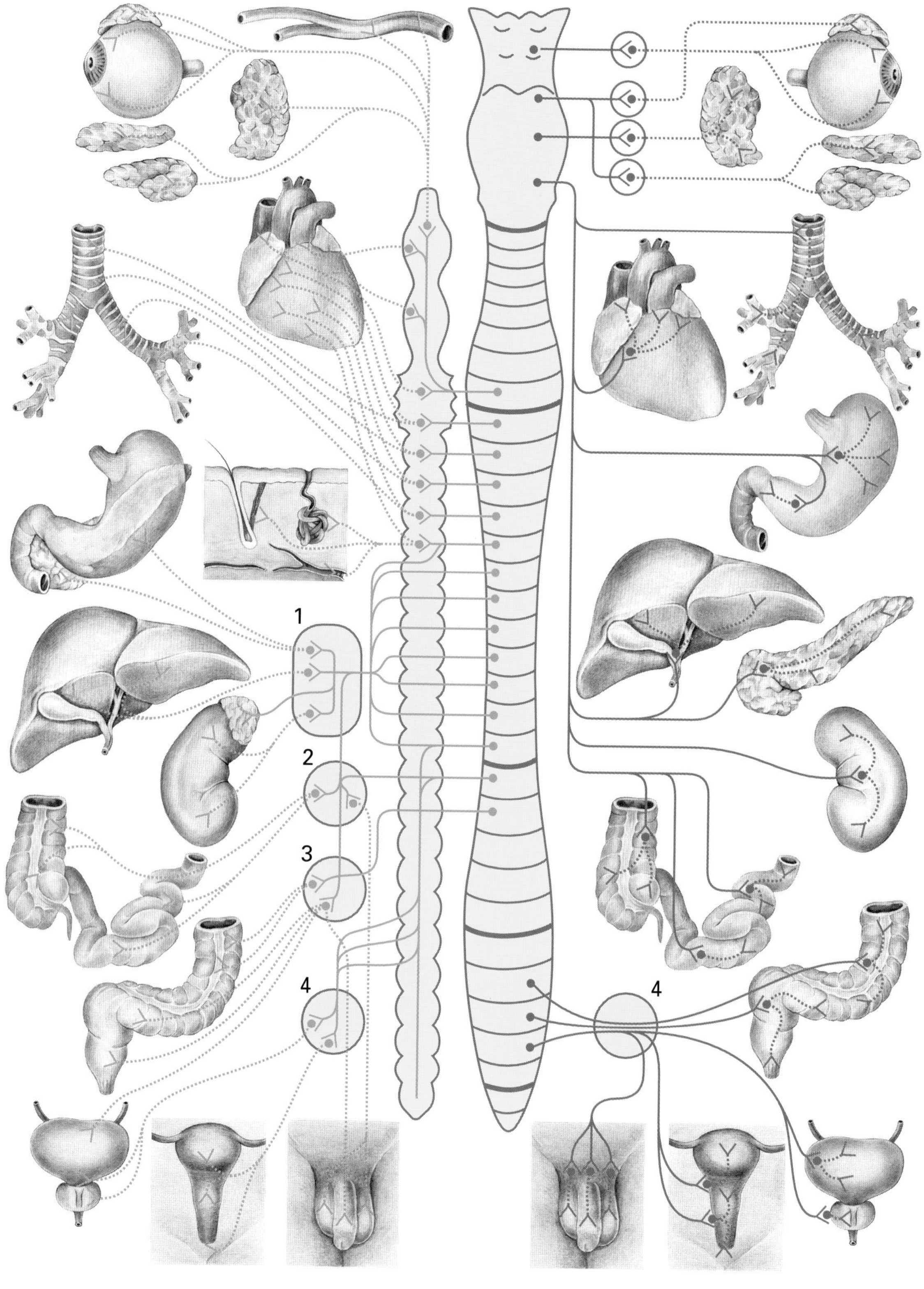

24 Autonomic nervous system

Origins, essential circuitry, and peripheral innervation of the sympathetic (**orange**, on the left side of the picture) and parasympathetic (**brown**, on the right) nervous systems. The interrupted lines indicate postganglionic nerve fibers.

1, celiac ganglia
2, superior mesenteric ganglion
3, inferior mesenteric ganglion
4, inferior hypogastric plexus.

Schematic representation, ventral aspect

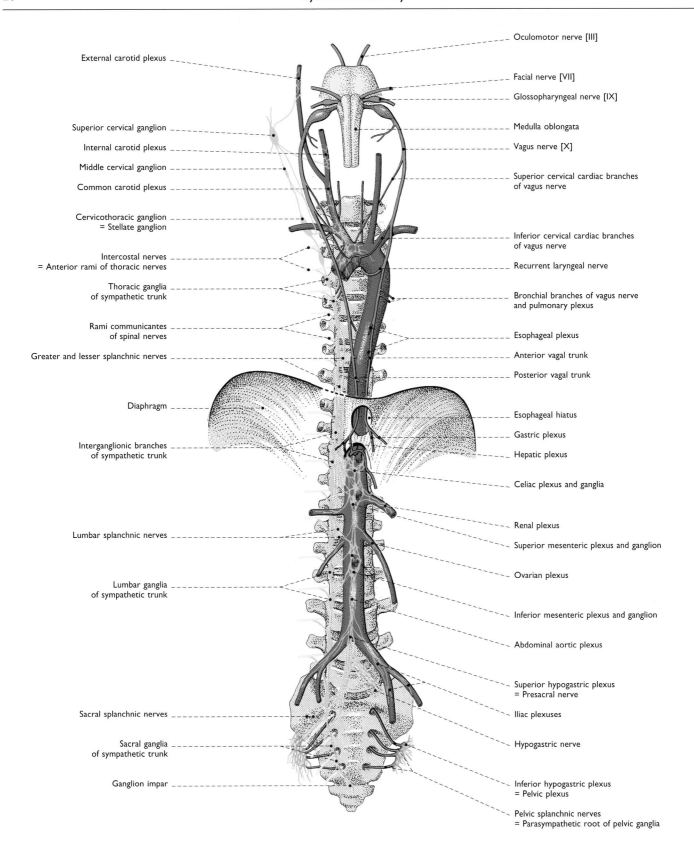

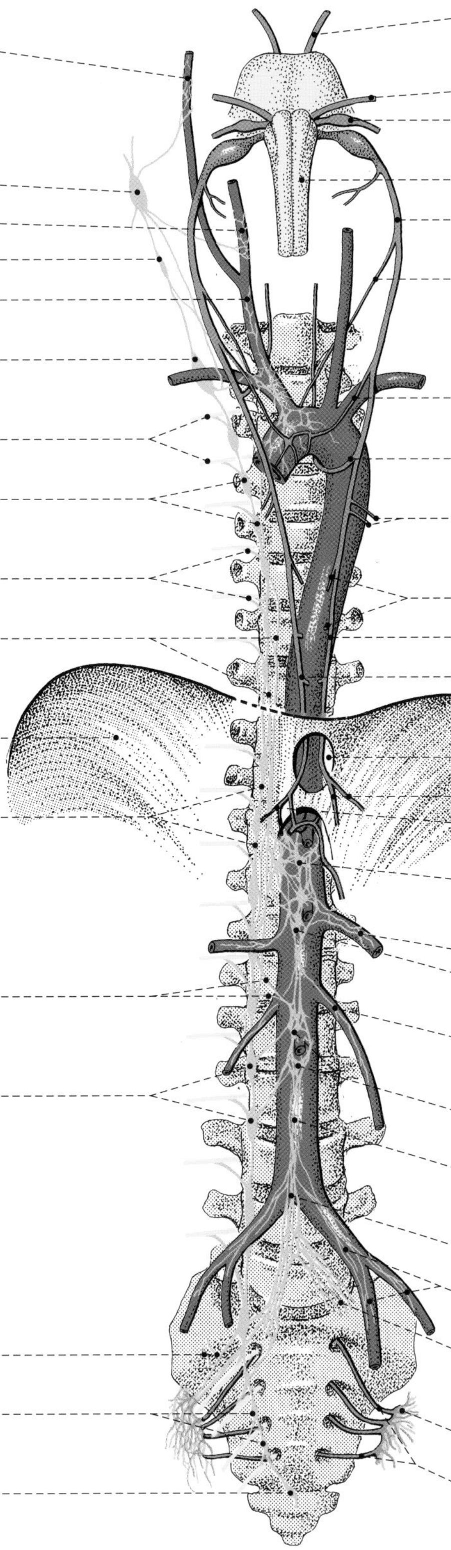
Oculomotor nerve [III]
External carotid plexus
Facial nerve [VII]
Glossopharyngeal nerve [IX]
Superior cervical ganglion
Medulla oblongata
Internal carotid plexus
Vagus nerve [X]
Middle cervical ganglion
Common carotid plexus
Superior cervical cardiac branches of vagus nerve
Cervicothoracic ganglion = Stellate ganglion
Inferior cervical cardiac branches of vagus nerve
Intercostal nerves = Anterior rami of thoracic nerves
Recurrent laryngeal nerve
Thoracic ganglia of sympathetic trunk
Bronchial branches of vagus nerve and pulmonary plexus
Rami communicantes of spinal nerves
Esophageal plexus
Greater and lesser splanchnic nerves
Anterior vagal trunk
Posterior vagal trunk
Diaphragm
Esophageal hiatus
Gastric plexus
Interganglionic branches of sympathetic trunk
Hepatic plexus
Celiac plexus and ganglia
Renal plexus
Lumbar splanchnic nerves
Superior mesenteric plexus and ganglion
Ovarian plexus
Lumbar ganglia of sympathetic trunk
Inferior mesenteric plexus and ganglion
Abdominal aortic plexus
Superior hypogastric plexus = Presacral nerve
Sacral splanchnic nerves
Iliac plexuses
Sacral ganglia of sympathetic trunk
Hypogastric nerve
Ganglion impar
Inferior hypogastric plexus = Pelvic plexus
Pelvic splanchnic nerves = Parasympathetic root of pelvic ganglia

25 Autonomic division of the peripheral nervous system (25%)

Peripheral sympathetic (**orange**) and parasympathetic (**brown**) nerves and ganglia. The sympathetic components are shown only on the left side of the picture. Ventral aspect

Body Wall

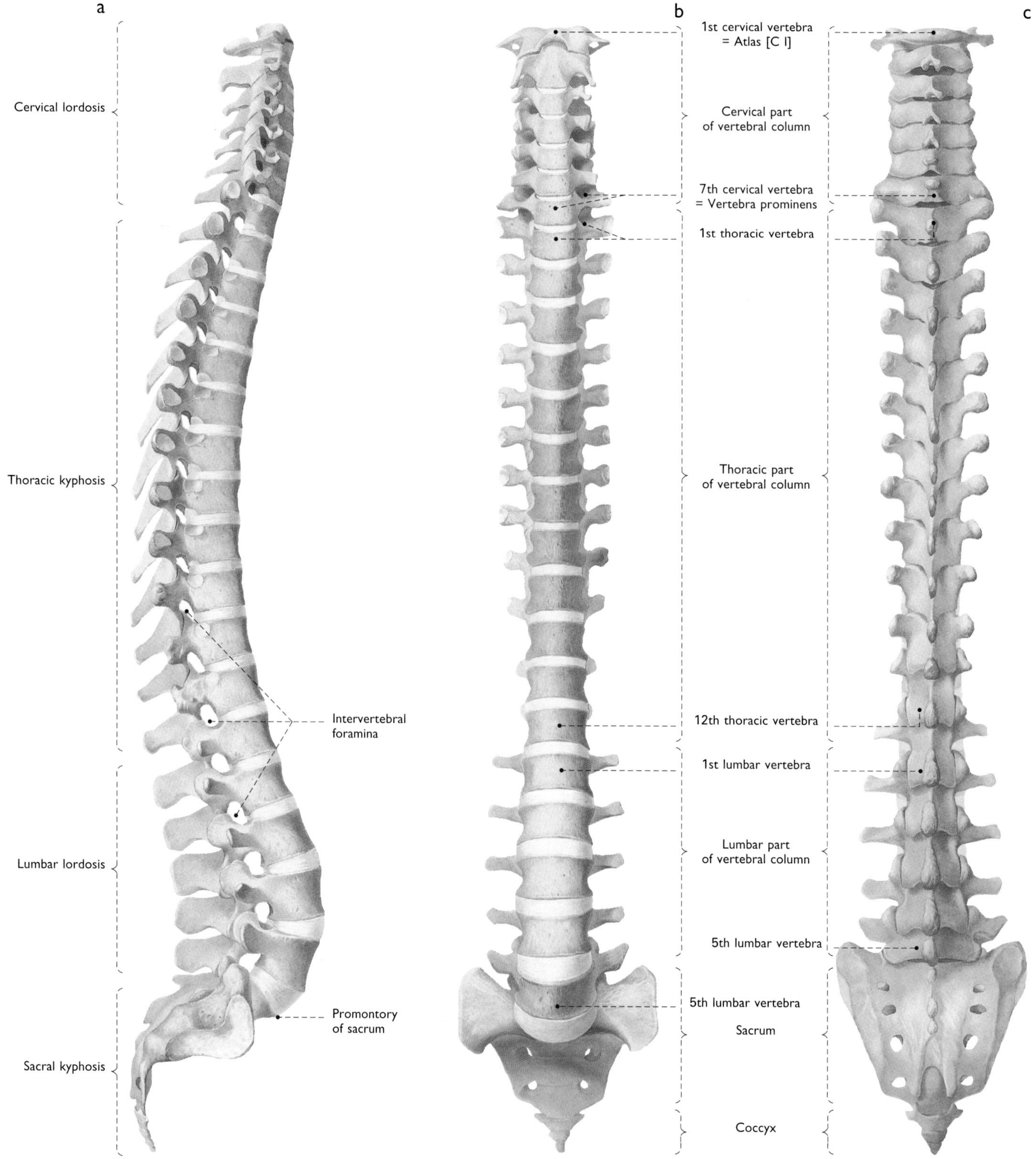
a
Cervical lordosis
Thoracic kyphosis
Lumbar lordosis
Sacral kyphosis
Intervertebral foramina
Promontory of sacrum
b
c
1st cervical vertebra = Atlas [C I]
Cervical part of vertebral column
7th cervical vertebra = Vertebra prominens
1st thoracic vertebra
Thoracic part of vertebral column
12th thoracic vertebra
1st lumbar vertebra
Lumbar part of vertebral column
5th lumbar vertebra
5th lumbar vertebra
Sacrum
Coccyx

28 Vertebral column (30%)

a Right lateral aspect
b Ventral aspect
c Dorsal aspect

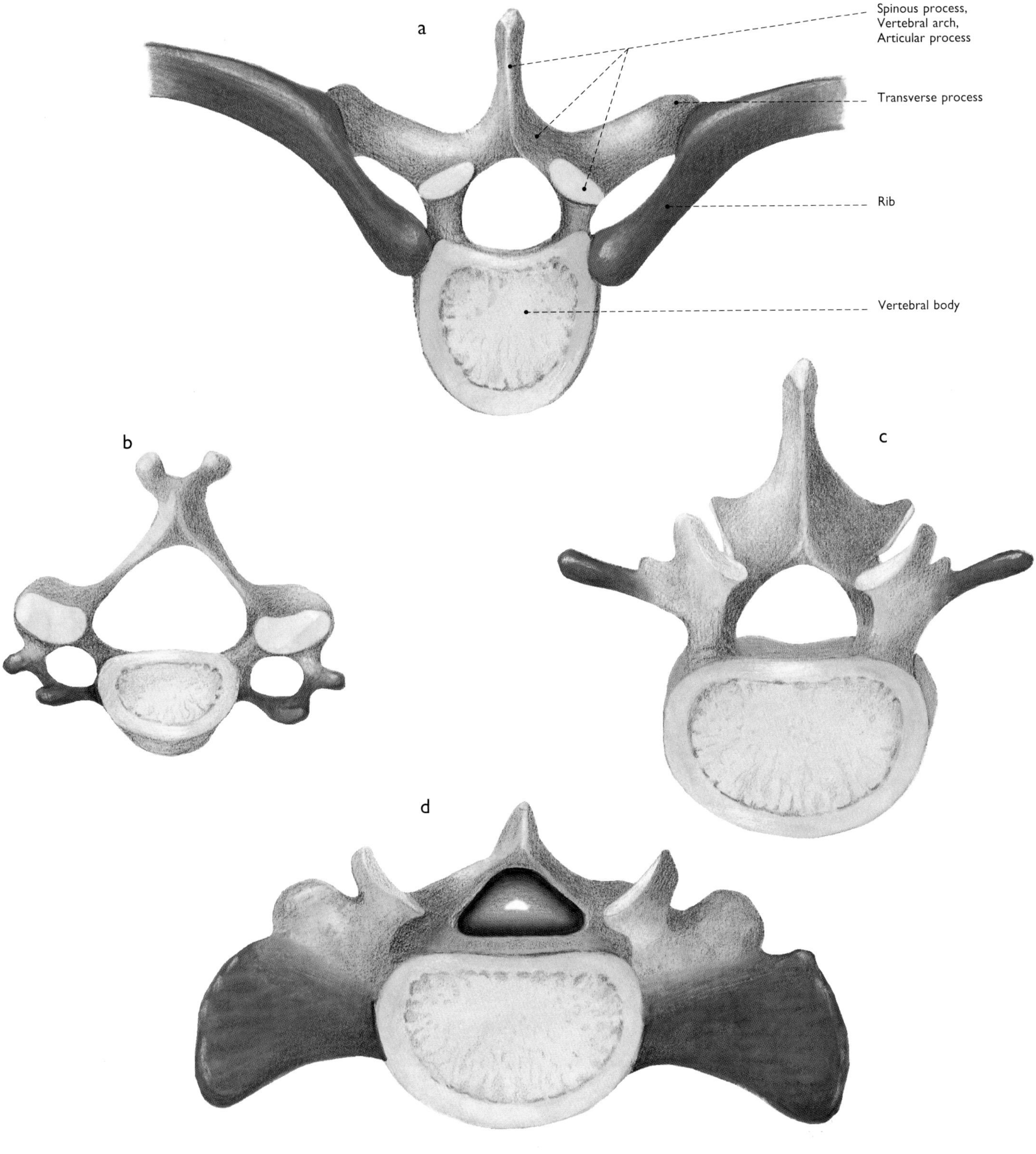
a
Spinous process,
Vertebral arch,
Articular process
Transverse process
Rib
Vertebral body
b
c
d

29 Homology of parts of vertebrae

Homologous parts of vertebrae are represented by the same color.
Cranial aspect

a Thoracic vertebra with ribs
b Cervical vertebra
c Lumbar vertebra
d Sacrum

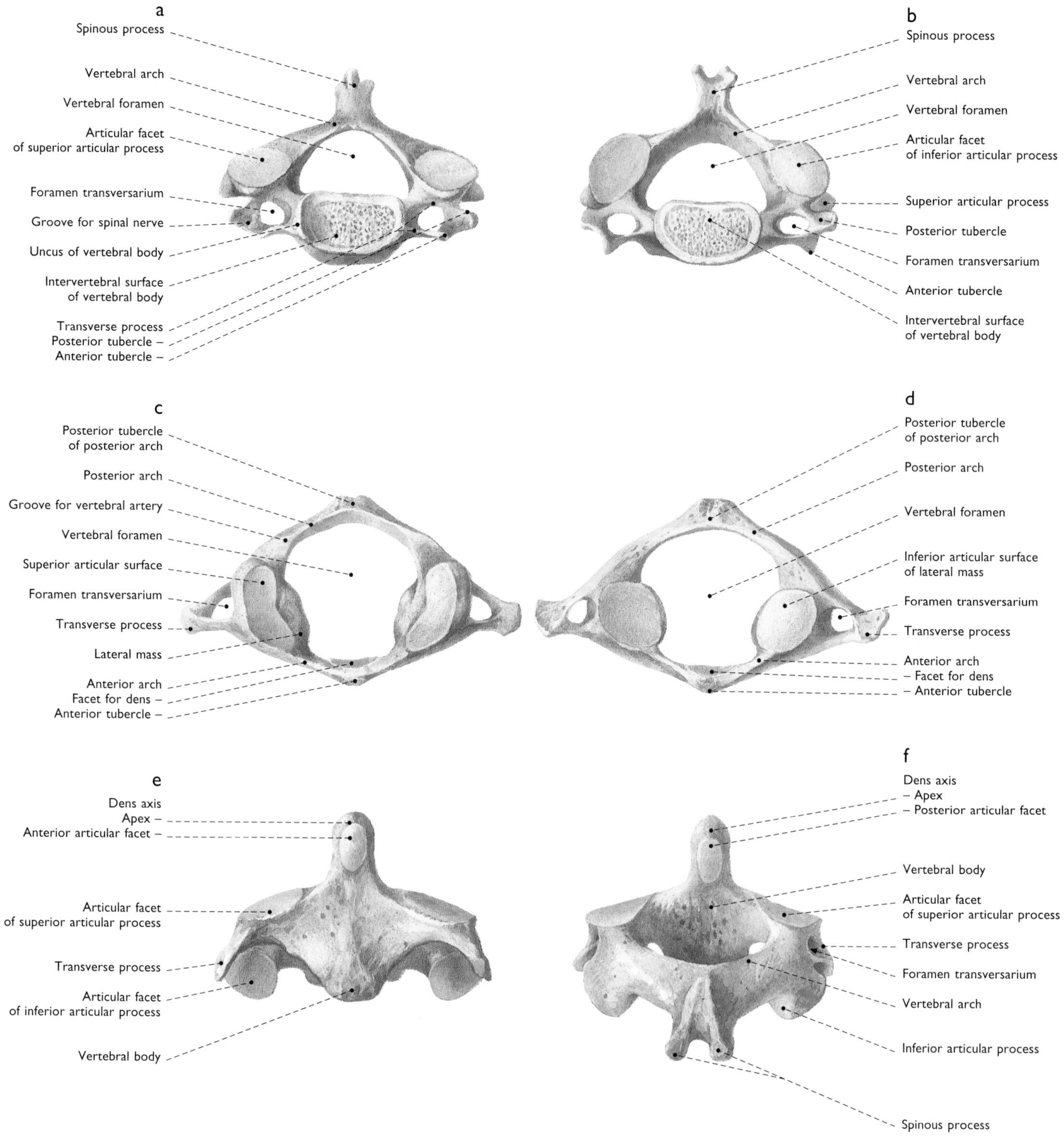
a
Spinous process
Vertebral arch
Vertebral foramen
Articular facet
of superior articular process
Foramen transversarium
Groove for spinal nerve
Uncus of vertebral body
Intervertebral surface
of vertebral body
Transverse process
Posterior tubercle –
Anterior tubercle –
b
Spinous process
Vertebral arch
Vertebral foramen
Articular facet
of inferior articular process
Superior articular process
Posterior tubercle
Foramen transversarium
Anterior tubercle
Intervertebral surface
of vertebral body
c
Posterior tubercle
of posterior arch
Posterior arch
Groove for vertebral artery
Vertebral foramen
Superior articular surface
Foramen transversarium
Transverse process
Lateral mass
Anterior arch
Facet for dens –
Anterior tubercle –
d
Posterior tubercle
of posterior arch
Posterior arch
Vertebral foramen
Inferior articular surface
of lateral mass
Foramen transversarium
Transverse process
Anterior arch
– Facet for dens
– Anterior tubercle
e
Dens axis
Apex –
Anterior articular facet –
Articular facet
of superior articular process
Transverse process
Articular facet
of inferior articular process
Vertebral body
f
Dens axis
– Apex
– Posterior articular facet
Vertebral body
Articular facet
of superior articular process
Transverse process
Foramen transversarium
Vertebral arch
Inferior articular process
Spinous process

30 Cervical vertebrae (90%)

a, b Middle cervical vertebra
a Cranial aspect
b Caudal aspect
c, d First cervical vertebra = atlas [C I]
c Cranial aspect
d Caudal aspect
e, f Second cervical vertebra = axis [C II]
e Ventral aspect
f Dorsal aspect

a

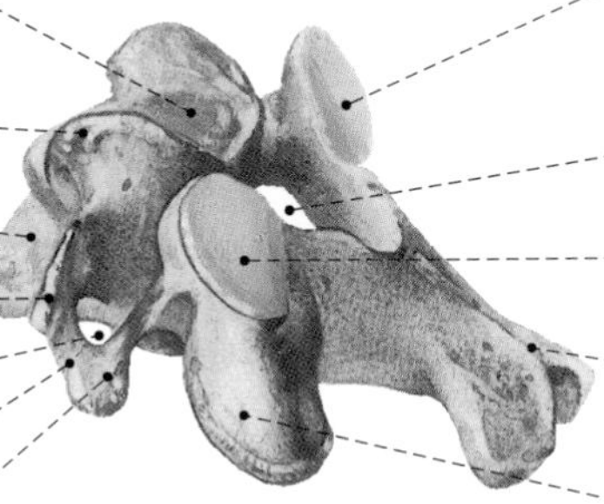
Intervertebral surface
of vertebral body
Uncus of vertebral body
= Uncinate process
Vertebral body
Anterior tubercle
Foramen transversarium
Groove for spinal nerve
Posterior tubercle
Articular facet
of right superior articular process
Vertebral foramen
Articular facet
of left superior articular process
Spinous process
Left inferior articular process

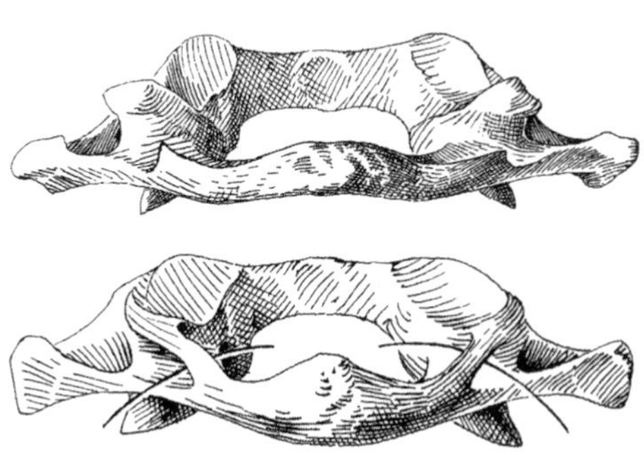
b
c

d

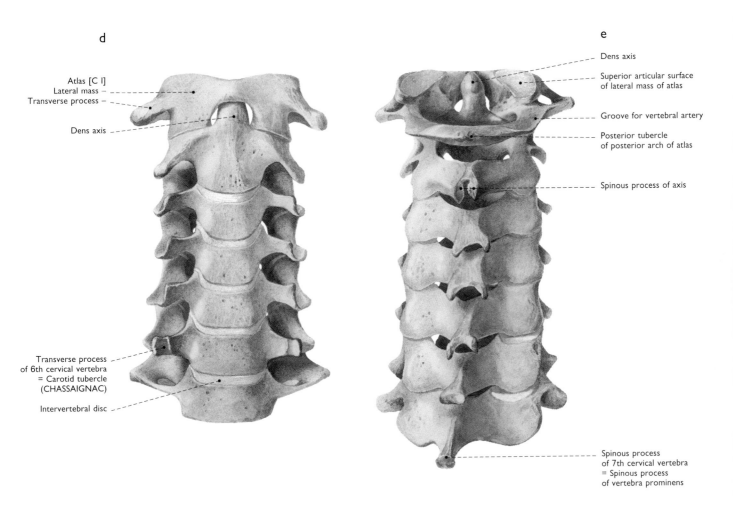

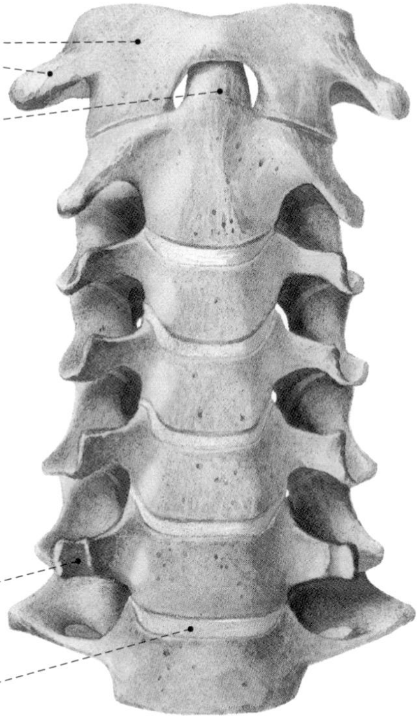
Atlas [C I]
Lateral mass
Transverse process
Dens axis
Transverse process
of 6th cervical vertebra
= Carotid tubercle
(CHASSAIGNAC)
Intervertebral disc

e

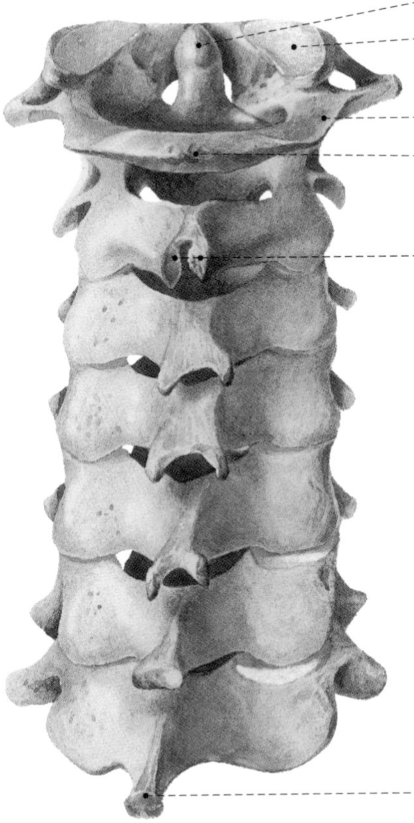
Dens axis
Superior articular surface
of lateral mass of atlas
Groove for vertebral artery
Posterior tubercle
of posterior arch of atlas
Spinous process of axis
Spinous process
of 7th cervical vertebra
= Spinous process
of vertebra prominens

31 Cervical vertebrae and cervical spine

a Middle cervical vertebra (90%), left lateral aspect
b, c First cervical vertebra = atlas [C I], dorsal aspect
b Deep groove for the vertebral artery on both sides
c Canal for the vertebral artery on both sides
d, e Cervical spine with intervertebral discs (100%)
d Ventral aspect
e Dorsal aspect

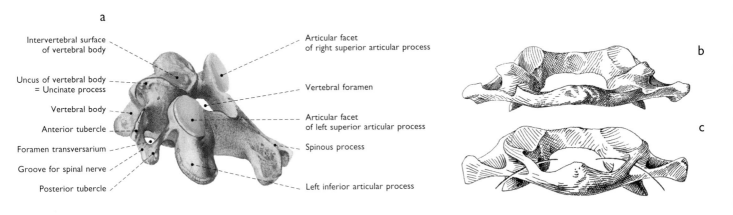

a

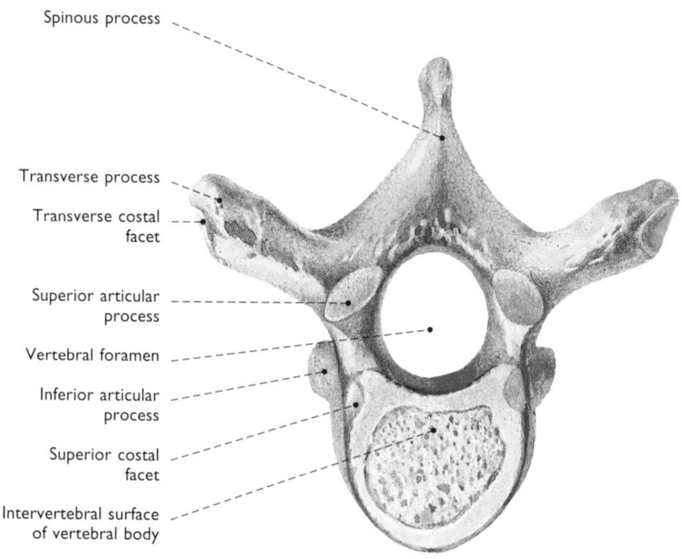
Spinous process
Transverse process
Transverse costal facet
Superior articular process
Vertebral foramen
Inferior articular process
Superior costal facet
Intervertebral surface of vertebral body

b

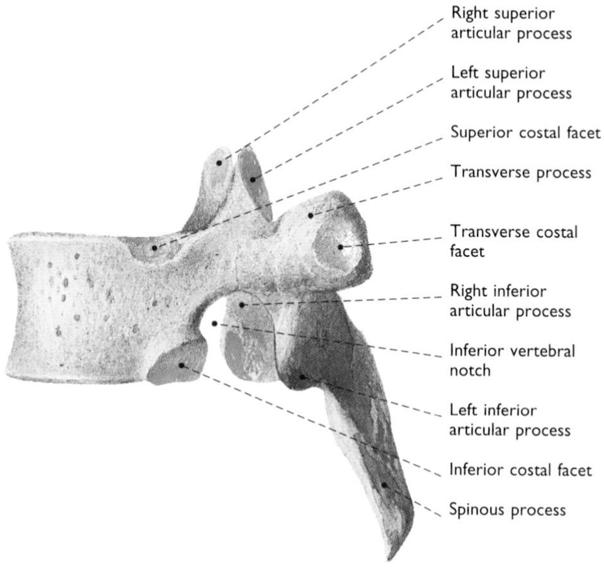
Right superior articular process
Left superior articular process
Superior costal facet
Transverse process
Transverse costal facet
Right inferior articular process
Inferior vertebral notch
Left inferior articular process
Inferior costal facet
Spinous process

c

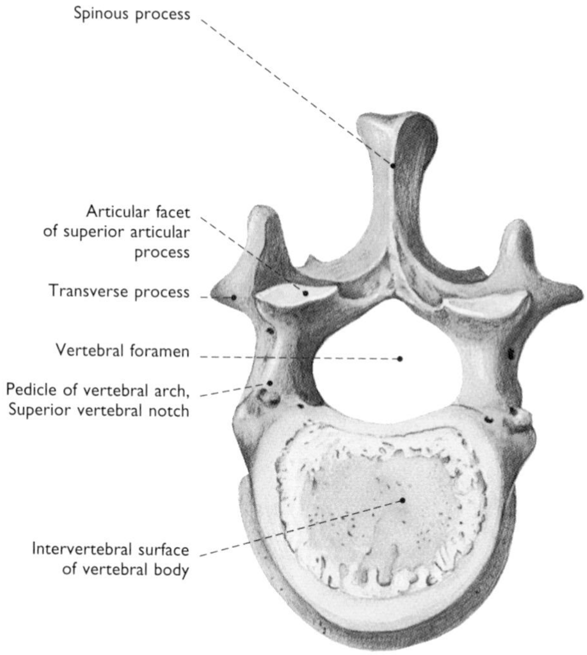
Spinous process
Articular facet of superior articular process
Transverse process
Vertebral foramen
Pedicle of vertebral arch, Superior vertebral notch
Intervertebral surface of vertebral body

d

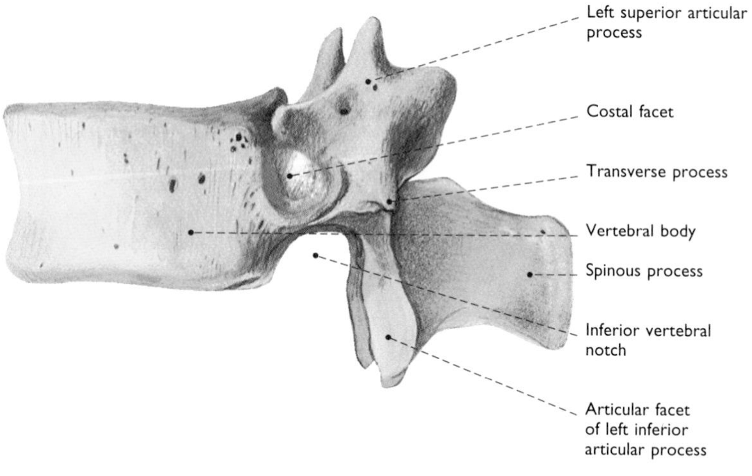
Left superior articular process
Costal facet
Transverse process
Vertebral body
Spinous process
Inferior vertebral notch
Articular facet of left inferior articular process

32 Thoracic vertebrae (100%)

a, b Sixth thoracic vertebra
 a Cranial aspect
 b Left lateral aspect
c, d Twelfth thoracic vertebra
 c Cranial aspect
 d Left lateral aspect

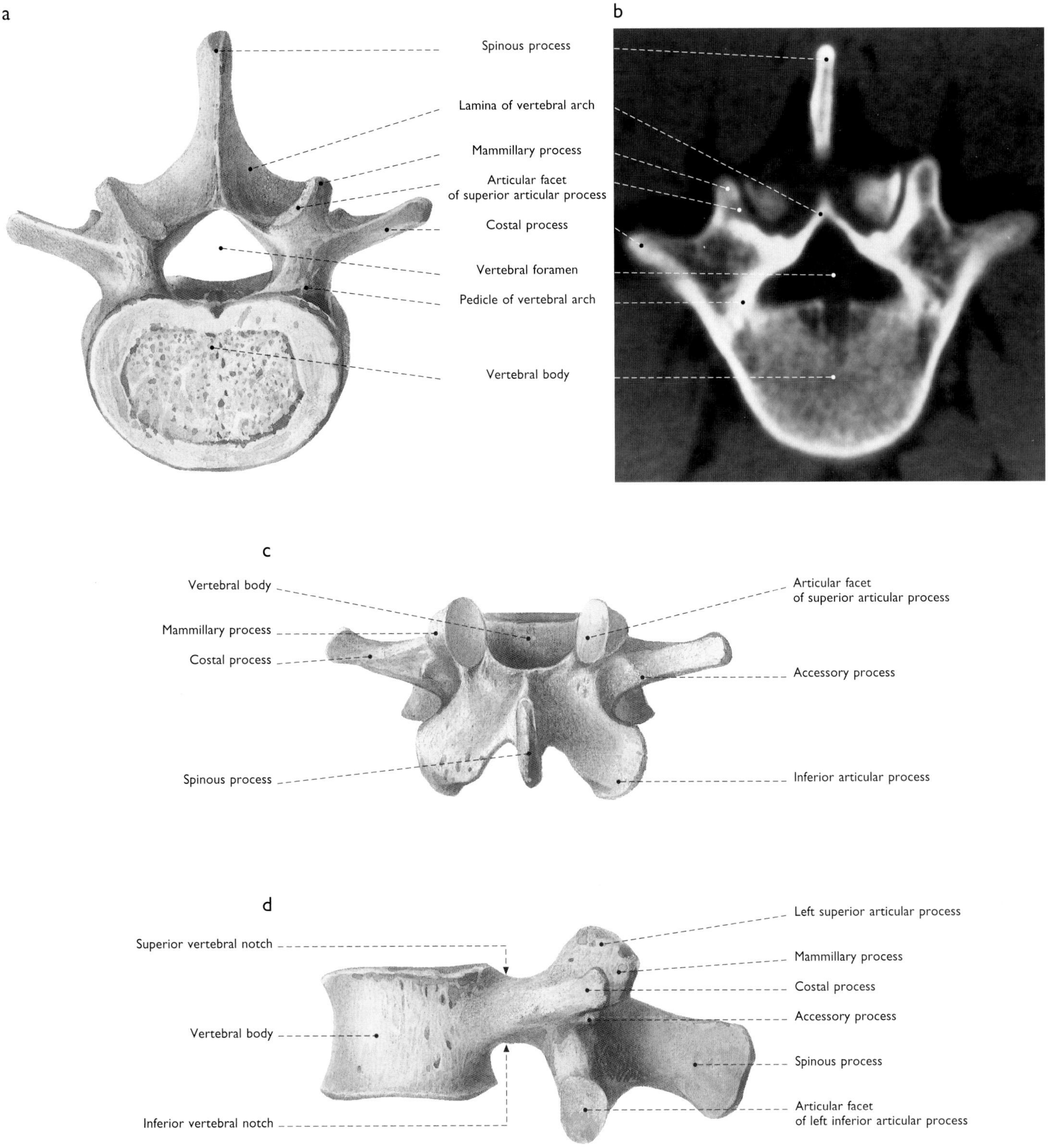
a
b
Spinous process
Lamina of vertebral arch
Mammillary process
Articular facet
of superior articular process
Costal process
Vertebral foramen
Pedicle of vertebral arch
Vertebral body
c
Vertebral body
Mammillary process
Costal process
Spinous process
Articular facet
of superior articular process
Accessory process
Inferior articular process
d
Superior vertebral notch
Vertebral body
Inferior vertebral notch
Left superior articular process
Mammillary process
Costal process
Accessory process
Spinous process
Articular facet
of left inferior articular process

33 Middle lumbar vertebra (100%)

a Cranial aspect
b Axial (transverse) computed tomogram (CT)
c Dorsal aspect
d Left lateral aspect

a

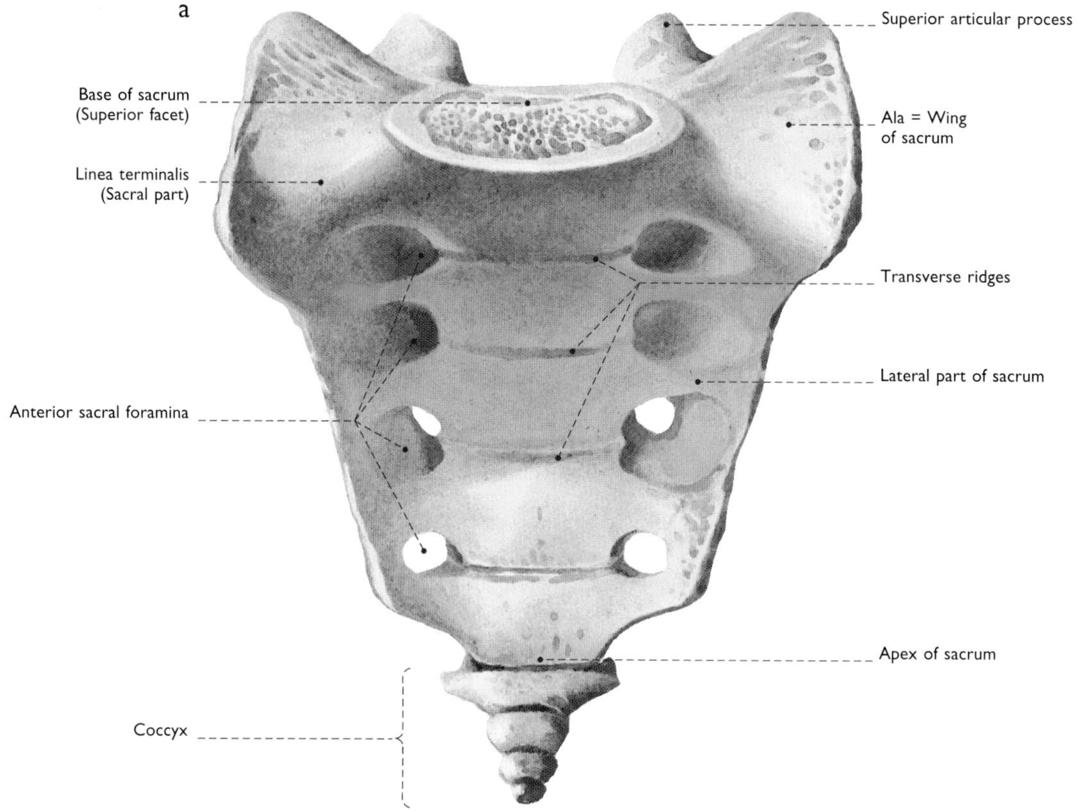
Superior articular process
Base of sacrum
(Superior facet)
Ala = Wing
of sacrum
Linea terminalis
(Sacral part)
Transverse ridges
Lateral part of sacrum
Anterior sacral foramina
Apex of sacrum
Coccyx

b

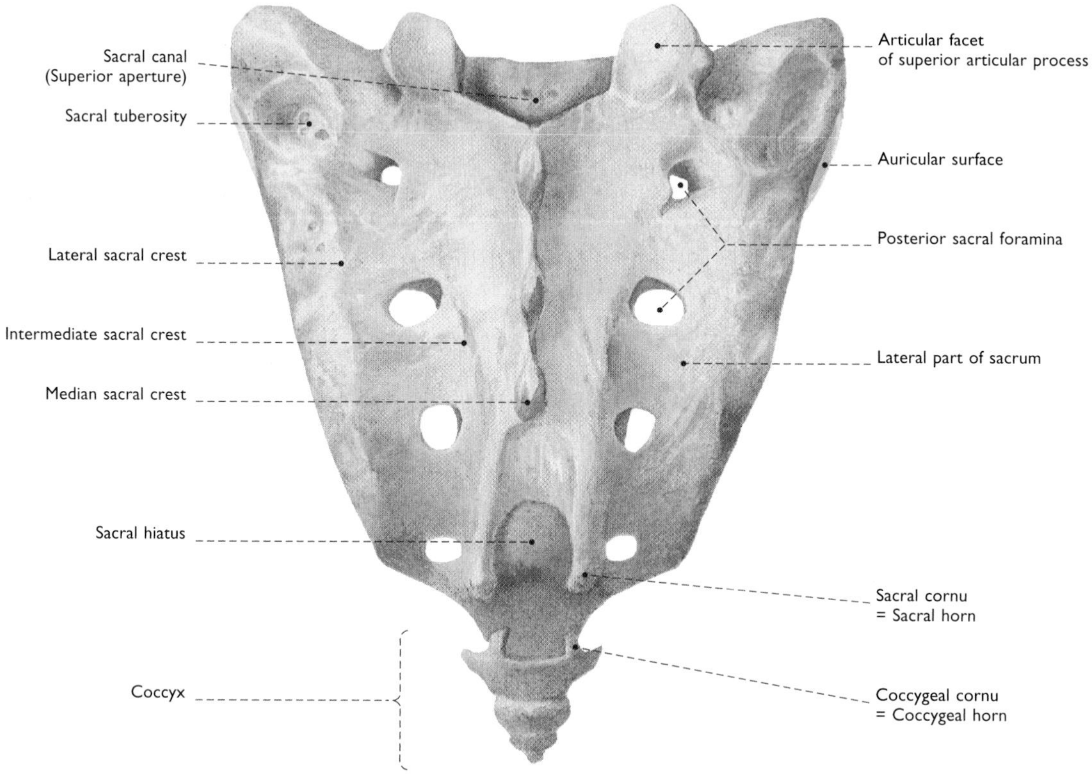
Sacral canal
(Superior aperture)
Articular facet
of superior articular process
Sacral tuberosity
Auricular surface
Posterior sacral foramina
Lateral sacral crest
Intermediate sacral crest
Lateral part of sacrum
Median sacral crest
Sacral hiatus
Sacral cornu
= Sacral horn
Coccyx
Coccygeal cornu
= Coccygeal horn

34 Sacrum and coccyx (80%)

a Ventral aspect
b Dorsal aspect

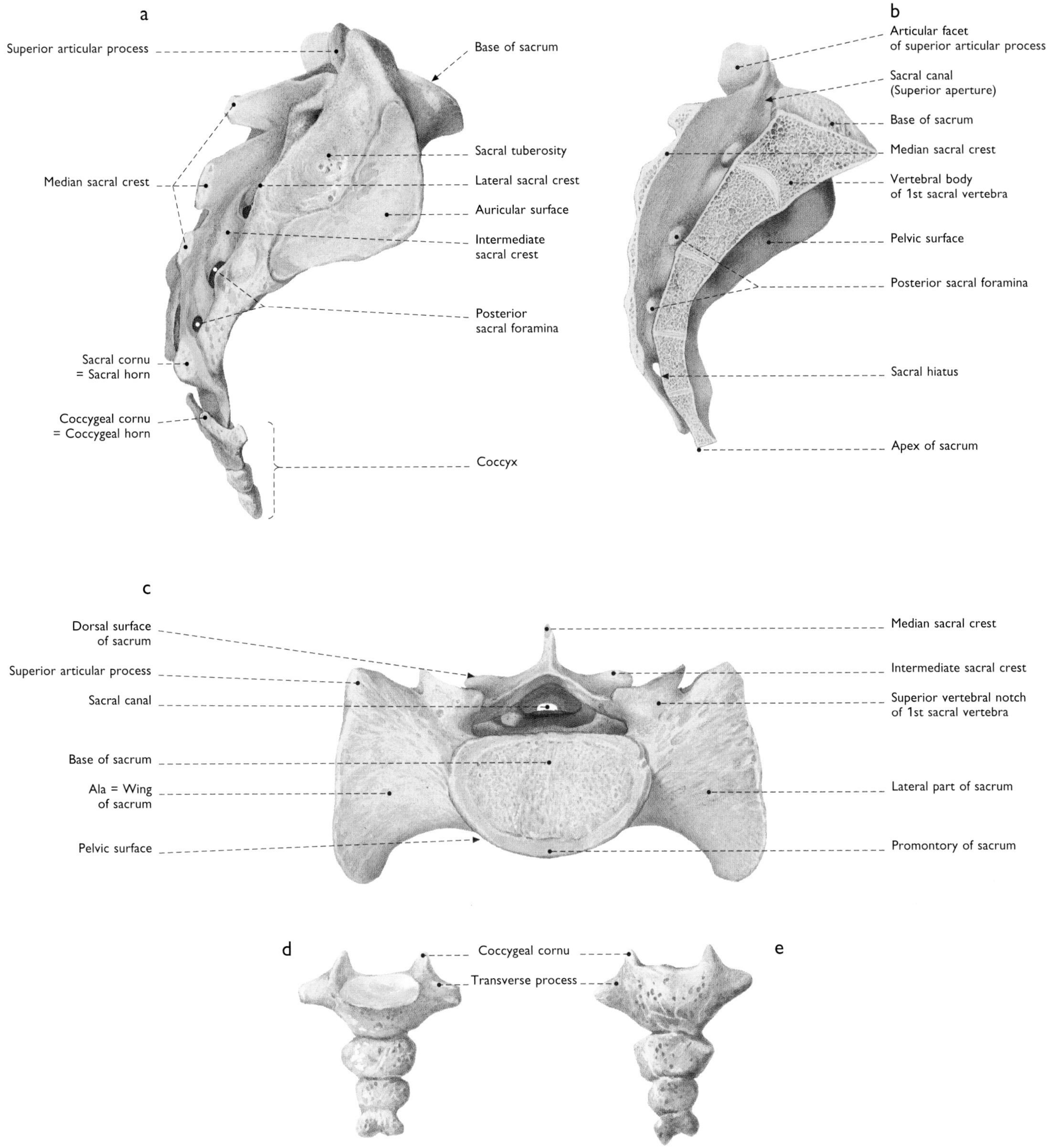
a
Superior articular process
Base of sacrum
Median sacral crest
Sacral tuberosity
Lateral sacral crest
Auricular surface
Intermediate sacral crest
Posterior sacral foramina
Sacral cornu = Sacral horn
Coccygeal cornu = Coccygeal horn
Coccyx
b
Articular facet of superior articular process
Sacral canal (Superior aperture)
Base of sacrum
Median sacral crest
Vertebral body of 1st sacral vertebra
Pelvic surface
Posterior sacral foramina
Sacral hiatus
Apex of sacrum
c
Dorsal surface of sacrum
Superior articular process
Sacral canal
Base of sacrum
Ala = Wing of sacrum
Pelvic surface
Median sacral crest
Intermediate sacral crest
Superior vertebral notch of 1st sacral vertebra
Lateral part of sacrum
Promontory of sacrum
d
e
Coccygeal cornu
Transverse process

35 Sacrum and coccyx

a–c Sacrum
a Right lateral aspect (60%)
b Median section, medial aspect of the left half (60%)
c Cranial aspect (70%)
d, e Coccyx (80%)
d Ventral aspect
e Dorsal aspect

a

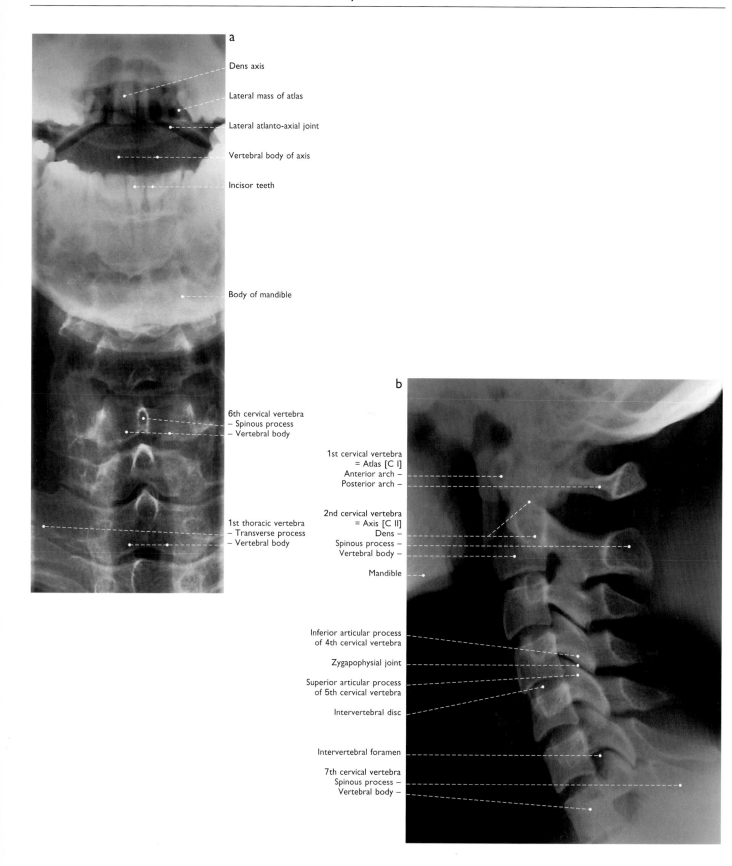

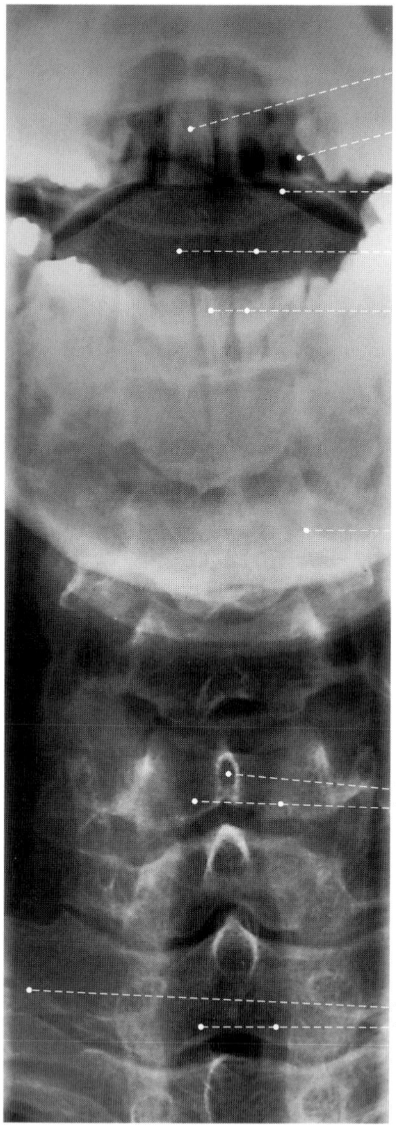
Dens axis
Lateral mass of atlas
Lateral atlanto-axial joint
Vertebral body of axis
Incisor teeth
Body of mandible
6th cervical vertebra
– Spinous process
– Vertebral body
1st thoracic vertebra
– Transverse process
– Vertebral body

b

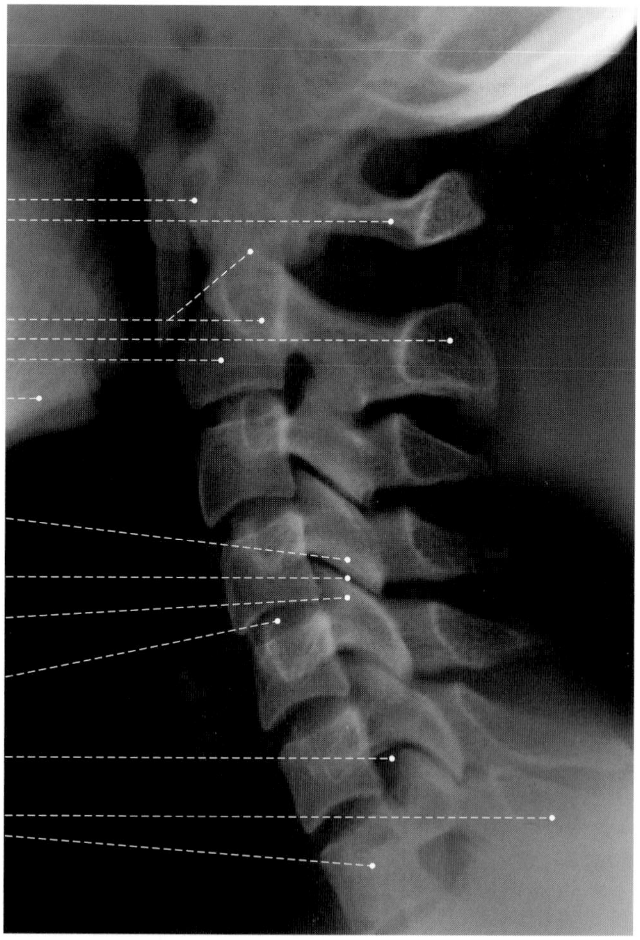
1st cervical vertebra
= Atlas [C I]
Anterior arch –
Posterior arch –
2nd cervical vertebra
= Axis [C II]
Dens –
Spinous process –
Vertebral body –
Mandible
Inferior articular process
of 4th cervical vertebra
Zygapophysial joint
Superior articular process
of 5th cervical vertebra
Intervertebral disc
Intervertebral foramen
7th cervical vertebra
Spinous process –
Vertebral body –

36 Cervical spine (100%)

a Anteroposterior radiograph
b Lateral radiograph

a

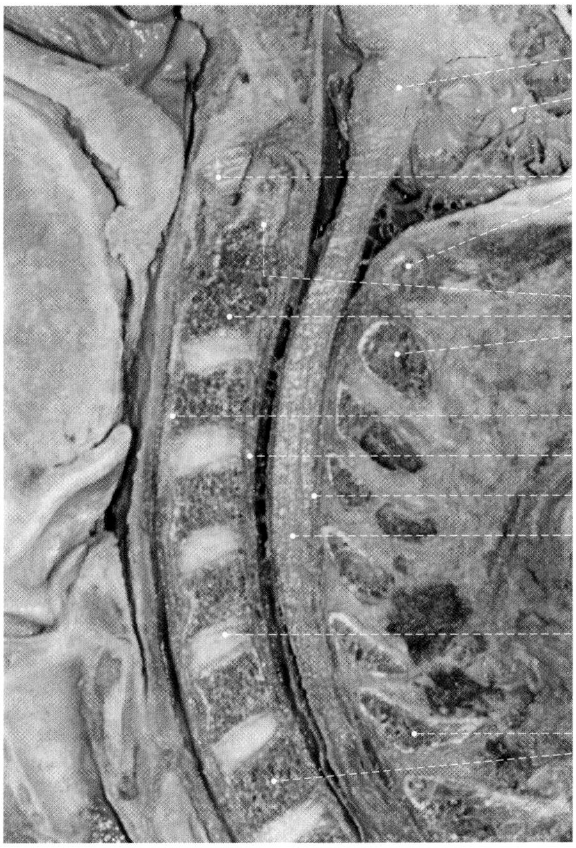
Medulla oblongata
Cerebellum
1st cervical vertebra = Atlas [C I]
– Anterior arch
– Posterior arch
2nd cervical vertebra = Axis [C II]
– Dens
– Vertebral body
– Spinous process
Anterior longitudinal ligament
Posterior longitudinal ligament
Ligamentum flavum
Spinal cord
Intervertebral disc
7th cervical vertebra
= Vertebra prominens
– Spinous process
– Vertebral body

b

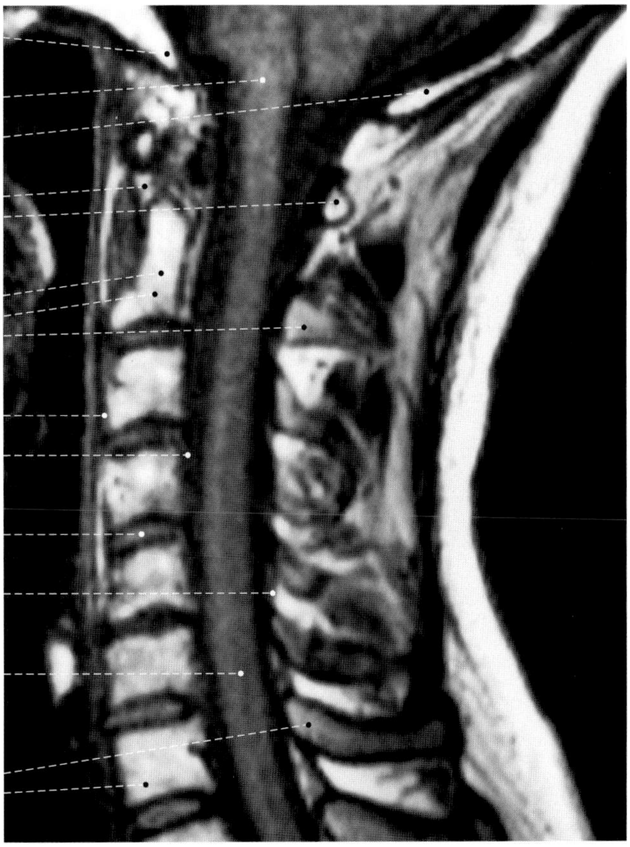
Basilar part of occipital bone
Medulla oblongata
Squamous part of occipital bone
1st cervical vertebra = Atlas [C I]
Anterior arch –
Posterior arch –
2nd cervical vertebra = Axis [C II]
Dens –
Vertebral body –
Spinous process –
Anterior longitudinal ligament
Posterior longitudinal ligament
Intervertebral disc
Ligamentum flavum
Spinal cord
7th cervical vertebra
= Vertebra prominens
Spinous process –
Vertebral body –

37 Cervical spine (90%)

Midsagittal section

a Anatomical section

b Magnetic resonance image (MRI, T_1-weighted)

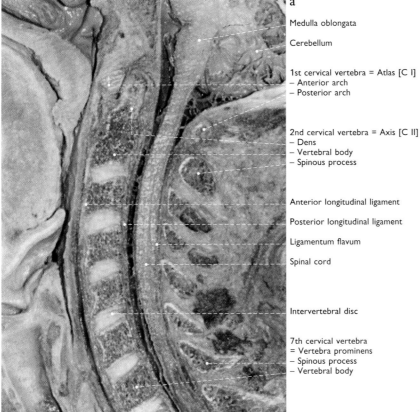

a

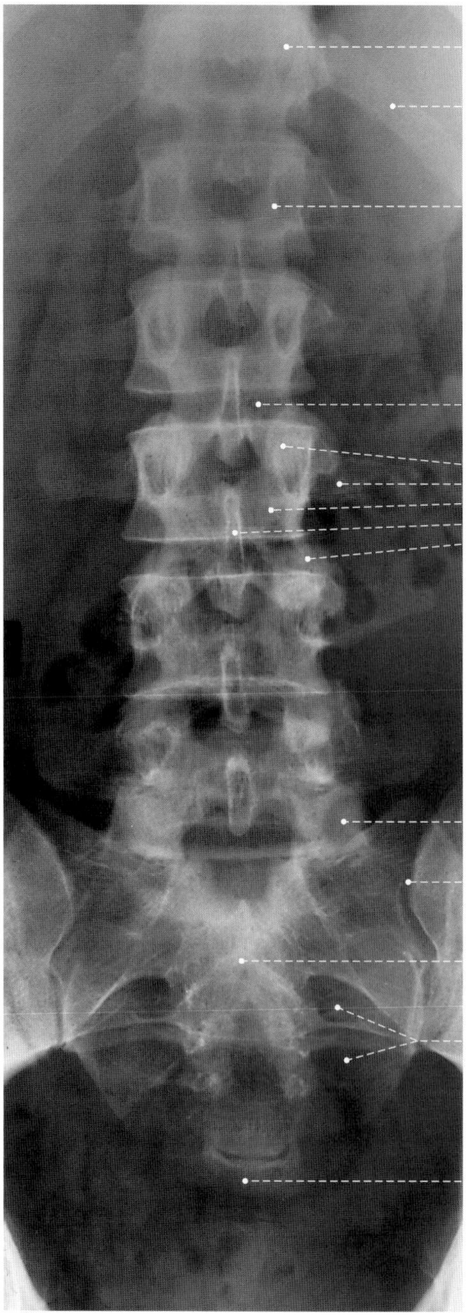
12th thoracic vertebra
12th rib
1st lumbar vertebra
Intervertebral disc
3rd lumbar vertebra
– Superior articular process
– Costal process
– Vertebral body
– Spinous process
– Inferior articular process
Superior articular process of sacrum
Sacro-iliac joint
Sacrum
Anterior sacral foramina
1st coccygeal vertebra

b

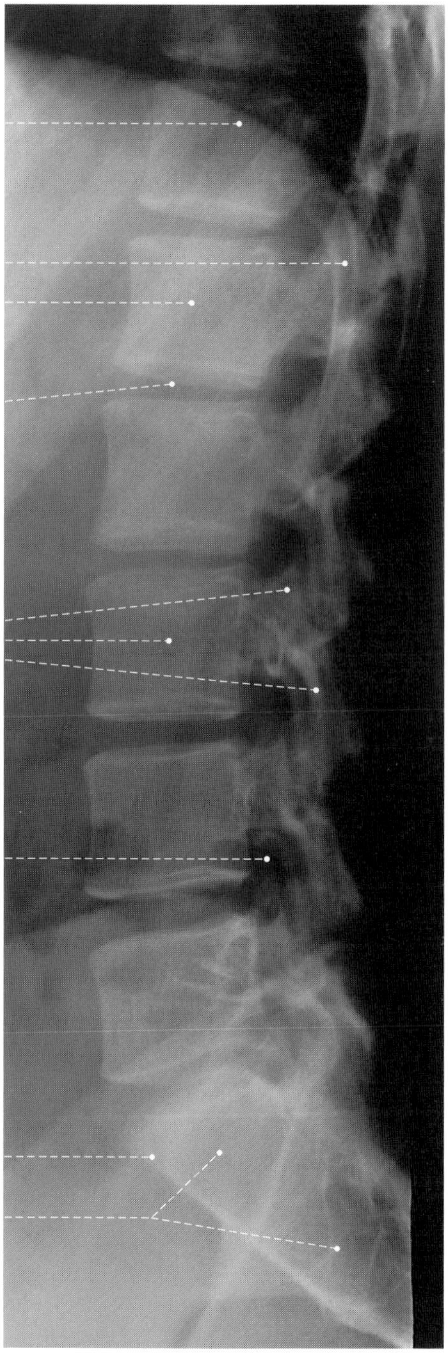
12th thoracic vertebra
12th rib
1st lumbar vertebra
Intervertebral disc
3rd lumbar vertebra
Superior articular process –
Vertebral body –
Inferior articular process –
Intervertebral foramen
Promontory of sacrum
Sacrum

38 Lumbar spine, sacrum, and coccyx (50%)

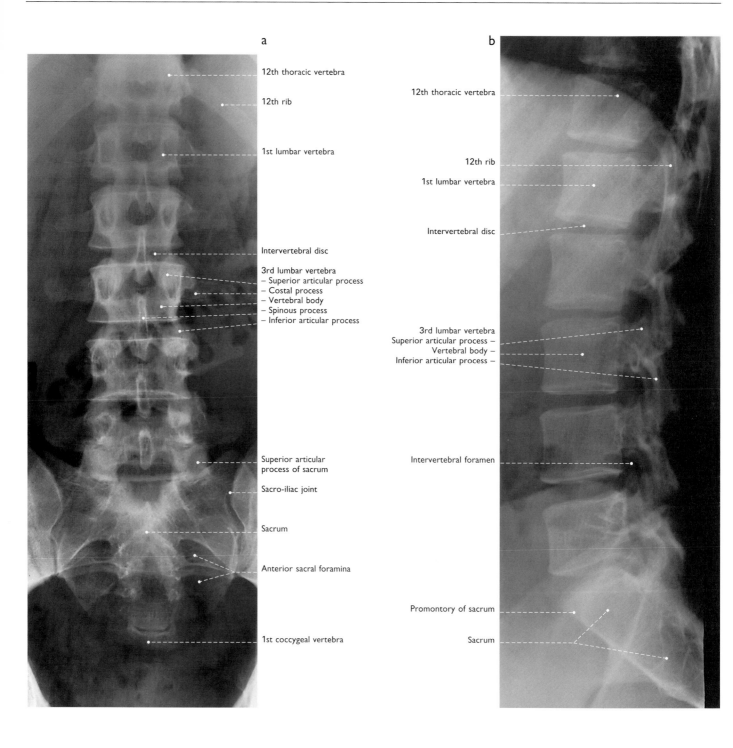

a Anteroposterior radiograph
b Lateral radiograph

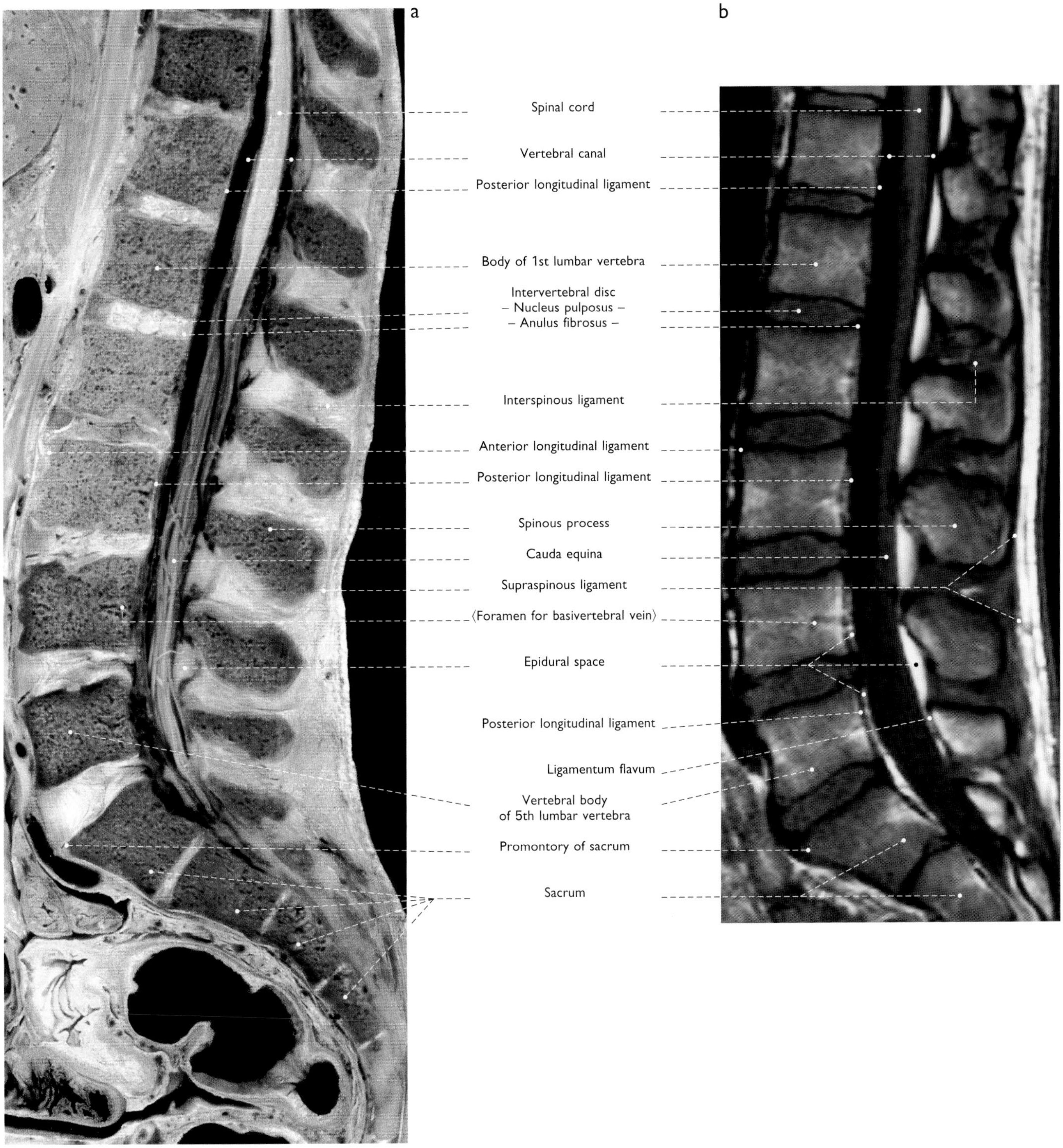
a
b
Spinal cord
Vertebral canal
Posterior longitudinal ligament
Body of 1st lumbar vertebra
Intervertebral disc
– Nucleus pulposus –
– Anulus fibrosus –
Interspinous ligament
Anterior longitudinal ligament
Posterior longitudinal ligament
Spinous process
Cauda equina
Supraspinous ligament
⟨Foramen for basivertebral vein⟩
Epidural space
Posterior longitudinal ligament
Ligamentum flavum
Vertebral body
of 5th lumbar vertebra
Promontory of sacrum
Sacrum

39 Lumbar spine, sacrum, and coccyx (50%)

Midsagittal section
a Anatomical section
b Magnetic resonance image (MRI, T_1-weighted)

a

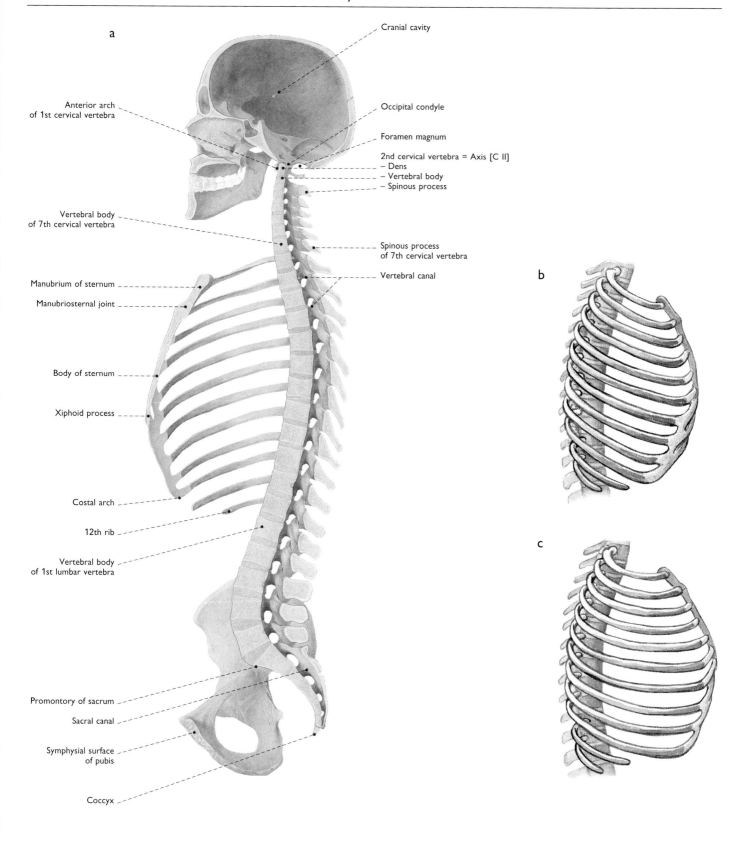

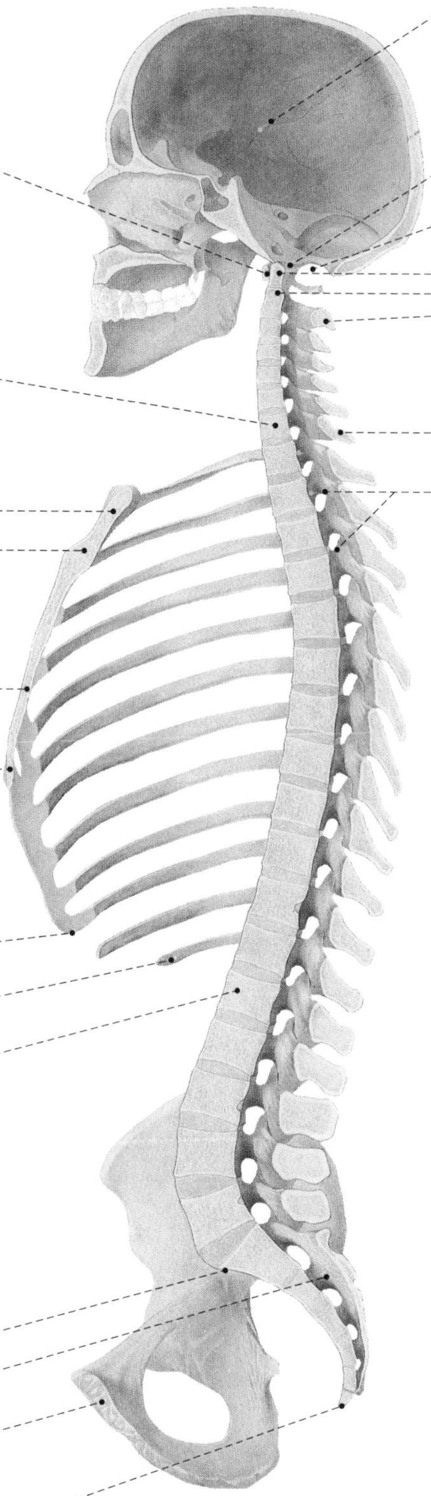
Cranial cavity
Anterior arch
of 1st cervical vertebra
Occipital condyle
Foramen magnum
2nd cervical vertebra = Axis [C II]
– Dens
– Vertebral body
– Spinous process
Vertebral body
of 7th cervical vertebra
Spinous process
of 7th cervical vertebra
Vertebral canal
Manubrium of sternum
Manubriosternal joint
Body of sternum
Xiphoid process
Costal arch
12th rib
Vertebral body
of 1st lumbar vertebra
Promontory of sacrum
Sacral canal
Symphysial surface
of pubis
Coccyx

b

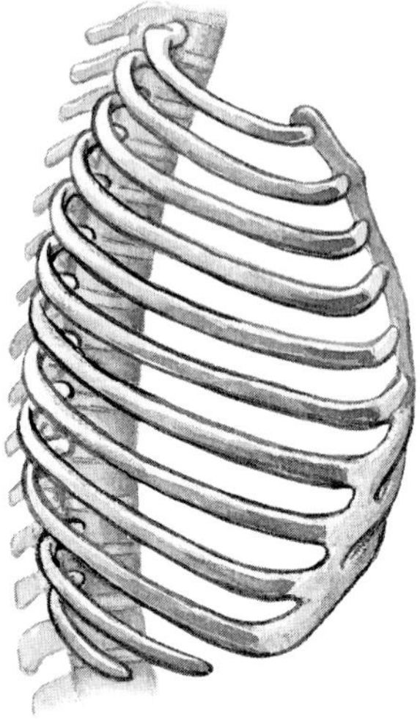

c

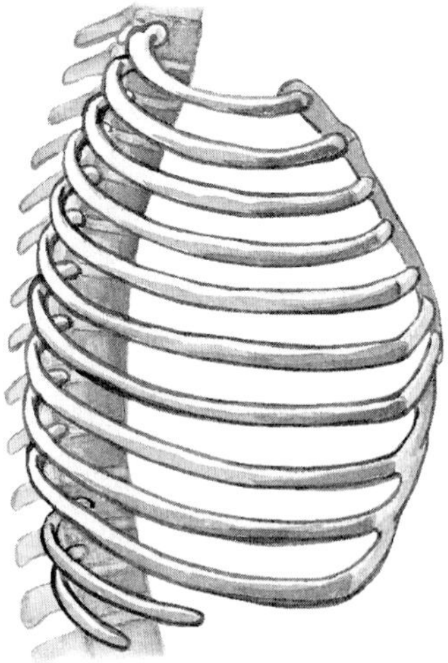

40 Axial skeleton and hip bone

a Median section (25%), medial aspect
b, c Alterations of the shape of thorax during respiration, right lateral aspect
b Phase of expiration
c Phase of inspiration

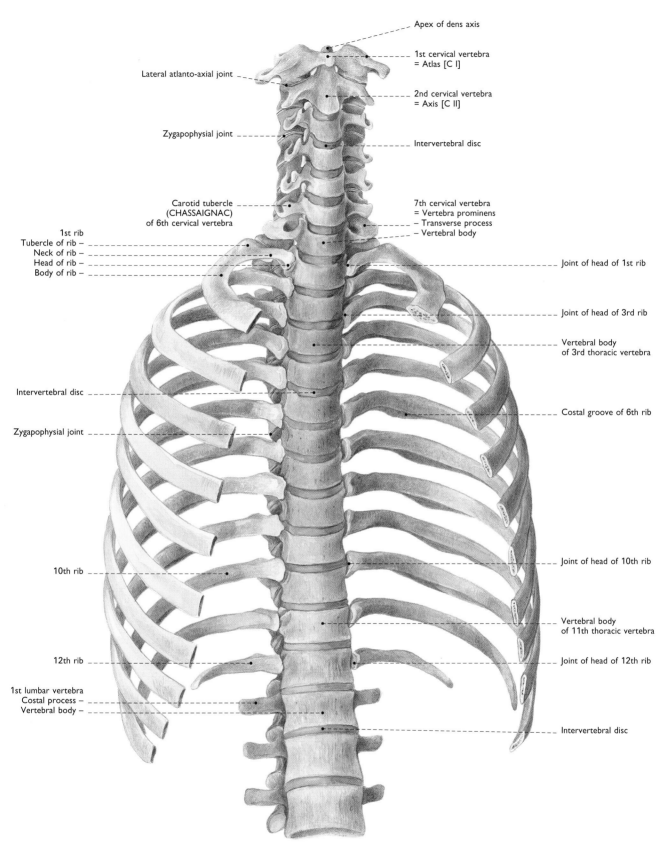

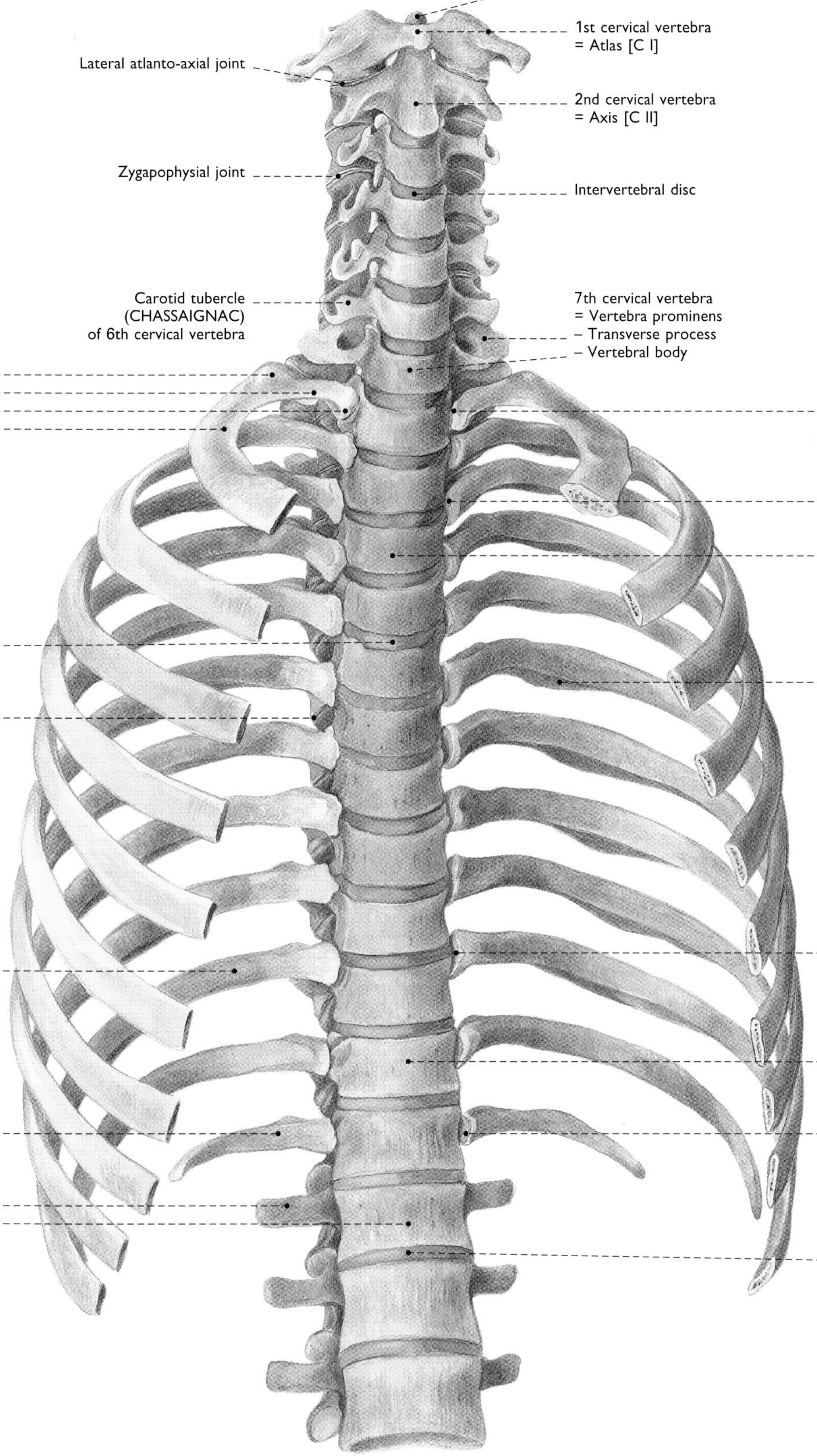
Apex of dens axis
1st cervical vertebra
= Atlas [C I]
Lateral atlanto-axial joint
2nd cervical vertebra
= Axis [C II]
Zygapophysial joint
Intervertebral disc
Carotid tubercle
(CHASSAIGNAC)
of 6th cervical vertebra
7th cervical vertebra
= Vertebra prominens
– Transverse process
– Vertebral body
1st rib
Tubercle of rib –
Neck of rib –
Head of rib –
Body of rib –
Joint of head of 1st rib
Joint of head of 3rd rib
Vertebral body
of 3rd thoracic vertebra
Intervertebral disc
Costal groove of 6th rib
Zygapophysial joint
Joint of head of 10th rib
10th rib
Vertebral body
of 11th thoracic vertebra
12th rib
Joint of head of 12th rib
1st lumbar vertebra
Costal process –
Vertebral body –
Intervertebral disc

41 Thorax (45%)

The sternum and the costal cartilages were removed in order to reveal the joints of costal heads.
Ventral aspect

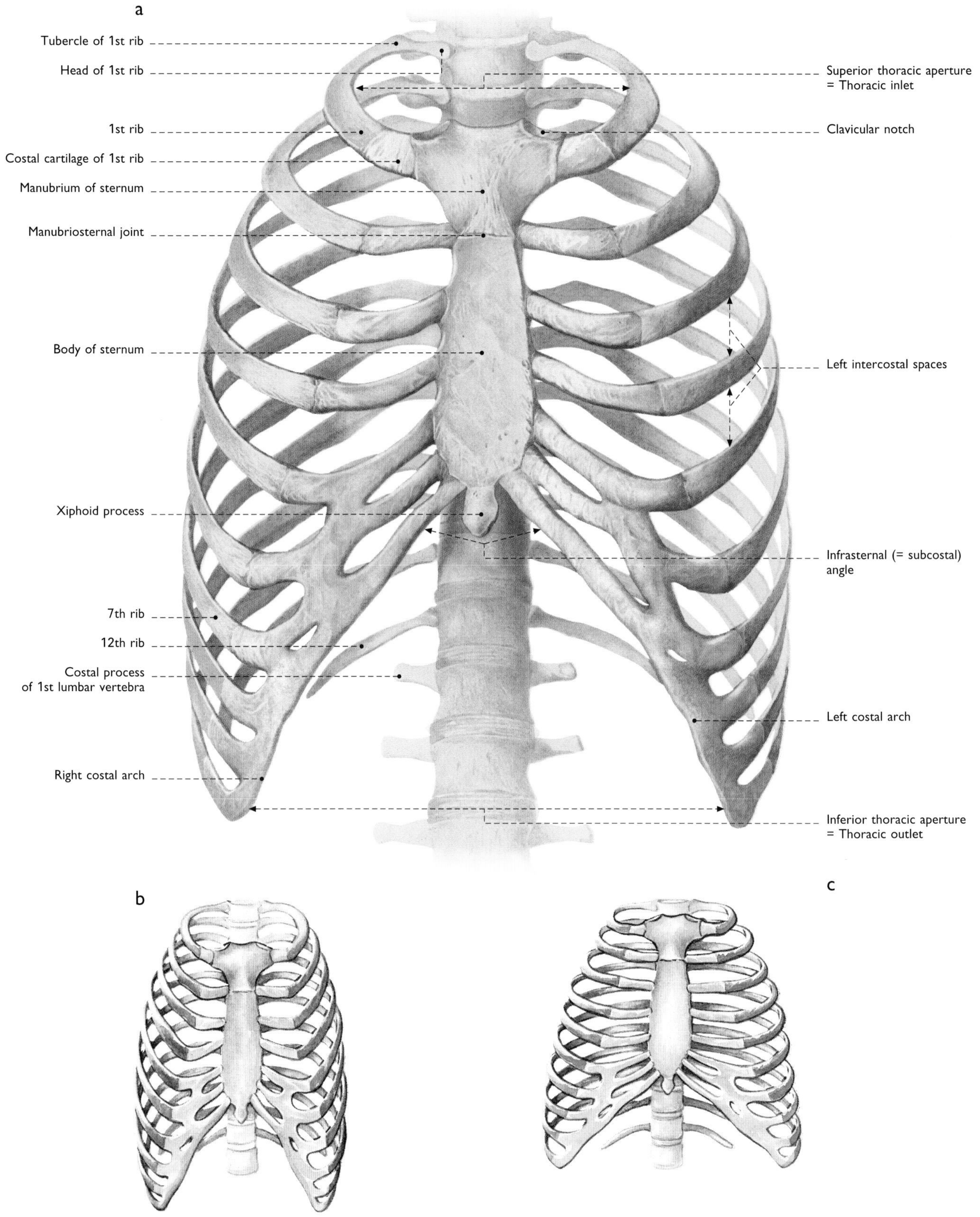
a
Tubercle of 1st rib
Head of 1st rib
1st rib
Costal cartilage of 1st rib
Manubrium of sternum
Manubriosternal joint
Body of sternum
Xiphoid process
7th rib
12th rib
Costal process
of 1st lumbar vertebra
Right costal arch
Superior thoracic aperture
= Thoracic inlet
Clavicular notch
Left intercostal spaces
Infrasternal (= subcostal)
angle
Left costal arch
Inferior thoracic aperture
= Thoracic outlet
b
c

42 Thorax

a Ventral aspect (45%)

b, c Alterations of the shape of thorax during respiration, ventral aspect

b Phase of expiration

c Phase of inspiration

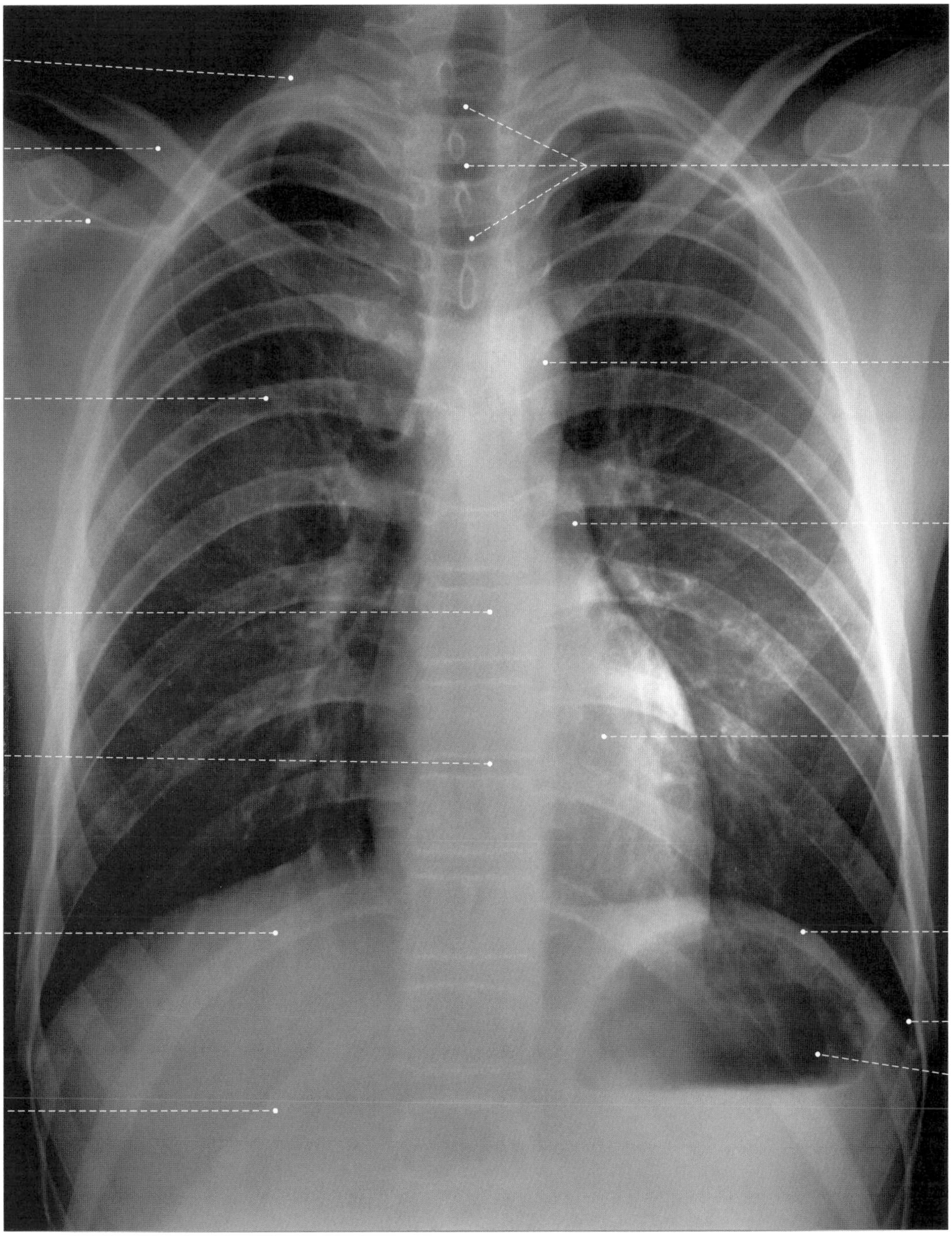
1st rib
Right clavicle
Scapula
6th rib
Vertebral body of 8th thoracic vertebra
Intervertebral disc
11th rib
12th rib
Trachea
Arch of aorta = Aortic arch
Pulmonary trunk
Heart
Diaphragm
Costodiaphragmatic recess
Fundus of stomach

43 Thorax (50%)

Postero-anterior radiograph of the thorax and the shoulder girdle. The arms are elevated. Ventral aspect

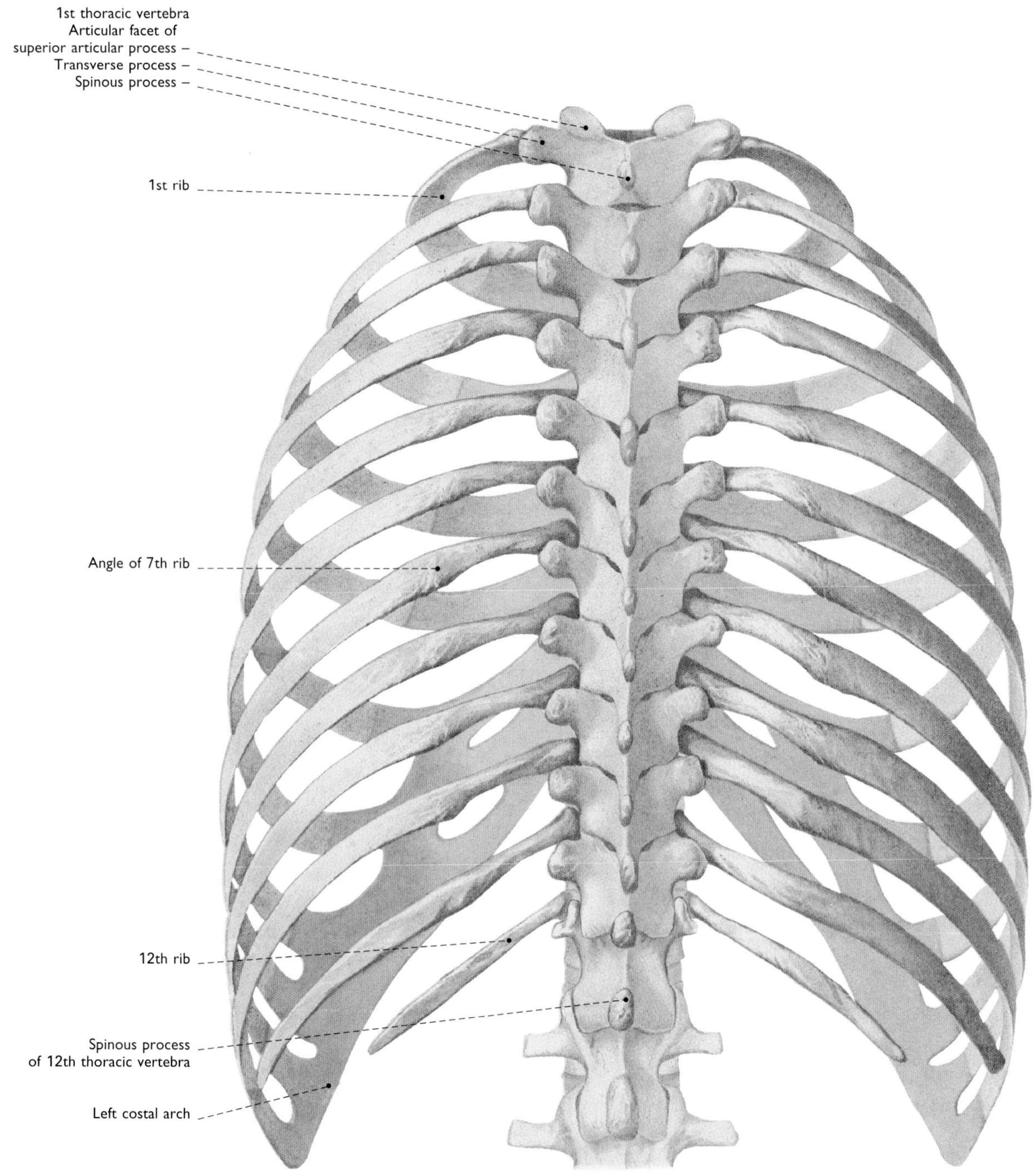
1st thoracic vertebra
Articular facet of
superior articular process
Transverse process
Spinous process
1st rib
Angle of 7th rib
12th rib
Spinous process
of 12th thoracic vertebra
Left costal arch

44 Thorax (50%)
Dorsal aspect

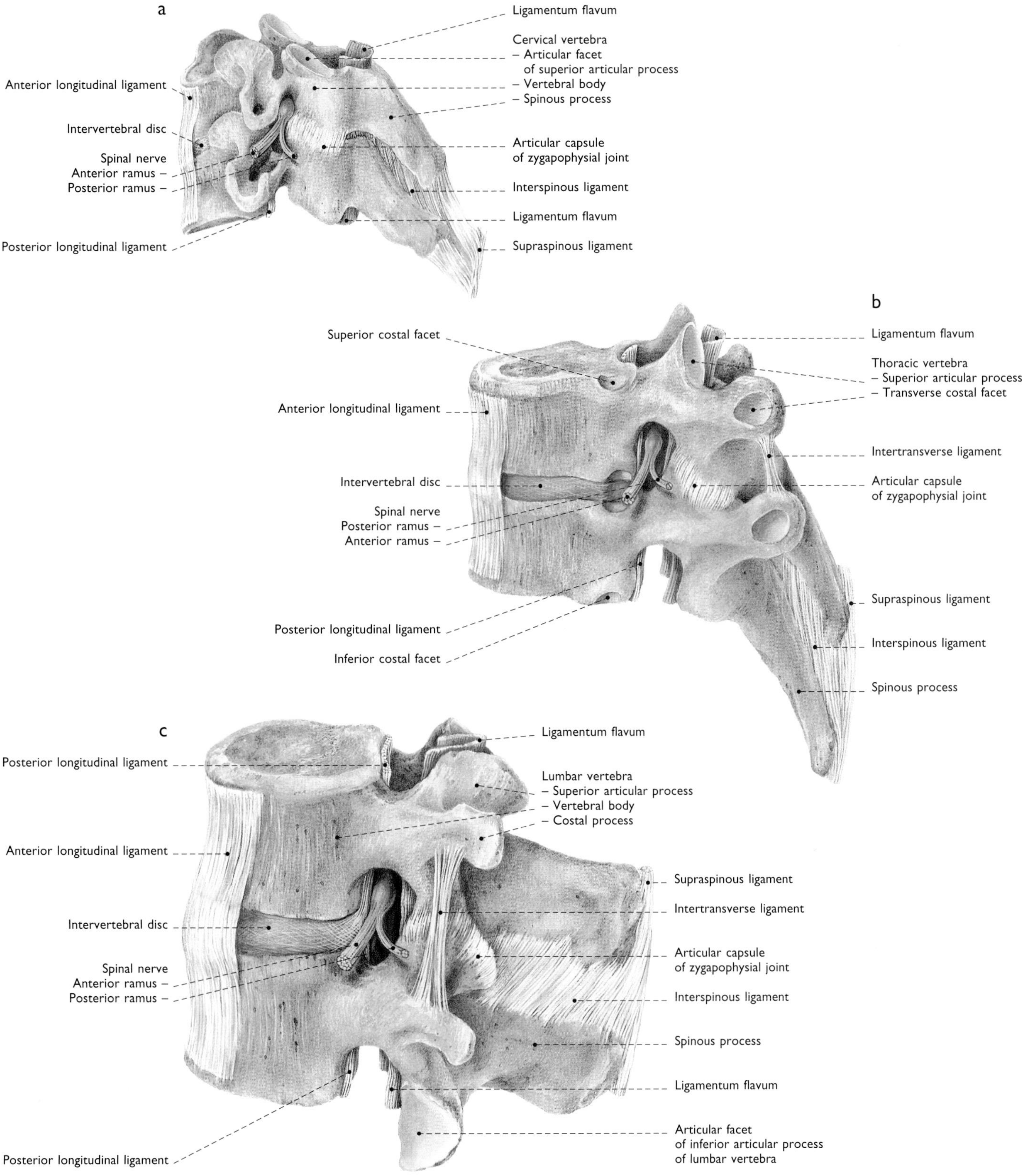
a
Ligamentum flavum
Cervical vertebra
– Articular facet
of superior articular process
– Vertebral body
– Spinous process
Anterior longitudinal ligament
Intervertebral disc
Spinal nerve
Anterior ramus –
Posterior ramus –
Articular capsule
of zygapophysial joint
Interspinous ligament
Ligamentum flavum
Supraspinous ligament
Posterior longitudinal ligament
b
Superior costal facet
Ligamentum flavum
Thoracic vertebra
– Superior articular process
– Transverse costal facet
Anterior longitudinal ligament
Intertransverse ligament
Intervertebral disc
Articular capsule
of zygapophysial joint
Spinal nerve
Posterior ramus –
Anterior ramus –
Supraspinous ligament
Posterior longitudinal ligament
Interspinous ligament
Inferior costal facet
Spinous process
c
Ligamentum flavum
Posterior longitudinal ligament
Lumbar vertebra
– Superior articular process
– Vertebral body
– Costal process
Anterior longitudinal ligament
Supraspinous ligament
Intertransverse ligament
Intervertebral disc
Articular capsule
of zygapophysial joint
Spinal nerve
Anterior ramus –
Posterior ramus –
Interspinous ligament
Spinous process
Ligamentum flavum
Articular facet
of inferior articular process
of lumbar vertebra
Posterior longitudinal ligament

49 Motor segments of the vertebral column (100%)

Left lateral aspect

a Cervical motor segment with spinal nerve
b Thoracic motor segment with spinal nerve
c Lumbar motor segment with spinal nerve

a

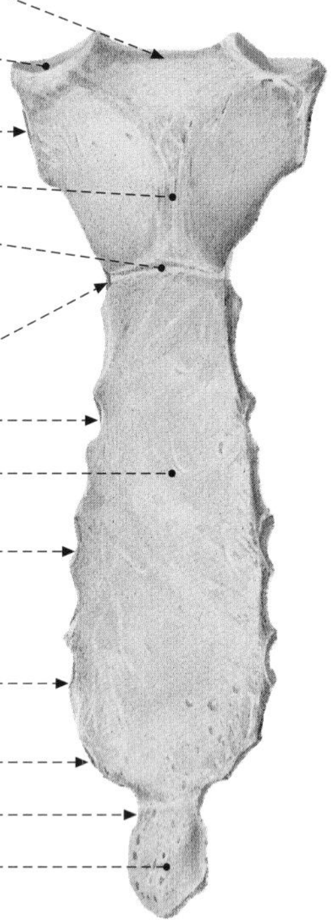
Jugular notch
= Suprasternal notch
Clavicular notch
Notch for 1st rib
Manubrium of sternum
Manubriosternal joint,
Sternal angle
(LOUIS)
Notch for 2nd rib
Notch for 3rd rib
Body of sternum
Notch for 4th rib
Notch for 5th rib
Notch for 6th rib
Notch for 7th rib
Xiphoid process

b

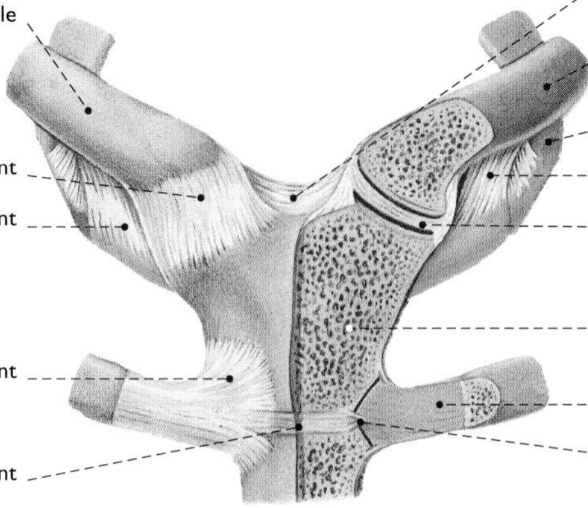
Clavicle
Anterior sternoclavicular ligament
Costoclavicular ligament
Radiate sternocostal ligament
Manubriosternal joint
Interclavicular ligament
Clavicle
1st rib
Costoclavicular ligament
Articular disc
of sternoclavicular joint
Manubrium of sternum
Costal cartilage of 2nd rib
Sternocostal joint,
Intra-articular
sternocostal ligament

c

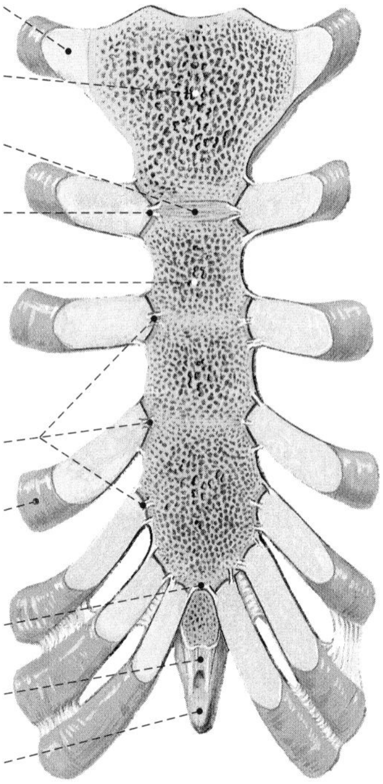
Synchondrosis
of 1st rib
Manubrium
of sternum
Manubriosternal
joint
Intra-articular
sternocostal ligament
Body of sternum
Sternocostal
joints
Costal cartilage
of 4th rib
Xiphisternal
joint
Costoxiphoid
ligaments
Xiphoid process

d

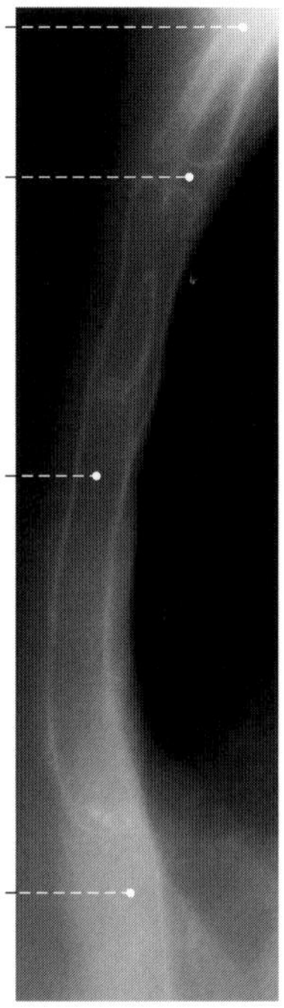
Manubrium
of sternum
Manubriosternal
joint
Body of sternum
Xiphoid process

e

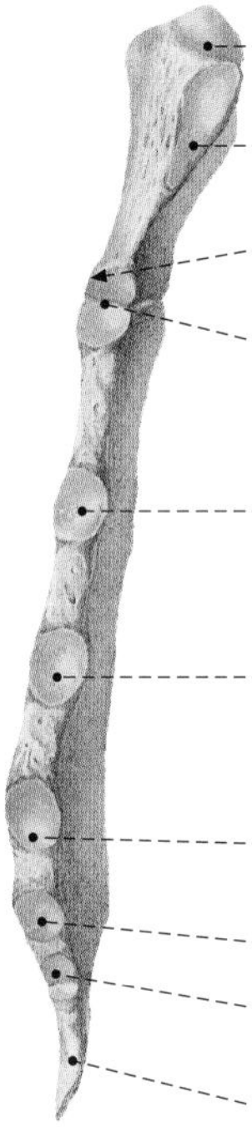
Clavicular notch
Notch for 1st rib
Sternal angle
(LOUIS)
Manubriosternal
joint
Notch for 3rd rib
Notch for 4th rib
Notch for 5th rib
Notch for 6th rib
Notch for 7th rib
Xiphoid process

50 Sternum and joints

a Sternum (45%), ventral aspect

b Sternoclavicular joint (70%), ventral aspect.
The sternoclavicular and sternocostal joints were exposed on the left side of the body by a frontal section.

c Sternocostal joints (45%), exposed by a frontal section, ventral aspect

d, e Sternum (50%)

d Lateral radiograph

e Left lateral aspect

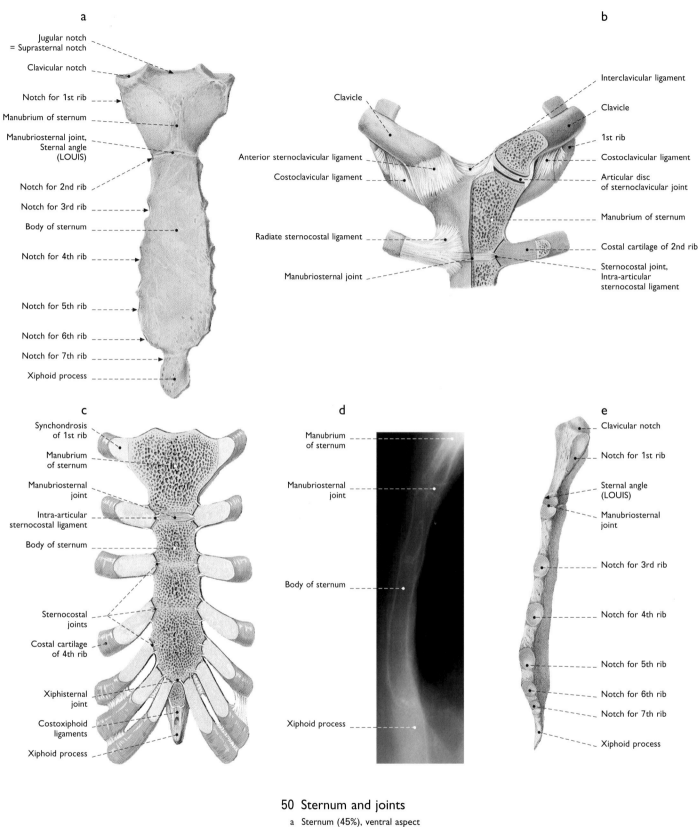

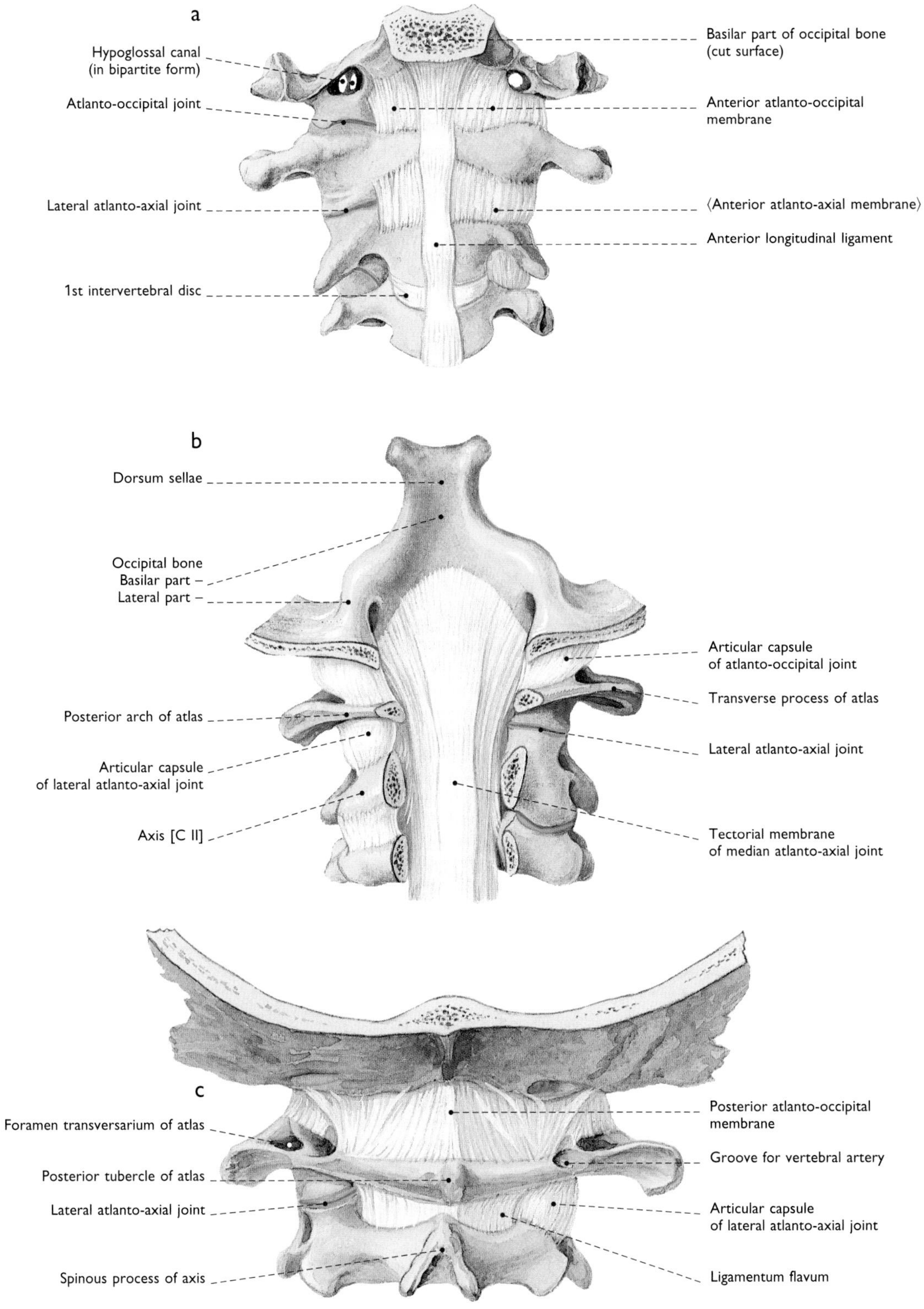
a
Hypoglossal canal
(in bipartite form)
Atlanto-occipital joint
Lateral atlanto-axial joint
1st intervertebral disc
Basilar part of occipital bone
(cut surface)
Anterior atlanto-occipital
membrane
⟨Anterior atlanto-axial membrane⟩
Anterior longitudinal ligament
b
Dorsum sellae
Occipital bone
Basilar part –
Lateral part –
Posterior arch of atlas
Articular capsule
of lateral atlanto-axial joint
Axis [C II]
Articular capsule
of atlanto-occipital joint
Transverse process of atlas
Lateral atlanto-axial joint
Tectorial membrane
of median atlanto-axial joint
c
Foramen transversarium of atlas
Posterior tubercle of atlas
Lateral atlanto-axial joint
Spinous process of axis
Posterior atlanto-occipital
membrane
Groove for vertebral artery
Articular capsule
of lateral atlanto-axial joint
Ligamentum flavum

51 Atlanto-occipital and atlanto-axial joints

a Ventral aspect (90%)

b Dorsal aspect (90%) after removal of the posterior part of the occipital bone and the arches of the upper cervical vertebrae. The vertebral canal was opened.

c Dorsal aspect with remaining vertebral arches (110%)

a

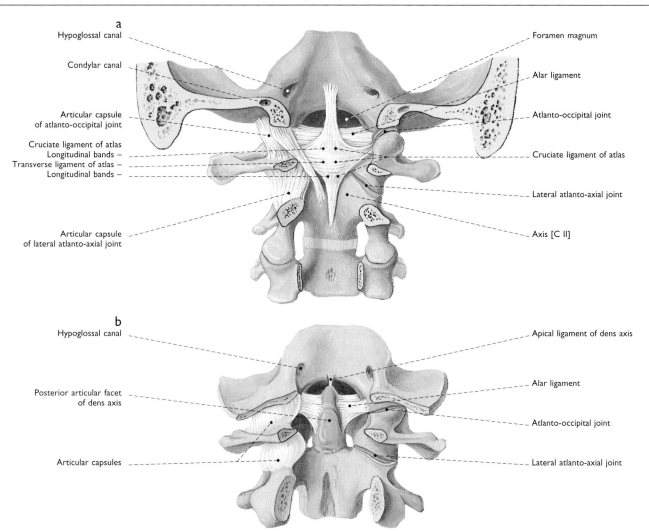

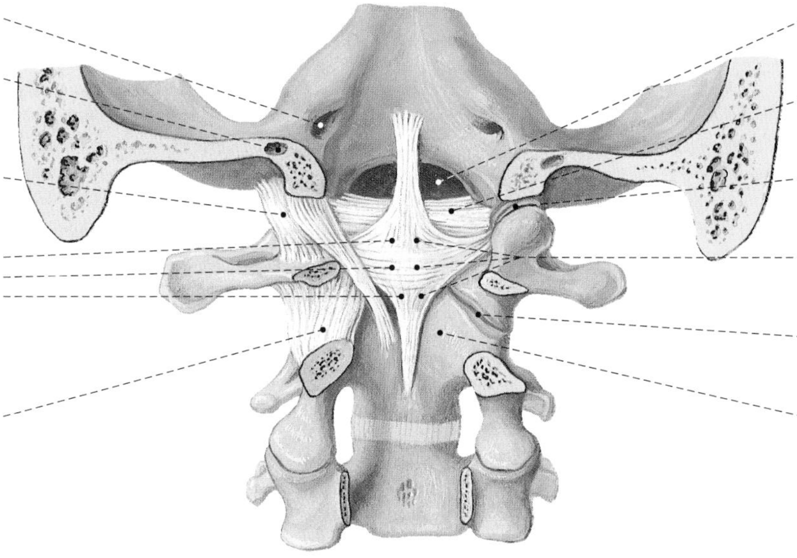
Hypoglossal canal
Condylar canal
Articular capsule of atlanto-occipital joint
Cruciate ligament of atlas
Longitudinal bands –
Transverse ligament of atlas –
Longitudinal bands –
Articular capsule of lateral atlanto-axial joint
Foramen magnum
Alar ligament
Atlanto-occipital joint
Cruciate ligament of atlas
Lateral atlanto-axial joint
Axis [C II]

b

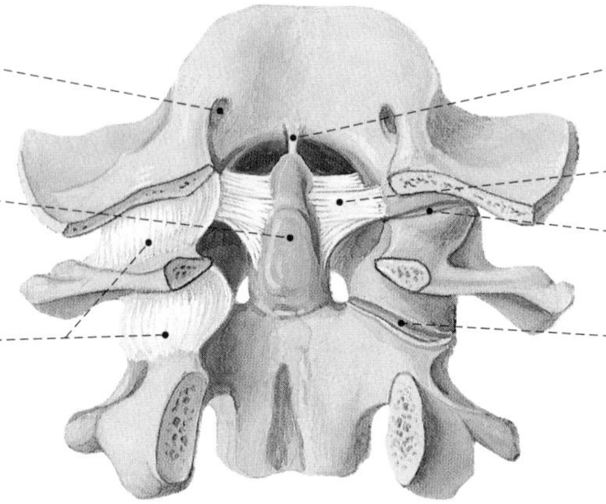
Hypoglossal canal
Posterior articular facet of dens axis
Articular capsules
Apical ligament of dens axis
Alar ligament
Atlanto-occipital joint
Lateral atlanto-axial joint

c

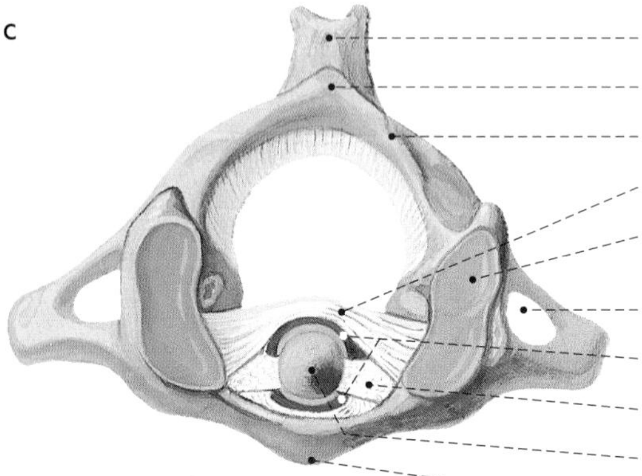
Spinous process of axis
Posterior tubercle of atlas
Posterior arch of atlas
Transverse ligament of atlas
Superior articular surface of atlas
Foramen transversarium
Median atlanto-axial joint
Alar ligament
Dens axis
Anterior tubercle of atlas

d

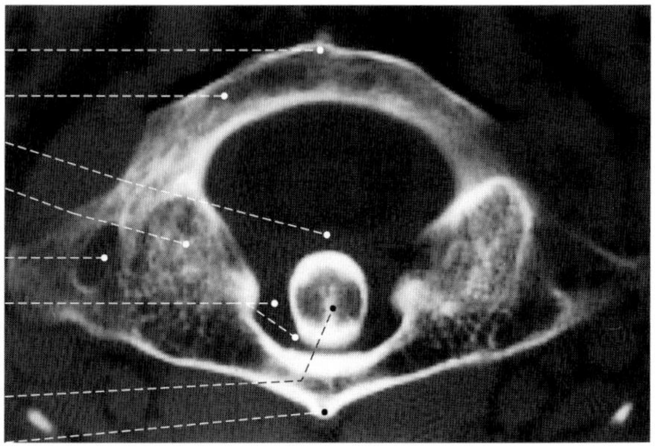

52 Atlanto-occipital and atlanto-axial joints (100%)

a Dorsal aspect after removal of the posterior part of the occipital bone and the arches of the upper cervical vertebrae. The vertebral canal was opened.
b Dorsal aspect after additional removal of the cruciate ligament of atlas
c Cranial aspect of the median atlanto-axial joint
d Axial (transverse) computed tomogram (CT) of the atlas and the median atlanto-axial joint

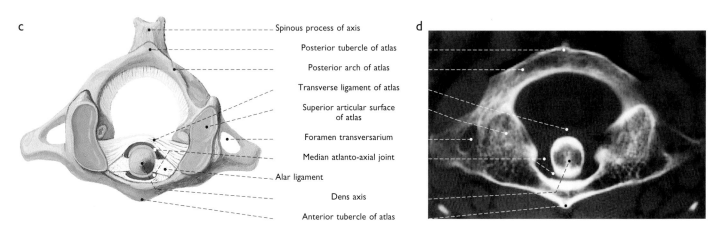

a

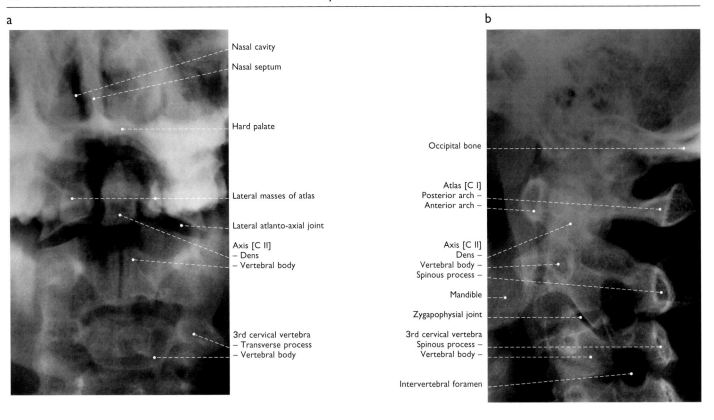

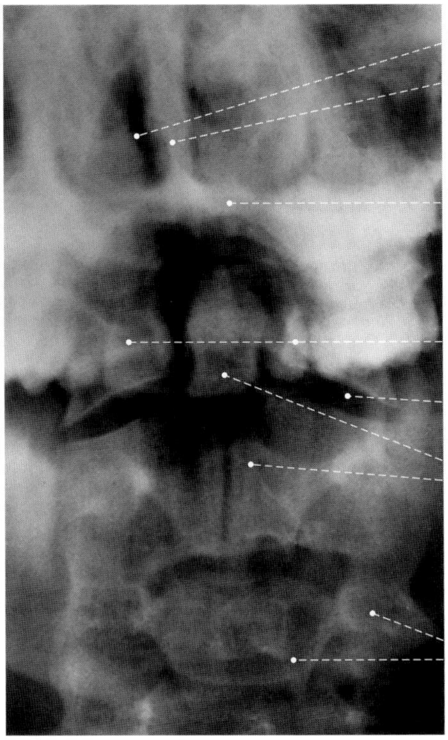
Nasal cavity
Nasal septum
Hard palate
Lateral masses of atlas
Lateral atlanto-axial joint
Axis [C II]
– Dens
– Vertebral body
3rd cervical vertebra
– Transverse process
– Vertebral body

b

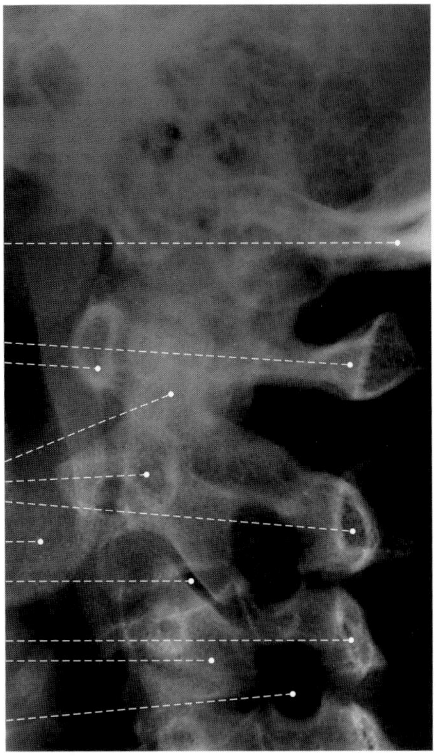
Occipital bone
Atlas [C I]
Posterior arch –
Anterior arch –
Axis [C II]
Dens –
Vertebral body –
Spinous process –
Mandible
Zygapophysial joint
3rd cervical vertebra
Spinous process –
Vertebral body –
Intervertebral foramen

c

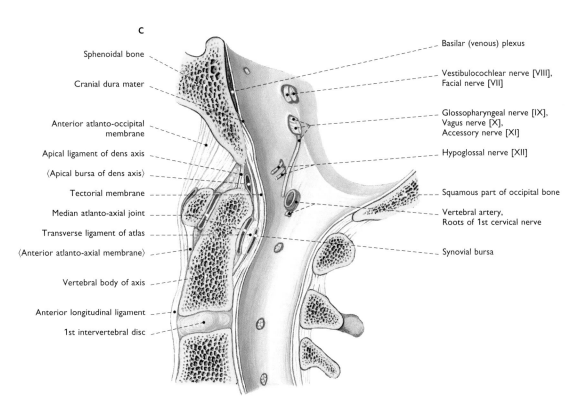

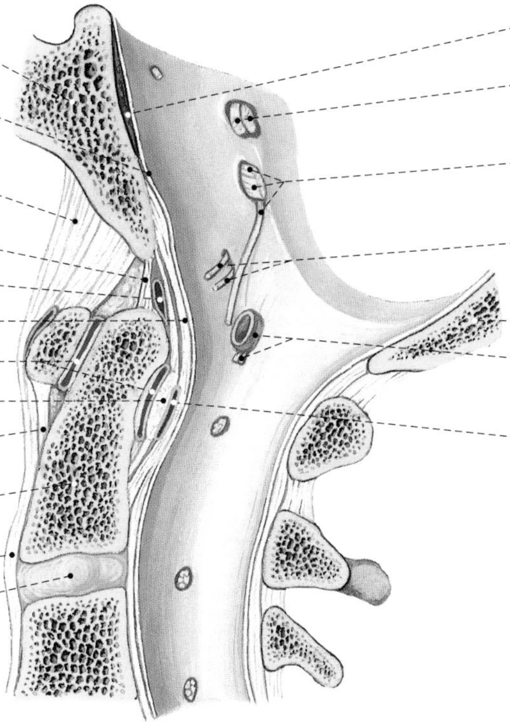
Sphenoidal bone
Cranial dura mater
Anterior atlanto-occipital membrane
Apical ligament of dens axis
⟨Apical bursa of dens axis⟩
Tectorial membrane
Median atlanto-axial joint
Transverse ligament of atlas
⟨Anterior atlanto-axial membrane⟩
Vertebral body of axis
Anterior longitudinal ligament
1st intervertebral disc
Basilar (venous) plexus
Vestibulocochlear nerve [VIII],
Facial nerve [VII]
Glossopharyngeal nerve [IX],
Vagus nerve [X],
Accessory nerve [XI]
Hypoglossal nerve [XII]
Squamous part of occipital bone
Vertebral artery,
Roots of 1st cervical nerve
Synovial bursa

53 Median atlanto-axial joint

a Anteroposterior radiograph of the upper cervical spine (mouth opened) (70%)
b Lateral radiograph of the upper cervical spine (70%)
c Medial aspect of a median section through the occipital bone and the upper cervical vertebrae (90%)

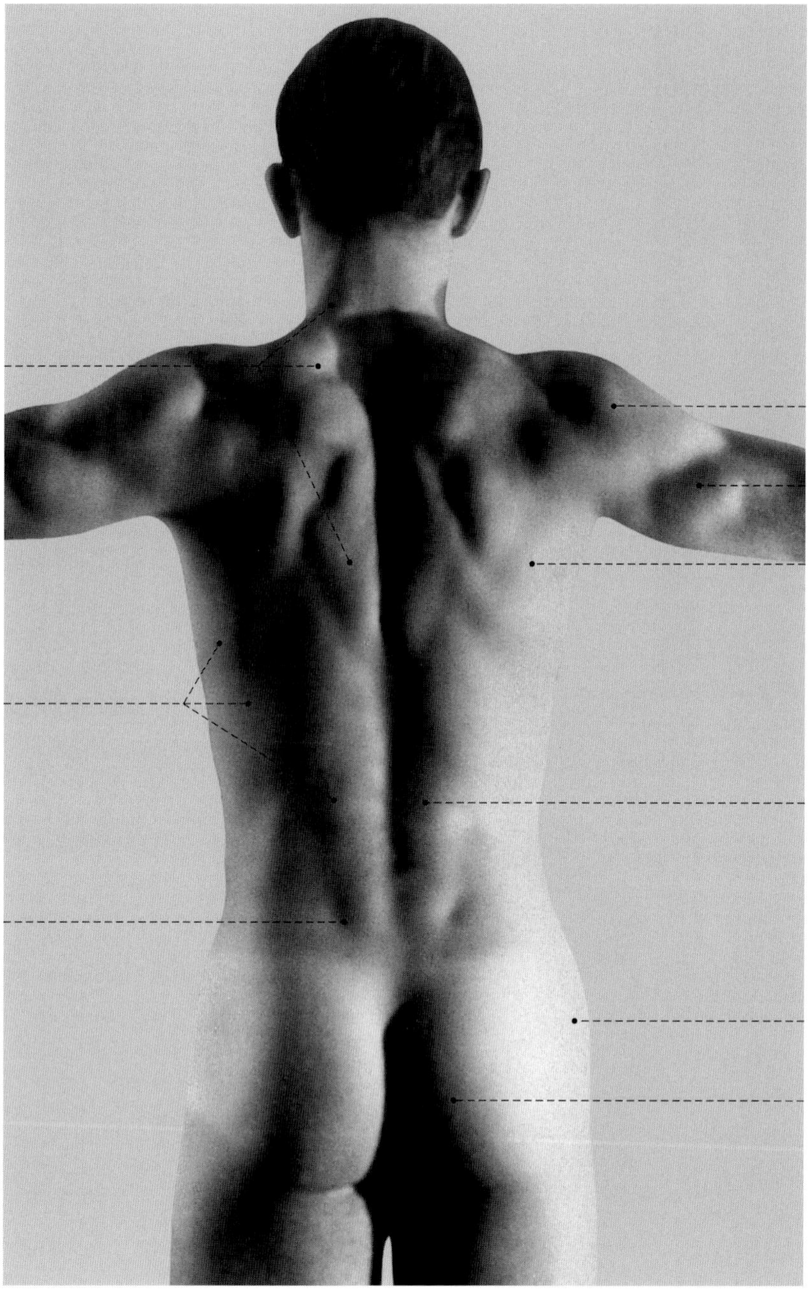
Trapezius muscle
Deltoid muscle
Triceps brachii muscle
Teres major muscle
Latissimus dorsi muscle
Erector spinae muscle
Posterior superior iliac spine
Gluteus medius muscle
Gluteus maximus muscle

54 Surface anatomy of the back of a male (20%)
Dorsal aspect

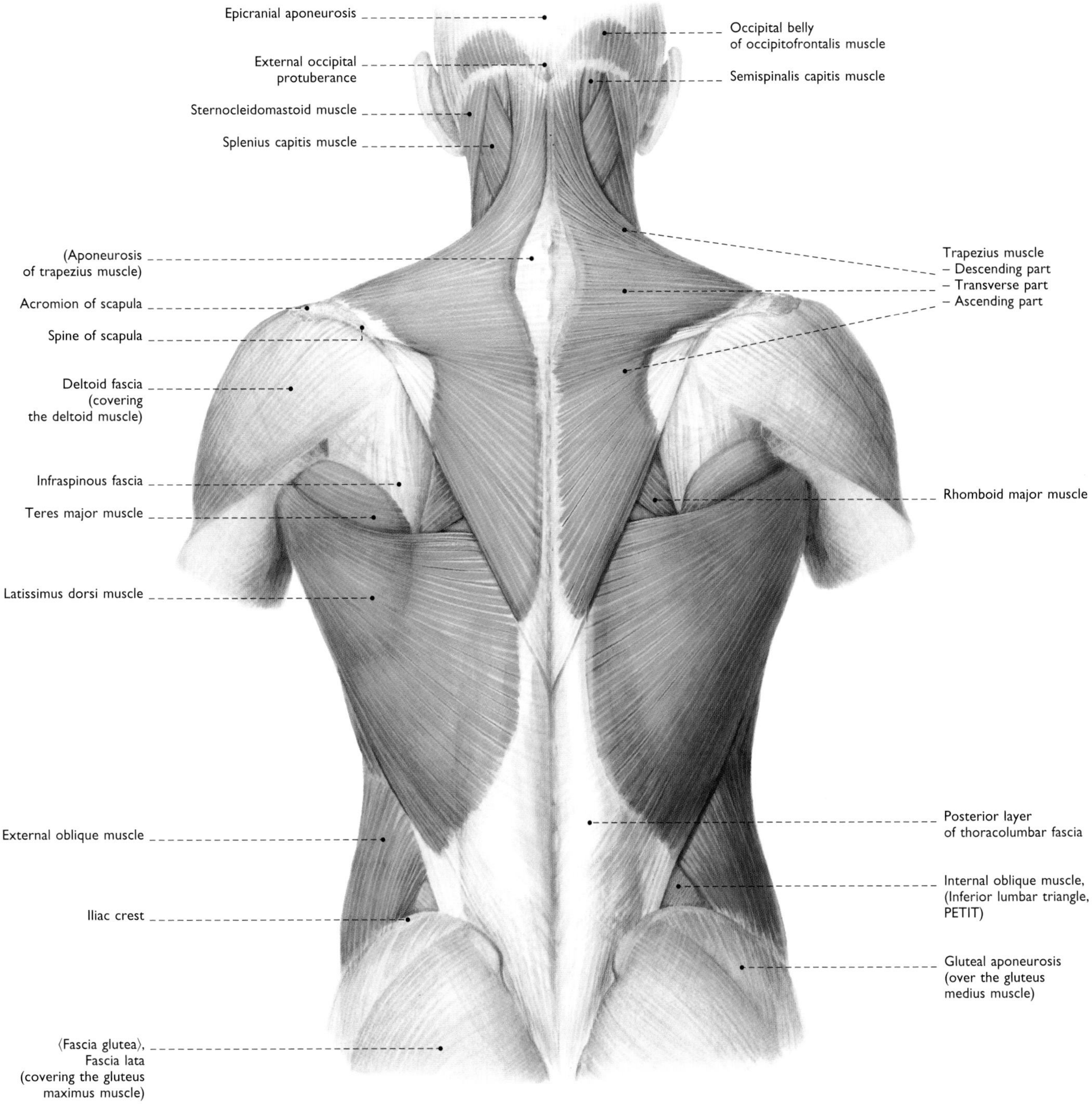
Epicranial aponeurosis
External occipital protuberance
Sternocleidomastoid muscle
Splenius capitis muscle
(Aponeurosis of trapezius muscle)
Acromion of scapula
Spine of scapula
Deltoid fascia (covering the deltoid muscle)
Infraspinous fascia
Teres major muscle
Latissimus dorsi muscle
External oblique muscle
Iliac crest
⟨Fascia glutea⟩, Fascia lata (covering the gluteus maximus muscle)
Occipital belly of occipitofrontalis muscle
Semispinalis capitis muscle
Trapezius muscle
– Descending part
– Transverse part
– Ascending part
Rhomboid major muscle
Posterior layer of thoracolumbar fascia
Internal oblique muscle, (Inferior lumbar triangle, PETIT)
Gluteal aponeurosis (over the gluteus medius muscle)

55 Muscles of the back (25%)

Superficial layer

a

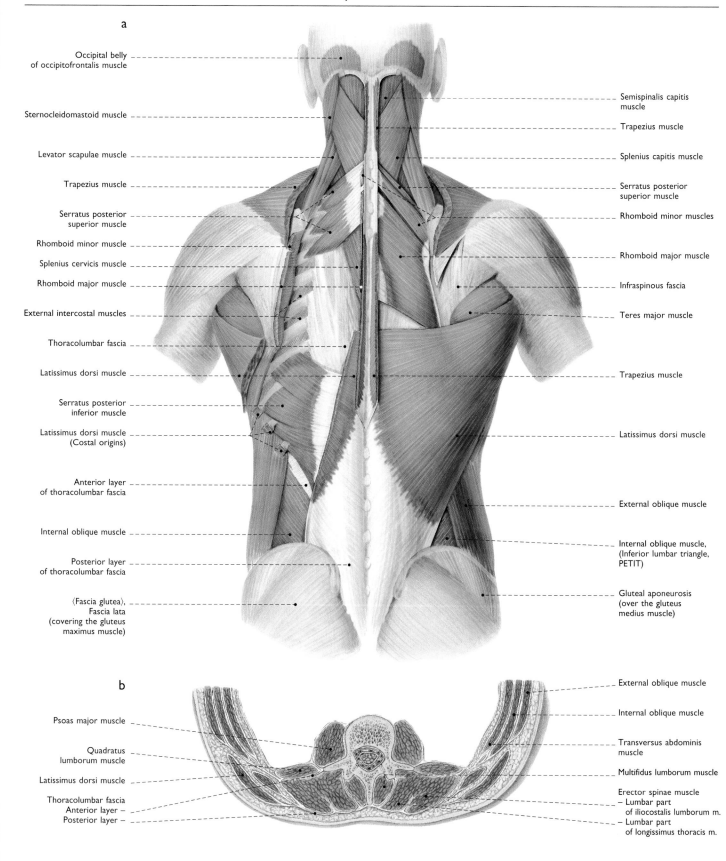

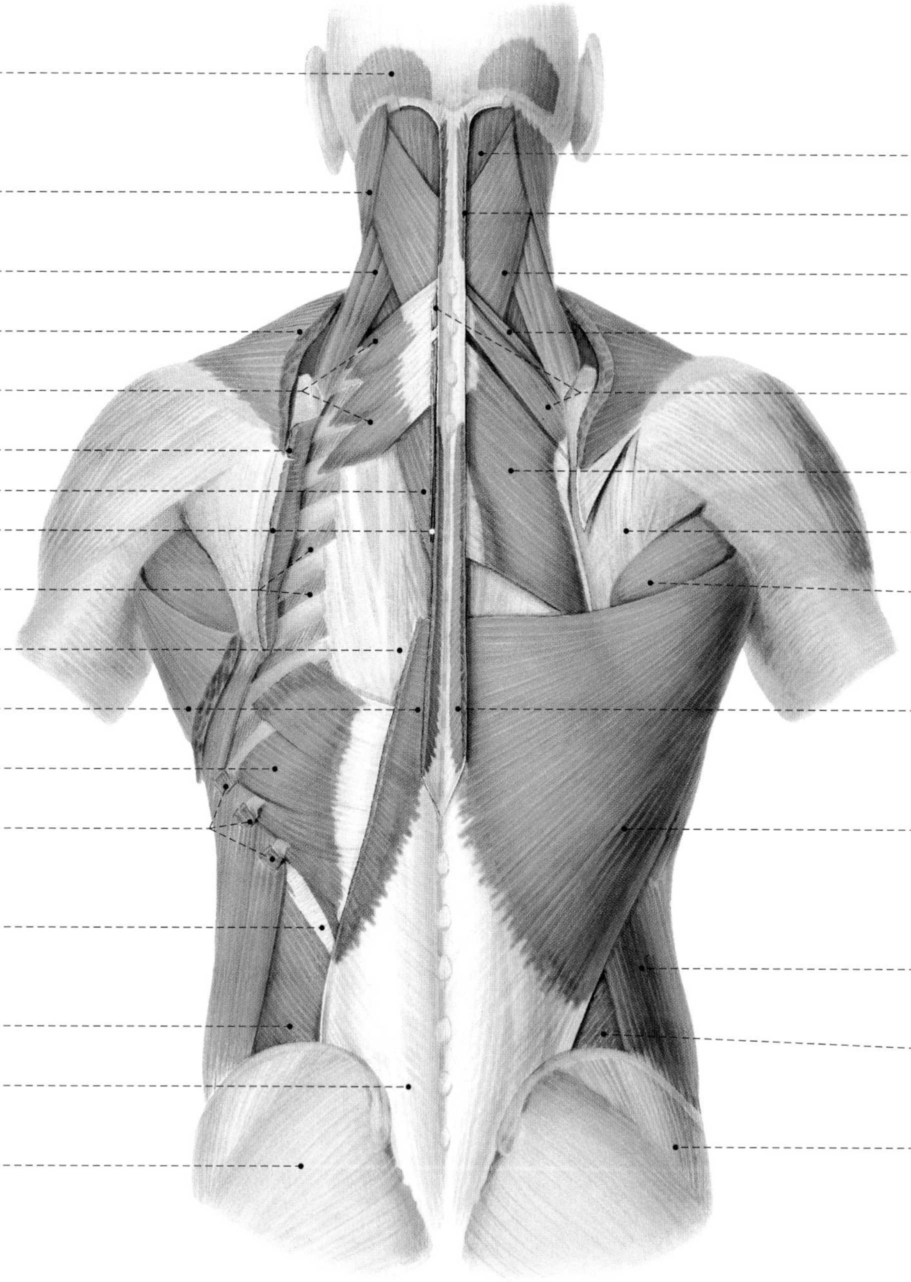
Occipital belly of occipitofrontalis muscle
Sternocleidomastoid muscle
Levator scapulae muscle
Trapezius muscle
Serratus posterior superior muscle
Rhomboid minor muscle
Splenius cervicis muscle
Rhomboid major muscle
External intercostal muscles
Thoracolumbar fascia
Latissimus dorsi muscle
Serratus posterior inferior muscle
Latissimus dorsi muscle (Costal origins)
Anterior layer of thoracolumbar fascia
Internal oblique muscle
Posterior layer of thoracolumbar fascia
⟨Fascia glutea⟩, Fascia lata (covering the gluteus maximus muscle)
Semispinalis capitis muscle
Trapezius muscle
Splenius capitis muscle
Serratus posterior superior muscle
Rhomboid minor muscles
Rhomboid major muscle
Infraspinous fascia
Teres major muscle
Trapezius muscle
Latissimus dorsi muscle
External oblique muscle
Internal oblique muscle, (Inferior lumbar triangle, PETIT)
Gluteal aponeurosis (over the gluteus medius muscle)

b

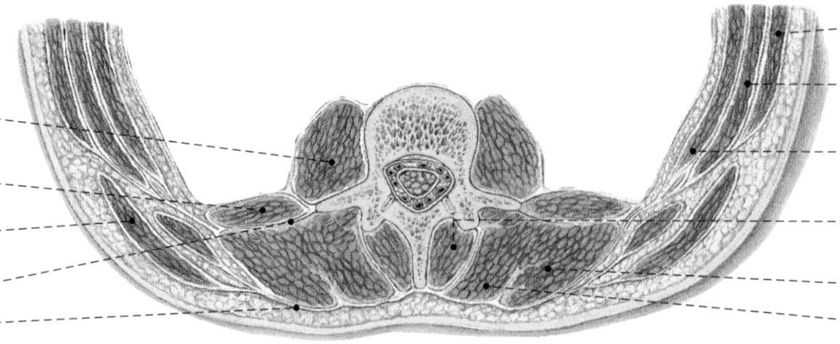
Psoas major muscle
Quadratus lumborum muscle
Latissimus dorsi muscle
Thoracolumbar fascia
Anterior layer –
Posterior layer –
External oblique muscle
Internal oblique muscle
Transversus abdominis muscle
Multifidus lumborum muscle
Erector spinae muscle
– Lumbar part of iliocostalis lumborum m.
– Lumbar part of longissimus thoracis m.

56 Muscles of the back

a Deeper layer (25%)

b Schematized transverse (axial) section through the posterior and lateral abdominal wall in the lumbar region (35%)

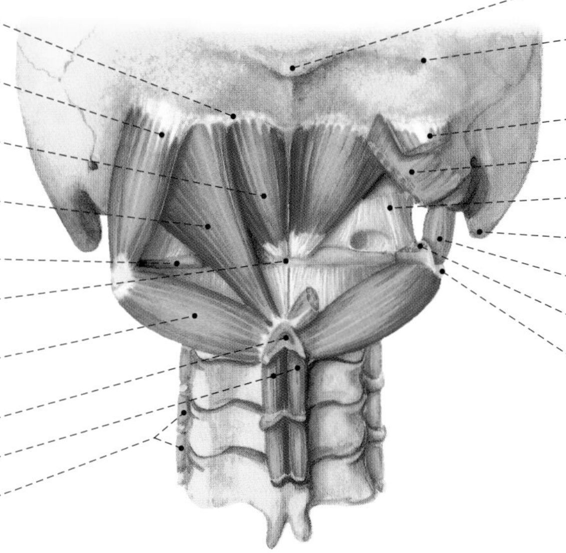
a
Inferior nuchal line
Obliquus capitis superior muscle
Rectus capitis posterior minor muscle
Rectus capitis posterior major muscle
Posterior arch of atlas
Posterior tubercle of atlas
Obliquus capitis inferior muscle
Spinous process of axis
Interspinales cervicis muscles
Posterior cervical intertransversarii muscles
External occipital protuberance
Superior nuchal line
Obliquus capitis superior muscle (cut)
Rectus capitis posterior major muscle
Posterior atlanto-occipital membrane
Mastoid process
Rectus capitis lateralis muscle
Obliquus capitis superior muscle (cut)
Transverse process of atlas

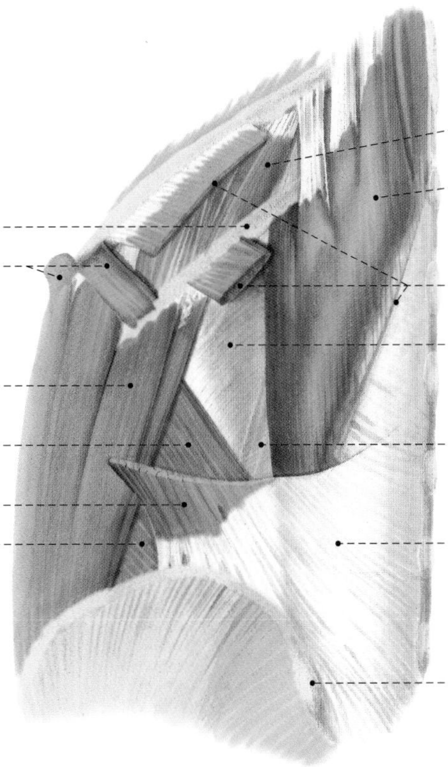
b
11th external intercostal muscle
Erector spinae muscle
12th rib
Latissimus dorsi muscle (Costal origins)
Serratus posterior inferior muscle
Anterior layer of thoracolumbar fascia = Quadratus lumborum fascia
External oblique muscle
Internal oblique muscle
Quadratus lumborum muscle
Latissimus dorsi muscle
(Inferior lumbar triangle, PETIT)
Posterior layer of thoracolumbar fascia
Posterior superior iliac spine

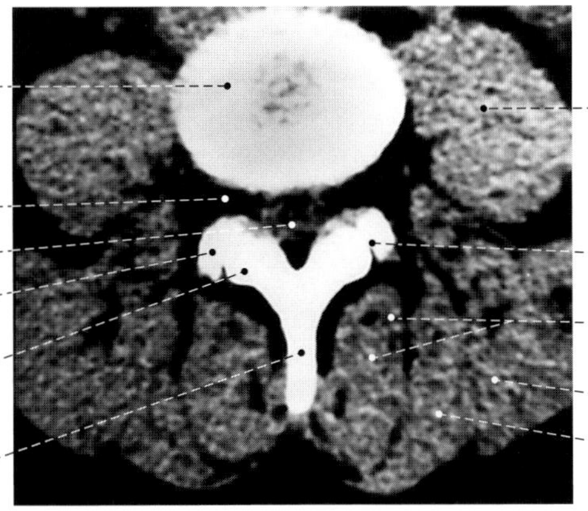
c
Vertebral body
Intervertebral foramen
Cauda equina
Superior articular process
Inferior articular process
Spinous process
Psoas major muscle
Zygapophysial joint (Joint between articular processes)
Multifidus lumborum muscle
Erector spinae muscle
– Lumbar part of iliocostalis lumborum muscle
– Lumbar part of longissimus thoracis muscle

57 Deep muscles of the neck and muscles of the lumbar region

a Deep muscles of the neck (50%), dorsal aspect

b Muscles of the lumbar region (40%), left dorsolateral aspect. The latissimus dorsi and serratus posterior inferior muscles were partially removed.

c Axial (transverse) computed tomogram (CT) of the fifth lumbar vertebra with adjacent muscles (40%)

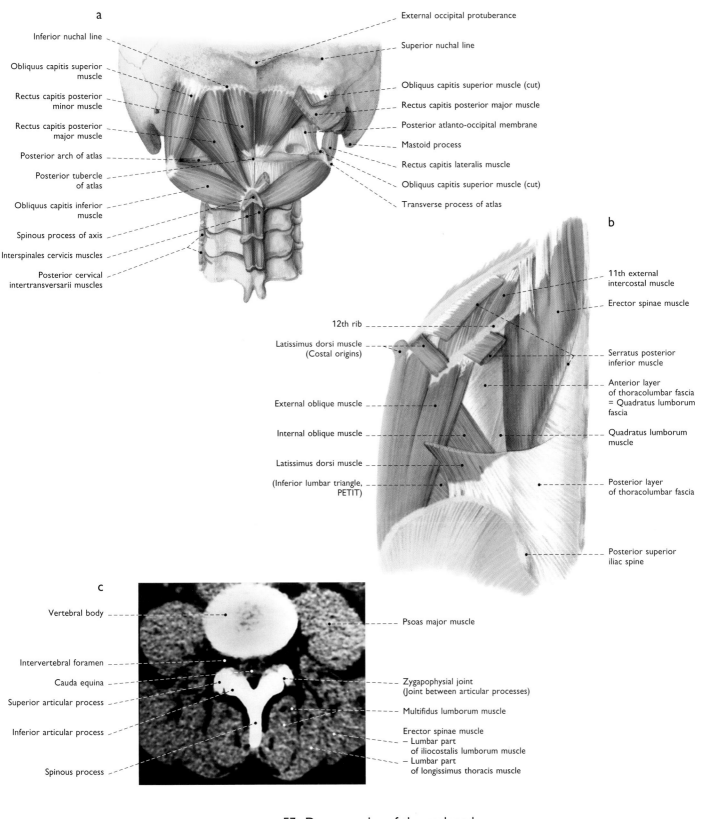

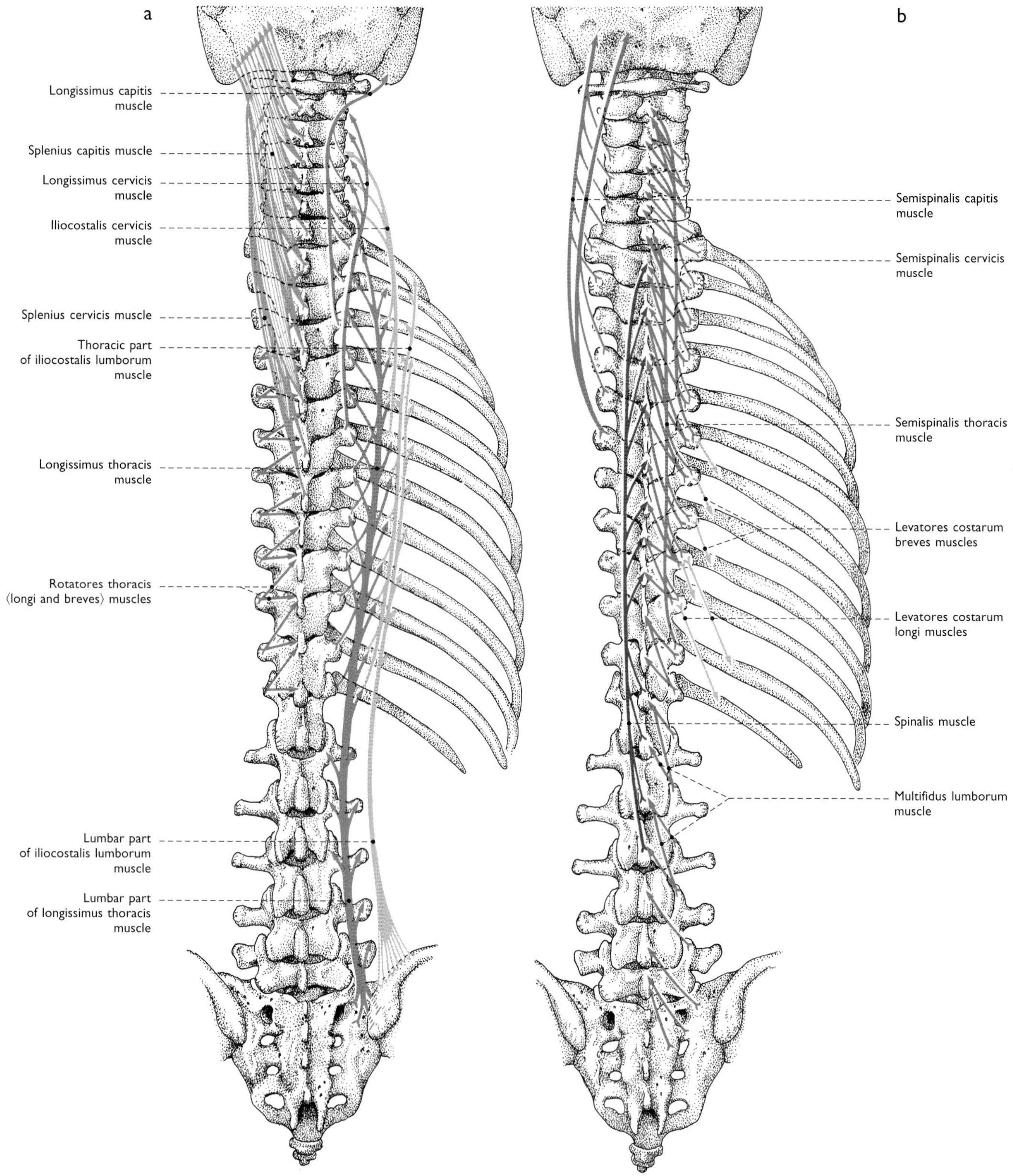
a
Longissimus capitis muscle
Splenius capitis muscle
Longissimus cervicis muscle
Iliocostalis cervicis muscle
Splenius cervicis muscle
Thoracic part of iliocostalis lumborum muscle
Longissimus thoracis muscle
Rotatores thoracis ⟨longi and breves⟩ muscles
Lumbar part of iliocostalis lumborum muscle
Lumbar part of longissimus thoracis muscle
b
Semispinalis capitis muscle
Semispinalis cervicis muscle
Semispinalis thoracis muscle
Levatores costarum breves muscles
Levatores costarum longi muscles
Spinalis muscle
Multifidus lumborum muscle

58 Muscles of the back proper (30%)

Schematic course
The muscles of the medial tract of the erector spinae are colored in red to brown, the muscles of the lateral tract in blue, the splenii and levatores costarum muscles are given in green.

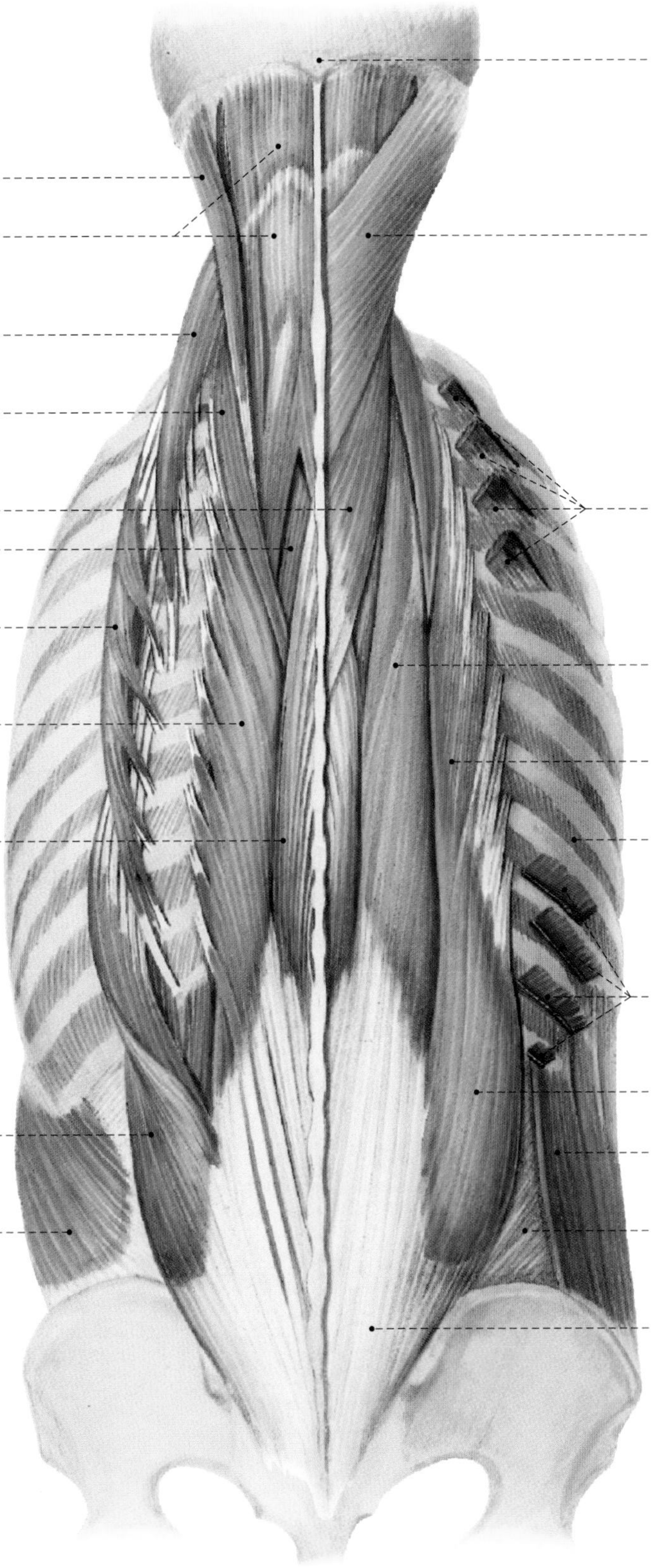
External occipital protuberance
Longissimus capitis muscle
Semispinalis capitis muscle
Splenius capitis muscle
Iliocostalis cervicis muscle
Longissimus cervicis muscle
Splenius cervicis muscle
Semispinalis thoracis muscle
Serratus posterior superior muscle
Thoracic part of iliocostalis lumborum muscle
Longissimus thoracis muscle
Longissimus thoracis muscle
Thoracic part of iliocostalis lumborum muscle
Spinalis muscle
External intercostal muscle
Serratus posterior inferior muscle
Lumbar part of iliocostalis lumborum muscle
Lumbar part of iliocostalis lumborum muscle
External oblique muscle
Internal oblique muscle
(Inferior lumbar triangle, PETIT), Internal oblique muscle
Erector spinae muscle

59 Muscles of the back proper (30%)
Superficial layer

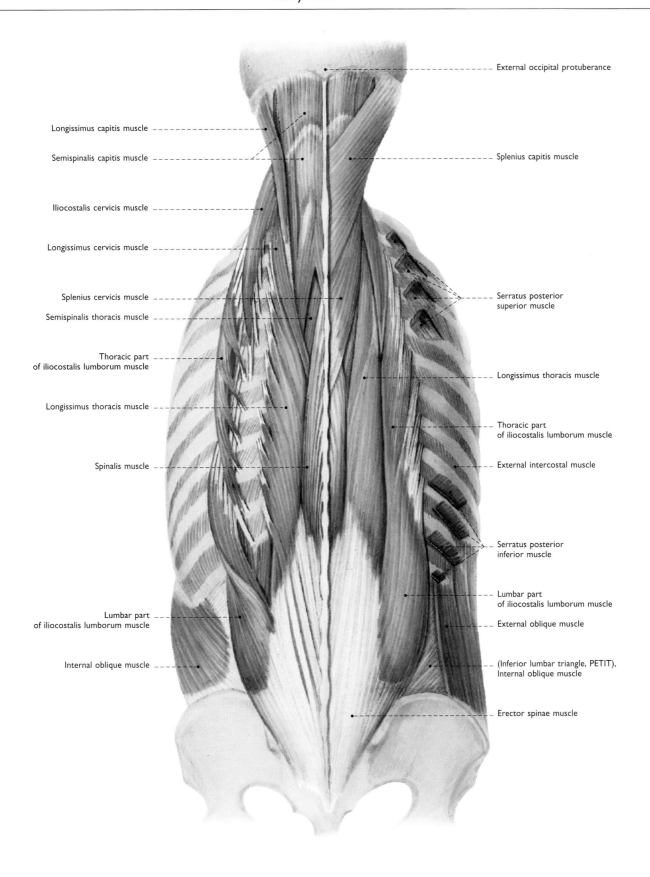

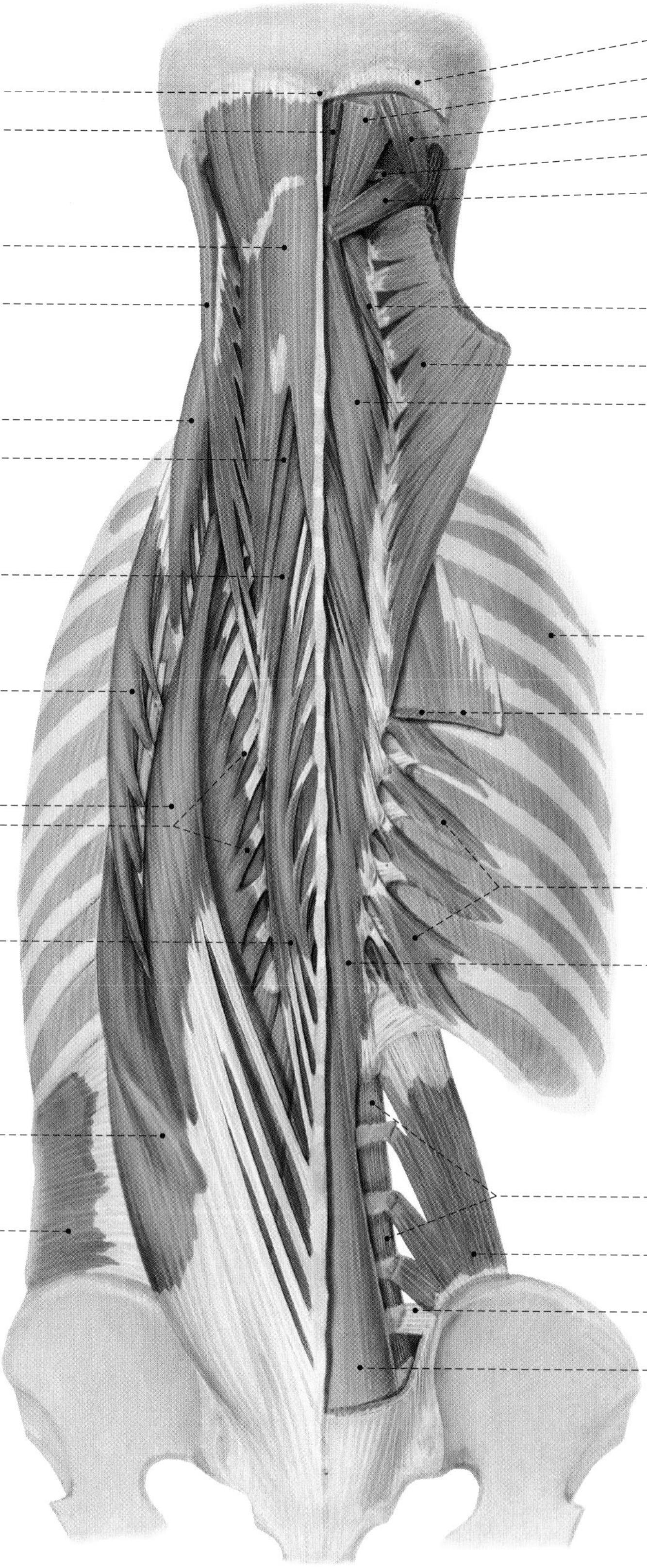
External occipital protuberance
Rectus capitis posterior minor muscle
Semispinalis capitis muscle
Longissimi capitis and cervicis muscles
Iliocostalis cervicis muscle
Semispinalis cervicis muscle
Semispinalis thoracis muscle
Thoracic part of iliocostalis lumborum muscle
Longissimus thoracis muscle
(Medial insertions)
Spinalis muscle
Lumbar part of iliocostalis lumborum muscle
Transversus abdominis muscle
Semispinalis capitis muscle
Rectus capitis posterior major muscle
Obliquus capitis superior muscle
Posterior arch of atlas
Obliquus capitis inferior muscle
Multifidus cervicis muscle
Semispinalis capitis muscle
Semispinalis cervicis muscle
External intercostal muscle
Longissimus thoracis muscle, Thoracic part of iliocostalis lumborum muscle
Levatores costarum longi and breves muscles
Multifidus thoracis muscle
Lateral lumbar intertransversarii muscles
Quadratus lumborum muscle
Iliolumbar ligament
Multifidus lumborum muscle

60 Muscles of the back proper (30%)

Deeper layer

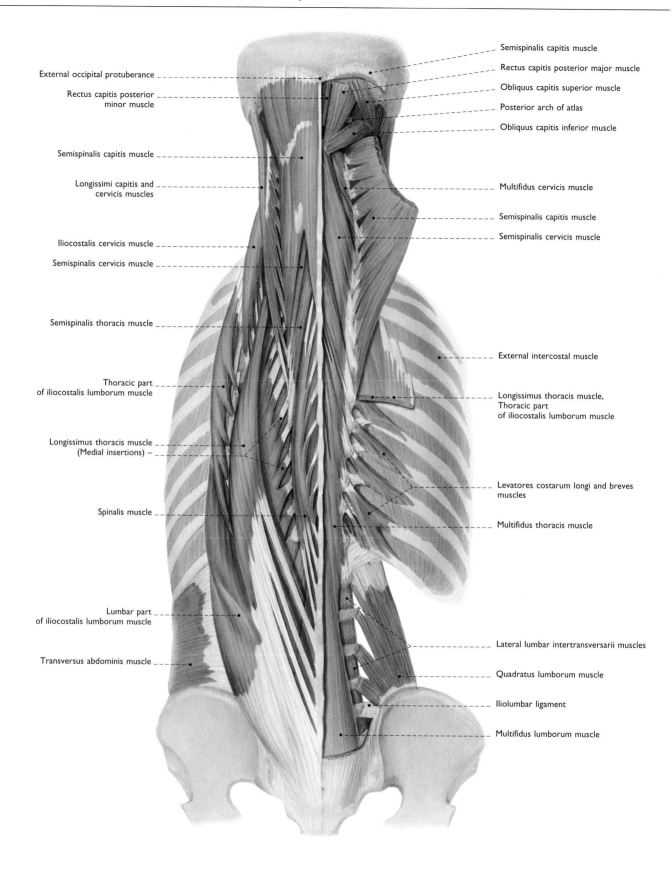

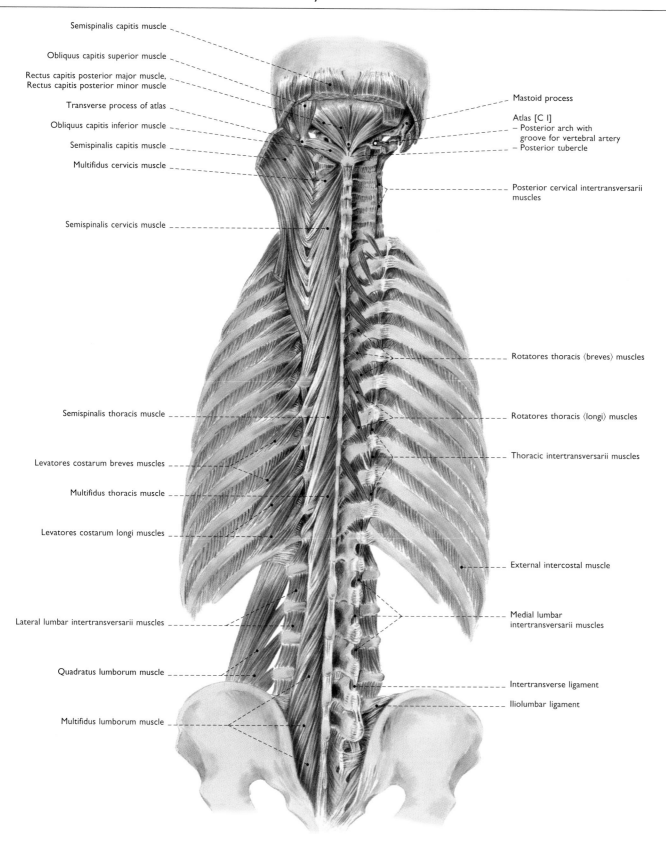

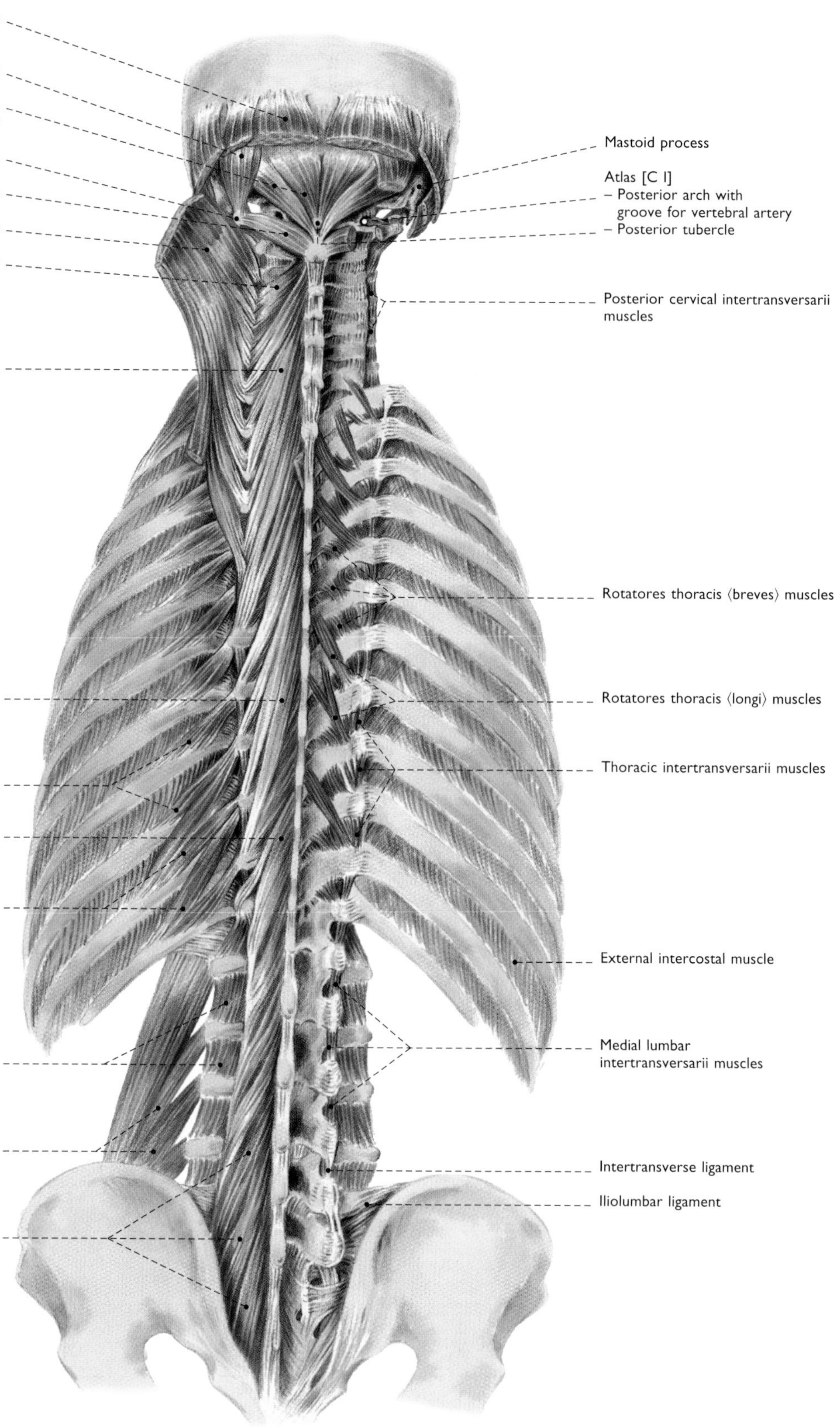
Semispinalis capitis muscle
Obliquus capitis superior muscle
Rectus capitis posterior major muscle,
Rectus capitis posterior minor muscle
Transverse process of atlas
Obliquus capitis inferior muscle
Semispinalis capitis muscle
Multifidus cervicis muscle
Semispinalis cervicis muscle
Semispinalis thoracis muscle
Levatores costarum breves muscles
Multifidus thoracis muscle
Levatores costarum longi muscles
Lateral lumbar intertransversarii muscles
Quadratus lumborum muscle
Multifidus lumborum muscle
Mastoid process
Atlas [C I]
– Posterior arch with groove for vertebral artery
– Posterior tubercle
Posterior cervical intertransversarii muscles
Rotatores thoracis ⟨breves⟩ muscles
Rotatores thoracis ⟨longi⟩ muscles
Thoracic intertransversarii muscles
External intercostal muscle
Medial lumbar intertransversarii muscles
Intertransverse ligament
Iliolumbar ligament

61 Muscles of the back proper (30%)

Deep layer

a

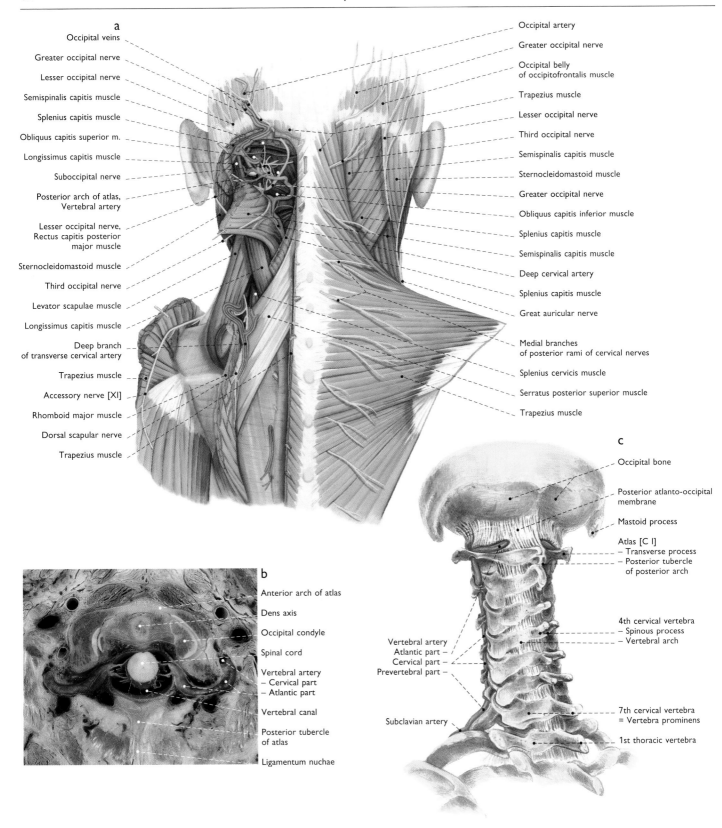

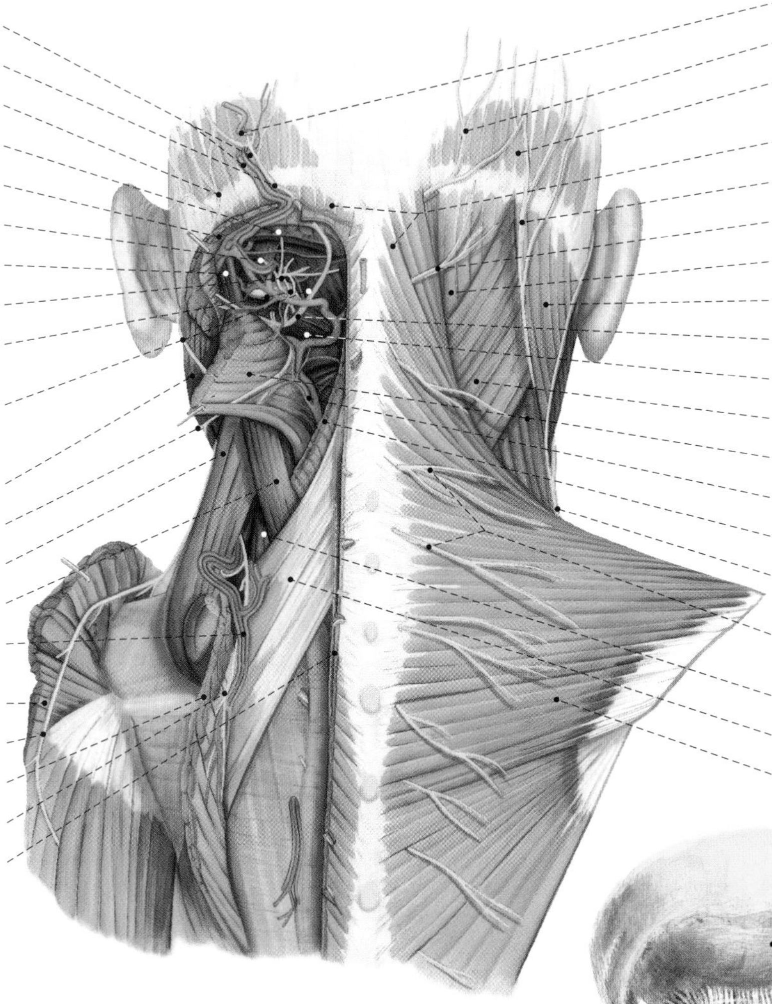
Occipital veins
Greater occipital nerve
Lesser occipital nerve
Semispinalis capitis muscle
Splenius capitis muscle
Obliquus capitis superior m.
Longissimus capitis muscle
Suboccipital nerve
Posterior arch of atlas, Vertebral artery
Lesser occipital nerve, Rectus capitis posterior major muscle
Sternocleidomastoid muscle
Third occipital nerve
Levator scapulae muscle
Longissimus capitis muscle
Deep branch of transverse cervical artery
Trapezius muscle
Accessory nerve [XI]
Rhomboid major muscle
Dorsal scapular nerve
Trapezius muscle
Occipital artery
Greater occipital nerve
Occipital belly of occipitofrontalis muscle
Trapezius muscle
Lesser occipital nerve
Third occipital nerve
Semispinalis capitis muscle
Sternocleidomastoid muscle
Greater occipital nerve
Obliquus capitis inferior muscle
Splenius capitis muscle
Semispinalis capitis muscle
Deep cervical artery
Splenius capitis muscle
Great auricular nerve
Medial branches of posterior rami of cervical nerves
Splenius cervicis muscle
Serratus posterior superior muscle
Trapezius muscle

b

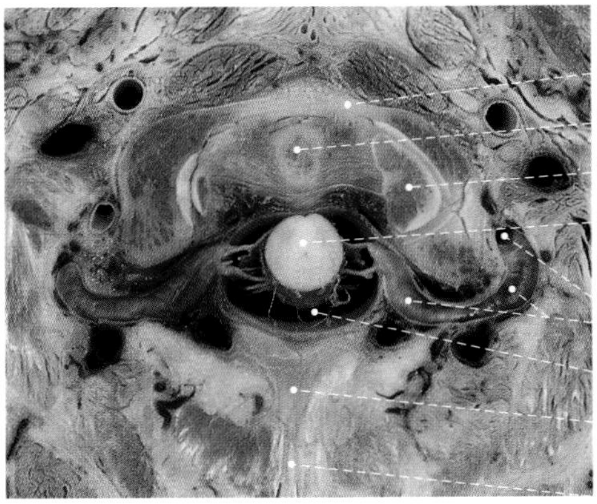
Anterior arch of atlas
Dens axis
Occipital condyle
Spinal cord
Vertebral artery
– Cervical part
– Atlantic part
Vertebral canal
Posterior tubercle of atlas
Ligamentum nuchae

c

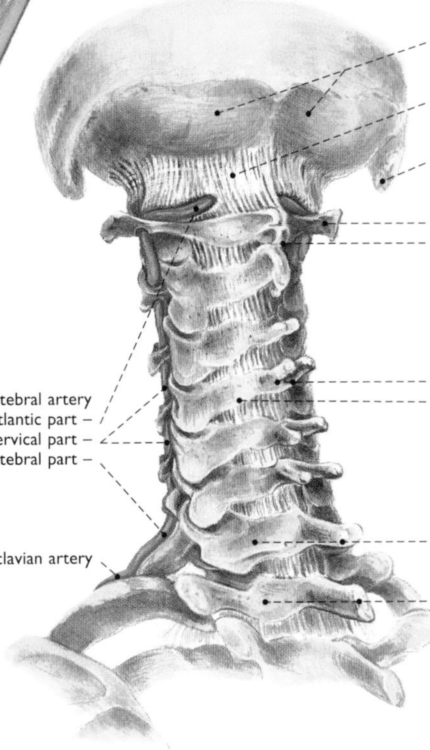
Occipital bone
Posterior atlanto-occipital membrane
Mastoid process
Atlas [C I]
– Transverse process
– Posterior tubercle of posterior arch
4th cervical vertebra
– Spinous process
– Vertebral arch
Vertebral artery
Atlantic part –
Cervical part –
Prevertebral part –
Subclavian artery
7th cervical vertebra = Vertebra prominens
1st thoracic vertebra

62 Neck and shoulder regions

a Right, superficial layer; left, deeper layer (40%). Dorsal aspect
b Horizontal (axial) section at the level of the first cervical vertebra (= atlas, C I) (60%). Cranial aspect
c Course of the vertebral artery (60%). Left dorsolateral aspect

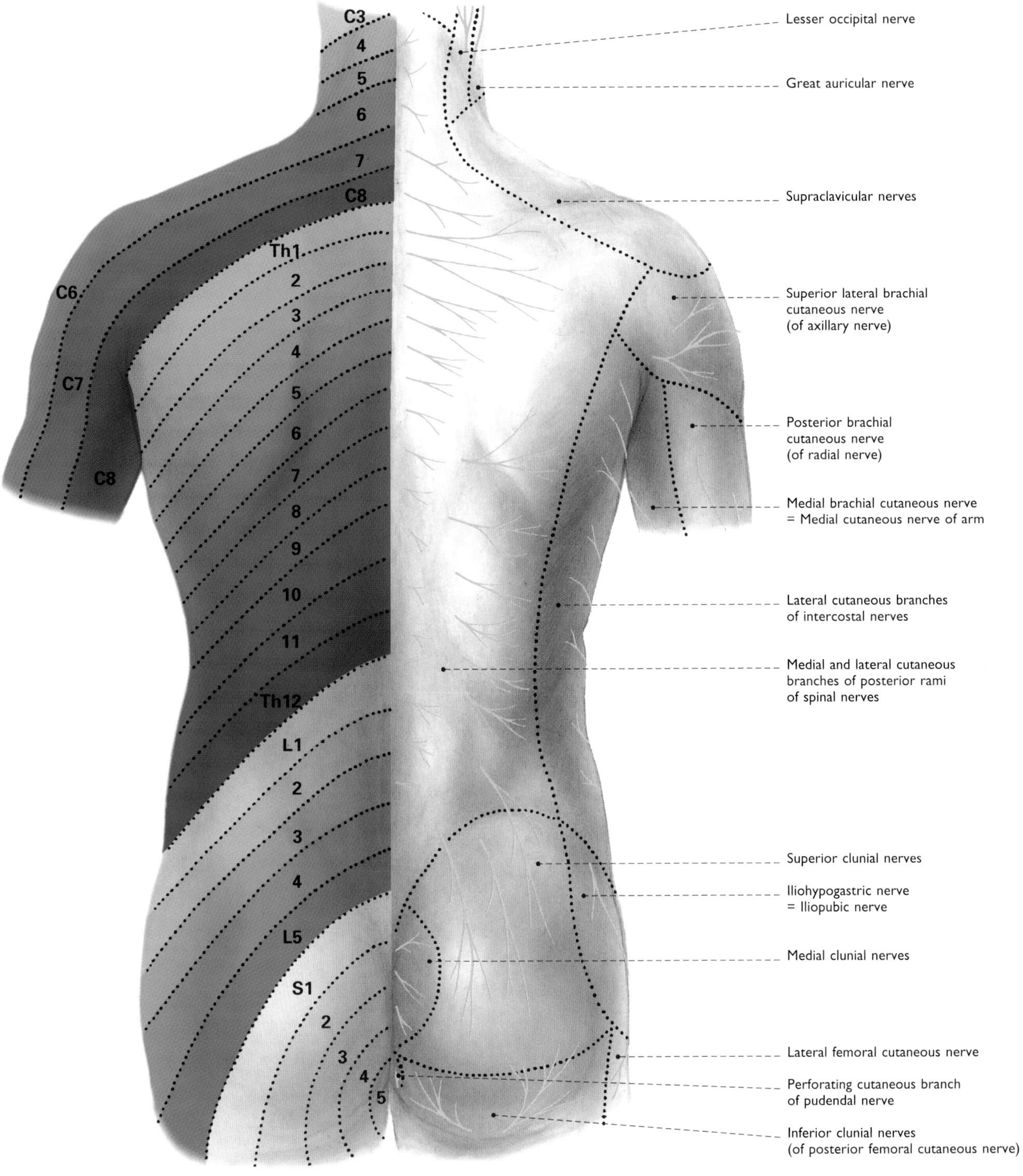
C3
4
5
6
7
C8
Th1
2
3
4
5
6
7
8
9
10
11
Th12
L1
2
3
4
L5
S1
2
3
4
5
C6
C7
C8
Lesser occipital nerve
Great auricular nerve
Supraclavicular nerves
Superior lateral brachial cutaneous nerve (of axillary nerve)
Posterior brachial cutaneous nerve (of radial nerve)
Medial brachial cutaneous nerve = Medial cutaneous nerve of arm
Lateral cutaneous branches of intercostal nerves
Medial and lateral cutaneous branches of posterior rami of spinal nerves
Superior clunial nerves
Iliohypogastric nerve = Iliopubic nerve
Medial clunial nerves
Lateral femoral cutaneous nerve
Perforating cutaneous branch of pudendal nerve
Inferior clunial nerves (of posterior femoral cutaneous nerve)

63 Cutaneous and segmental innervation of the dorsal body wall (25%)

Schematic representation

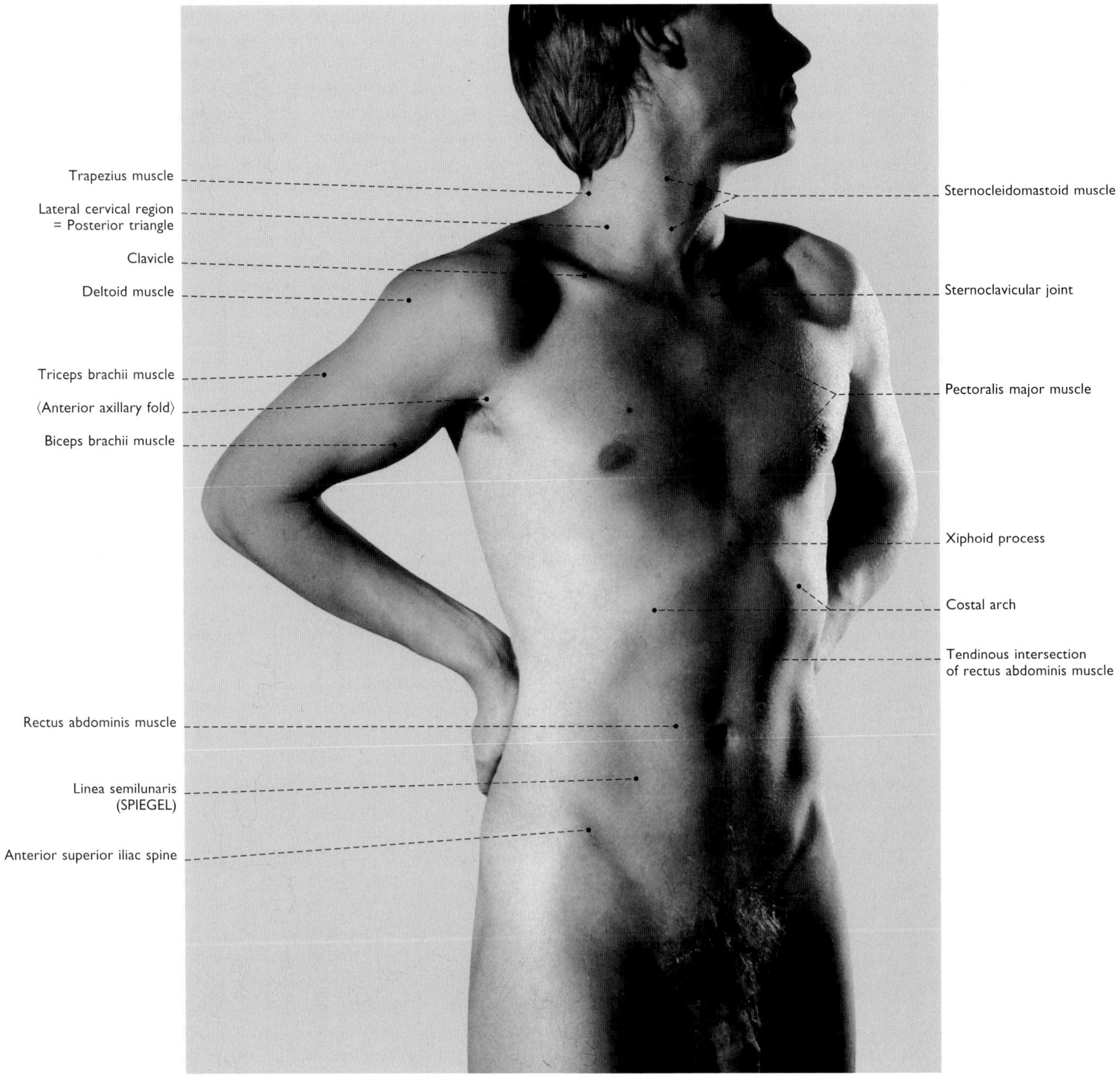
Trapezius muscle
Lateral cervical region
= Posterior triangle
Clavicle
Deltoid muscle
Triceps brachii muscle
⟨Anterior axillary fold⟩
Biceps brachii muscle
Rectus abdominis muscle
Linea semilunaris
(SPIEGEL)
Anterior superior iliac spine
Sternocleidomastoid muscle
Sternoclavicular joint
Pectoralis major muscle
Xiphoid process
Costal arch
Tendinous intersection
of rectus abdominis muscle

64 Surface anatomy of the thorax and abdomen of a male (20%)

Ventral aspect

a

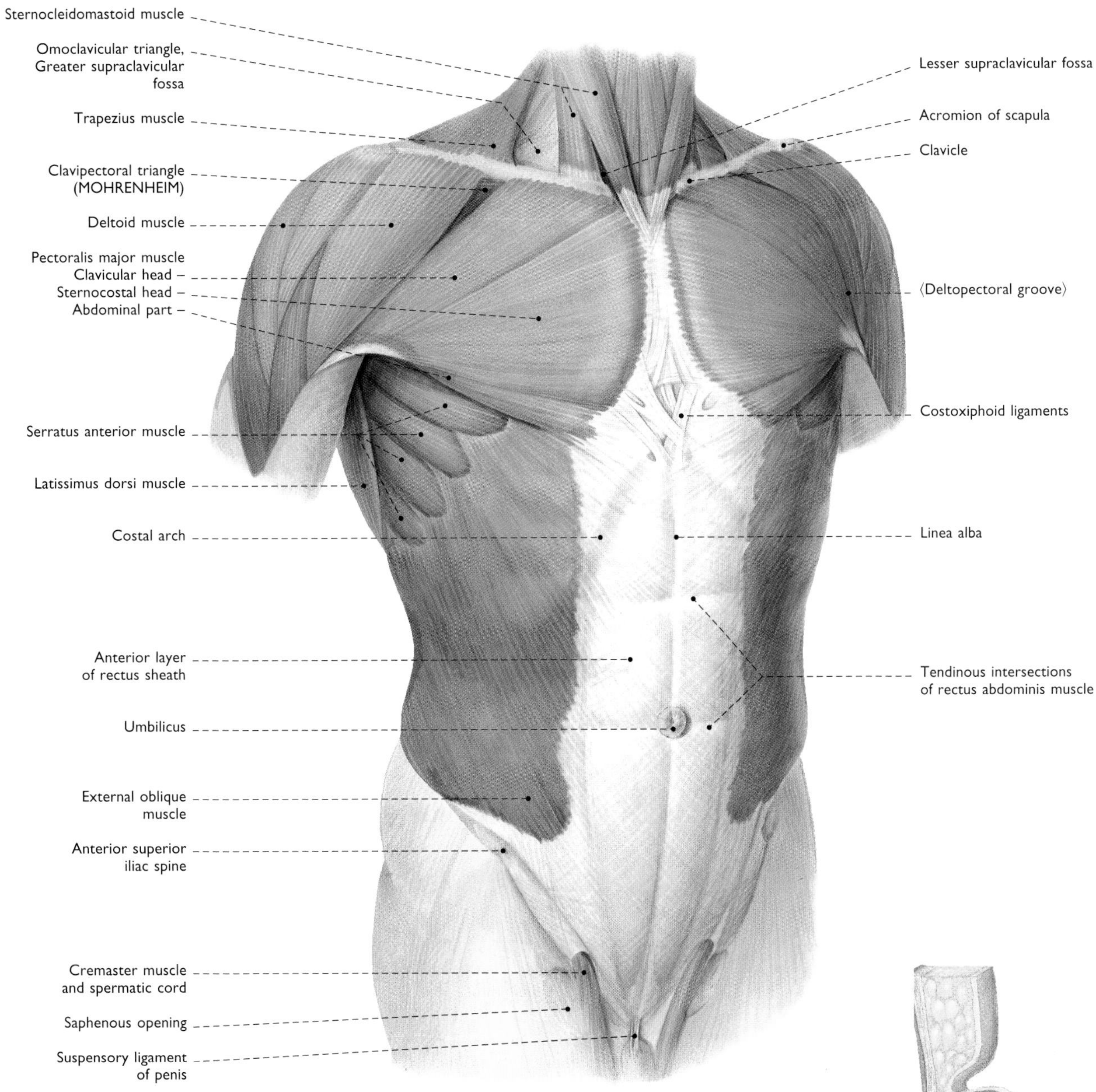
Sternocleidomastoid muscle
Omoclavicular triangle, Greater supraclavicular fossa
Trapezius muscle
Clavipectoral triangle (MOHRENHEIM)
Deltoid muscle
Pectoralis major muscle
Clavicular head –
Sternocostal head –
Abdominal part –
Serratus anterior muscle
Latissimus dorsi muscle
Costal arch
Anterior layer of rectus sheath
Umbilicus
External oblique muscle
Anterior superior iliac spine
Cremaster muscle and spermatic cord
Saphenous opening
Suspensory ligament of penis
Lesser supraclavicular fossa
Acromion of scapula
Clavicle
⟨Deltopectoral groove⟩
Costoxiphoid ligaments
Linea alba
Tendinous intersections of rectus abdominis muscle

b

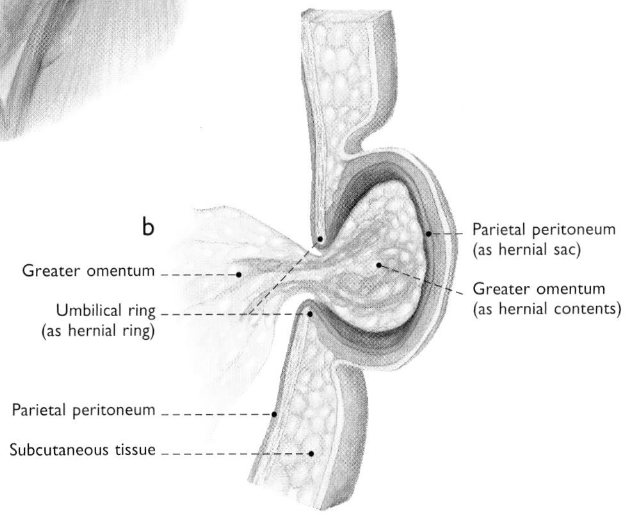
Greater omentum
Umbilical ring (as hernial ring)
Parietal peritoneum
Subcutaneous tissue
Parietal peritoneum (as hernial sac)
Greater omentum (as hernial contents)

65 Ventral muscles of the trunk

a Superficial layer (25%)
b Schematic representation of an umbilical hernia

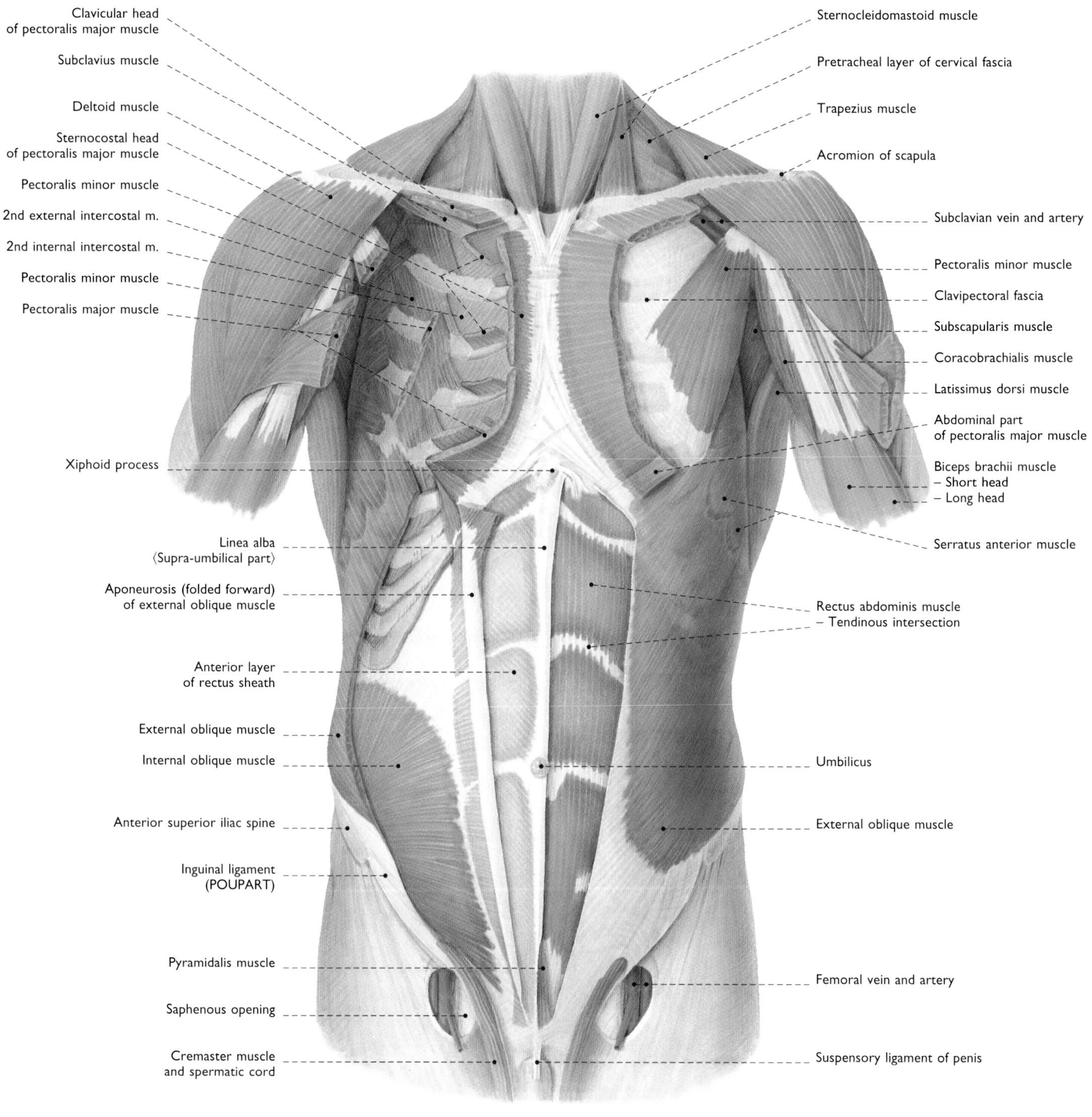
Clavicular head of pectoralis major muscle
Subclavius muscle
Deltoid muscle
Sternocostal head of pectoralis major muscle
Pectoralis minor muscle
2nd external intercostal m.
2nd internal intercostal m.
Pectoralis minor muscle
Pectoralis major muscle
Xiphoid process
Linea alba ⟨Supra-umbilical part⟩
Aponeurosis (folded forward) of external oblique muscle
Anterior layer of rectus sheath
External oblique muscle
Internal oblique muscle
Anterior superior iliac spine
Inguinal ligament (POUPART)
Pyramidalis muscle
Saphenous opening
Cremaster muscle and spermatic cord
Sternocleidomastoid muscle
Pretracheal layer of cervical fascia
Trapezius muscle
Acromion of scapula
Subclavian vein and artery
Pectoralis minor muscle
Clavipectoral fascia
Subscapularis muscle
Coracobrachialis muscle
Latissimus dorsi muscle
Abdominal part of pectoralis major muscle
Biceps brachii muscle
– Short head
– Long head
Serratus anterior muscle
Rectus abdominis muscle
– Tendinous intersection
Umbilicus
External oblique muscle
Femoral vein and artery
Suspensory ligament of penis

66 Ventral muscles of the trunk (25%)

Deeper layer

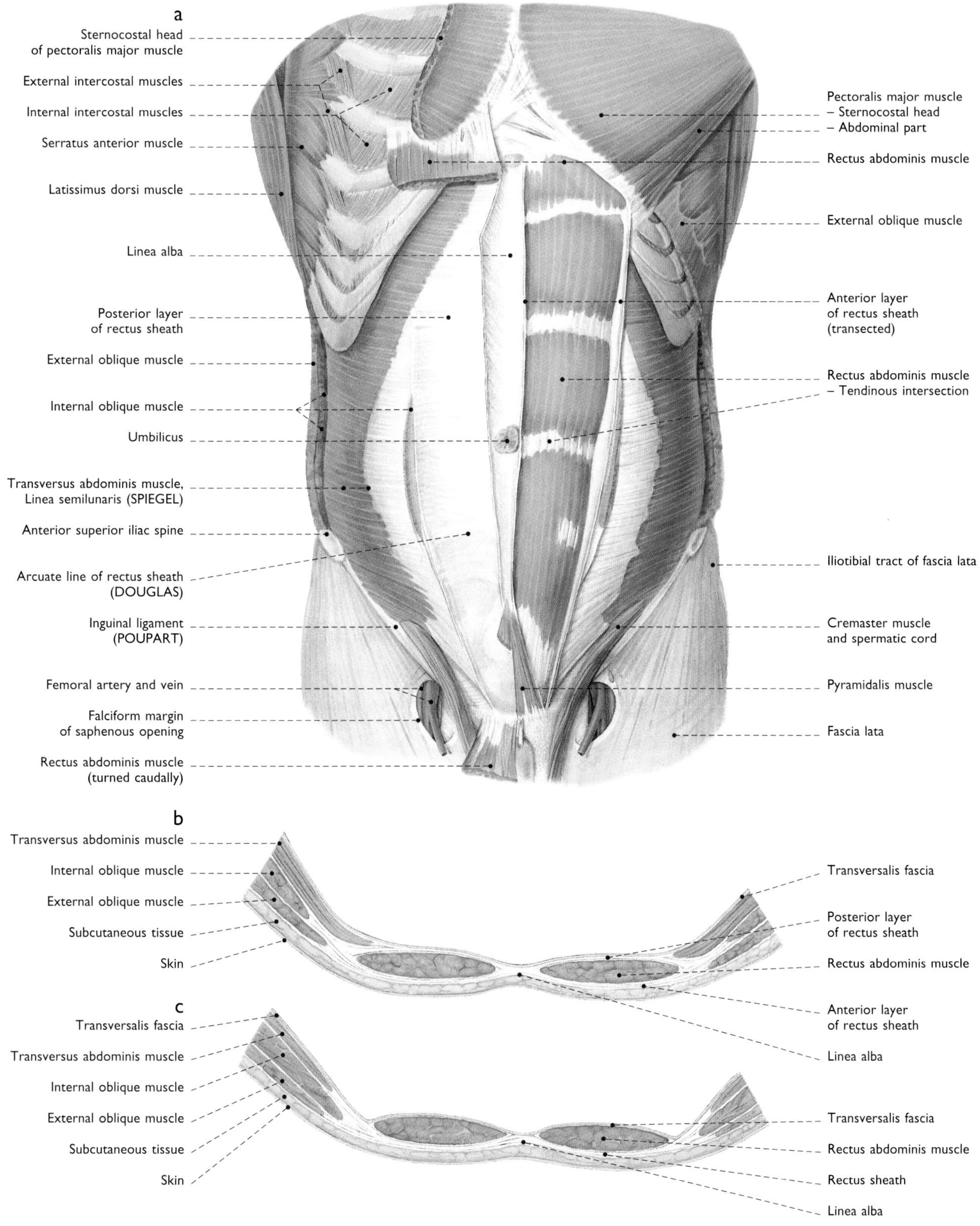
a
Sternocostal head of pectoralis major muscle
External intercostal muscles
Internal intercostal muscles
Serratus anterior muscle
Latissimus dorsi muscle
Linea alba
Posterior layer of rectus sheath
External oblique muscle
Internal oblique muscle
Umbilicus
Transversus abdominis muscle, Linea semilunaris (SPIEGEL)
Anterior superior iliac spine
Arcuate line of rectus sheath (DOUGLAS)
Inguinal ligament (POUPART)
Femoral artery and vein
Falciform margin of saphenous opening
Rectus abdominis muscle (turned caudally)
Pectoralis major muscle
– Sternocostal head
– Abdominal part
Rectus abdominis muscle
External oblique muscle
Anterior layer of rectus sheath (transected)
Rectus abdominis muscle
– Tendinous intersection
Iliotibial tract of fascia lata
Cremaster muscle and spermatic cord
Pyramidalis muscle
Fascia lata
b
Transversus abdominis muscle
Internal oblique muscle
External oblique muscle
Subcutaneous tissue
Skin
Transversalis fascia
Posterior layer of rectus sheath
Rectus abdominis muscle
Anterior layer of rectus sheath
Linea alba
c
Transversalis fascia
Transversus abdominis muscle
Internal oblique muscle
External oblique muscle
Subcutaneous tissue
Skin
Transversalis fascia
Rectus abdominis muscle
Rectus sheath
Linea alba

67 Muscles of the abdomen

a Deepest layer (30%)
b, c Schematized transverse sections through the anterior abdominal wall (50%)
b above the umbilical region
c below the arcuate line of rectus sheath

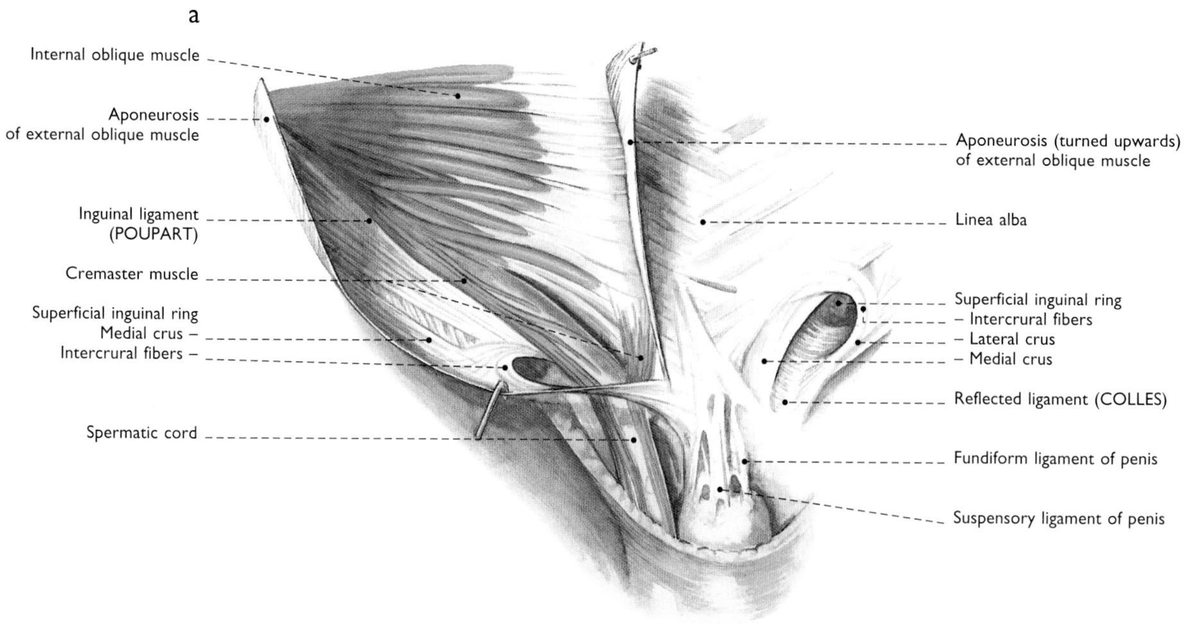
a
Internal oblique muscle
Aponeurosis of external oblique muscle
Inguinal ligament (POUPART)
Cremaster muscle
Superficial inguinal ring
Medial crus –
Intercrural fibers –
Spermatic cord
Aponeurosis (turned upwards) of external oblique muscle
Linea alba
Superficial inguinal ring
– Intercrural fibers
– Lateral crus
– Medial crus
Reflected ligament (COLLES)
Fundiform ligament of penis
Suspensory ligament of penis

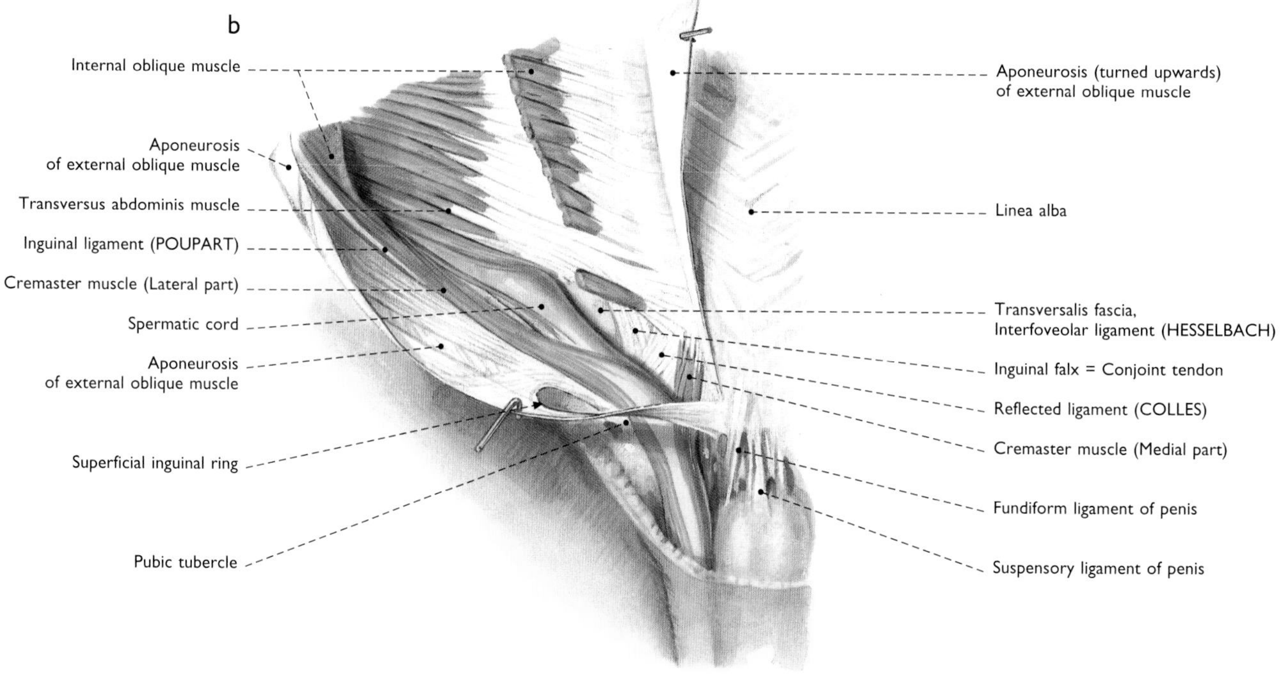
b
Internal oblique muscle
Aponeurosis of external oblique muscle
Transversus abdominis muscle
Inguinal ligament (POUPART)
Cremaster muscle (Lateral part)
Spermatic cord
Aponeurosis of external oblique muscle
Superficial inguinal ring
Pubic tubercle
Aponeurosis (turned upwards) of external oblique muscle
Linea alba
Transversalis fascia, Interfoveolar ligament (HESSELBACH)
Inguinal falx = Conjoint tendon
Reflected ligament (COLLES)
Cremaster muscle (Medial part)
Fundiform ligament of penis
Suspensory ligament of penis

68 Inguinal region of a male (60%)

a Superficial layer
b Deep layer
a, b The two portions of the dissected aponeurosis of the external oblique muscle were retracted on the right side of the body. In fig. b, the internal oblique muscle was additionally removed partially. On the left side of the body in fig. a, the spermatic cord was taken away to demonstrate the inguinal canal.

a

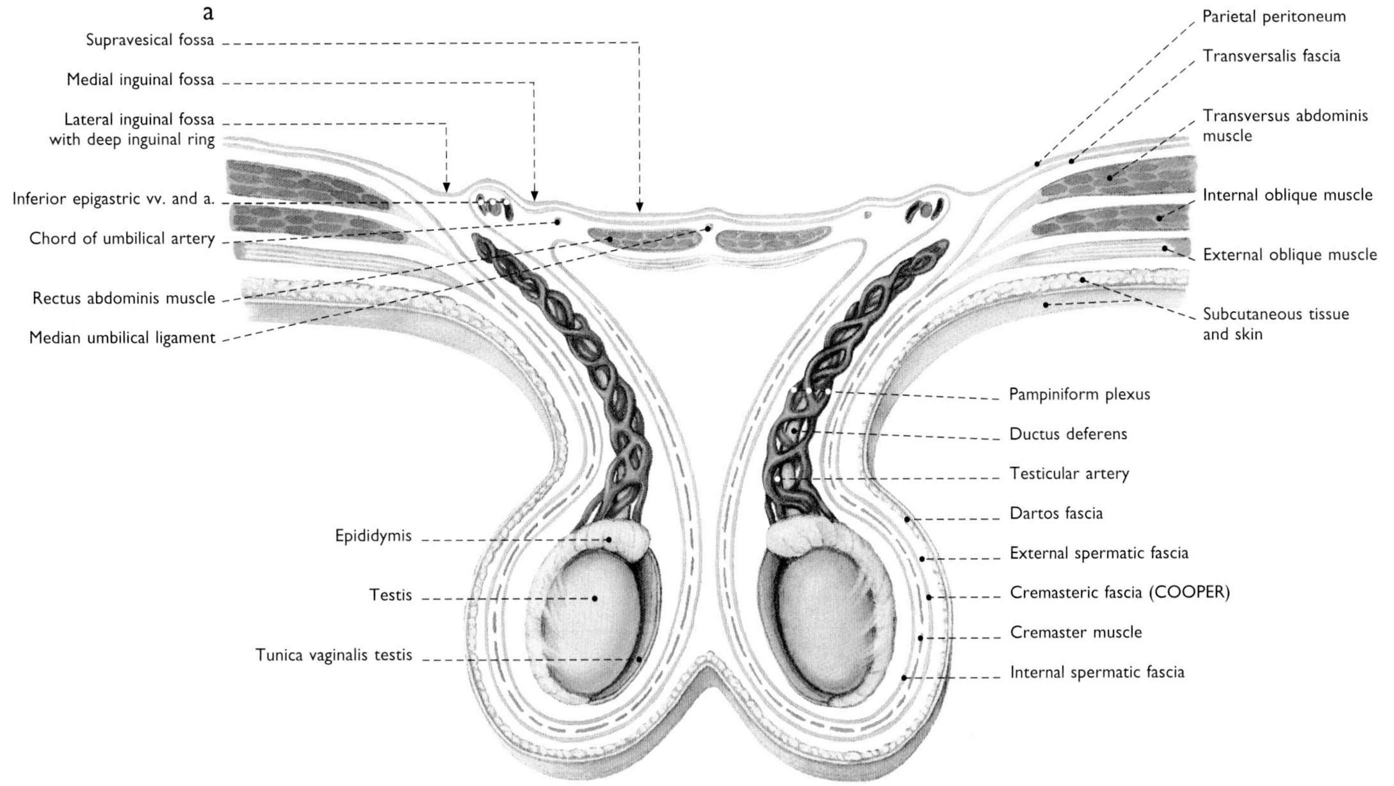
Supravesical fossa
Medial inguinal fossa
Lateral inguinal fossa with deep inguinal ring
Inferior epigastric vv. and a.
Chord of umbilical artery
Rectus abdominis muscle
Median umbilical ligament
Parietal peritoneum
Transversalis fascia
Transversus abdominis muscle
Internal oblique muscle
External oblique muscle
Subcutaneous tissue and skin
Pampiniform plexus
Ductus deferens
Testicular artery
Dartos fascia
External spermatic fascia
Cremasteric fascia (COOPER)
Cremaster muscle
Internal spermatic fascia
Epididymis
Testis
Tunica vaginalis testis

b

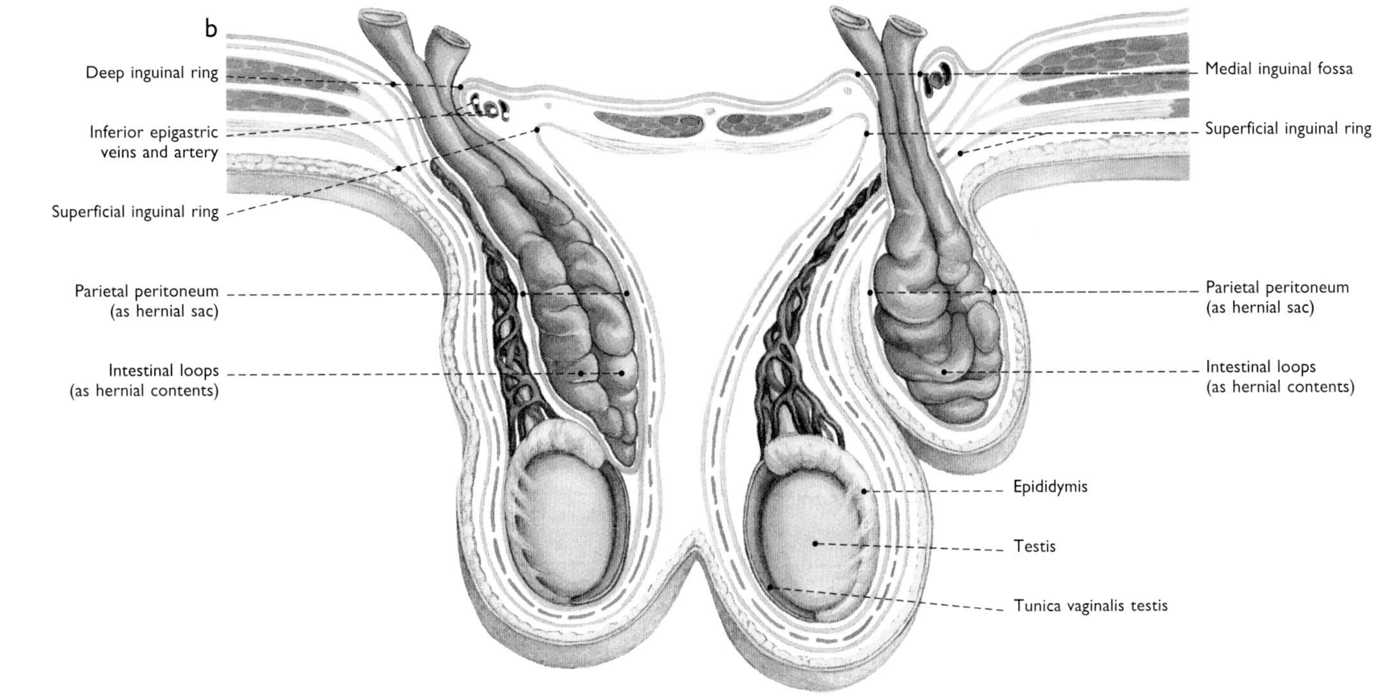
Deep inguinal ring
Inferior epigastric veins and artery
Superficial inguinal ring
Parietal peritoneum (as hernial sac)
Intestinal loops (as hernial contents)
Medial inguinal fossa
Superficial inguinal ring
Parietal peritoneum (as hernial sac)
Intestinal loops (as hernial contents)
Epididymis
Testis
Tunica vaginalis testis

69 Inguinal region of a male

a, b Schematized sections through the anterior abdominal wall on the level of the inguinal canal and through the scrotum (according to BENNINGHOFF, 1985). Ventral aspect

a Normal situation

b Inguinal herniae. On the right side of the body, a lateral indirect hernia through the inguinal canal; the inner hernial ring is the deep inguinal ring lateral to the inferior epigastric vessels.
On the left side of the body, a medial direct hernia; the inner hernial ring is the medial inguinal fossa medial to the inferior epigastric vessels.

a

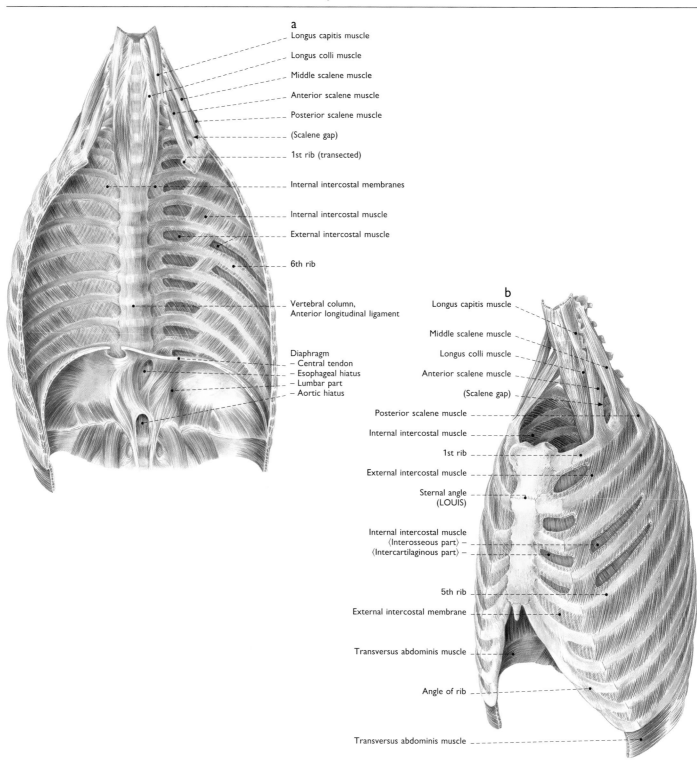

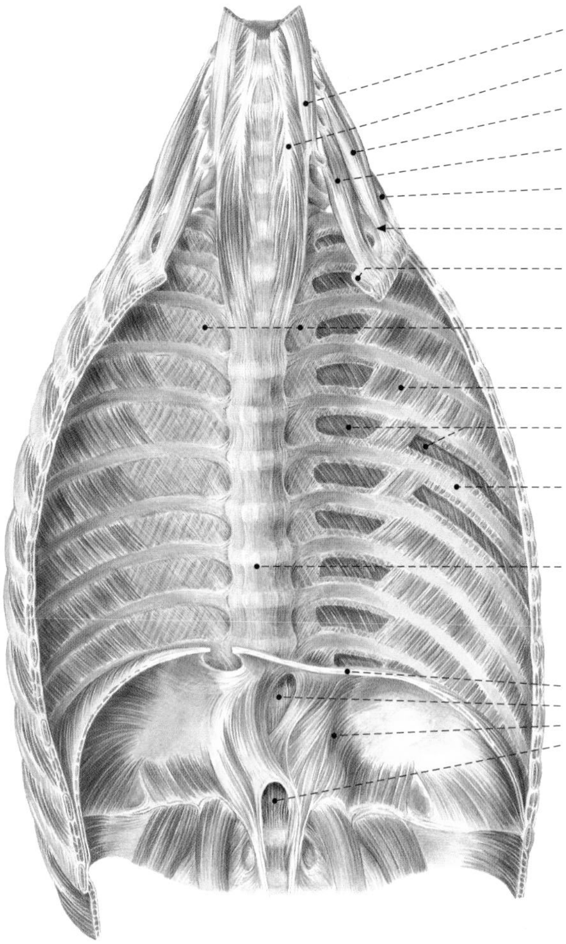
Longus capitis muscle
Longus colli muscle
Middle scalene muscle
Anterior scalene muscle
Posterior scalene muscle
(Scalene gap)
1st rib (transected)
Internal intercostal membranes
Internal intercostal muscle
External intercostal muscle
6th rib
Vertebral column,
Anterior longitudinal ligament
Diaphragm
– Central tendon
– Esophageal hiatus
– Lumbar part
– Aortic hiatus

b

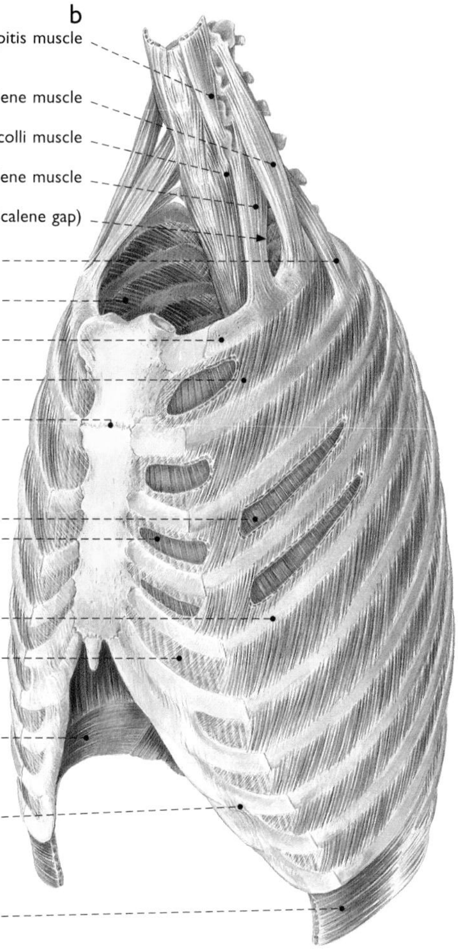
Longus capitis muscle
Middle scalene muscle
Longus colli muscle
Anterior scalene muscle
(Scalene gap)
Posterior scalene muscle
Internal intercostal muscle
1st rib
External intercostal muscle
Sternal angle
(LOUIS)
Internal intercostal muscle
⟨Interosseous part⟩ –
⟨Intercartilaginous part⟩ –
5th rib
External intercostal membrane
Transversus abdominis muscle
Angle of rib
Transversus abdominis muscle

70 Muscles of the thorax (30%)

a Internal aspect of the posterior chest wall with intercostal muscles. On the left side of the body, the internal intercostal membrane and the internal intercostal muscle were opened at several sites in order to demonstrate the external intercostal muscle lying externally. Ventral aspect

b Lateral and anterior chest wall with intercostal muscles. On the left side of the body, the internal intercostal muscle can be recognized in the windows cut into the external intercostal membrane and the external intercostal muscle. Left ventrolateral aspect

a

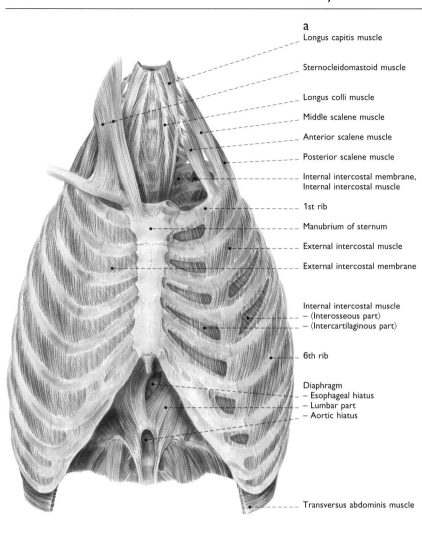

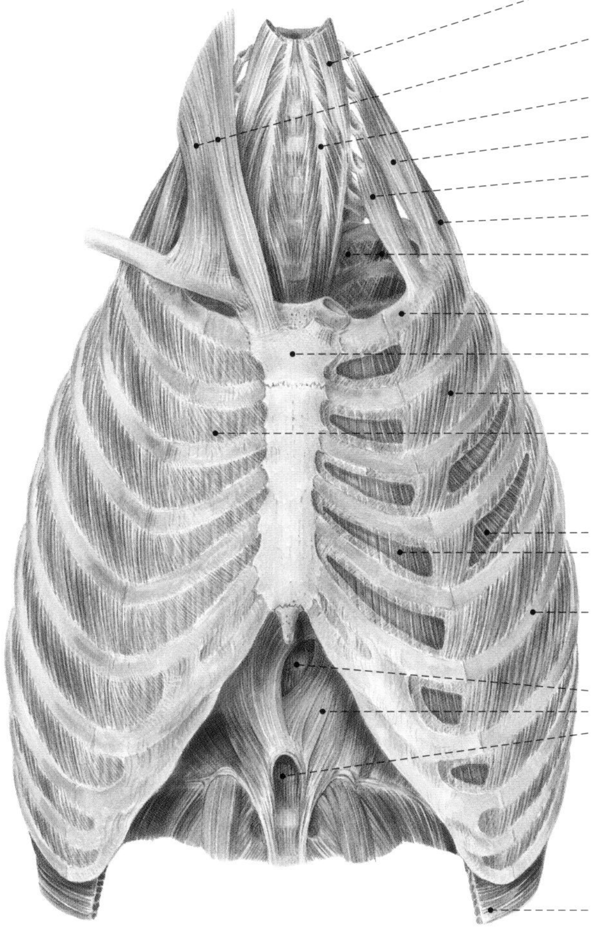
Longus capitis muscle
Sternocleidomastoid muscle
Longus colli muscle
Middle scalene muscle
Anterior scalene muscle
Posterior scalene muscle
Internal intercostal membrane,
Internal intercostal muscle
1st rib
Manubrium of sternum
External intercostal muscle
External intercostal membrane
Internal intercostal muscle
– ⟨Interosseous part⟩
– ⟨Intercartilaginous part⟩
6th rib
Diaphragm
– Esophageal hiatus
– Lumbar part
– Aortic hiatus
Transversus abdominis muscle

b

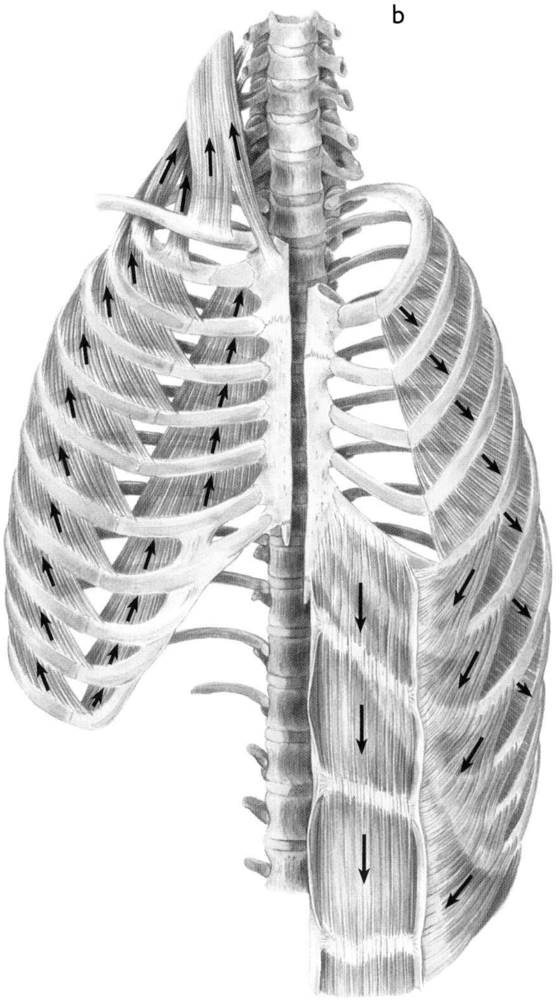

71 Muscles of the thorax (30%)

Ventral aspect

a Anterior chest wall with intercostal muscles. On the left side of the body, the external intercostal membrane and the external intercostal muscle were opened at several sites in order to show the internal intercostal muscle.

b Right side of the body, muscles of inspiration in case of thoracic breathing; left side of the body, muscles of forced expiration

a

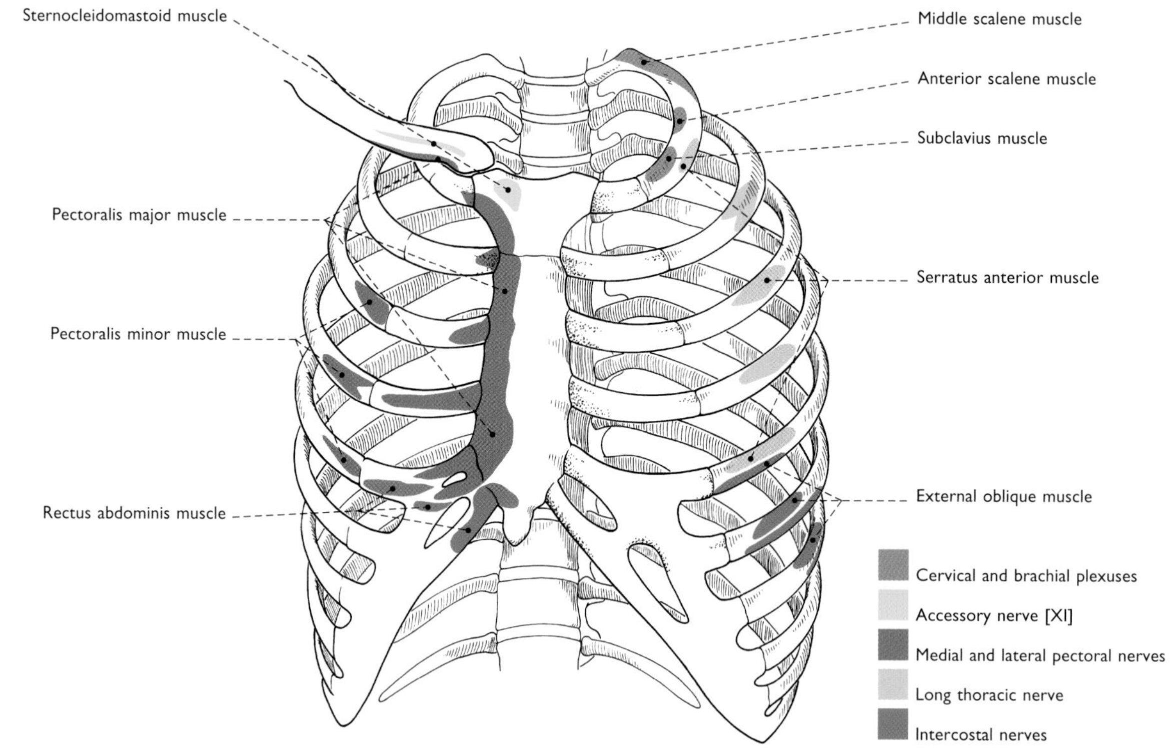
Sternocleidomastoid muscle
Pectoralis major muscle
Pectoralis minor muscle
Rectus abdominis muscle
Middle scalene muscle
Anterior scalene muscle
Subclavius muscle
Serratus anterior muscle
External oblique muscle
Cervical and brachial plexuses
Accessory nerve [XI]
Medial and lateral pectoral nerves
Long thoracic nerve
Intercostal nerves

b

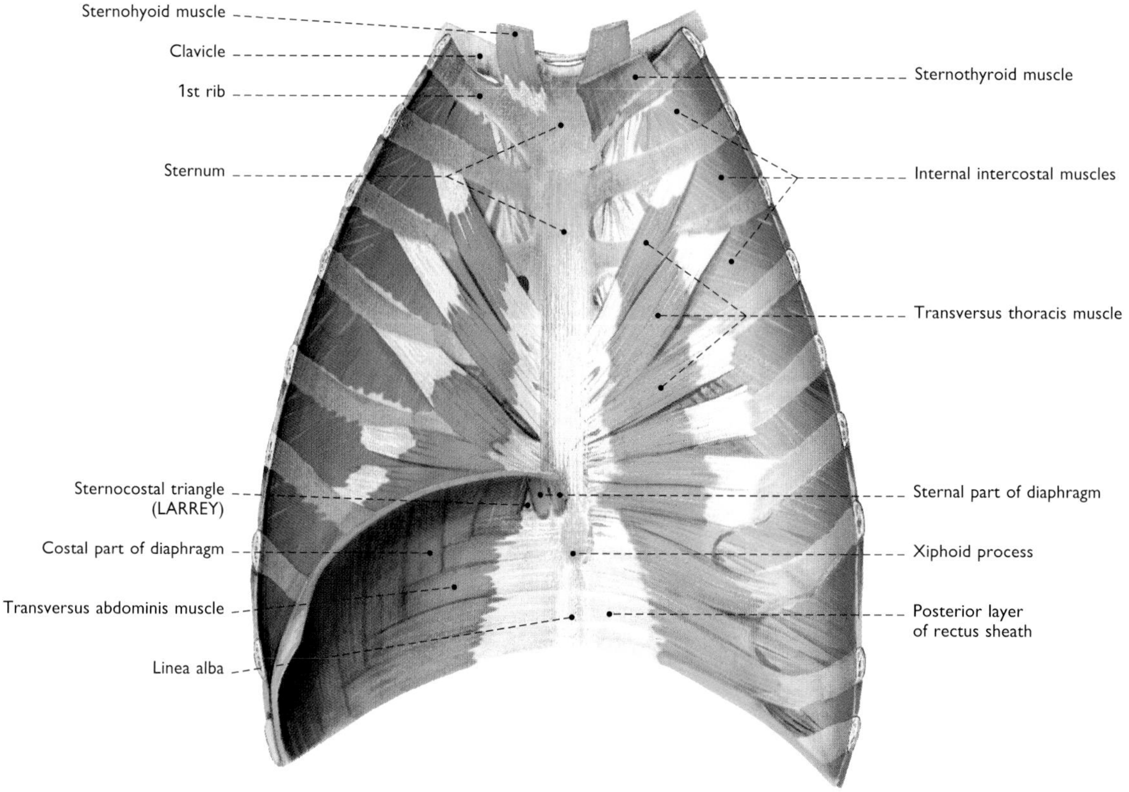
Sternohyoid muscle
Clavicle
1st rib
Sternum
Sternocostal triangle (LARREY)
Costal part of diaphragm
Transversus abdominis muscle
Linea alba
Sternothyroid muscle
Internal intercostal muscles
Transversus thoracis muscle
Sternal part of diaphragm
Xiphoid process
Posterior layer of rectus sheath

72 Ventral muscles of the trunk

a Muscle attachments on the ventrolateral thorax. The colors indicate the innervation.

b Internal aspect of the anterior chest wall and the genuine muscles of the thorax (35%)

a

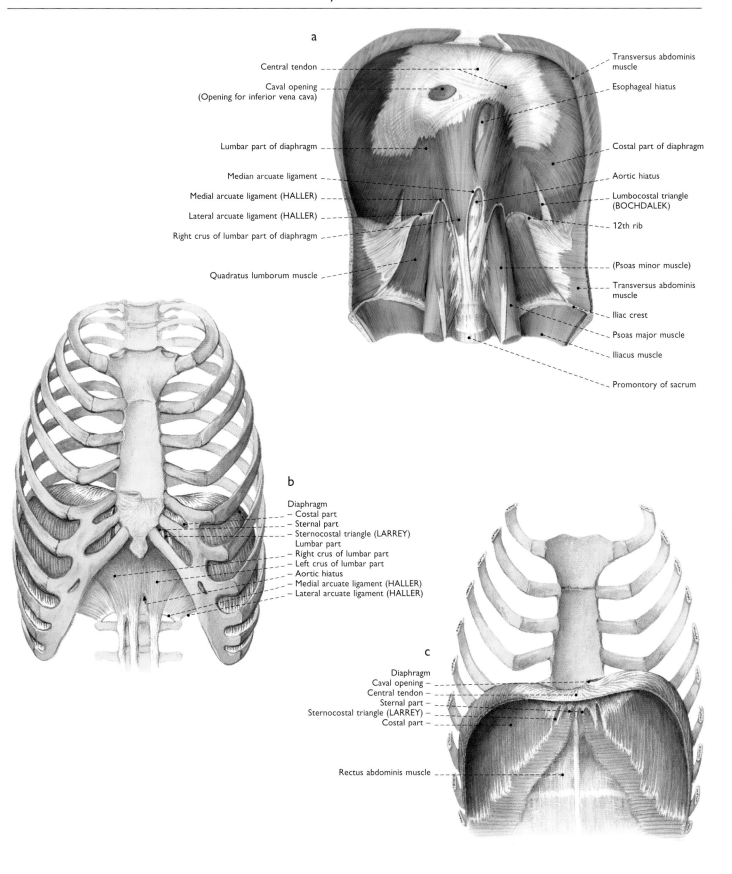

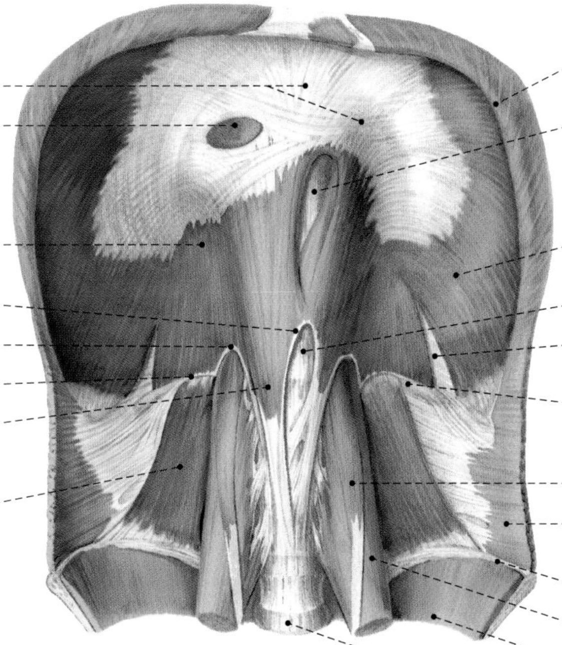
Central tendon
Caval opening
(Opening for inferior vena cava)
Lumbar part of diaphragm
Median arcuate ligament
Medial arcuate ligament (HALLER)
Lateral arcuate ligament (HALLER)
Right crus of lumbar part of diaphragm
Quadratus lumborum muscle
Transversus abdominis muscle
Esophageal hiatus
Costal part of diaphragm
Aortic hiatus
Lumbocostal triangle (BOCHDALEK)
12th rib
(Psoas minor muscle)
Transversus abdominis muscle
Iliac crest
Psoas major muscle
Iliacus muscle
Promontory of sacrum

b

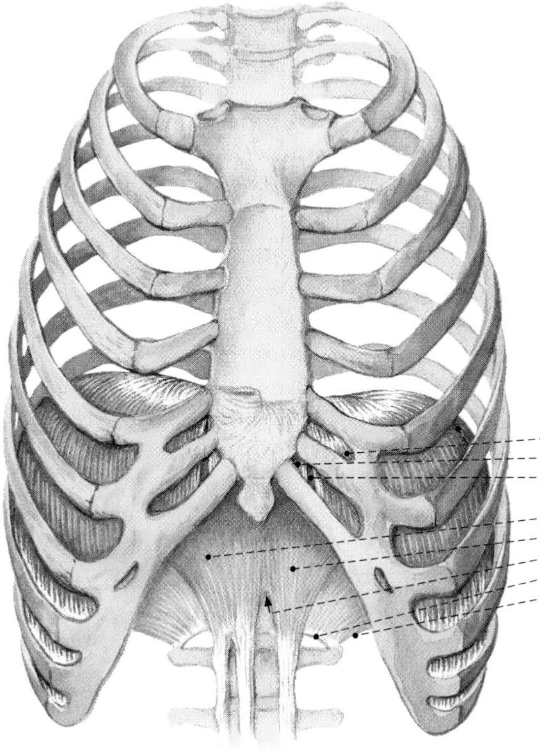
Diaphragm
– Costal part
– Sternal part
– Sternocostal triangle (LARREY)
Lumbar part
– Right crus of lumbar part
– Left crus of lumbar part
– Aortic hiatus
– Medial arcuate ligament (HALLER)
– Lateral arcuate ligament (HALLER)

c

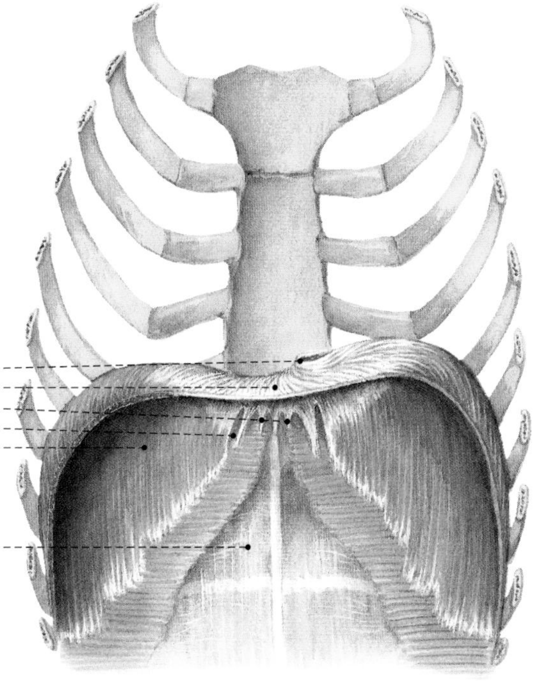
Diaphragm
Caval opening –
Central tendon –
Sternal part –
Sternocostal triangle (LARREY) –
Costal part –
Rectus abdominis muscle

73 Diaphragm (30%)

a Caudal aspect
b Ventral aspect
c Dorsal aspect

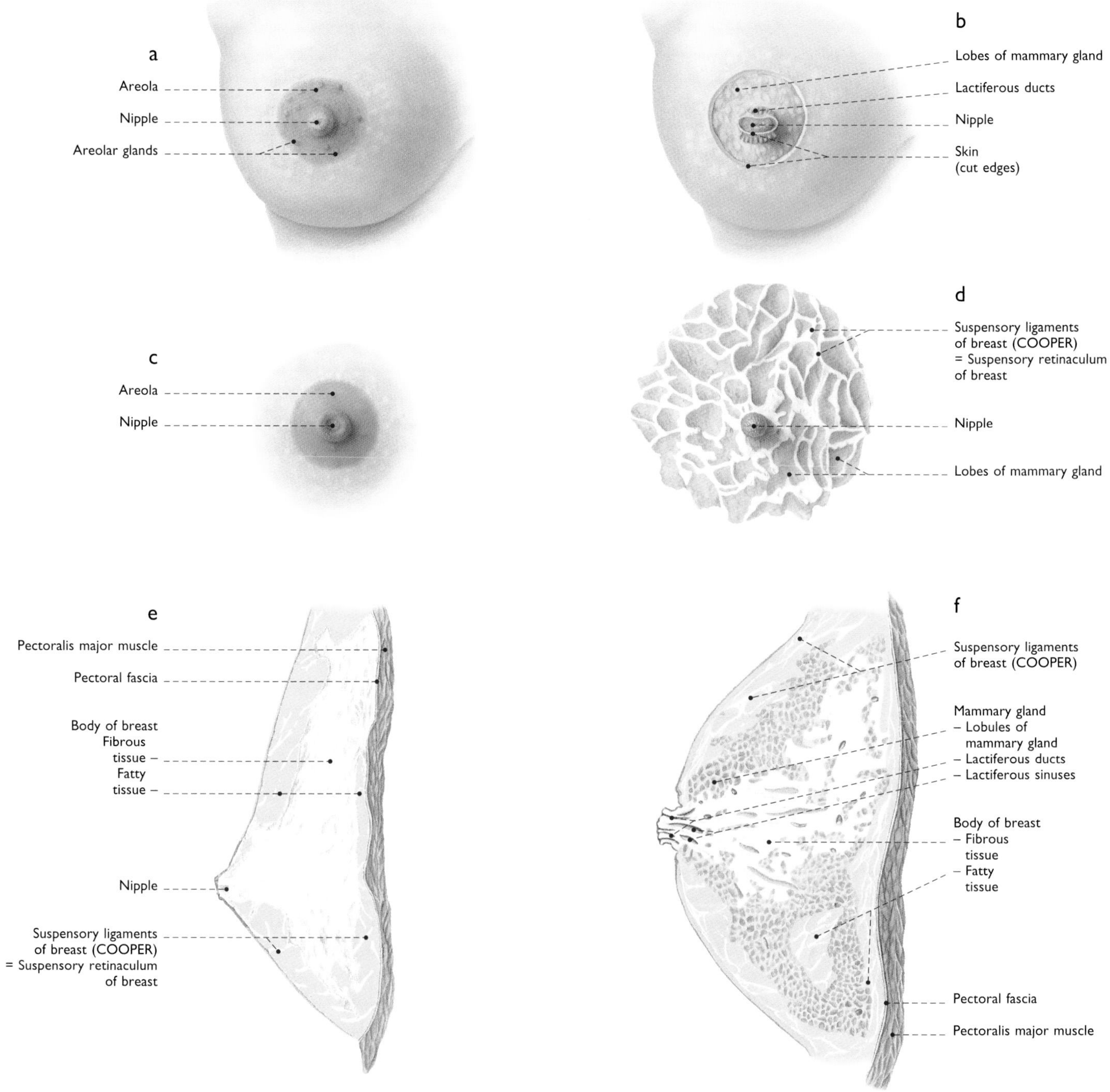
a
Areola
Nipple
Areolar glands
b
Lobes of mammary gland
Lactiferous ducts
Nipple
Skin
(cut edges)
c
Areola
Nipple
d
Suspensory ligaments of breast (COOPER) = Suspensory retinaculum of breast
Nipple
Lobes of mammary gland
e
Pectoralis major muscle
Pectoral fascia
Body of breast
Fibrous tissue –
Fatty tissue –
Nipple
Suspensory ligaments of breast (COOPER) = Suspensory retinaculum of breast
f
Suspensory ligaments of breast (COOPER)
Mammary gland
– Lobules of mammary gland
– Lactiferous ducts
– Lactiferous sinuses
Body of breast
– Fibrous tissue
– Fatty tissue
Pectoral fascia
Pectoralis major muscle

74 Breast

- a Ventral aspect (40%)
- b Ventral aspect (40%). The skin around the nipple was removed.
- c Depressed nipple (70%)
- d Parenchyma of the mammary gland after removal of the skin and the subcutaneous tissue (40%)
- e Sagittal section through the breast of a 16-year-old non-pregnant nullipara (60%)
- f Sagittal section through the breast of a 28-year-old woman immediately before lactation (60%)

a

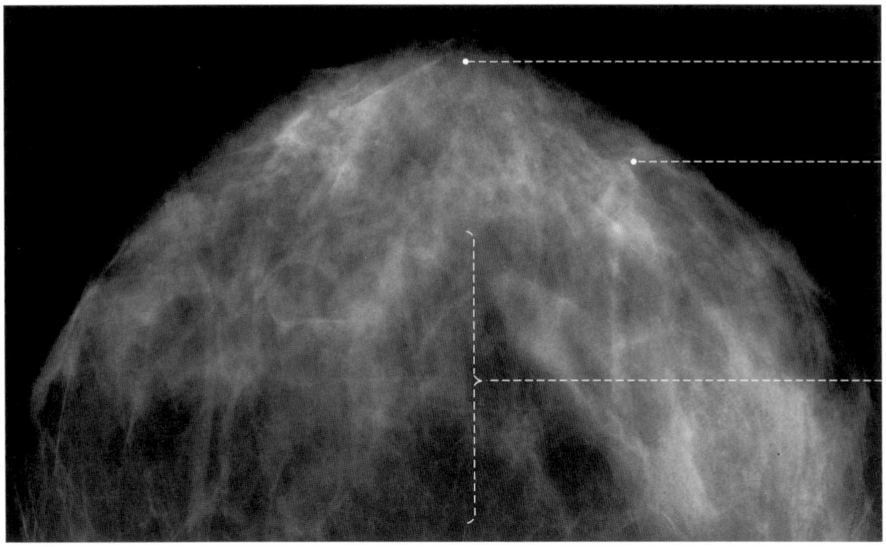
Nipple
Suspensory ligament of breast (COOPER) = Suspensory retinaculum of breast
Body of breast

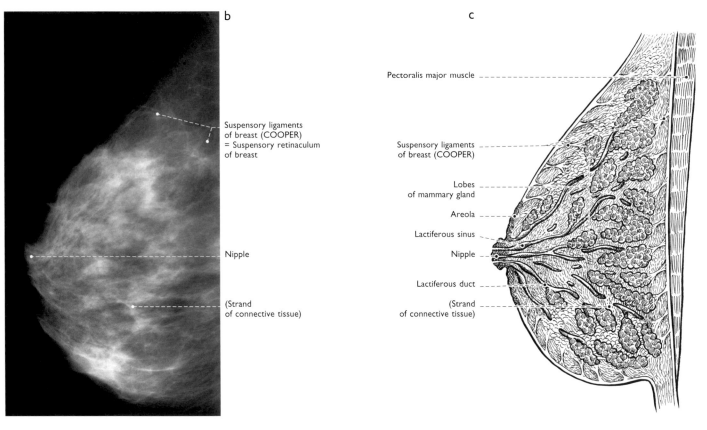

b

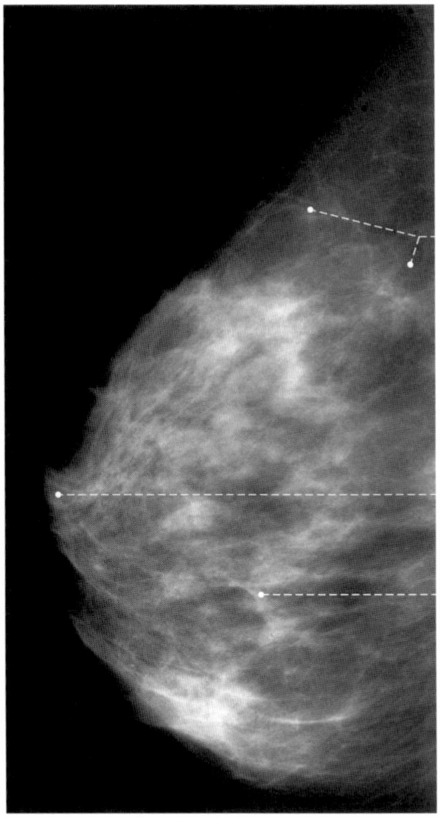
Suspensory ligaments of breast (COOPER) = Suspensory retinaculum of breast
Nipple
(Strand of connective tissue)

c

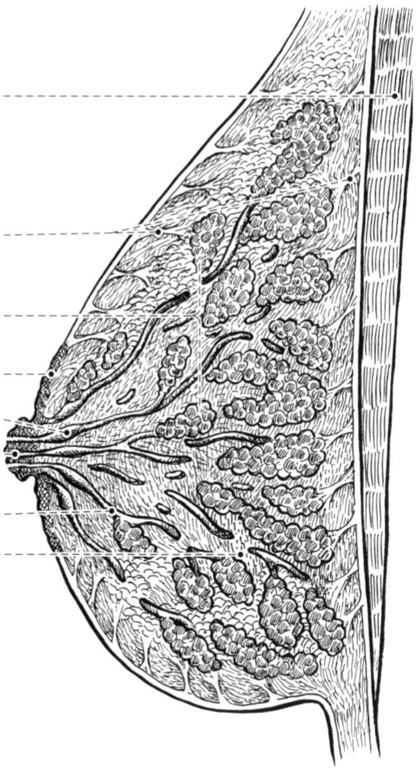
Pectoralis major muscle
Suspensory ligaments of breast (COOPER)
Lobes of mammary gland
Areola
Lactiferous sinus
Nipple
Lactiferous duct
(Strand of connective tissue)

75 Breast

a, b Mammograms
a Craniocaudal radiogram
b Lateral radiogram
c Construction of the breast, schematized representation of a sagittal section

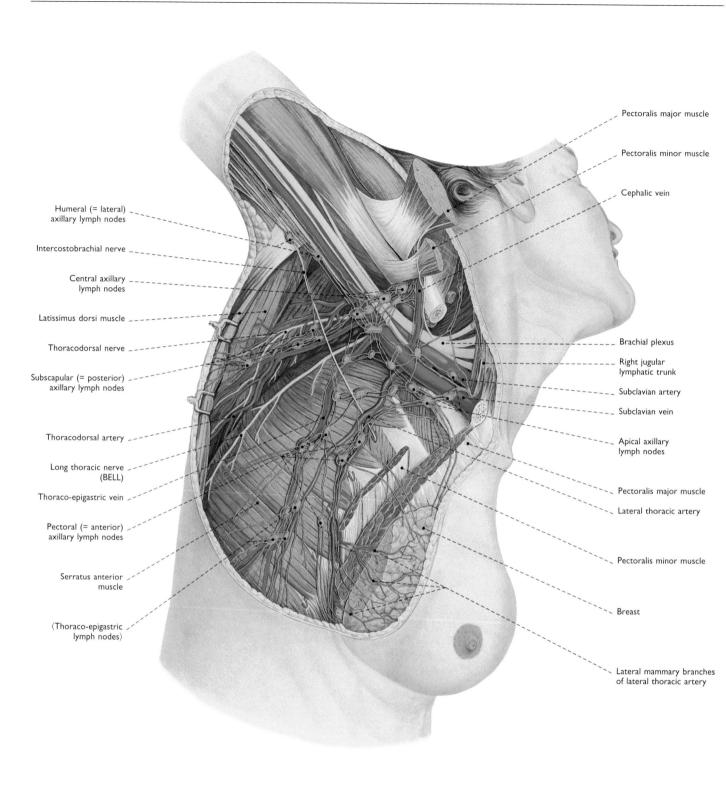

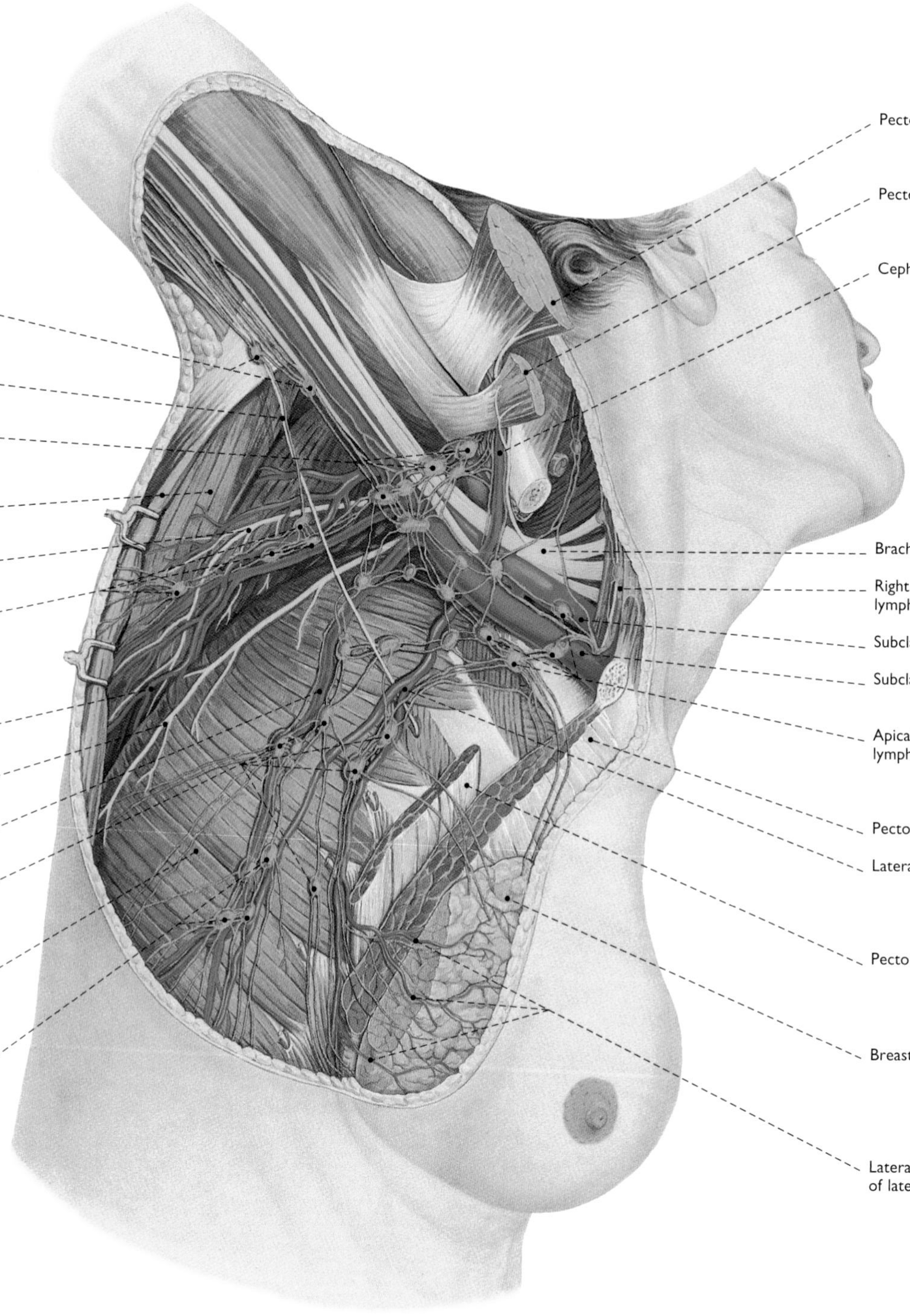
Pectoralis major muscle
Pectoralis minor muscle
Cephalic vein
Humeral (= lateral) axillary lymph nodes
Intercostobrachial nerve
Central axillary lymph nodes
Latissimus dorsi muscle
Thoracodorsal nerve
Subscapular (= posterior) axillary lymph nodes
Brachial plexus
Right jugular lymphatic trunk
Subclavian artery
Subclavian vein
Apical axillary lymph nodes
Thoracodorsal artery
Long thoracic nerve (BELL)
Thoraco-epigastric vein
Pectoral (= anterior) axillary lymph nodes
Serratus anterior muscle
⟨Thoraco-epigastric lymph nodes⟩
Pectoralis major muscle
Lateral thoracic artery
Pectoralis minor muscle
Breast
Lateral mammary branches of lateral thoracic artery

76 Lymphatic vessels and lymph nodes of the axilla and the anterior chest wall (50%)

Lateral aspect

a

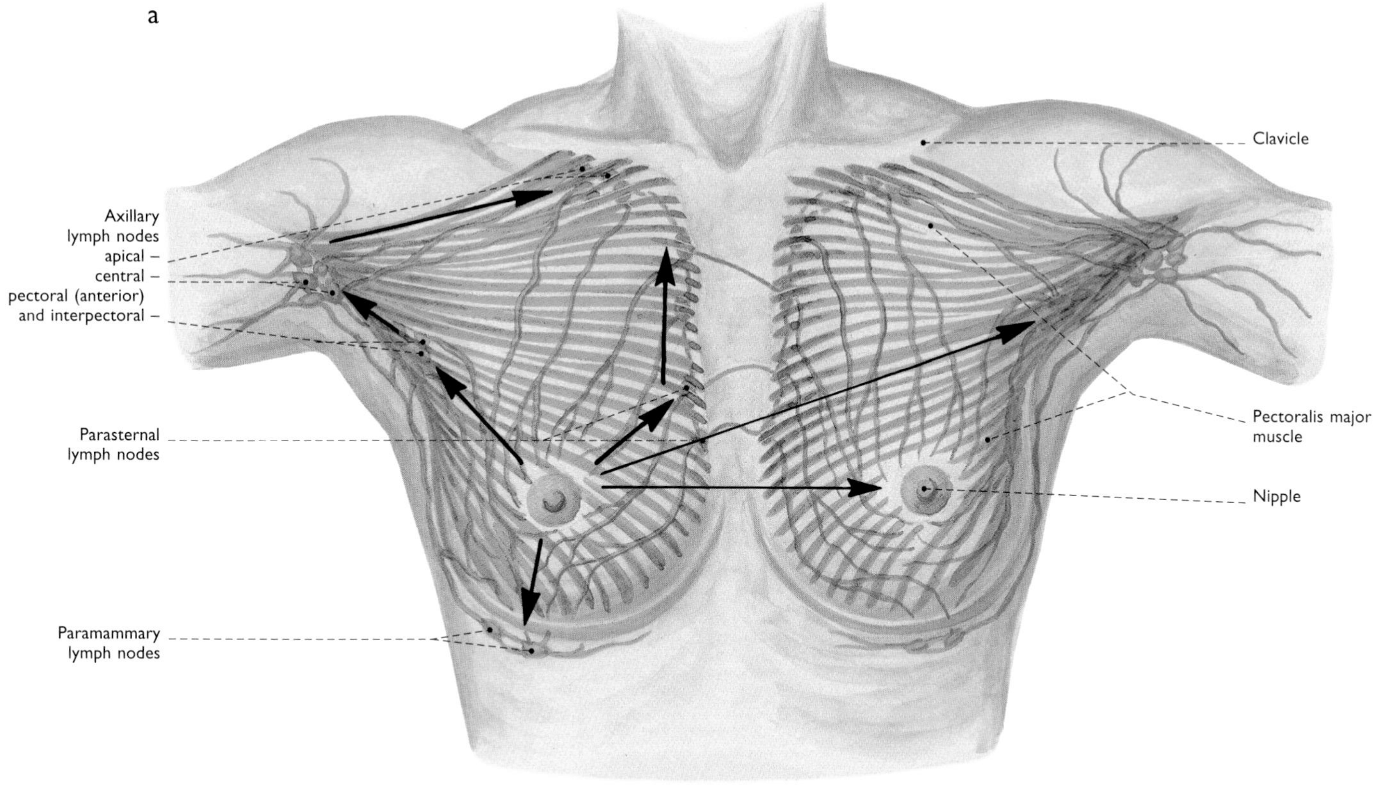
Axillary
lymph nodes
apical –
central –
pectoral (anterior)
and interpectoral –
Parasternal
lymph nodes
Paramammary
lymph nodes
Clavicle
Pectoralis major
muscle
Nipple

b

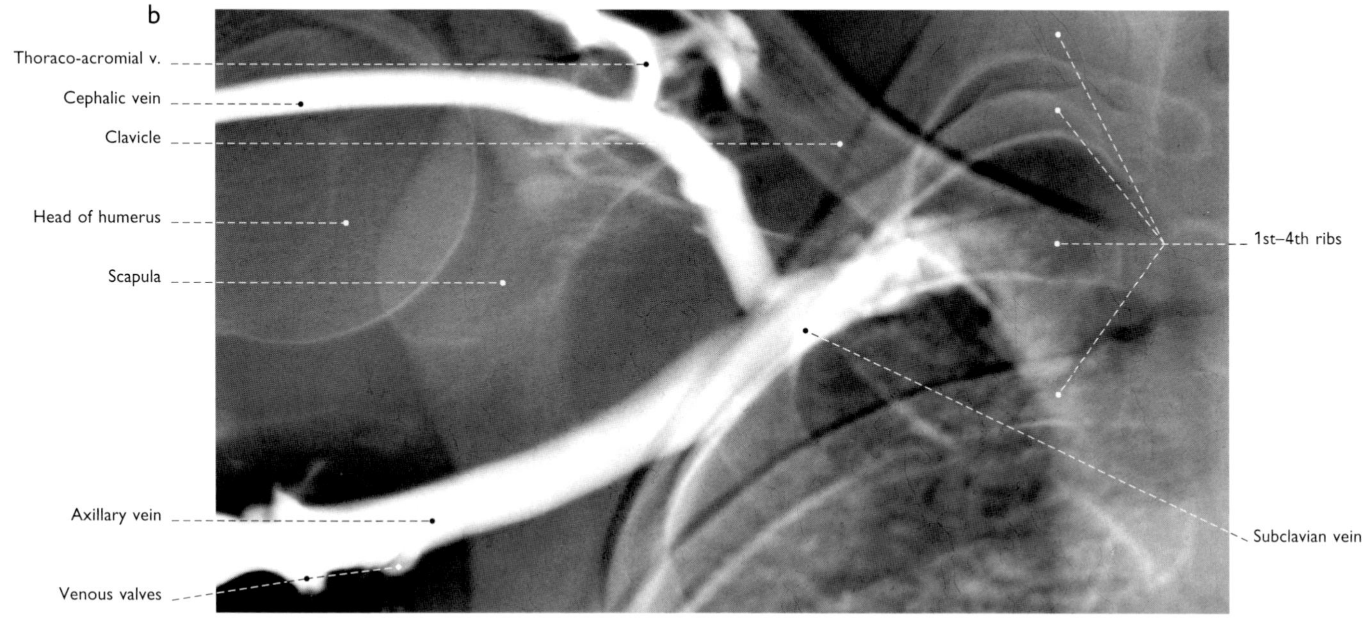
Thoraco-acromial v.
Cephalic vein
Clavicle
Head of humerus
Scapula
Axillary vein
Venous valves
1st–4th ribs
Subclavian vein

77 Lymphatic vessels, lymph nodes, and veins of the axilla and the anterior chest wall

a Schematic representation of the lymphatic drainage from the right breast (30%). The arrows illustrate the main ways of drainage.

b Venogram of the veins of the axilla after injection of contrast medium, postero-anterior radiogram (80%)

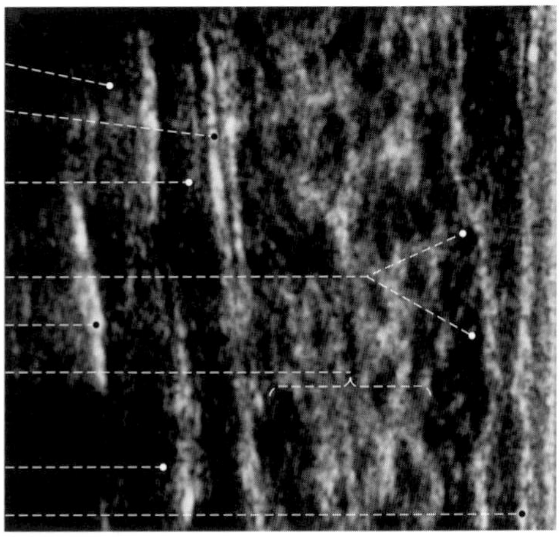
a
Rib
Pectoral fascia
Pectoralis major muscle
Suspensory ligaments of breast
Parietal pleura
Body of breast
Rib
Skin

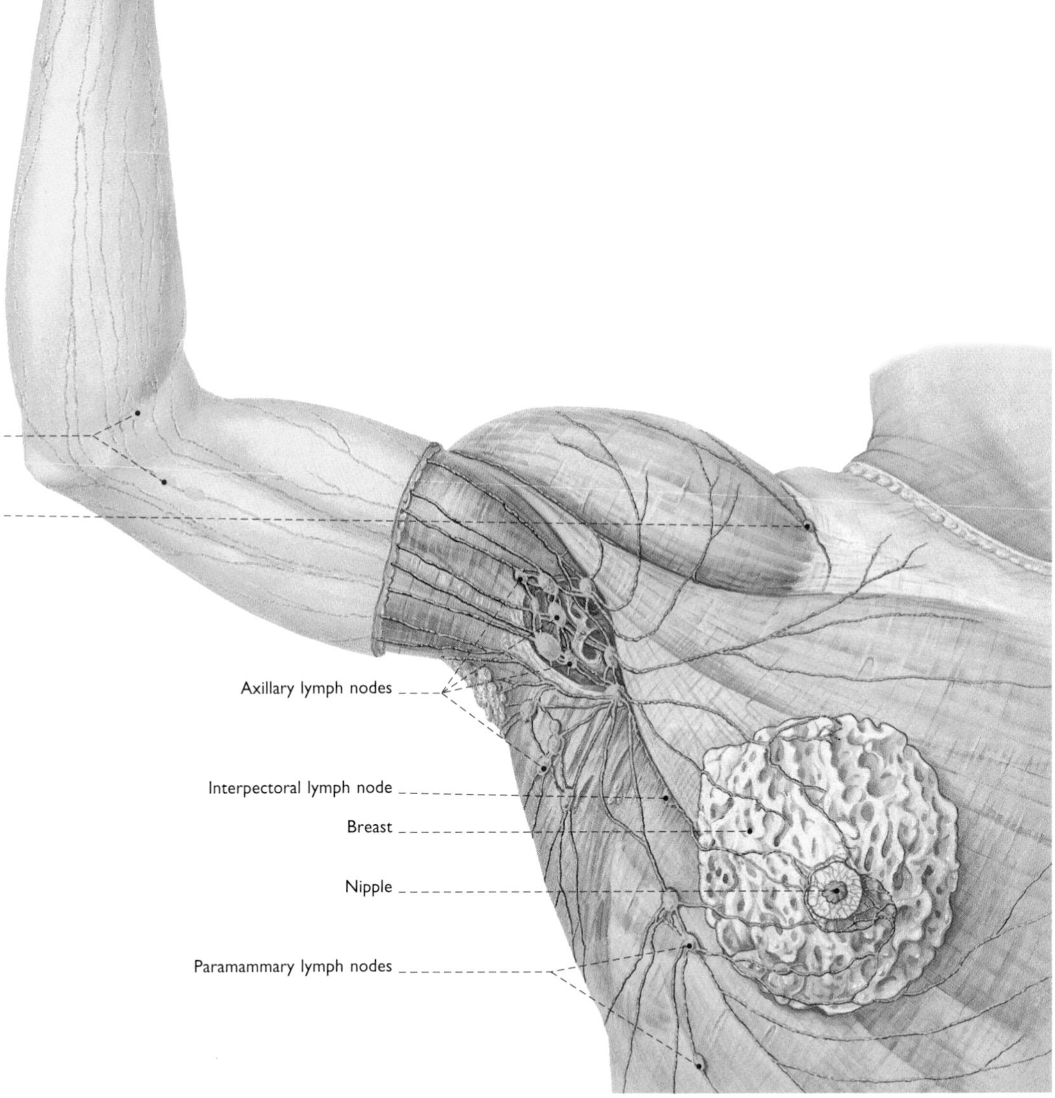
b
Cubital lymph nodes
Deltopectoral lymph node = Infraclavicular lymph node
Axillary lymph nodes
Interpectoral lymph node
Breast
Nipple
Paramammary lymph nodes

78 Breast, lymphatic vessels, and lymph nodes of the upper limb and the breast

a Sonogram (ultrasonic image) of the breast, sagittal section
b Lymphatic drainage from the upper limb and the breast (35%), ventral aspect

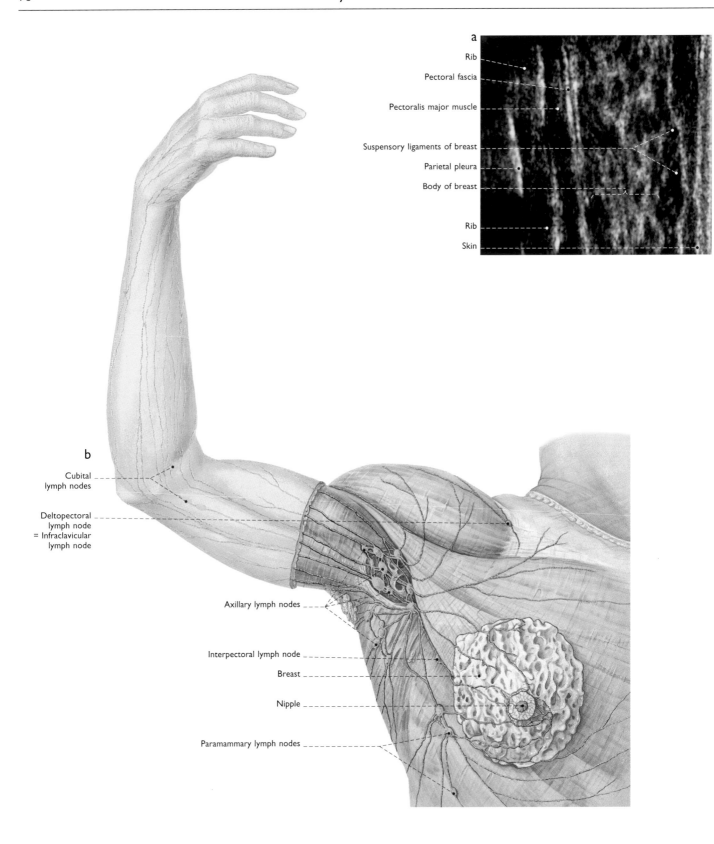

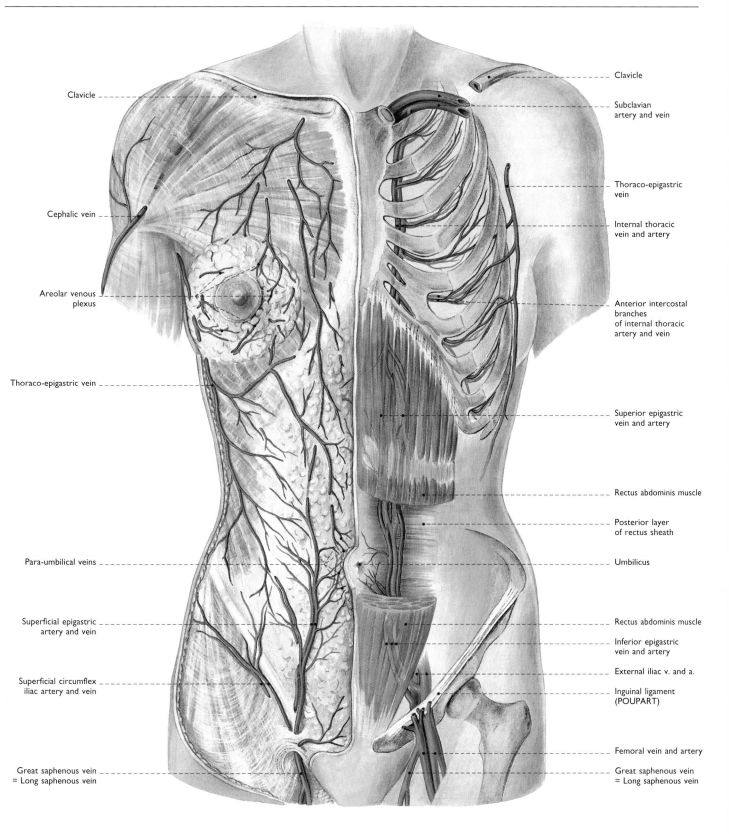

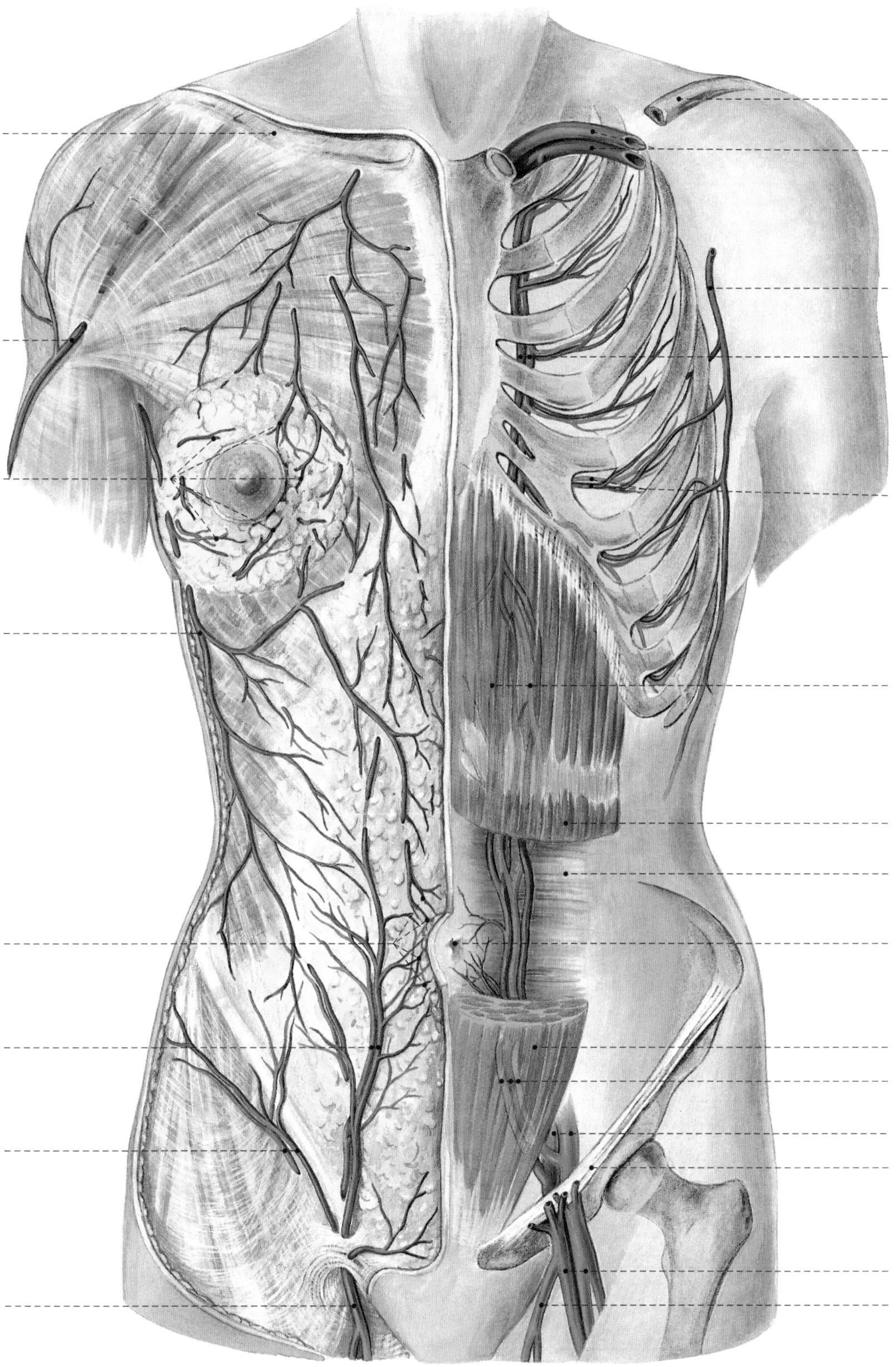
Clavicle
Cephalic vein
Areolar venous plexus
Thoraco-epigastric vein
Para-umbilical veins
Superficial epigastric artery and vein
Superficial circumflex iliac artery and vein
Great saphenous vein = Long saphenous vein
Clavicle
Subclavian artery and vein
Thoraco-epigastric vein
Internal thoracic vein and artery
Anterior intercostal branches of internal thoracic artery and vein
Superior epigastric vein and artery
Rectus abdominis muscle
Posterior layer of rectus sheath
Umbilicus
Rectus abdominis muscle
Inferior epigastric vein and artery
External iliac v. and a.
Inguinal ligament (POUPART)
Femoral vein and artery
Great saphenous vein = Long saphenous vein

79 Blood vessels of the ventral body wall (35%)

On the right side of the body, superficial vessels in the subcutaneous fatty tissue; on the left side of the body, deep vessels shining through the covering layers (the rectus abdominis muscle is cut above and below the umbilical region)

a

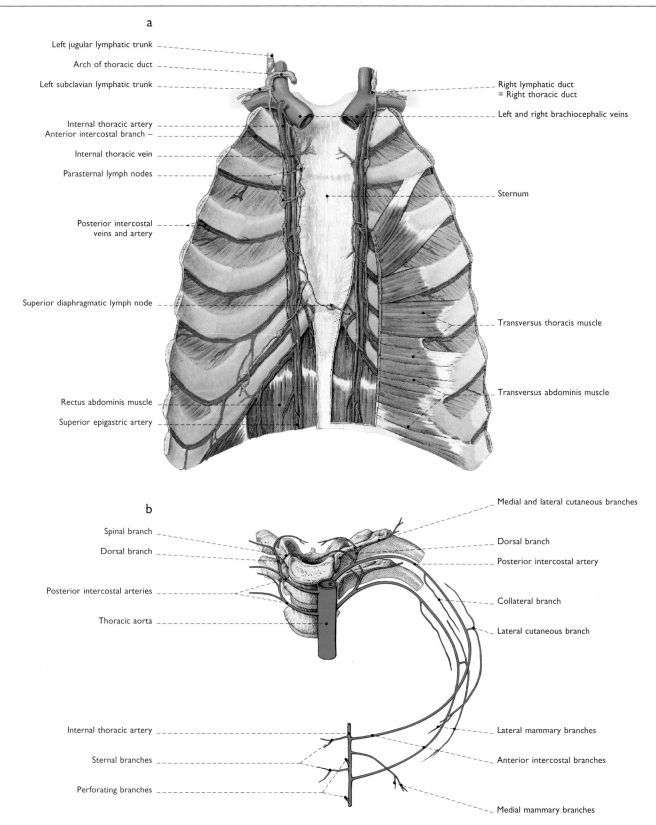

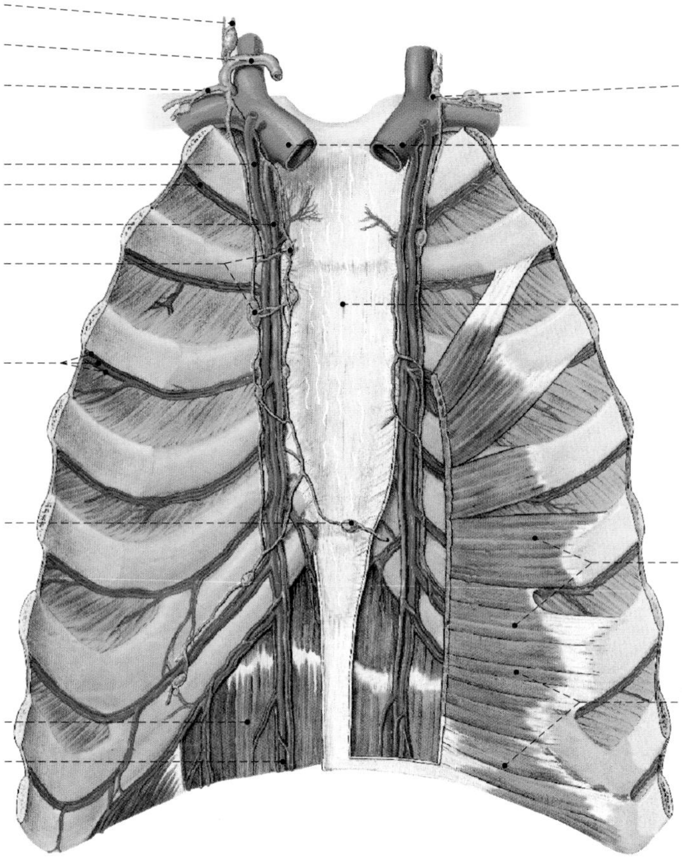
Left jugular lymphatic trunk
Arch of thoracic duct
Left subclavian lymphatic trunk
Internal thoracic artery
Anterior intercostal branch –
Internal thoracic vein
Parasternal lymph nodes
Posterior intercostal veins and artery
Superior diaphragmatic lymph node
Rectus abdominis muscle
Superior epigastric artery
Right lymphatic duct = Right thoracic duct
Left and right brachiocephalic veins
Sternum
Transversus thoracis muscle
Transversus abdominis muscle

b

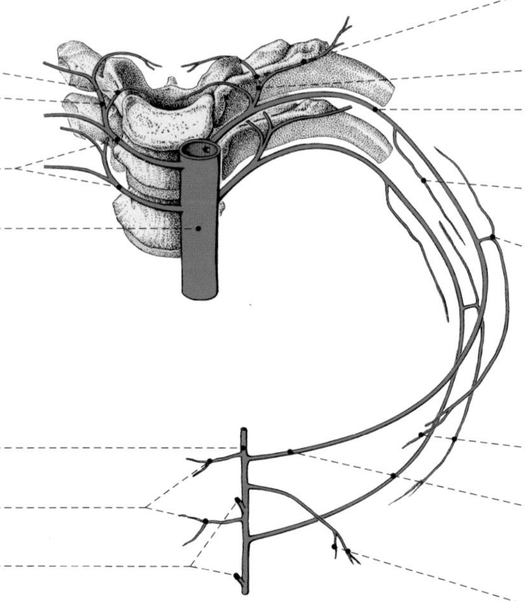
Spinal branch
Dorsal branch
Posterior intercostal arteries
Thoracic aorta
Internal thoracic artery
Sternal branches
Perforating branches
Medial and lateral cutaneous branches
Dorsal branch
Posterior intercostal artery
Collateral branch
Lateral cutaneous branch
Lateral mammary branches
Anterior intercostal branches
Medial mammary branches

80 Blood and lymphatic vessels of the thorax

a Internal aspect of the anterior chest wall (35%)

b Segmental arteries of the chest wall, cranioventral aspect of the left half (30%)

a

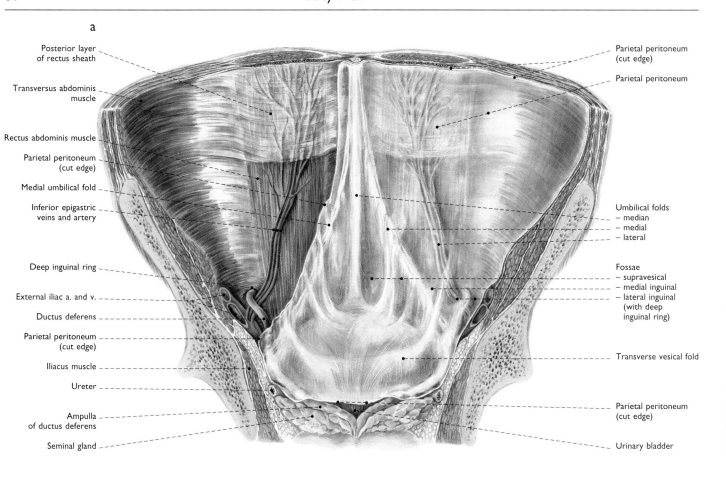

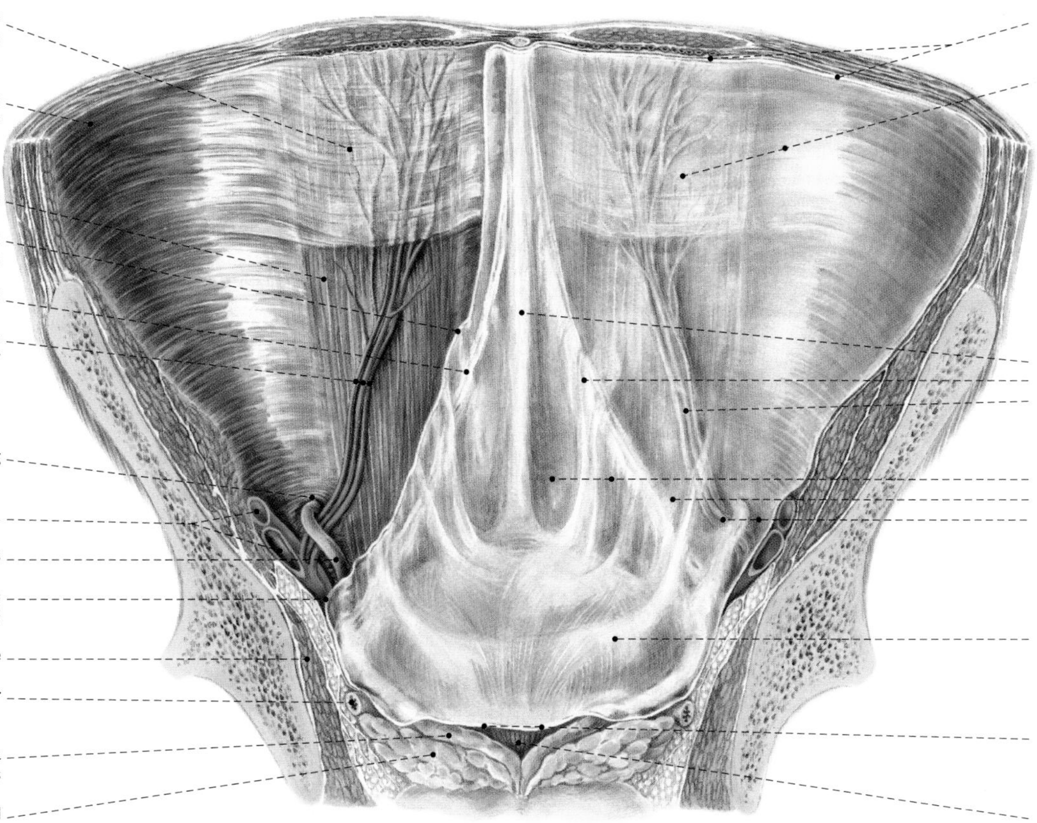
Posterior layer of rectus sheath
Transversus abdominis muscle
Rectus abdominis muscle
Parietal peritoneum (cut edge)
Medial umbilical fold
Inferior epigastric veins and artery
Deep inguinal ring
External iliac a. and v.
Ductus deferens
Parietal peritoneum (cut edge)
Iliacus muscle
Ureter
Ampulla of ductus deferens
Seminal gland
Parietal peritoneum (cut edge)
Parietal peritoneum
Umbilical folds
– median
– medial
– lateral
Fossae
– supravesical
– medial inguinal
– lateral inguinal (with deep inguinal ring)
Transverse vesical fold
Parietal peritoneum (cut edge)
Urinary bladder

b

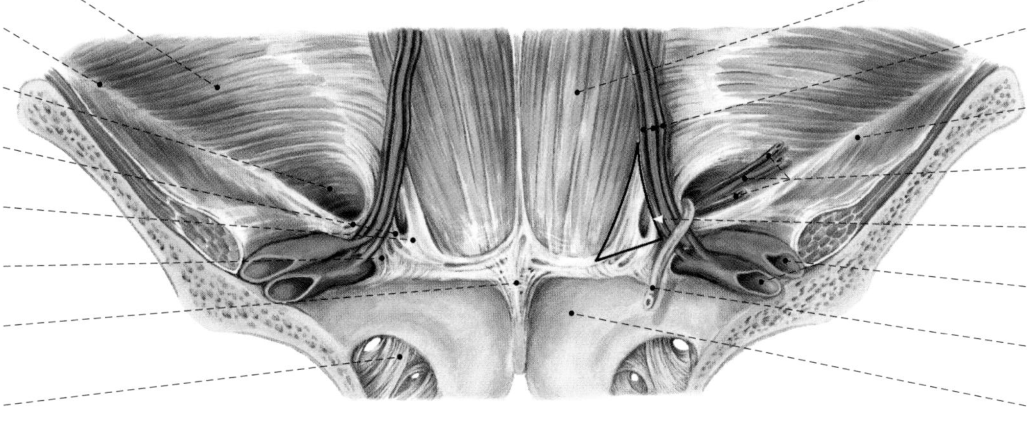
Transversus abdominis muscle
Inguinal ligament (POUPART)
Deep inguinal ring
Interfoveolar ligament (HESSELBACH)
Inguinal falx
Lacunar ligament (GIMBERNAT)
Posterior attachment of linea alba
Obturator membrane
Rectus abdominis muscle
Inferior epigastric veins and artery
Inguinal ligament (POUPART)
Testicular veins and artery
Inguinal triangle (HESSELBACH)
External iliac artery and vein
Ductus deferens
Pubis

81 Inner surface of the anterior abdominal wall (50%)

Dorsal aspect

a Area between the umbilical region and the lesser pelvis, covered completely by peritoneum on the right side, but only partially on the left side

b Inguinal and pubic regions without peritoneal covering; on the right, the ductus deferens is additionally shown.

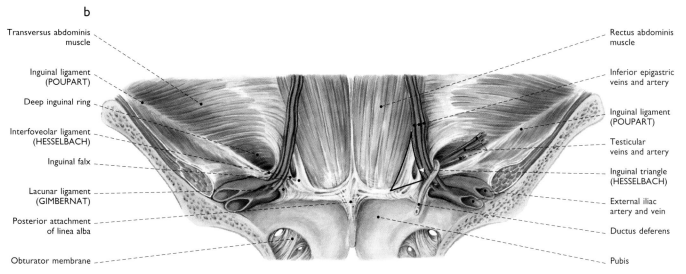

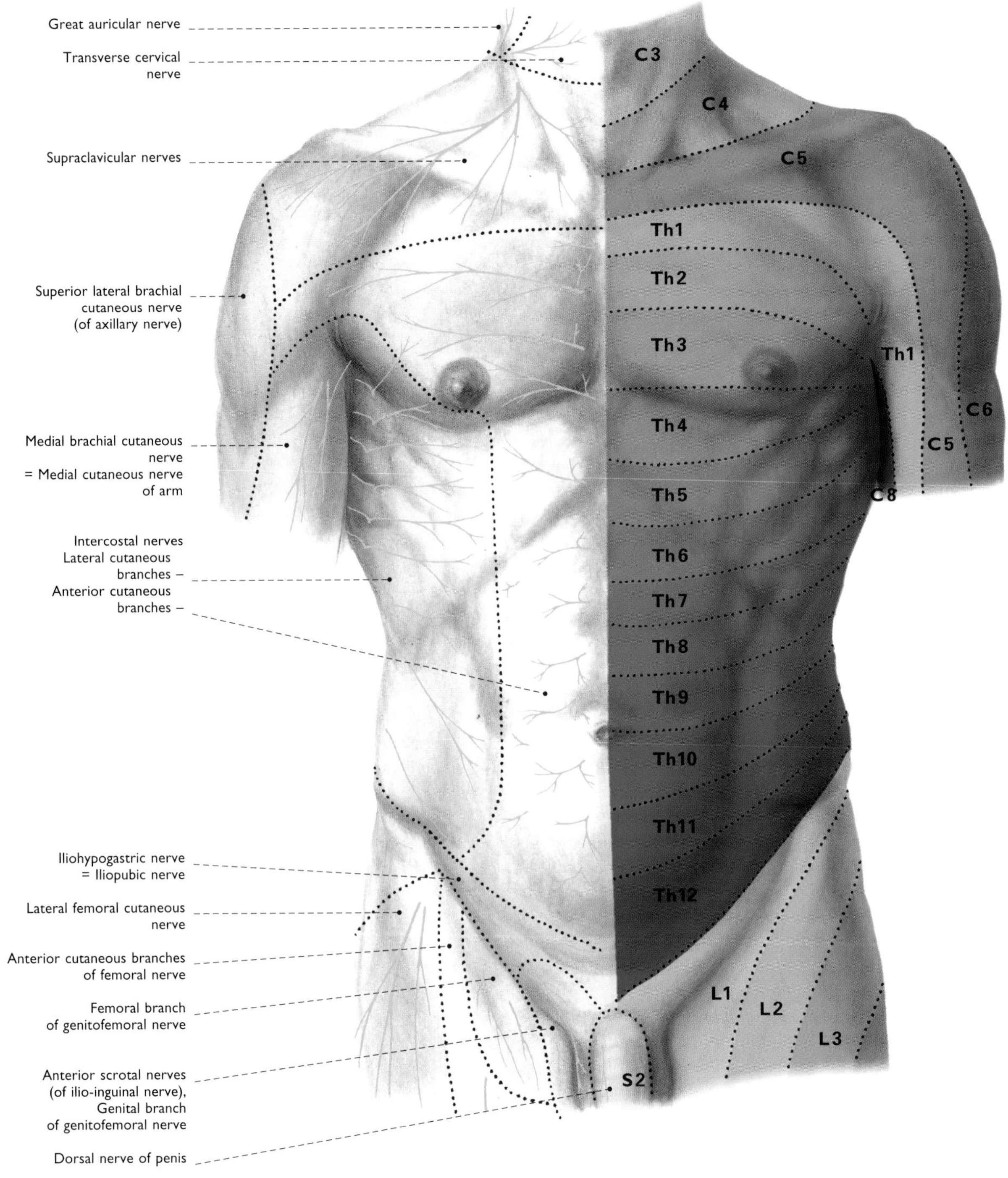
Great auricular nerve
Transverse cervical nerve
Supraclavicular nerves
Superior lateral brachial cutaneous nerve (of axillary nerve)
Medial brachial cutaneous nerve = Medial cutaneous nerve of arm
Intercostal nerves
Lateral cutaneous branches –
Anterior cutaneous branches –
Iliohypogastric nerve = Iliopubic nerve
Lateral femoral cutaneous nerve
Anterior cutaneous branches of femoral nerve
Femoral branch of genitofemoral nerve
Anterior scrotal nerves (of ilio-inguinal nerve), Genital branch of genitofemoral nerve
Dorsal nerve of penis
C3
C4
C5
Th1
Th2
Th3
Th1
C6
Th4
C5
Th5
C8
Th6
Th7
Th8
Th9
Th10
Th11
Th12
L1
L2
L3
S2

82 Cutaneous and segmental innervation of the ventral body wall (25%)

Schematic representation

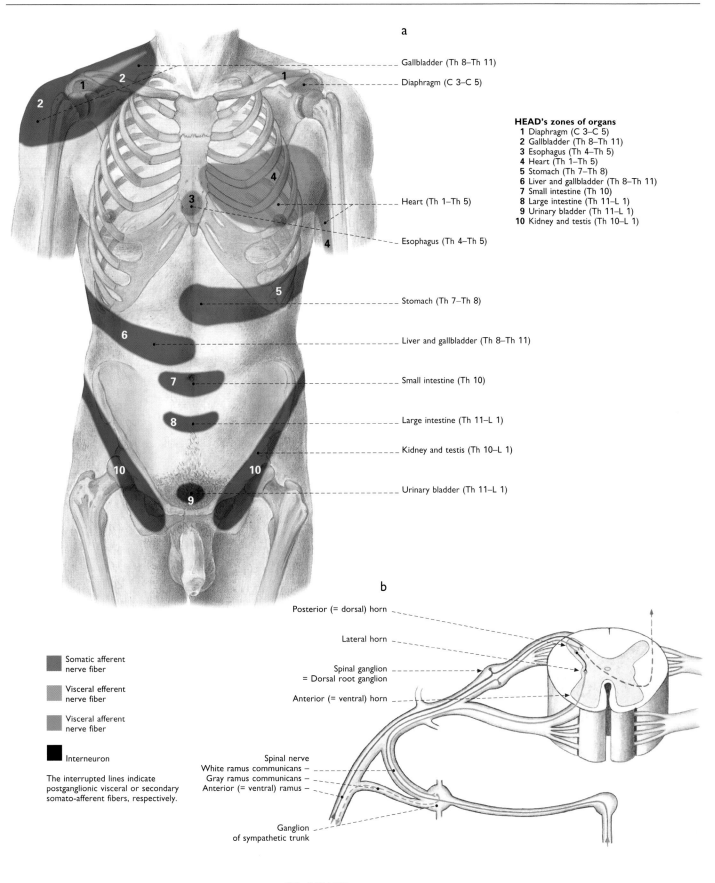

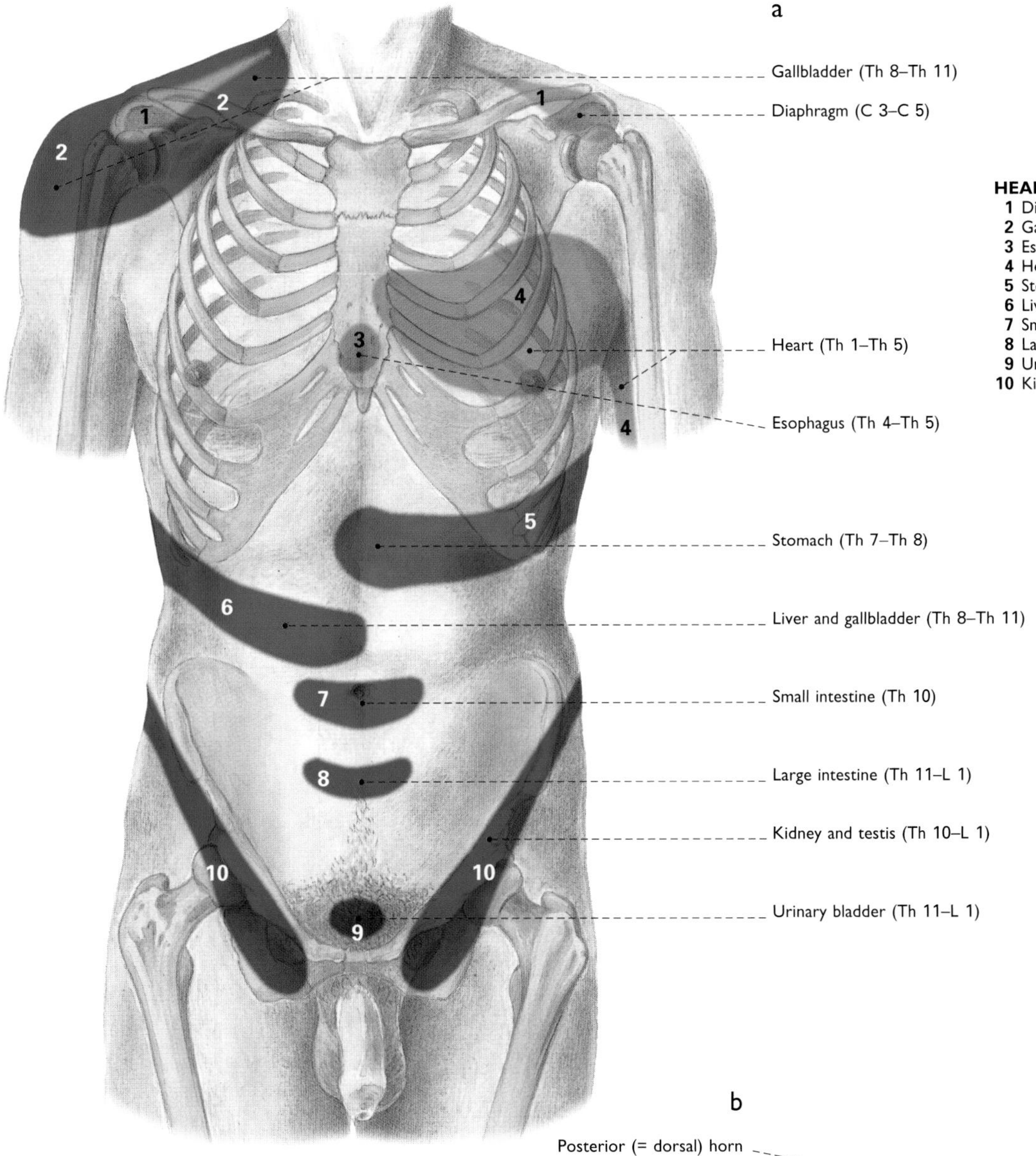
a
Gallbladder (Th 8–Th 11)
Diaphragm (C 3–C 5)
Heart (Th 1–Th 5)
Esophagus (Th 4–Th 5)
Stomach (Th 7–Th 8)
Liver and gallbladder (Th 8–Th 11)
Small intestine (Th 10)
Large intestine (Th 11–L 1)
Kidney and testis (Th 10–L 1)
Urinary bladder (Th 11–L 1)
1
2
3
4
5
6
7
8
9
10

HEAD's zones of organs
1 Diaphragm (C 3–C 5)
2 Gallbladder (Th 8–Th 11)
3 Esophagus (Th 4–Th 5)
4 Heart (Th 1–Th 5)
5 Stomach (Th 7–Th 8)
6 Liver and gallbladder (Th 8–Th 11)
7 Small intestine (Th 10)
8 Large intestine (Th 11–L 1)
9 Urinary bladder (Th 11–L 1)
10 Kidney and testis (Th 10–L 1)

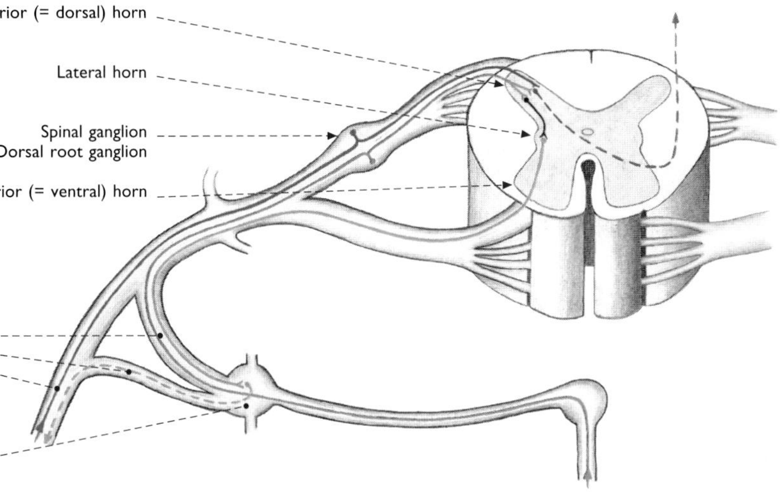
b
Posterior (= dorsal) horn
Lateral horn
Spinal ganglion
= Dorsal root ganglion
Anterior (= ventral) horn
Spinal nerve
White ramus communicans –
Gray ramus communicans –
Anterior (= ventral) ramus –
Ganglion
of sympathetic trunk

Somatic afferent nerve fiber

Visceral efferent nerve fiber

Visceral afferent nerve fiber

Interneuron

The interrupted lines indicate postganglionic visceral or secondary somato-afferent fibers, respectively.

83 HEAD's zones

a Zones of hyperalgesia of diverse inner organs at the body surface (20%)
b Scheme of circuitry of the radiated pain (HEAD's zones)

Upper Limb

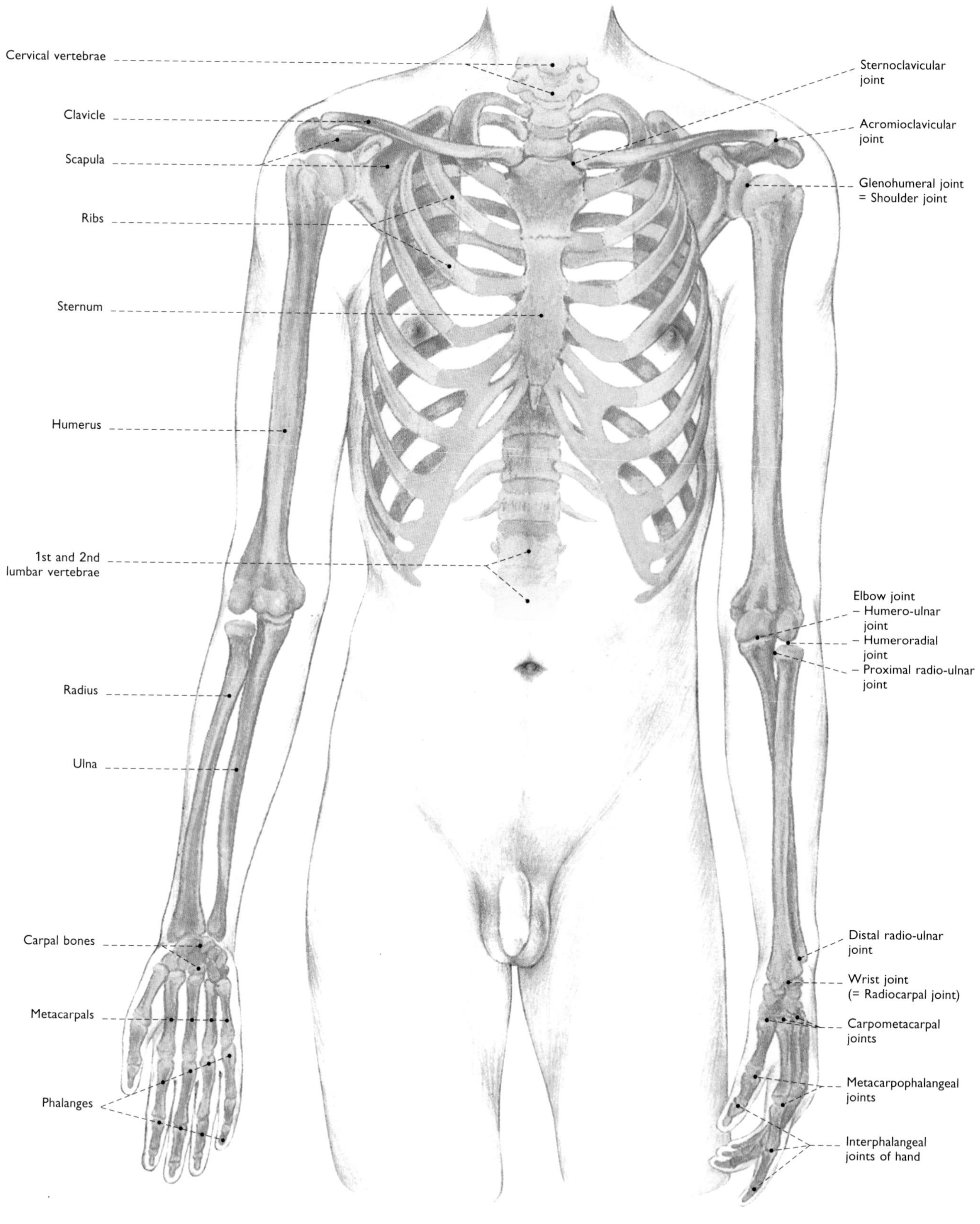
Cervical vertebrae
Clavicle
Scapula
Ribs
Sternum
Humerus
1st and 2nd lumbar vertebrae
Radius
Ulna
Carpal bones
Metacarpals
Phalanges
Sternoclavicular joint
Acromioclavicular joint
Glenohumeral joint = Shoulder joint
Elbow joint
– Humero-ulnar joint
– Humeroradial joint
– Proximal radio-ulnar joint
Distal radio-ulnar joint
Wrist joint (= Radiocarpal joint)
Carpometacarpal joints
Metacarpophalangeal joints
Interphalangeal joints of hand

86 Upper limbs and thorax (25%)
Ventral aspect

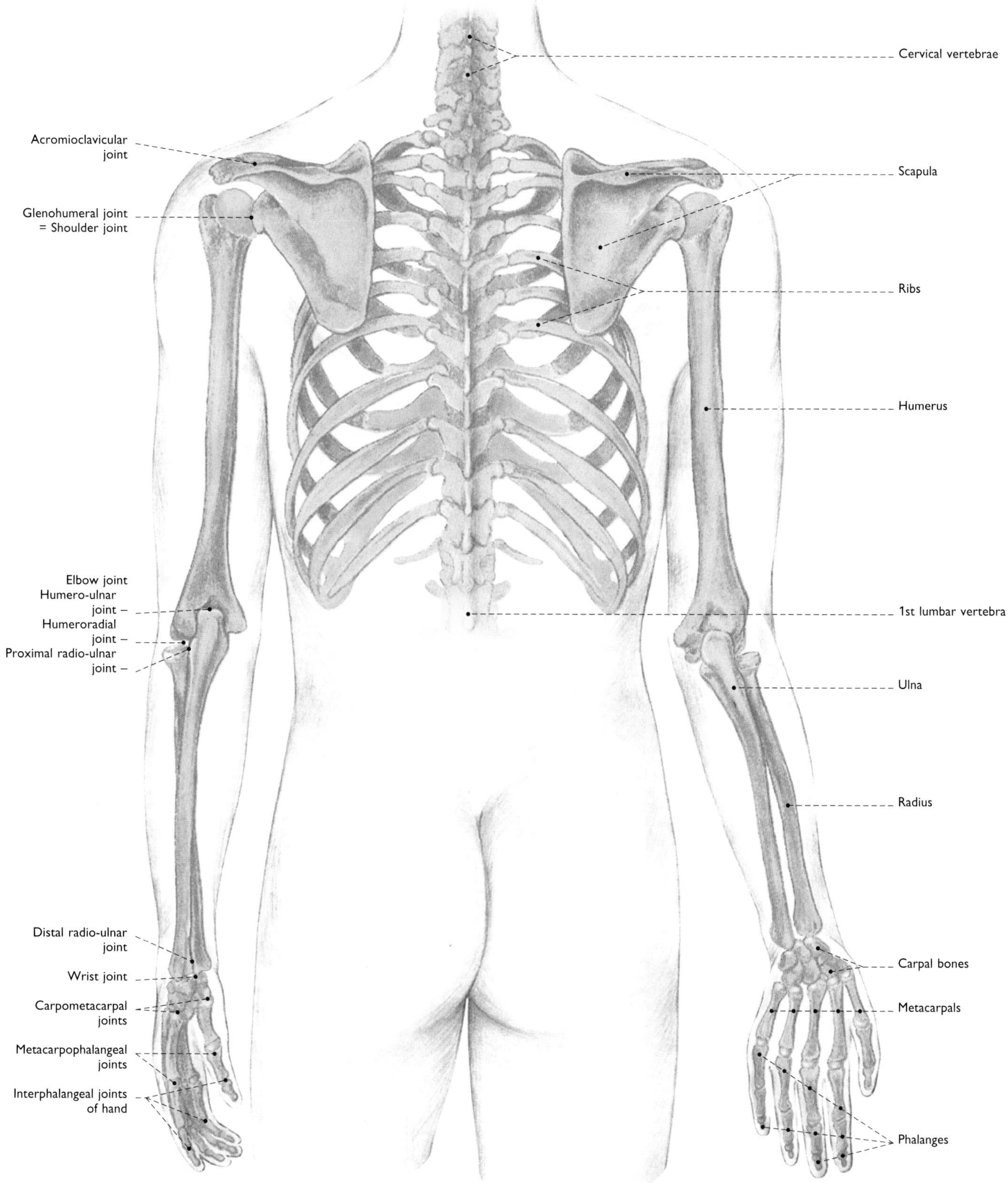
Cervical vertebrae
Acromioclavicular joint
Scapula
Glenohumeral joint = Shoulder joint
Ribs
Humerus
Elbow joint
Humero-ulnar joint –
Humeroradial joint –
Proximal radio-ulnar joint –
1st lumbar vertebra
Ulna
Radius
Distal radio-ulnar joint
Wrist joint
Carpometacarpal joints
Metacarpophalangeal joints
Interphalangeal joints of hand
Carpal bones
Metacarpals
Phalanges

87 Upper limbs and thorax (25%)

Dorsal aspect

a

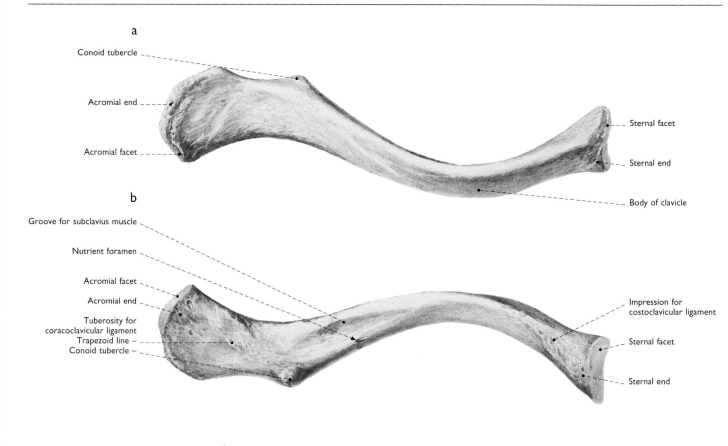

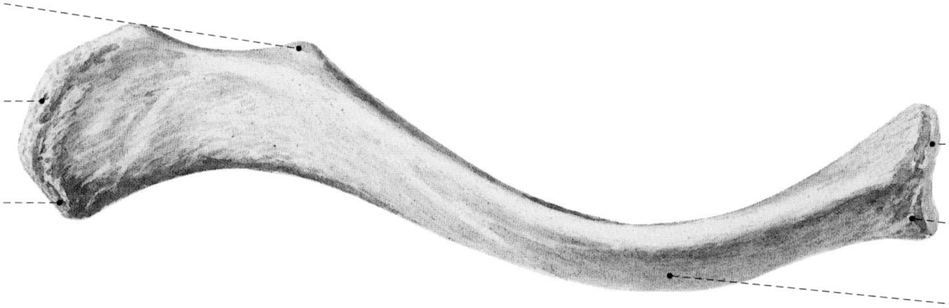
Conoid tubercle
Acromial end
Acromial facet
Sternal facet
Sternal end
Body of clavicle

b

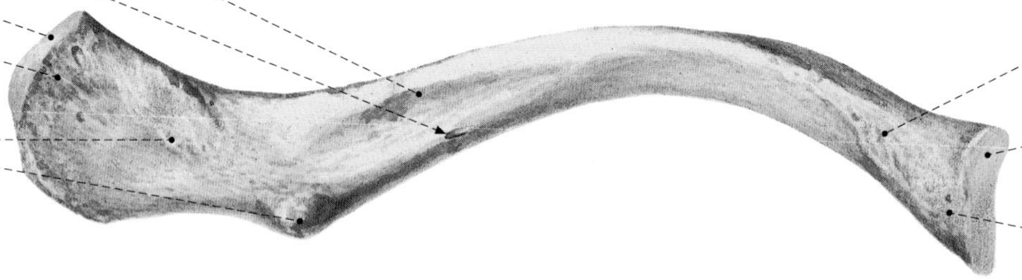
Groove for subclavius muscle
Nutrient foramen
Acromial facet
Acromial end
Tuberosity for coracoclavicular ligament
Trapezoid line
Conoid tubercle
Impression for costoclavicular ligament
Sternal facet
Sternal end

c

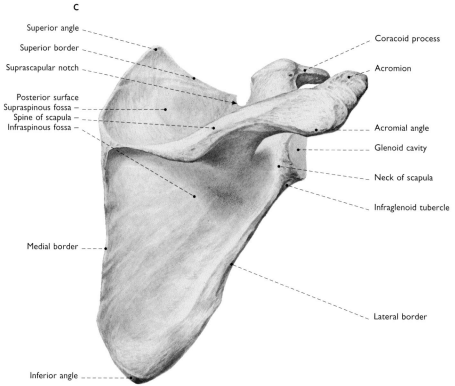

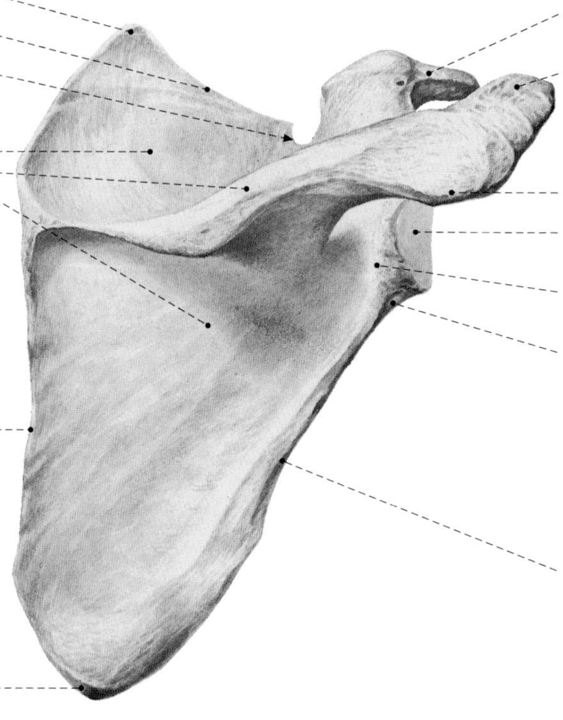
Superior angle
Superior border
Suprascapular notch
Posterior surface
Supraspinous fossa
Spine of scapula
Infraspinous fossa
Medial border
Inferior angle
Coracoid process
Acromion
Acromial angle
Glenoid cavity
Neck of scapula
Infraglenoid tubercle
Lateral border

88 Pectoral (= shoulder) girdle

a, b Right clavicle (90%)
a Superior aspect
b Inferior aspect
c Right scapula (50%), dorsal aspect

a

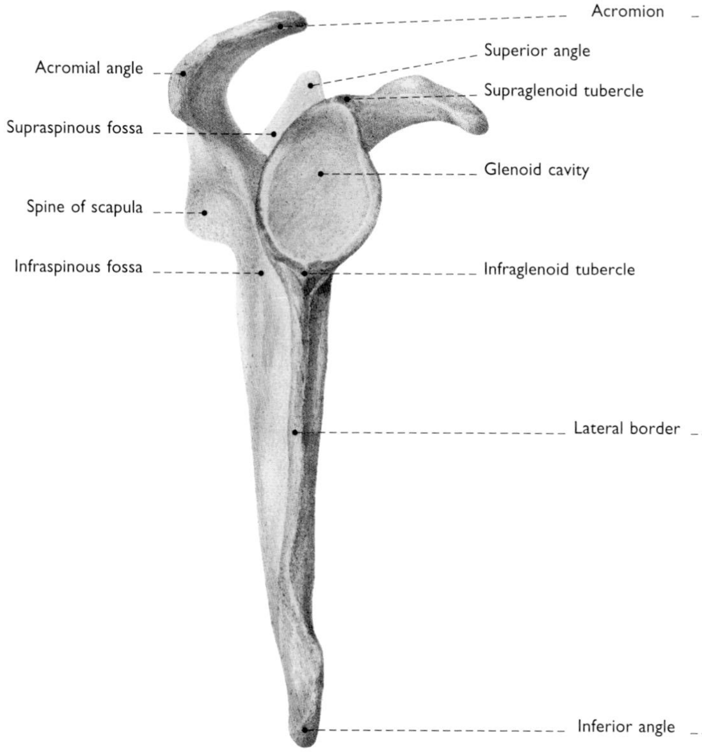
Acromion
Acromial angle
Superior angle
Supraglenoid tubercle
Supraspinous fossa
Glenoid cavity
Spine of scapula
Infraspinous fossa
Infraglenoid tubercle
Lateral border
Inferior angle

b

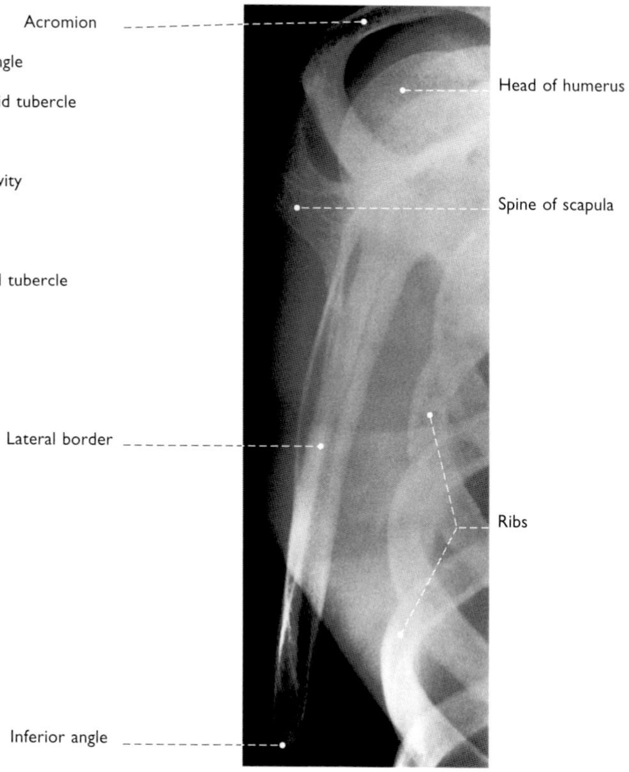
Head of humerus
Spine of scapula
Ribs

c

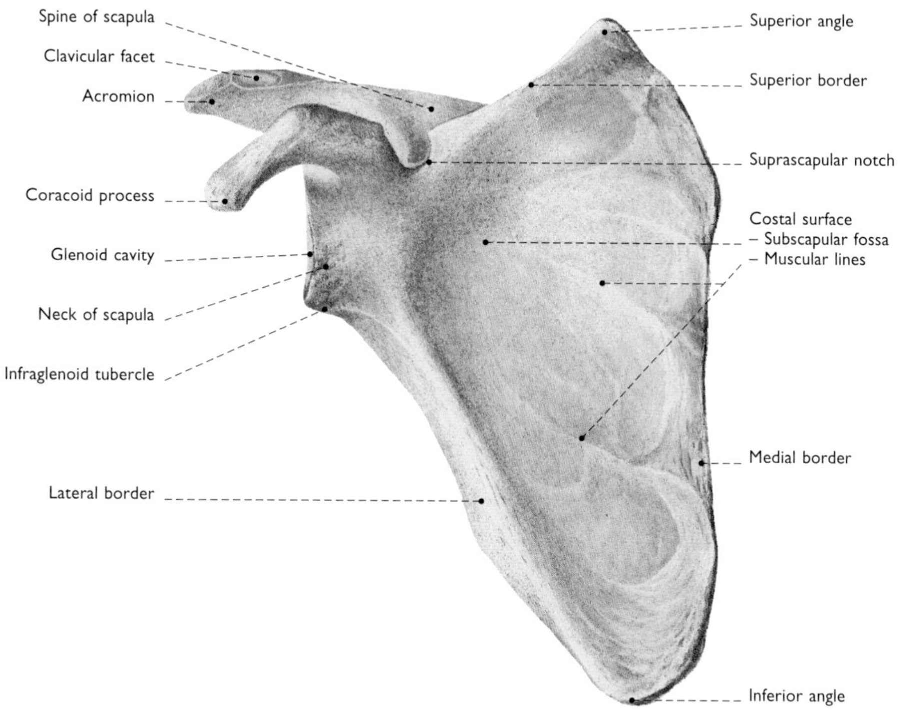
Spine of scapula
Clavicular facet
Acromion
Superior angle
Superior border
Suprascapular notch
Coracoid process
Costal surface
– Subscapular fossa
– Muscular lines
Glenoid cavity
Neck of scapula
Infraglenoid tubercle
Medial border
Lateral border
Inferior angle

89 Right scapula (50%)

a Lateral aspect
b Lateral radiograph
c Ventral aspect

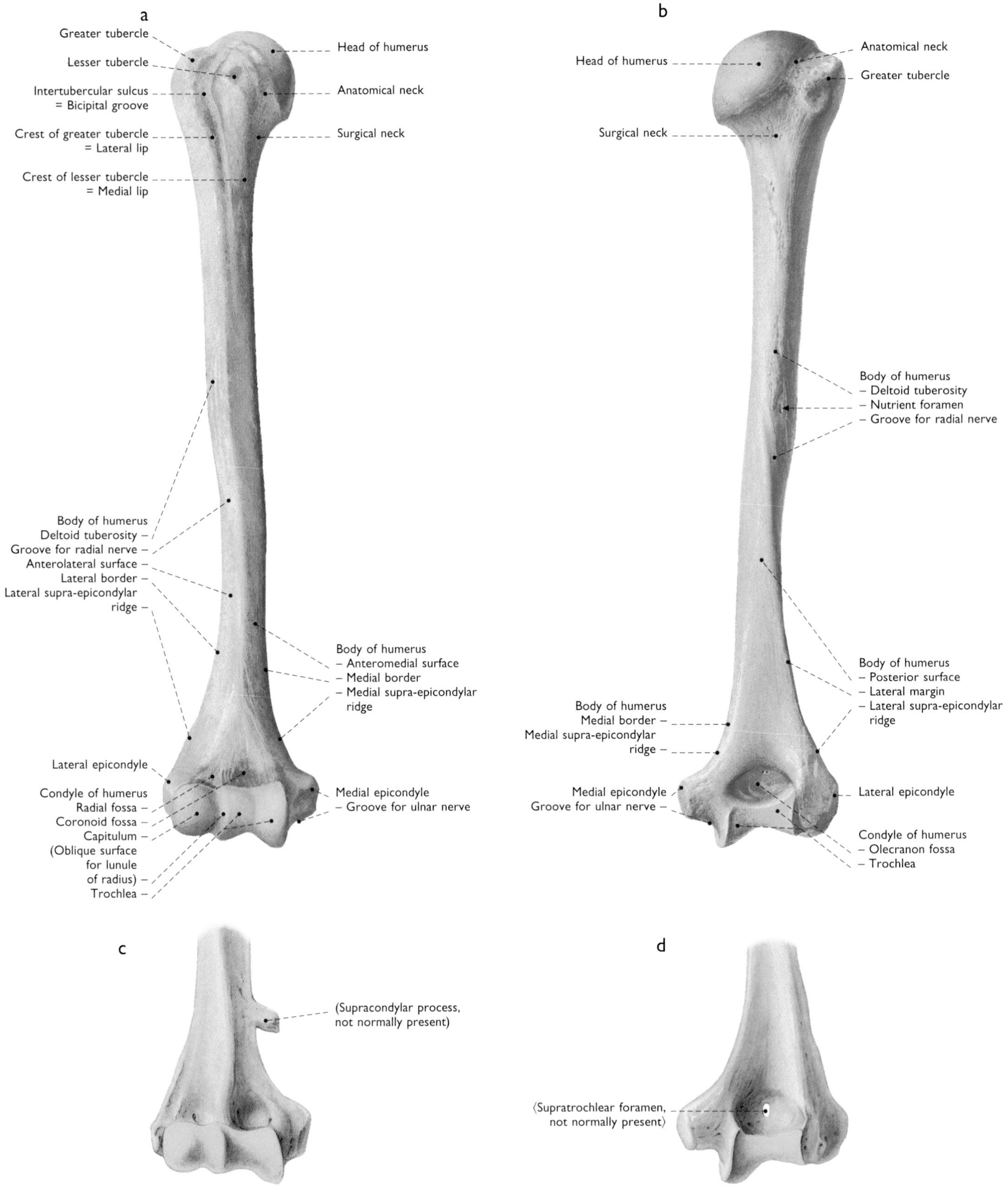
a
Greater tubercle
Lesser tubercle
Intertubercular sulcus
= Bicipital groove
Crest of greater tubercle
= Lateral lip
Crest of lesser tubercle
= Medial lip
Head of humerus
Anatomical neck
Surgical neck
Body of humerus
Deltoid tuberosity –
Groove for radial nerve –
Anterolateral surface –
Lateral border –
Lateral supra-epicondylar
ridge –
Body of humerus
– Anteromedial surface
– Medial border
– Medial supra-epicondylar
ridge
Lateral epicondyle
Condyle of humerus
Radial fossa –
Coronoid fossa –
Capitulum –
(Oblique surface
for lunule
of radius) –
Trochlea –
Medial epicondyle
– Groove for ulnar nerve
b
Head of humerus
Anatomical neck
Greater tubercle
Surgical neck
Body of humerus
– Deltoid tuberosity
– Nutrient foramen
– Groove for radial nerve
Body of humerus
– Posterior surface
– Lateral margin
– Lateral supra-epicondylar
ridge
Body of humerus
Medial border –
Medial supra-epicondylar
ridge –
Medial epicondyle
Groove for ulnar nerve –
Lateral epicondyle
Condyle of humerus
– Olecranon fossa
– Trochlea
c
(Supracondylar process,
not normally present)
d
⟨Supratrochlear foramen,
not normally present⟩

90 Right humerus (50%)

a Ventral aspect
b Dorsal aspect
c, d Distal part
c Ventral aspect
d Dorsal aspect

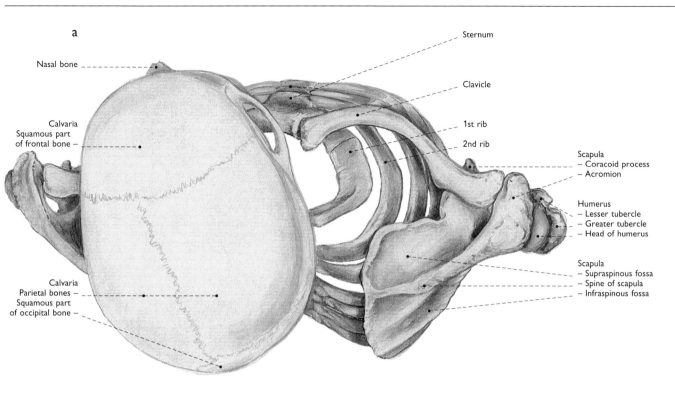

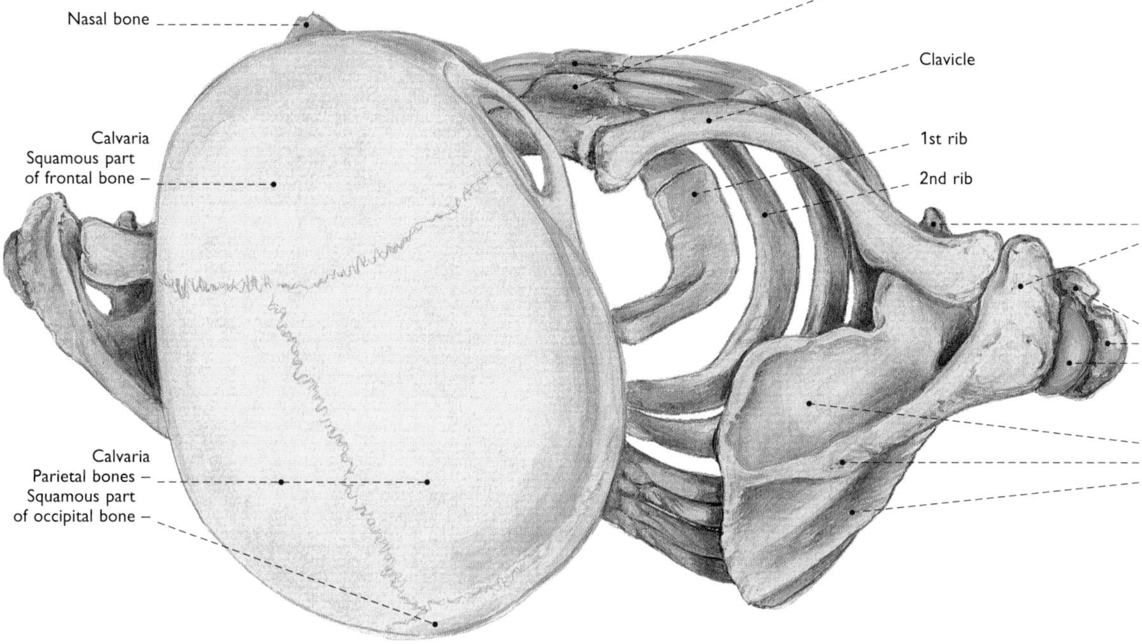
a
Nasal bone
Calvaria
Squamous part
of frontal bone
Calvaria
Parietal bones
Squamous part
of occipital bone
Sternum
Clavicle
1st rib
2nd rib
Scapula
– Coracoid process
– Acromion
Humerus
– Lesser tubercle
– Greater tubercle
– Head of humerus
Scapula
– Supraspinous fossa
– Spine of scapula
– Infraspinous fossa

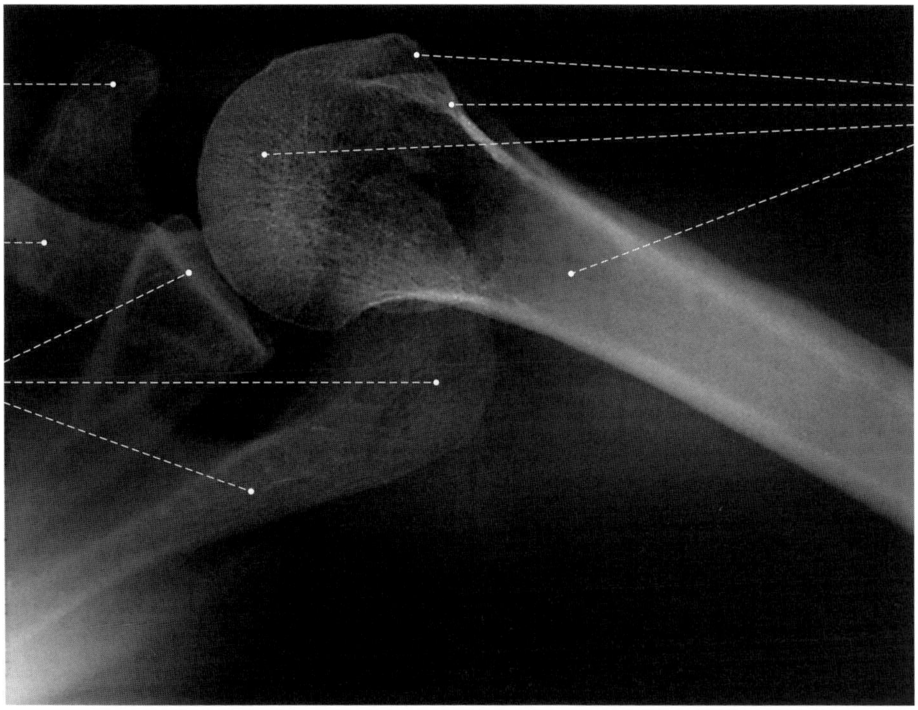
b
Scapula
Coracoid process
Clavicle
Scapula
Glenoid cavity
Acromion
Spine of scapula
Humerus
– Lesser tubercle
– Greater tubercle
– Head of humerus
– Body of humerus

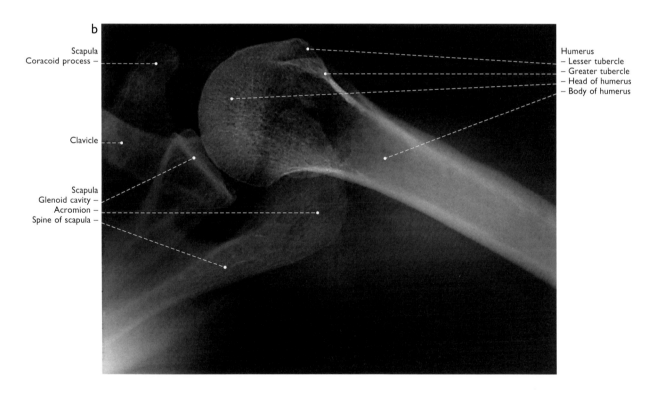

91 Right pectoral (= shoulder) girdle and humerus

a Superior aspect (45%)

b Supero-inferior (axial) radiograph, arm in abducted position

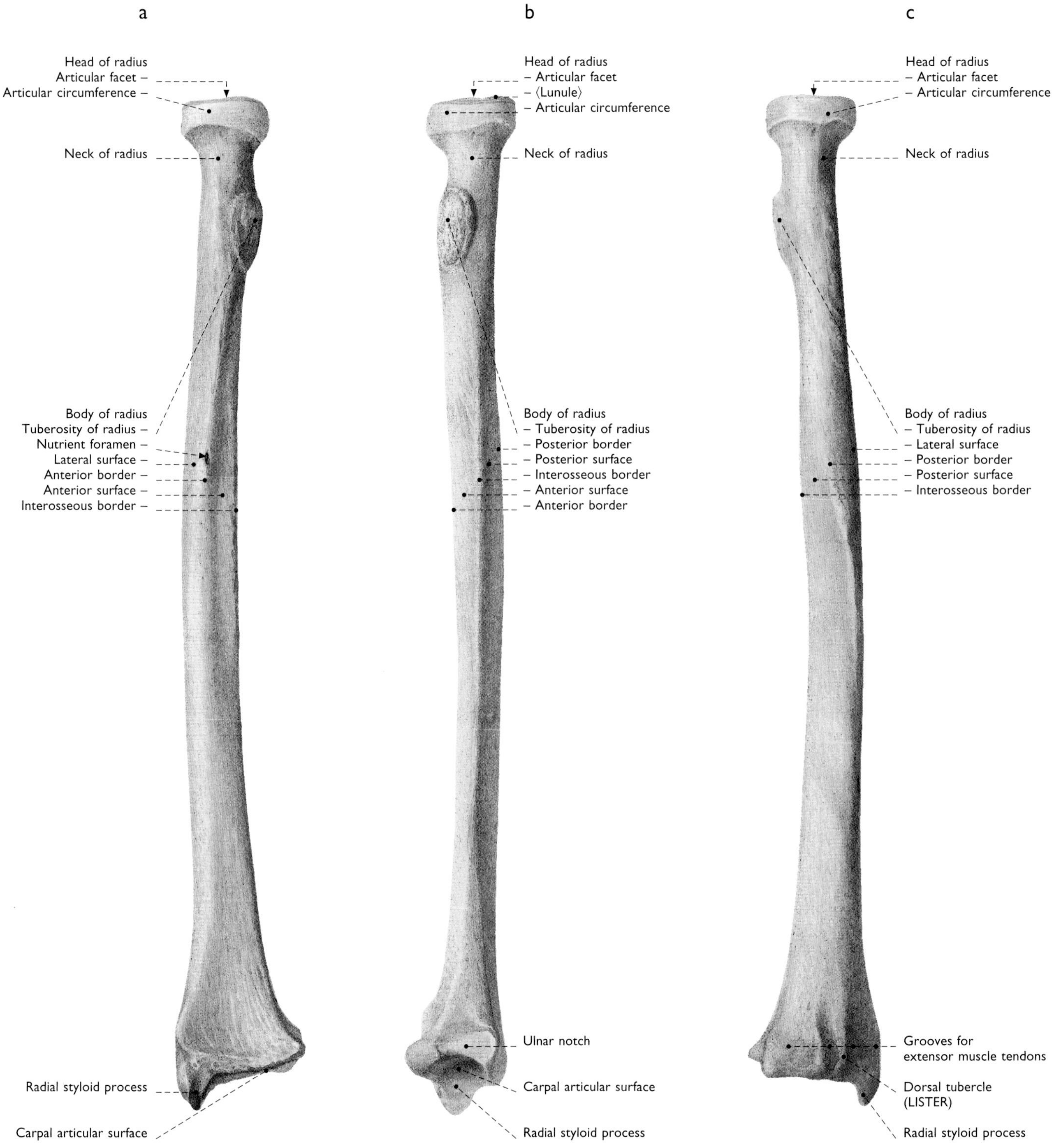
a
Head of radius
Articular facet –
Articular circumference –
Neck of radius
Body of radius
Tuberosity of radius –
Nutrient foramen –
Lateral surface –
Anterior border –
Anterior surface –
Interosseous border –
Radial styloid process
Carpal articular surface
b
Head of radius
– Articular facet
– ⟨Lunule⟩
– Articular circumference
Neck of radius
Body of radius
– Tuberosity of radius
– Posterior border
– Posterior surface
– Interosseous border
– Anterior surface
– Anterior border
Ulnar notch
Carpal articular surface
Radial styloid process
c
Head of radius
– Articular facet
– Articular circumference
Neck of radius
Body of radius
– Tuberosity of radius
– Lateral surface
– Posterior border
– Posterior surface
– Interosseous border
Grooves for
extensor muscle tendons
Dorsal tubercle
(LISTER)
Radial styloid process

92 Right radius (70%)

a Ventral aspect
b Medial aspect
c Dorsal aspect

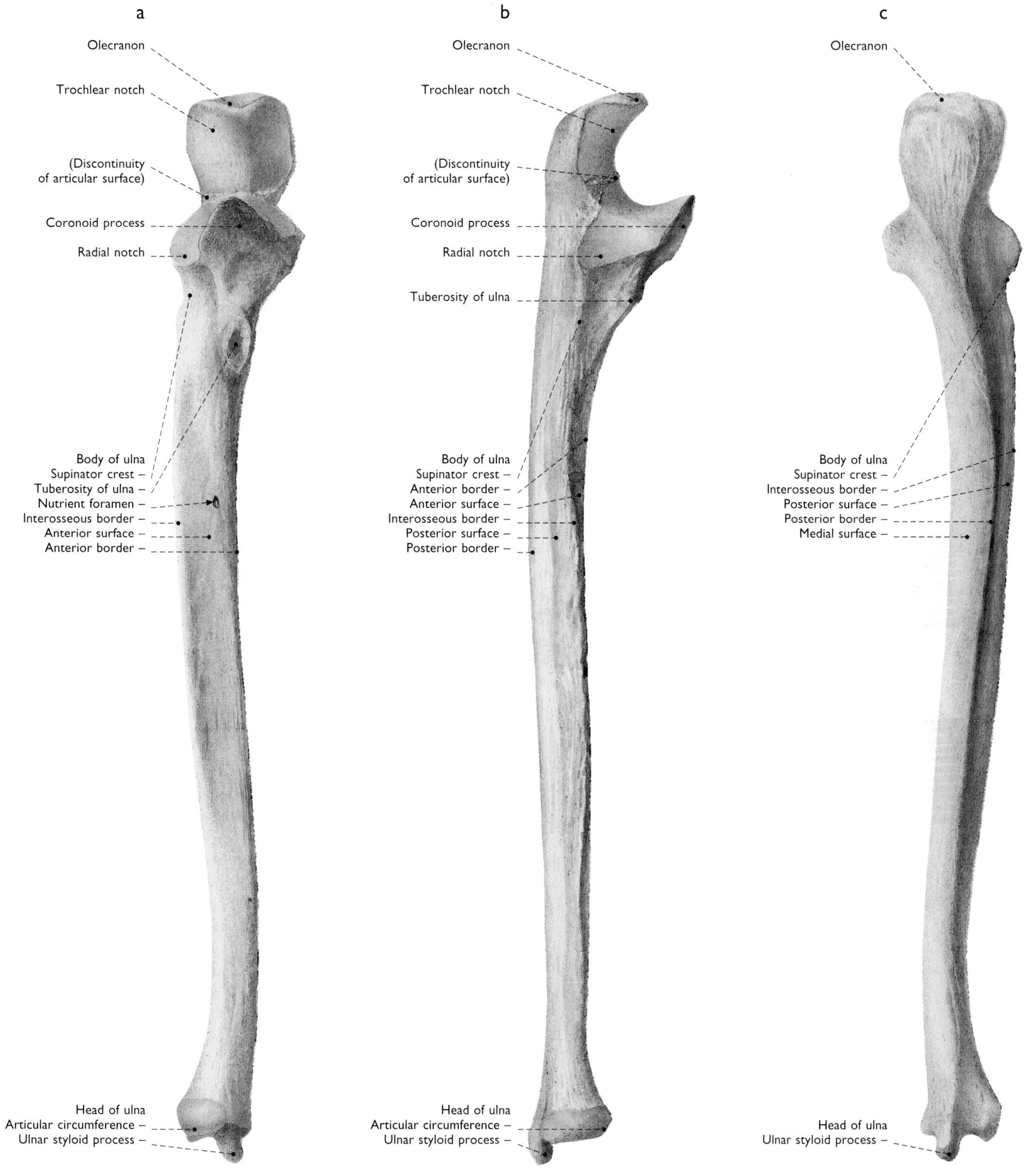
a
Olecranon
Trochlear notch
(Discontinuity of articular surface)
Coronoid process
Radial notch
Body of ulna
Supinator crest
Tuberosity of ulna
Nutrient foramen
Interosseous border
Anterior surface
Anterior border
Head of ulna
Articular circumference
Ulnar styloid process
b
Olecranon
Trochlear notch
(Discontinuity of articular surface)
Coronoid process
Radial notch
Tuberosity of ulna
Body of ulna
Supinator crest
Anterior border
Anterior surface
Interosseous border
Posterior surface
Posterior border
Head of ulna
Articular circumference
Ulnar styloid process
c
Olecranon
Body of ulna
Supinator crest
Interosseous border
Posterior surface
Posterior border
Medial surface
Head of ulna
Ulnar styloid process

93 Right ulna (70%)

a Ventral aspect
b Lateral aspect
c Dorsal aspect

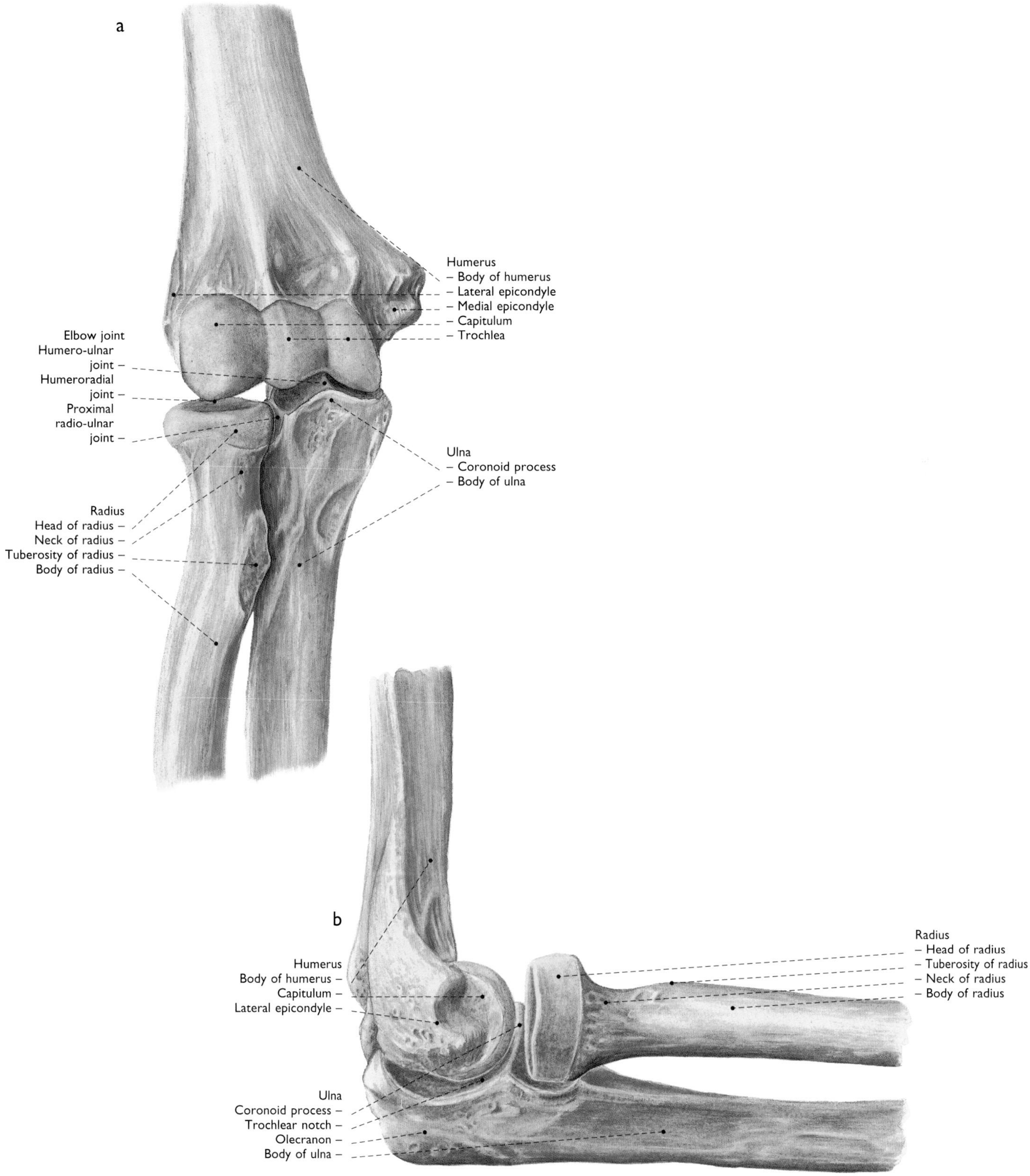
a
Humerus
– Body of humerus
– Lateral epicondyle
– Medial epicondyle
– Capitulum
– Trochlea
Elbow joint
Humero-ulnar joint –
Humeroradial joint –
Proximal radio-ulnar joint –
Ulna
– Coronoid process
– Body of ulna
Radius
Head of radius –
Neck of radius –
Tuberosity of radius –
Body of radius –
b
Radius
– Head of radius
– Tuberosity of radius
– Neck of radius
– Body of radius
Humerus
Body of humerus –
Capitulum –
Lateral epicondyle –
Ulna
Coronoid process –
Trochlear notch –
Olecranon –
Body of ulna –

94 Bones of the right elbow joint (90%)

a Ventral aspect
b Lateral (radial) aspect

a

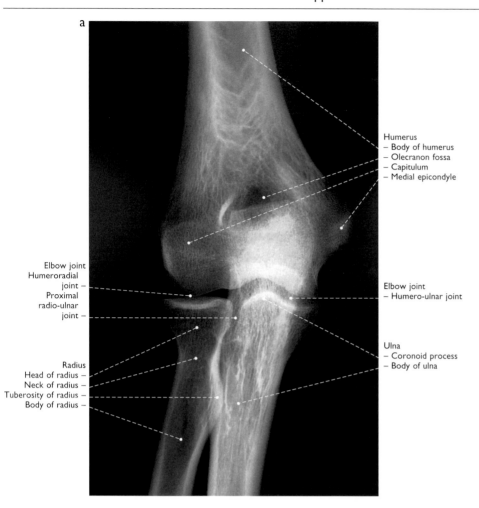

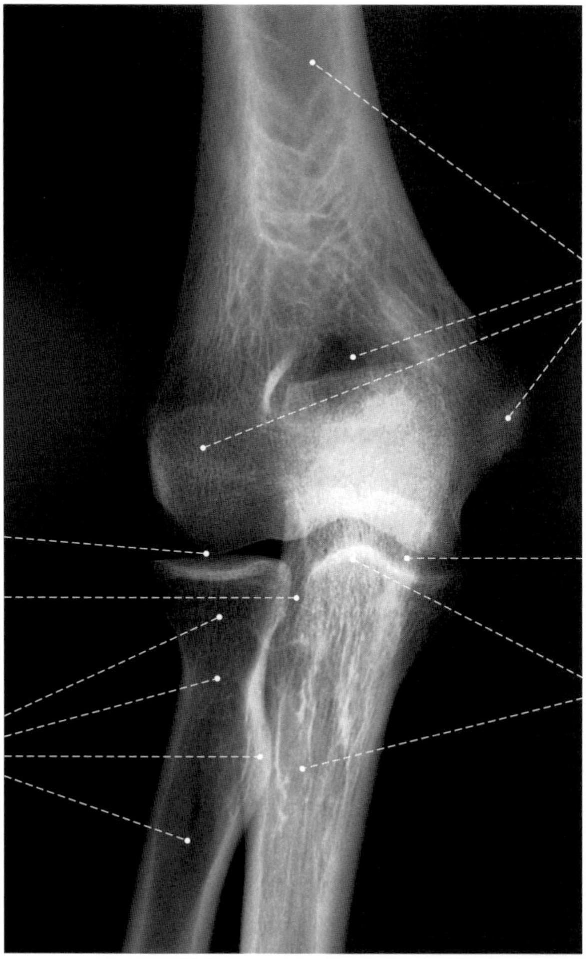
Humerus
– Body of humerus
– Olecranon fossa
– Capitulum
– Medial epicondyle
Elbow joint
Humeroradial joint –
Proximal radio-ulnar joint –
Elbow joint
– Humero-ulnar joint
Radius
Head of radius –
Neck of radius –
Tuberosity of radius –
Body of radius –
Ulna
– Coronoid process
– Body of ulna

b

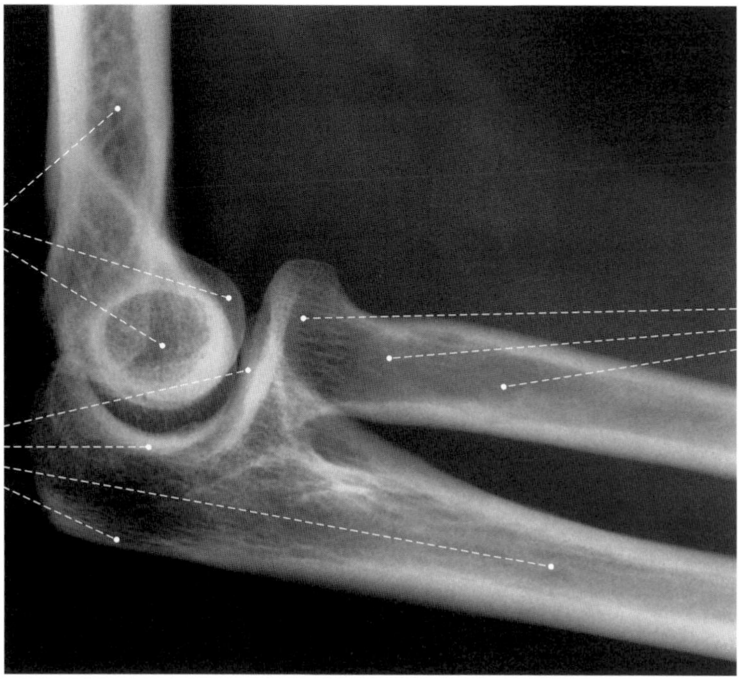
Humerus
Body of humerus –
Trochlea –
Capitulum –
Radius
– Head of radius
– Neck of radius
– Body of radius
Ulna
Coronoid process –
Trochlear notch –
Body of ulna –
Olecranon –

95 Right elbow joint (90%)

a Anteroposterior radiograph
b Radio-ulnar radiograph

a

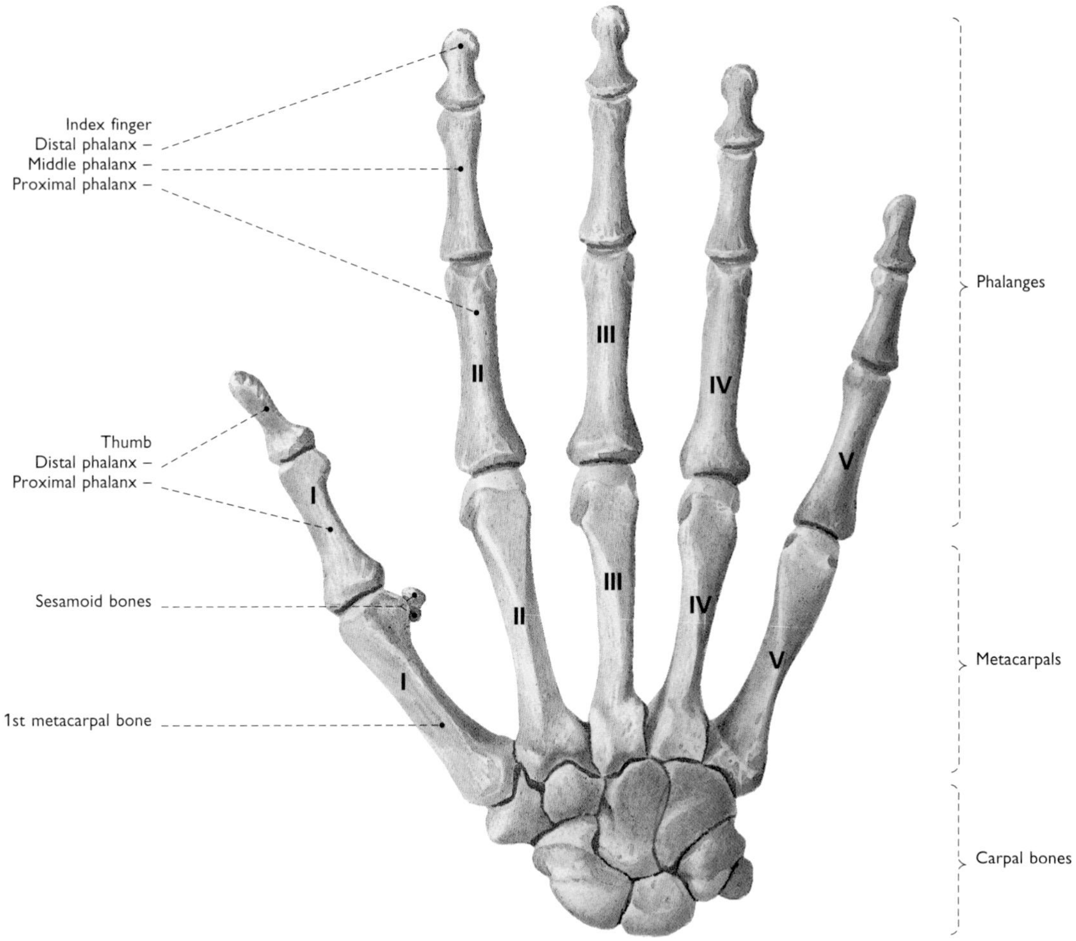
Index finger
Distal phalanx –
Middle phalanx –
Proximal phalanx –
Thumb
Distal phalanx –
Proximal phalanx –
Sesamoid bones
1st metacarpal bone
I
II
III
IV
V
Phalanges
Metacarpals
Carpal bones

b

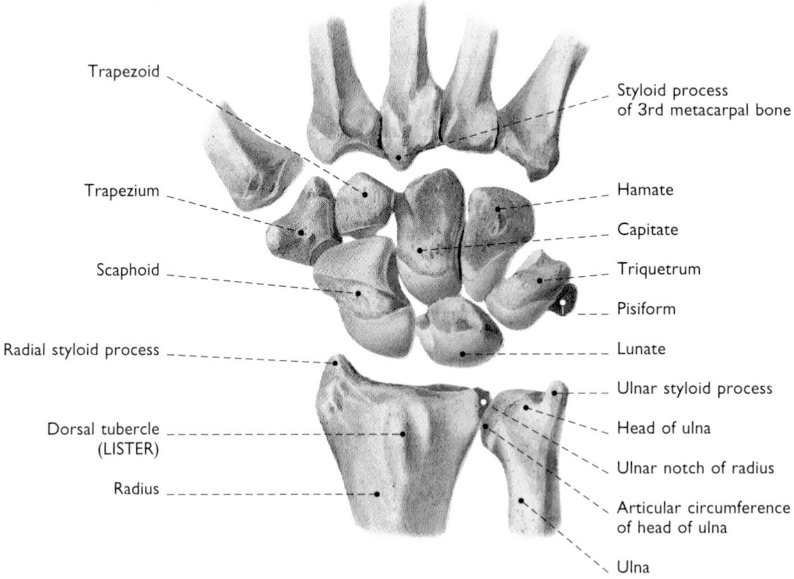
Trapezoid
Trapezium
Scaphoid
Radial styloid process
Dorsal tubercle
(LISTER)
Radius
Styloid process
of 3rd metacarpal bone
Hamate
Capitate
Triquetrum
Pisiform
Lunate
Ulnar styloid process
Head of ulna
Ulnar notch of radius
Articular circumference
of head of ulna
Ulna

96 Bones of the right hand

a Dorsal aspect (60%)
b Carpal bones (70%), dorsal aspect

a

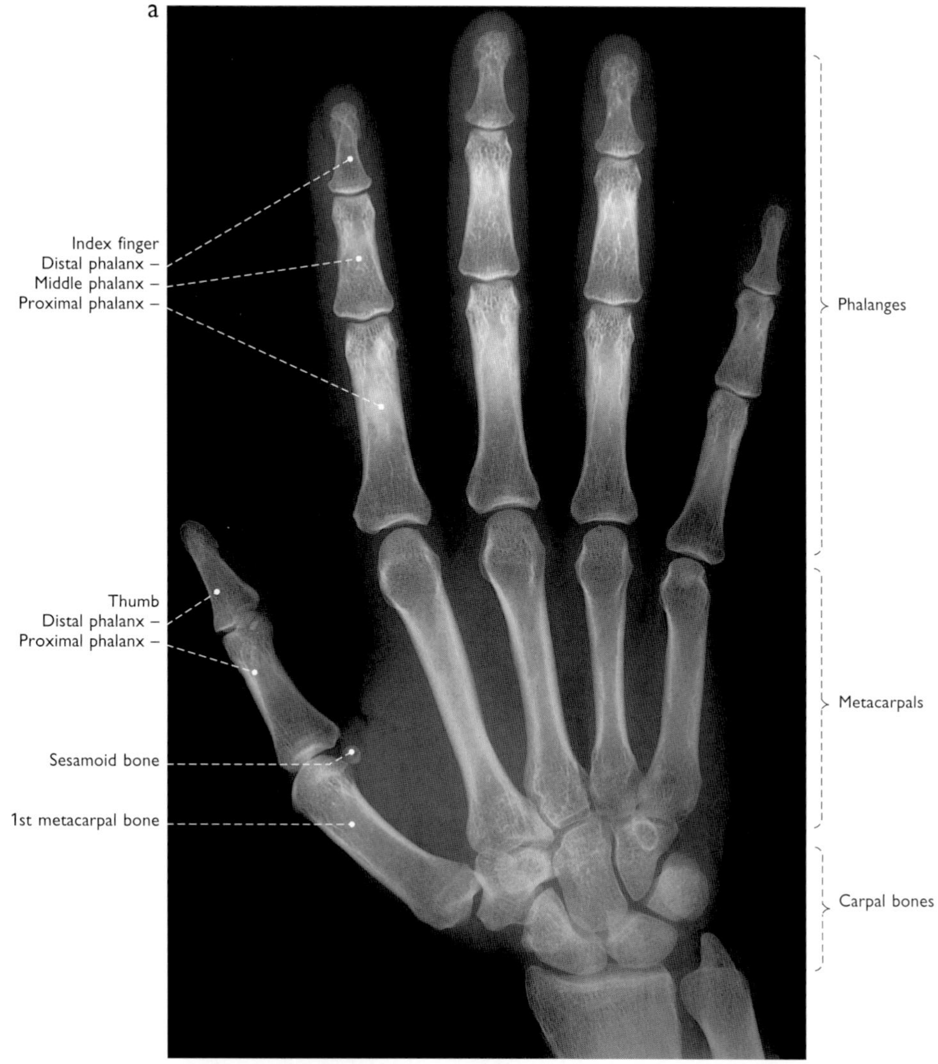

b

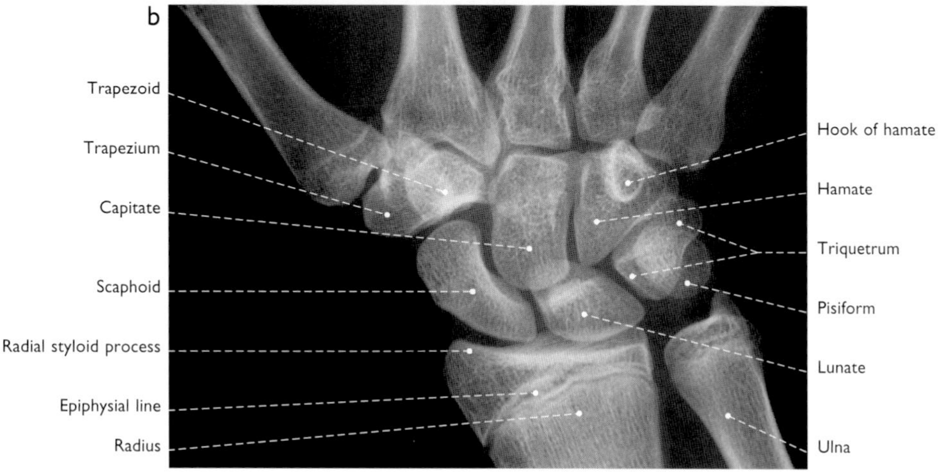

97 Bones of the right hand

a Dorsopalmar radiograph (60%)
b Carpal bones (80%), dorsopalmar radiograph

a

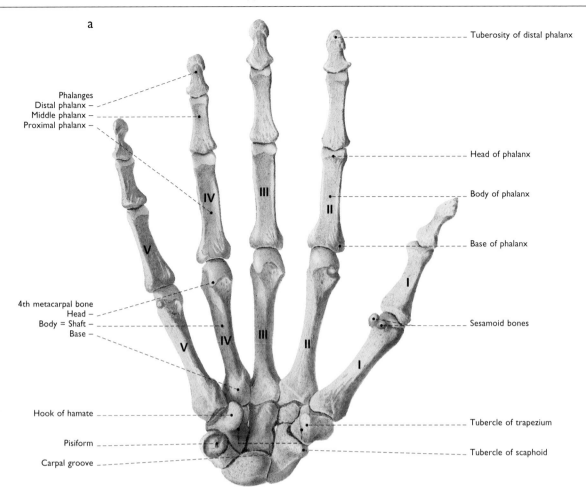

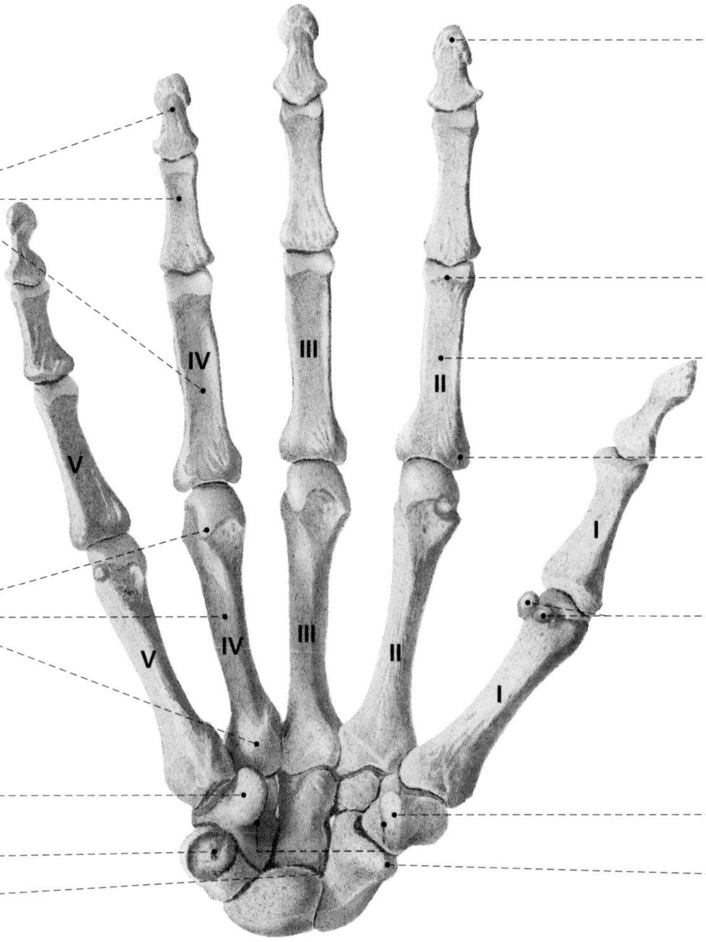
Phalanges
Distal phalanx
Middle phalanx
Proximal phalanx
4th metacarpal bone
Head
Body = Shaft
Base
Hook of hamate
Pisiform
Carpal groove
Tuberosity of distal phalanx
Head of phalanx
Body of phalanx
Base of phalanx
Sesamoid bones
Tubercle of trapezium
Tubercle of scaphoid
I
II
III
IV
V

b

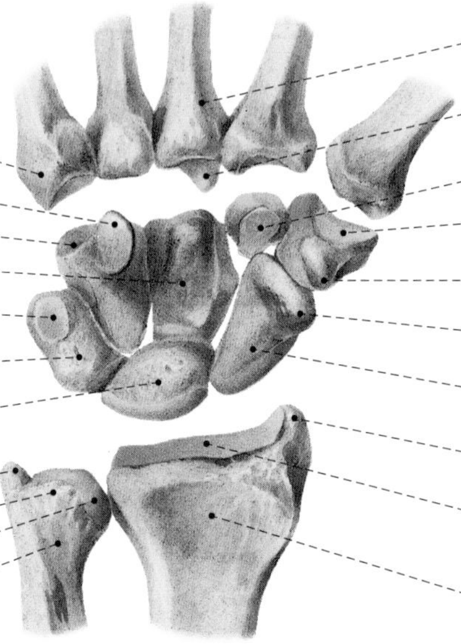
⟨Tubercle of 5th metacarpal bone⟩
Hook of hamate
Hamate
Capitate
Articular facet for pisiform
Triquetrum
Lunate
Ulnar styloid process
Head of ulna
Articular circumference
Ulna
3rd metacarpal bone
Styloid process of 3rd metacarpal bone
Trapezoid
Trapezium
Tubercle of trapezium
Tubercle of scaphoid
Scaphoid
Radial styloid process
Carpal articular surface
Radius

98 Bones of the right hand

a Palmar aspect (60%)
b Carpal bones (70%). The pisiform bone was removed. Palmar aspect

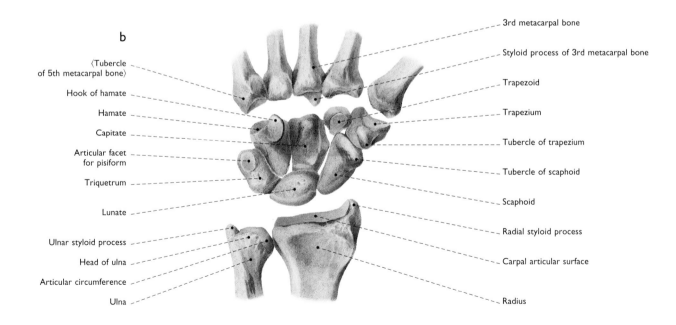

a

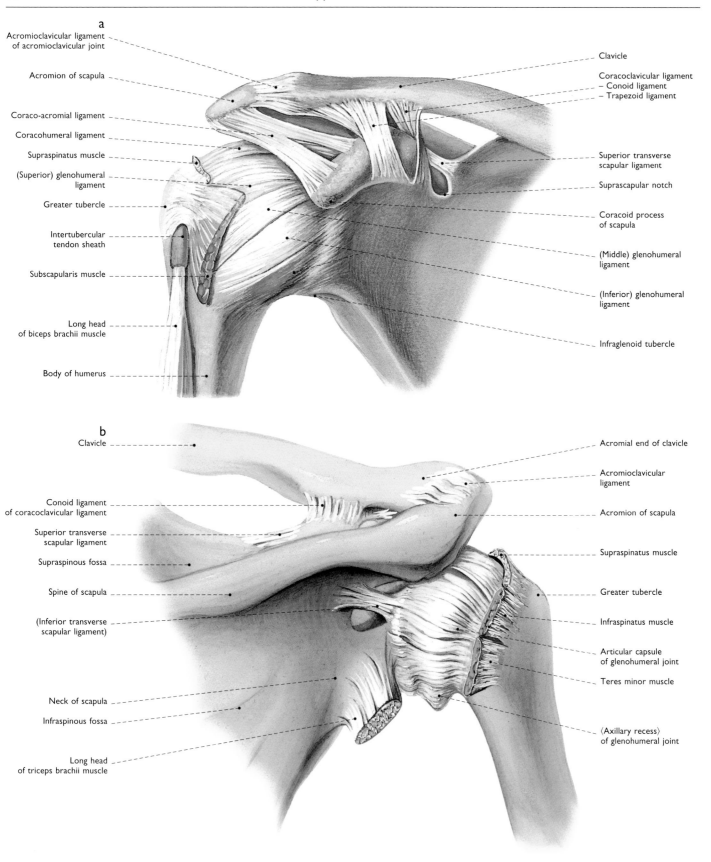

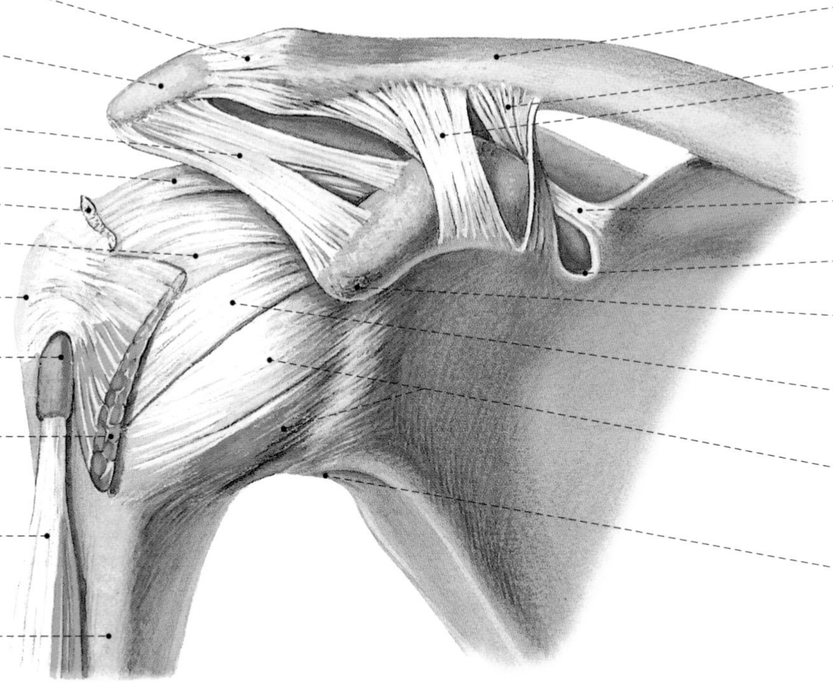
Acromioclavicular ligament of acromioclavicular joint
Acromion of scapula
Coraco-acromial ligament
Coracohumeral ligament
Supraspinatus muscle
(Superior) glenohumeral ligament
Greater tubercle
Intertubercular tendon sheath
Subscapularis muscle
Long head of biceps brachii muscle
Body of humerus
Clavicle
Coracoclavicular ligament
– Conoid ligament
– Trapezoid ligament
Superior transverse scapular ligament
Suprascapular notch
Coracoid process of scapula
(Middle) glenohumeral ligament
(Inferior) glenohumeral ligament
Infraglenoid tubercle

b

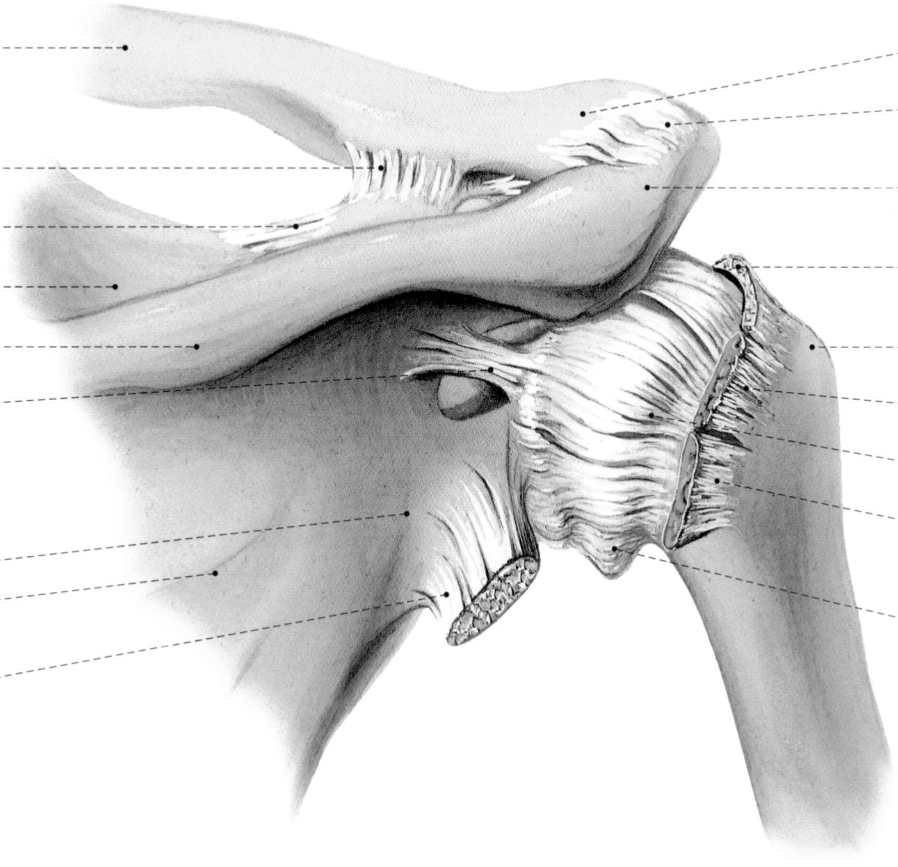
Clavicle
Conoid ligament of coracoclavicular ligament
Superior transverse scapular ligament
Supraspinous fossa
Spine of scapula
(Inferior transverse scapular ligament)
Neck of scapula
Infraspinous fossa
Long head of triceps brachii muscle
Acromial end of clavicle
Acromioclavicular ligament
Acromion of scapula
Supraspinatus muscle
Greater tubercle
Infraspinatus muscle
Articular capsule of glenohumeral joint
Teres minor muscle
⟨Axillary recess⟩ of glenohumeral joint

99 Right glenohumeral (= shoulder) joint (80%)

a Ventral aspect

b Dorsal aspect

a

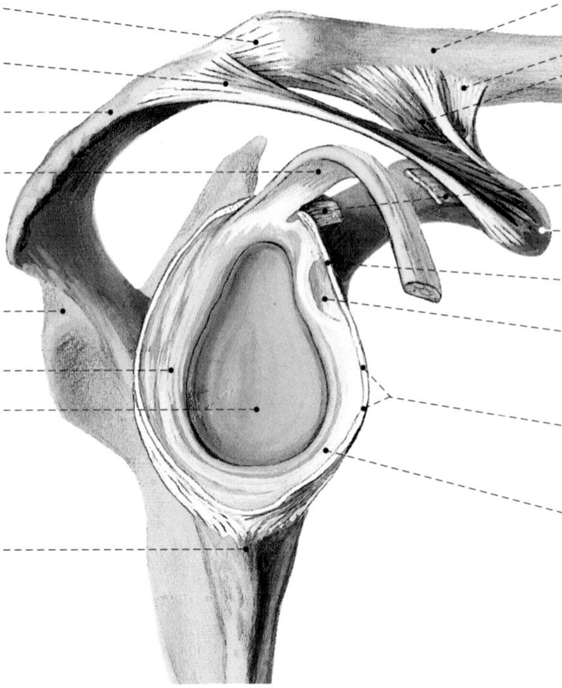
Acromioclavicular ligament of acromioclavicular joint
Coraco-acromial ligament
Acromion of scapula
Tendon of long head of biceps brachii muscle
Spine of scapula
Glenoid labrum
Glenoid cavity of scapula
Infraglenoid tubercle
Clavicle
Coracoclavicular ligament
– Conoid ligament
– Trapezoid ligament
Coracohumeral ligament (transected)
Coracoid process of scapula
(Superior) glenohumeral ligament
Communication with subtendinous bursa of subscapularis muscle
(Middle and inferior) glenohumeral ligaments
Articular capsule of glenohumeral joint

b

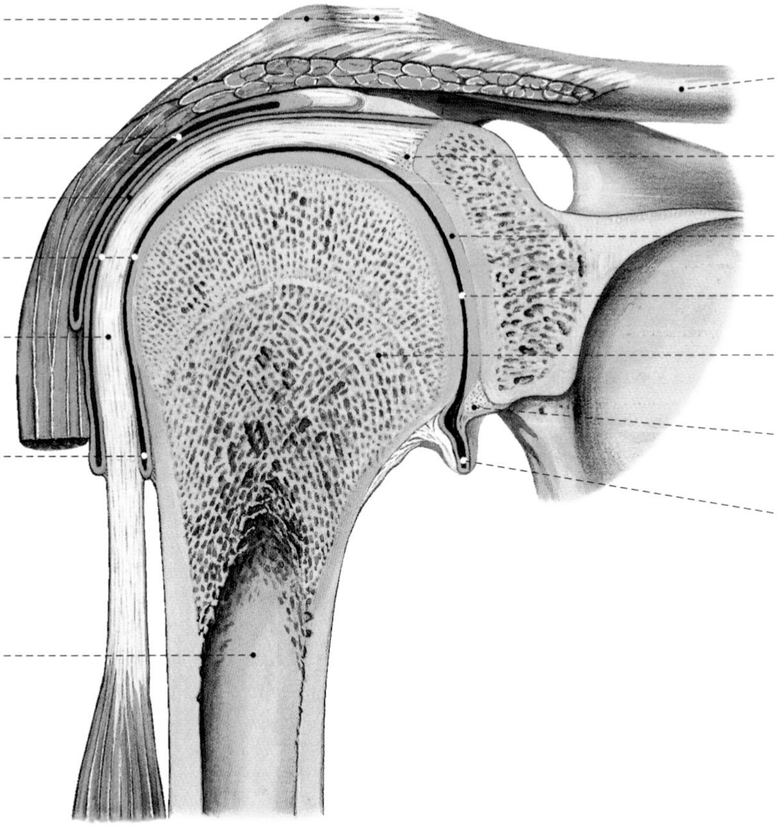
Acromion of scapula, Acromioclavicular ligament
Deltoid muscle
Subdeltoid and subacromial bursae (combined)
Articular capsule of glenohumeral joint
Articular cavity of glenohumeral joint
Tendon of long head of biceps brachii muscle
Intertubercular tendon sheath
Body of humerus
Clavicle
Glenoid labrum
Glenoid cavity of scapula
Articular cavity of glenohumeral joint
Head of humerus
Glenoid labrum
⟨Axillary recess⟩ of glenohumeral joint

100 Right glenohumeral (= shoulder) joint (100%)

a Shoulder joint socket and supra-articular ligaments, lateral aspect
b Frontal (coronal) section, ventral aspect

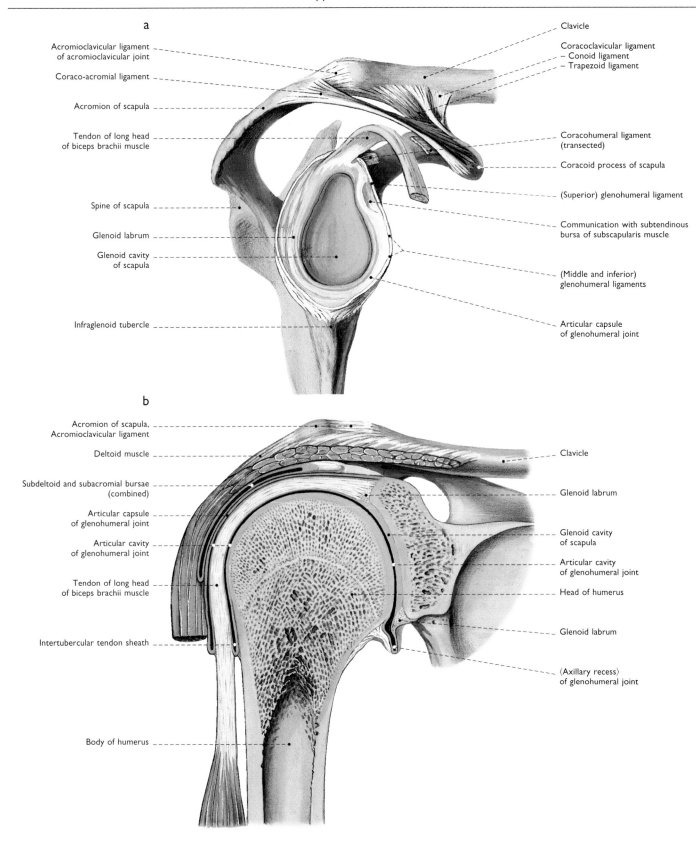

a

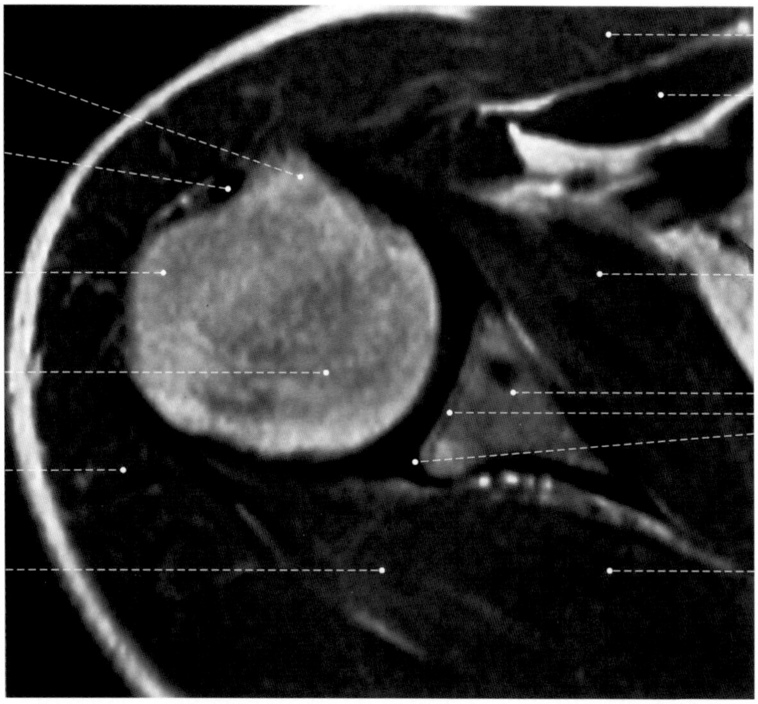
Lesser tubercle of humerus
Tendon of long head of biceps brachii muscle
Greater tubercle of humerus
Head of humerus
Deltoid muscle
Teres minor muscle
Pectoralis major muscle
Pectoralis minor muscle
Subscapularis muscle
Scapula
– Glenoid cavity
– Glenoid labrum
Infraspinatus muscle

b

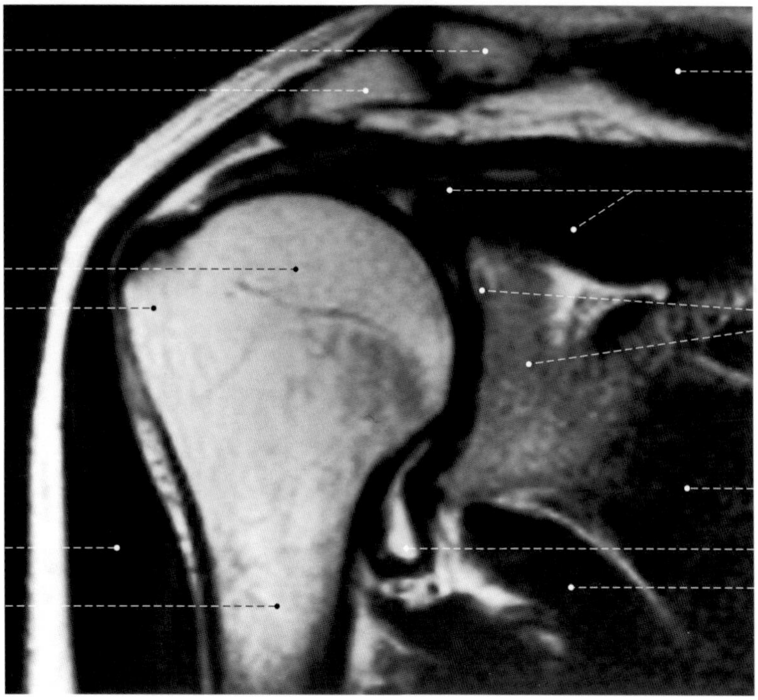
Acromial end of clavicle
Acromion of scapula
Head of humerus
Greater tubercle of humerus
Deltoid muscle
Body of humerus
Trapezius muscle
Supraspinatus muscle
Scapula
– Glenoid cavity
– Neck of scapula
Subscapularis muscle
⟨Axillary recess⟩
Teres major muscle

101 Right glenohumeral (= shoulder) joint (100%)

a Axial (transverse) magnetic resonance image (MRI, T_2-weighted), inferior aspect

b Coronal magnetic resonance image (MRI, T_2-weighted), ventral aspect

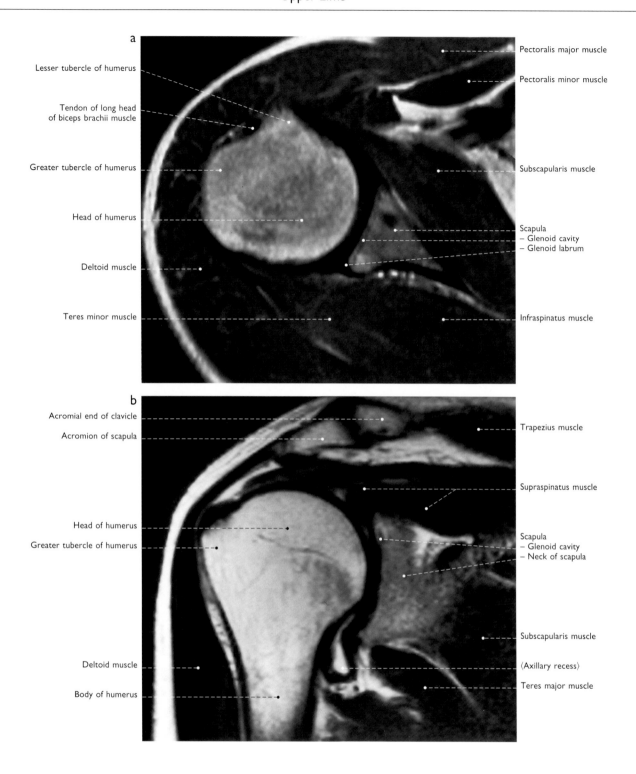

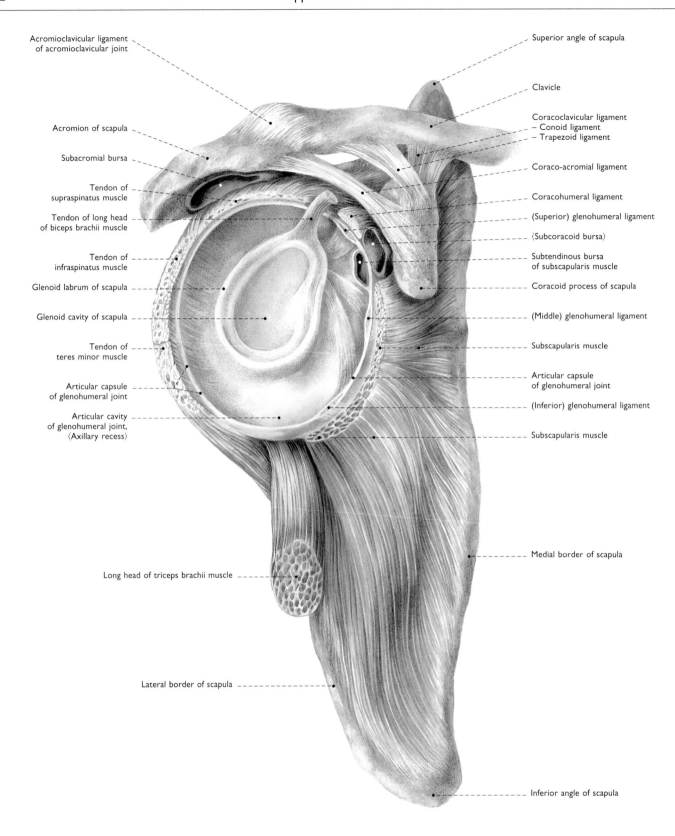

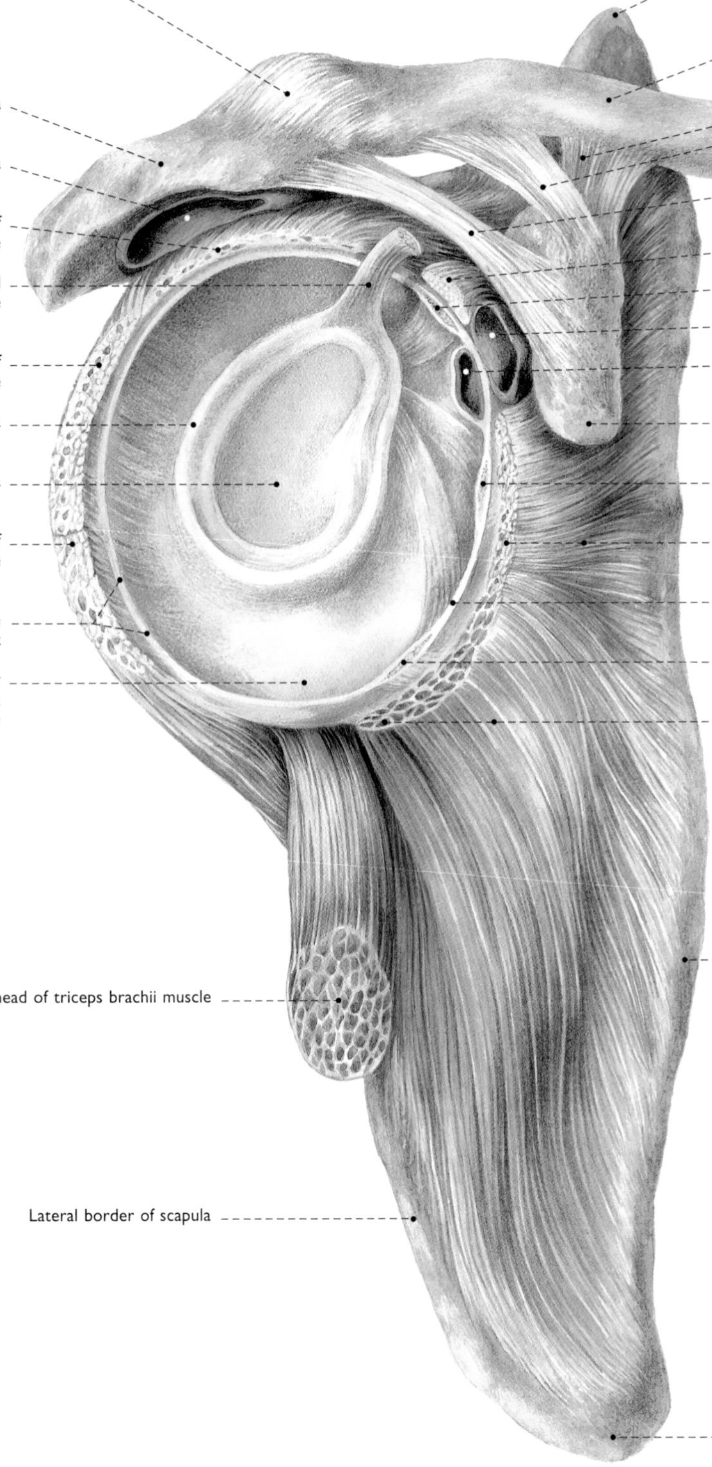
Acromioclavicular ligament of acromioclavicular joint
Acromion of scapula
Subacromial bursa
Tendon of supraspinatus muscle
Tendon of long head of biceps brachii muscle
Tendon of infraspinatus muscle
Glenoid labrum of scapula
Glenoid cavity of scapula
Tendon of teres minor muscle
Articular capsule of glenohumeral joint
Articular cavity of glenohumeral joint, ⟨Axillary recess⟩
Long head of triceps brachii muscle
Lateral border of scapula
Superior angle of scapula
Clavicle
Coracoclavicular ligament
– Conoid ligament
– Trapezoid ligament
Coraco-acromial ligament
Coracohumeral ligament
(Superior) glenohumeral ligament
⟨Subcoracoid bursa⟩
Subtendinous bursa of subscapularis muscle
Coracoid process of scapula
(Middle) glenohumeral ligament
Subscapularis muscle
Articular capsule of glenohumeral joint
(Inferior) glenohumeral ligament
Subscapularis muscle
Medial border of scapula
Inferior angle of scapula

102 Right glenohumeral (= shoulder) joint (100%)

Shoulder joint socket and articular capsule with ligaments and adjoining muscles ('rotator cuff'), lateral aspect

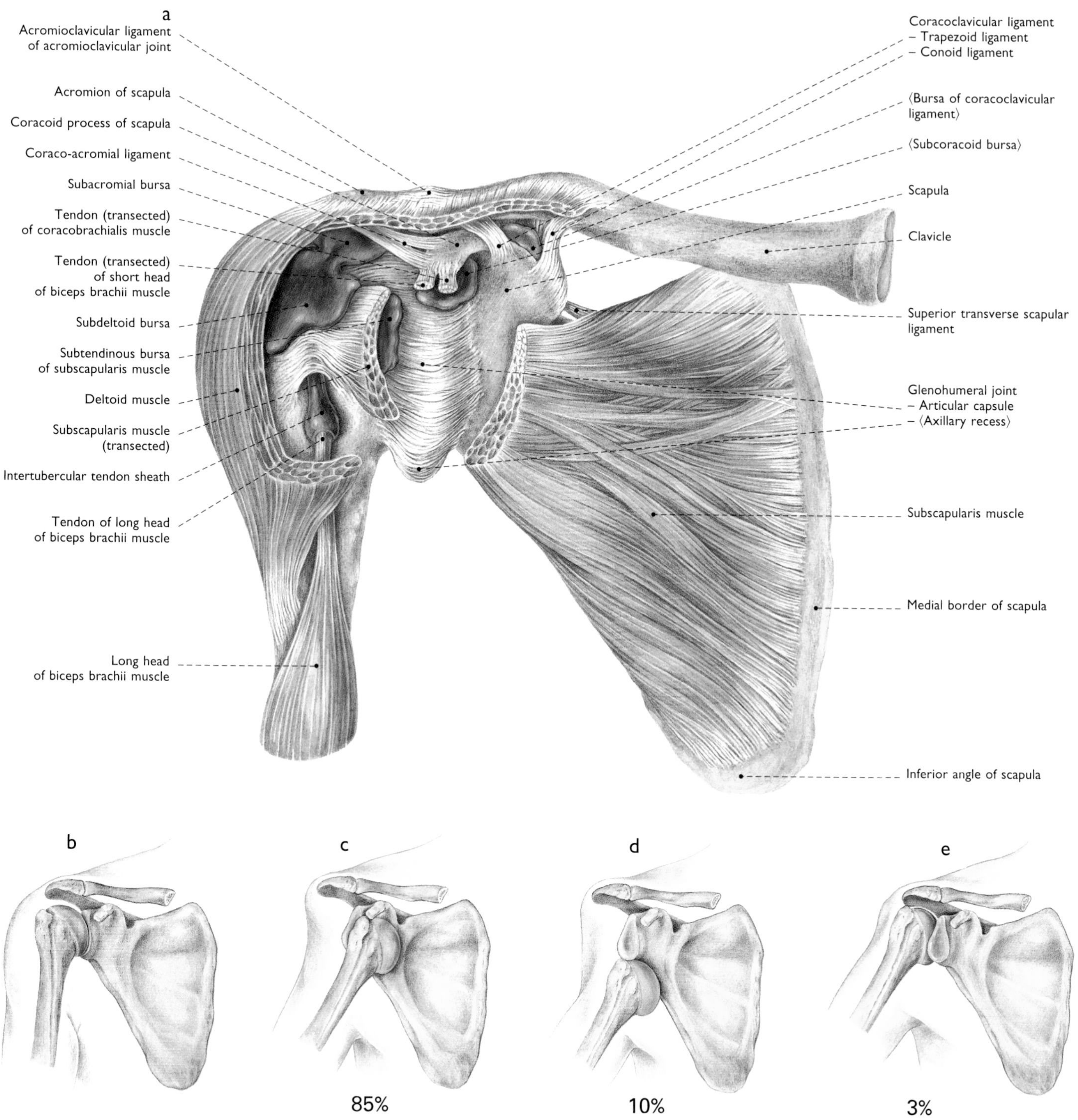
a
Acromioclavicular ligament of acromioclavicular joint
Acromion of scapula
Coracoid process of scapula
Coraco-acromial ligament
Subacromial bursa
Tendon (transected) of coracobrachialis muscle
Tendon (transected) of short head of biceps brachii muscle
Subdeltoid bursa
Subtendinous bursa of subscapularis muscle
Deltoid muscle
Subscapularis muscle (transected)
Intertubercular tendon sheath
Tendon of long head of biceps brachii muscle
Long head of biceps brachii muscle
Coracoclavicular ligament
– Trapezoid ligament
– Conoid ligament
⟨Bursa of coracoclavicular ligament⟩
⟨Subcoracoid bursa⟩
Scapula
Clavicle
Superior transverse scapular ligament
Glenohumeral joint
– Articular capsule
– ⟨Axillary recess⟩
Subscapularis muscle
Medial border of scapula
Inferior angle of scapula
b
c
d
e
85%
10%
3%

103 Right glenohumeral (= shoulder) joint

Ventral aspect

a Synovial bursae in the shoulder region (50%)

b–e Dislocations of the shoulder. The percentile numbers indicate the approximate frequency of occurrence.

b Normal situation

c Anterior dislocation of the head of humerus (subcoracoid luxation), most frequent type

d Inferior dislocation (axillary = subglenoid luxation)

e Posterior dislocation (subacromial luxation)

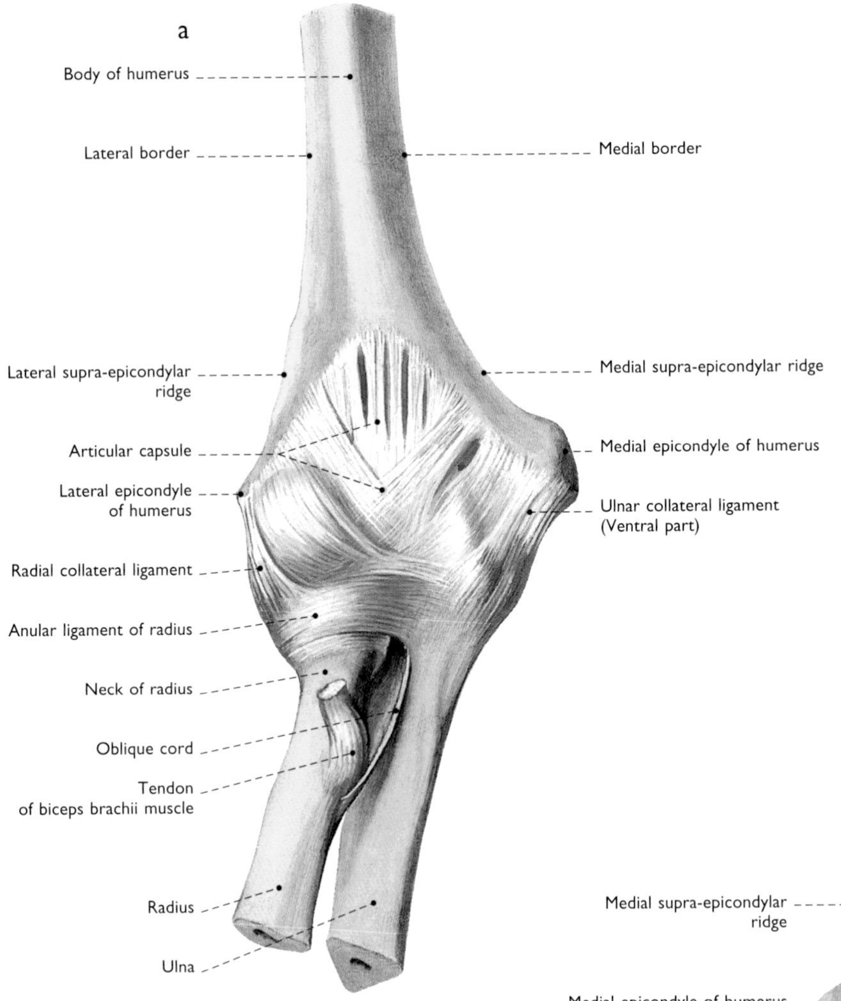
a
Body of humerus
Lateral border
Medial border
Lateral supra-epicondylar ridge
Medial supra-epicondylar ridge
Articular capsule
Medial epicondyle of humerus
Lateral epicondyle of humerus
Ulnar collateral ligament (Ventral part)
Radial collateral ligament
Anular ligament of radius
Neck of radius
Oblique cord
Tendon of biceps brachii muscle
Radius
Ulna

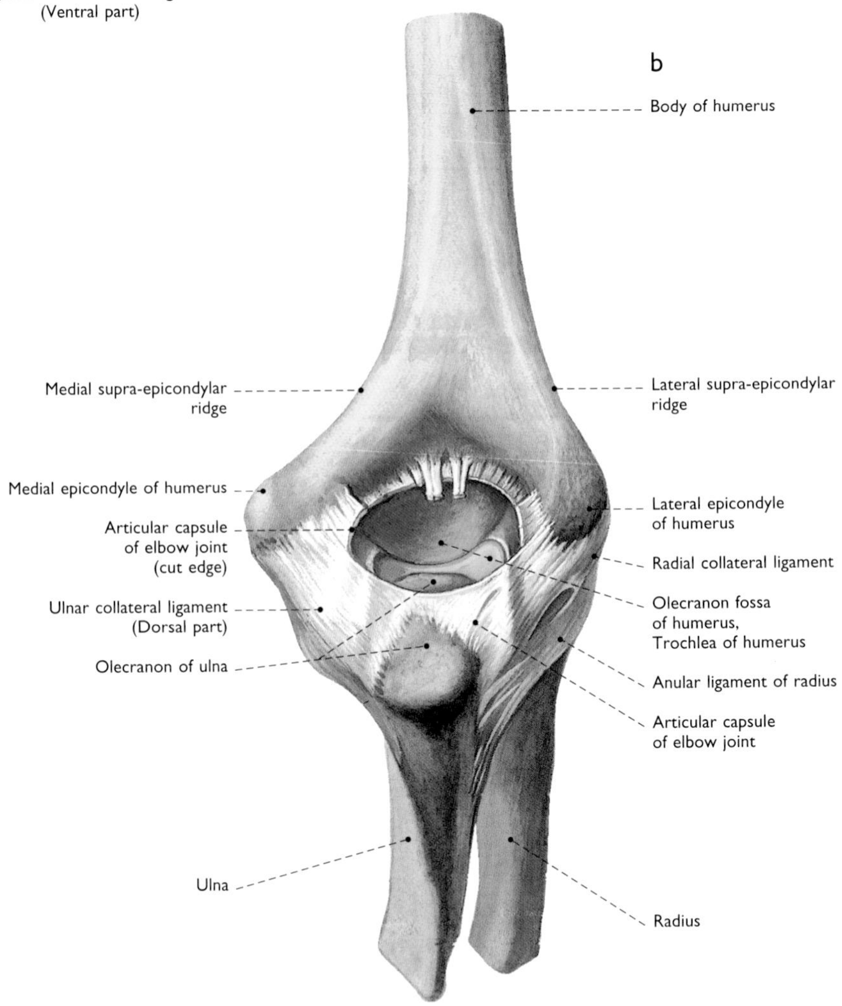
b
Body of humerus
Medial supra-epicondylar ridge
Lateral supra-epicondylar ridge
Medial epicondyle of humerus
Lateral epicondyle of humerus
Articular capsule of elbow joint (cut edge)
Radial collateral ligament
Olecranon fossa of humerus, Trochlea of humerus
Ulnar collateral ligament (Dorsal part)
Anular ligament of radius
Olecranon of ulna
Articular capsule of elbow joint
Ulna
Radius

104 Right elbow joint (85%)

a Ventral aspect
b Dorsal aspect

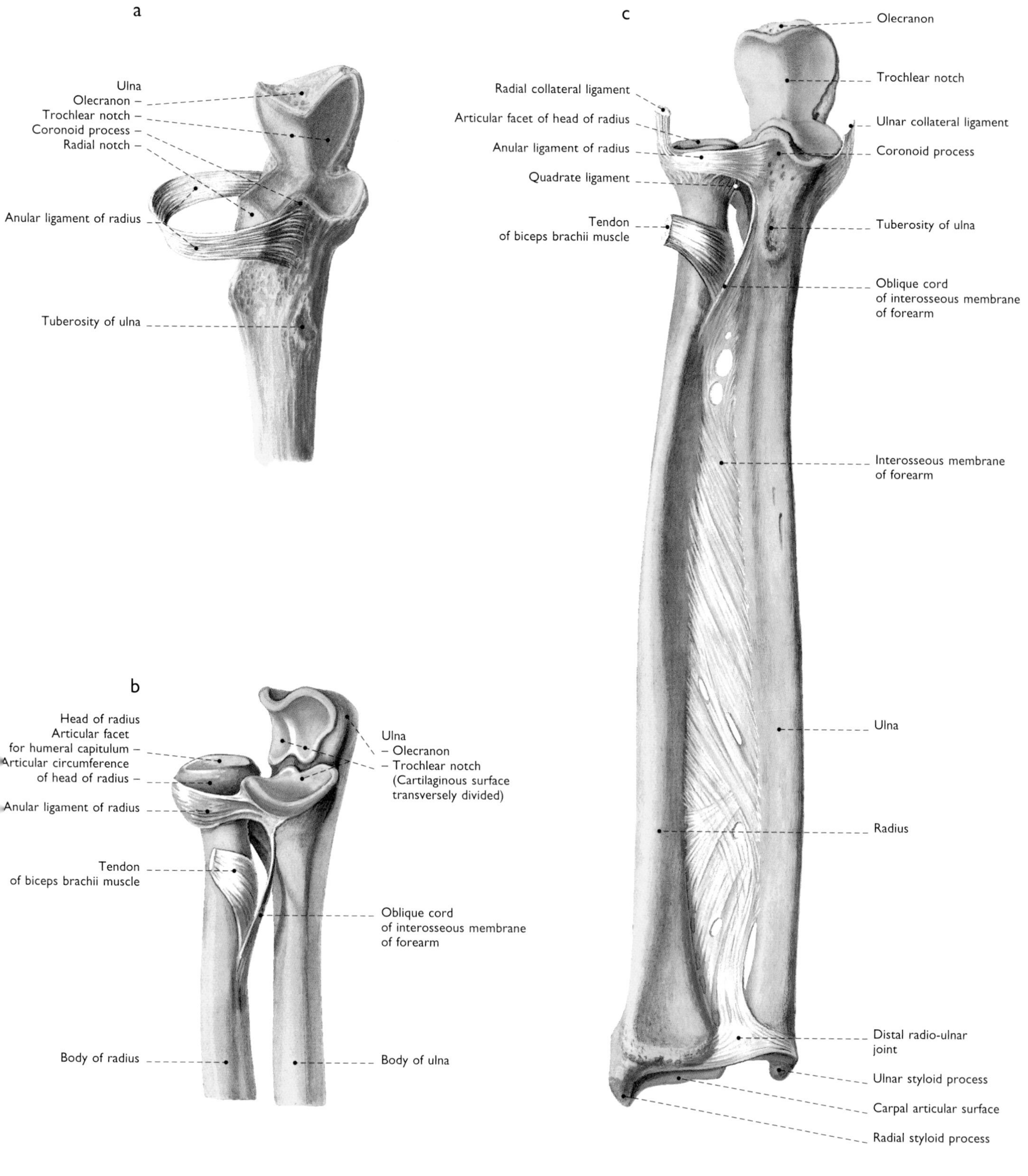
a
Ulna
Olecranon
Trochlear notch
Coronoid process
Radial notch
Anular ligament of radius
Tuberosity of ulna
b
Head of radius
Articular facet for humeral capitulum
Articular circumference of head of radius
Anular ligament of radius
Tendon of biceps brachii muscle
Body of radius
Ulna
– Olecranon
– Trochlear notch (Cartilaginous surface transversely divided)
Oblique cord of interosseous membrane of forearm
Body of ulna
c
Radial collateral ligament
Articular facet of head of radius
Anular ligament of radius
Quadrate ligament
Tendon of biceps brachii muscle
Olecranon
Trochlear notch
Ulnar collateral ligament
Coronoid process
Tuberosity of ulna
Oblique cord of interosseous membrane of forearm
Interosseous membrane of forearm
Ulna
Radius
Distal radio-ulnar joint
Ulnar styloid process
Carpal articular surface
Radial styloid process

105 Radio-ulnar joints of the right forearm

a Proximal end of ulna and anular ligament of radius (80%), ventral aspect
b Proximal radio-ulnar joint (70%), ventral aspect
c Forearm bones in supinated position (70%), ventral aspect

a

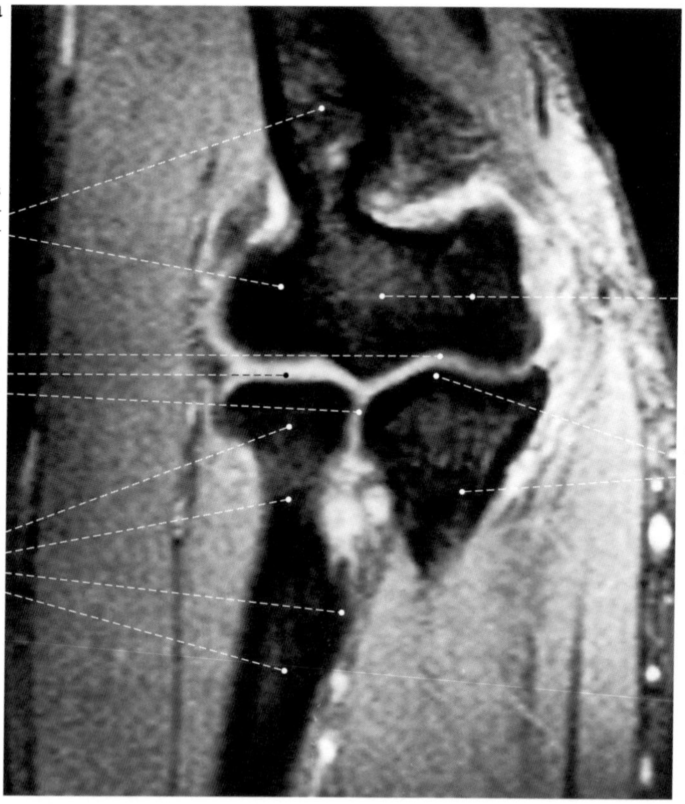
Humerus
Body of humerus –
Capitulum –
Elbow joint
Humero-ulnar joint –
Humeroradial joint –
Proximal radio-ulnar joint –
Radius
Head of radius –
Neck of radius –
Tuberosity of radius –
Body of radius –
Humerus
– Trochlea
Ulna
– Coronoid process
– Body of ulna

b

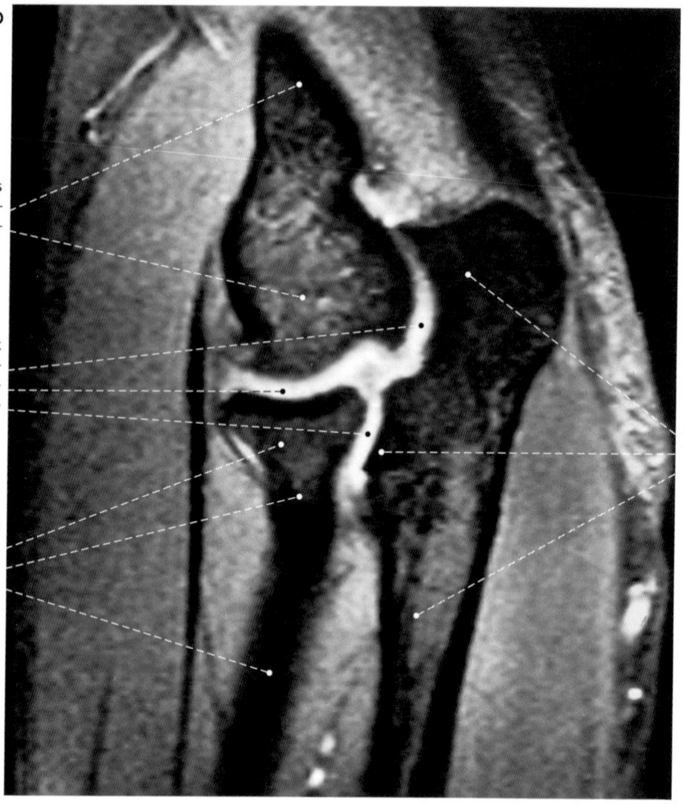
Humerus
Body of humerus –
Capitulum –
Elbow joint
Humero-ulnar joint –
Humeroradial joint –
Proximal radio-ulnar joint –
Radius
Head of radius –
Neck of radius –
Body of radius –
Ulna
– Olecranon
– Radial notch
– Body of ulna

106 Right elbow joint (100%)

Coronal magnetic resonance images (MRI, T_2-weighted)
a through the ventral part
b through the dorsal part
of the elbow joint, ventral aspect

a

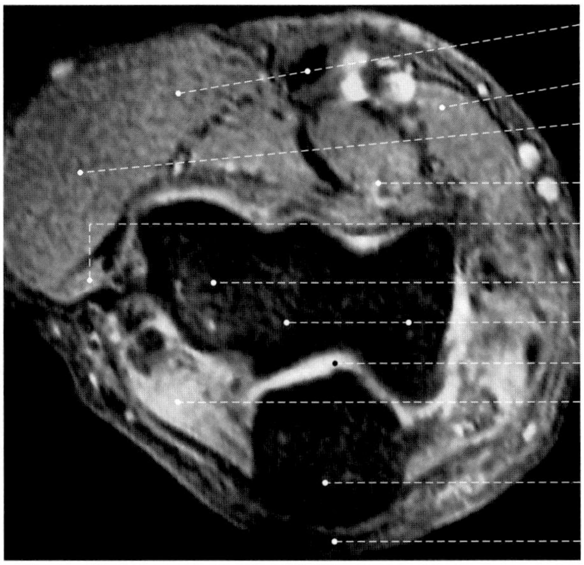

b

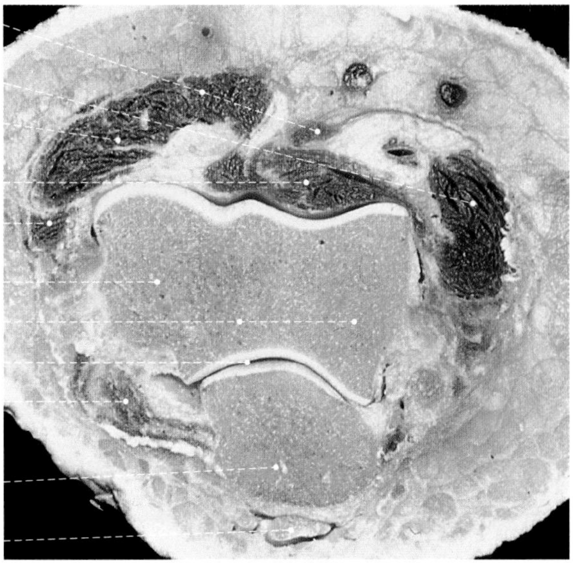
Brachioradialis muscle,
Tendon of biceps brachii m.
Pronator teres muscle
Extensor carpi radialis longus muscle
Brachialis muscle
Extensor carpi radialis brevis muscle
Capitulum of humerus
Trochlea of humerus
Humero-ulnar joint
Anconeus muscle
Olecranon of ulna
Tendon of triceps brachii m.

c

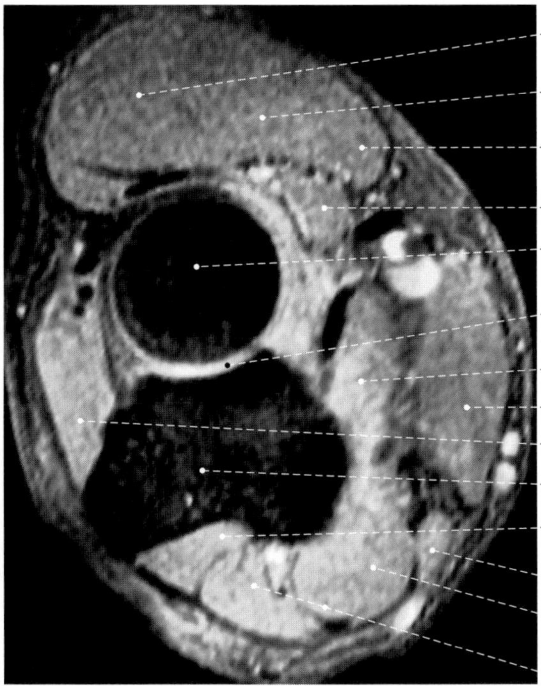

d

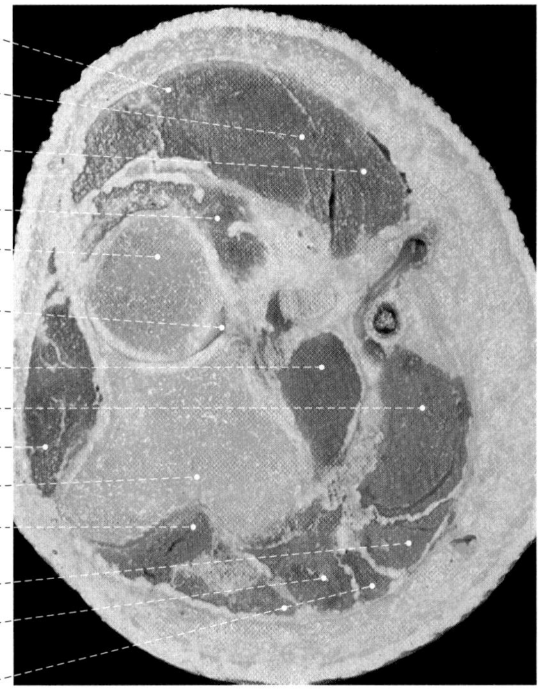
Extensor carpi radialis brevis muscle
Extensor carpi radialis longus muscle
Brachioradialis muscle
Supinator muscle
Head of radius
Proximal radio-ulnar joint
Brachialis muscle
Pronator teres muscle
Anconeus muscle
Body of ulna
Flexor digitorum profundus muscle
Flexor carpi radialis m.
Flexor digitorum superficialis muscle
Flexor carpi ulnaris muscle,
Palmaris longus muscle

107 Right elbow joint (90%)

a, b Axial (transverse) sections through the distal arm and the humero-ulnar joint

c, d Axial (transverse) sections through the proximal forearm and the proximal radio-ulnar joint

a, c Magnetic resonance images (MRI, T_2-weighted), distal aspect

b, d Anatomical sections, distal aspect

The pictures c and d are rotated by about 90° in relation to a and b.

a

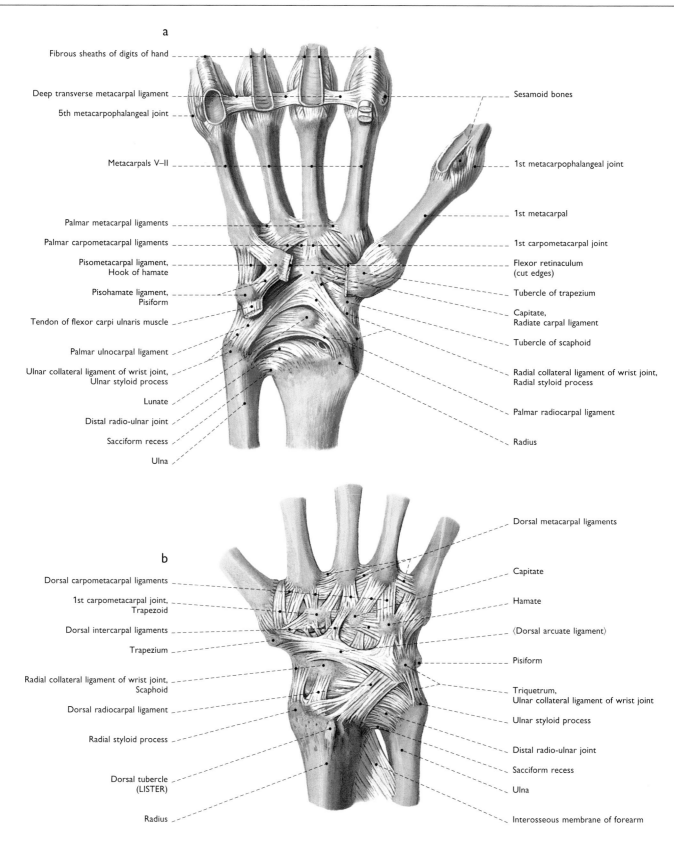

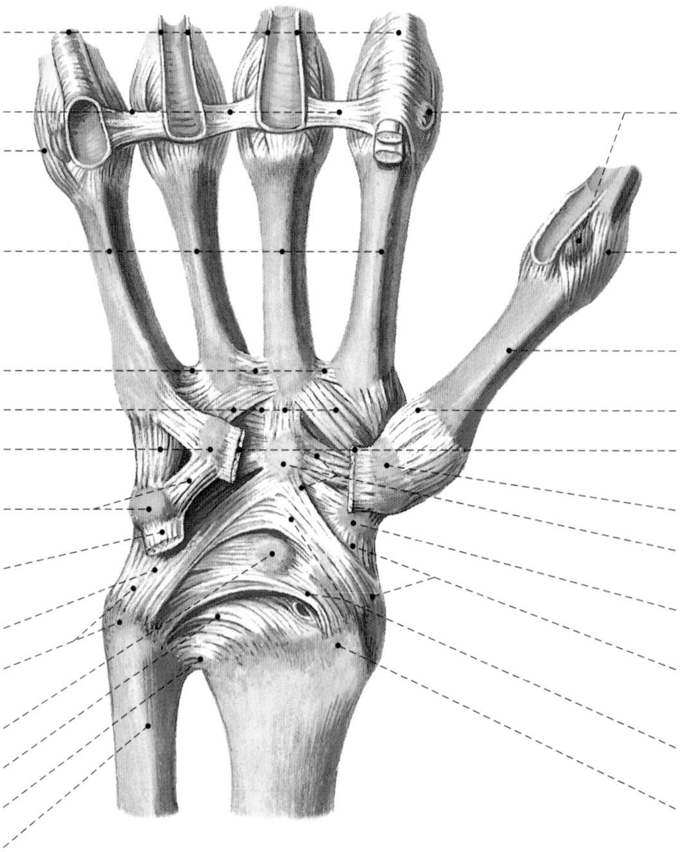
Fibrous sheaths of digits of hand
Deep transverse metacarpal ligament
5th metacarpophalangeal joint
Metacarpals V–II
Palmar metacarpal ligaments
Palmar carpometacarpal ligaments
Pisometacarpal ligament,
Hook of hamate
Pisohamate ligament,
Pisiform
Tendon of flexor carpi ulnaris muscle
Palmar ulnocarpal ligament
Ulnar collateral ligament of wrist joint,
Ulnar styloid process
Lunate
Distal radio-ulnar joint
Sacciform recess
Ulna
Sesamoid bones
1st metacarpophalangeal joint
1st metacarpal
1st carpometacarpal joint
Flexor retinaculum
(cut edges)
Tubercle of trapezium
Capitate,
Radiate carpal ligament
Tubercle of scaphoid
Radial collateral ligament of wrist joint,
Radial styloid process
Palmar radiocarpal ligament
Radius

b

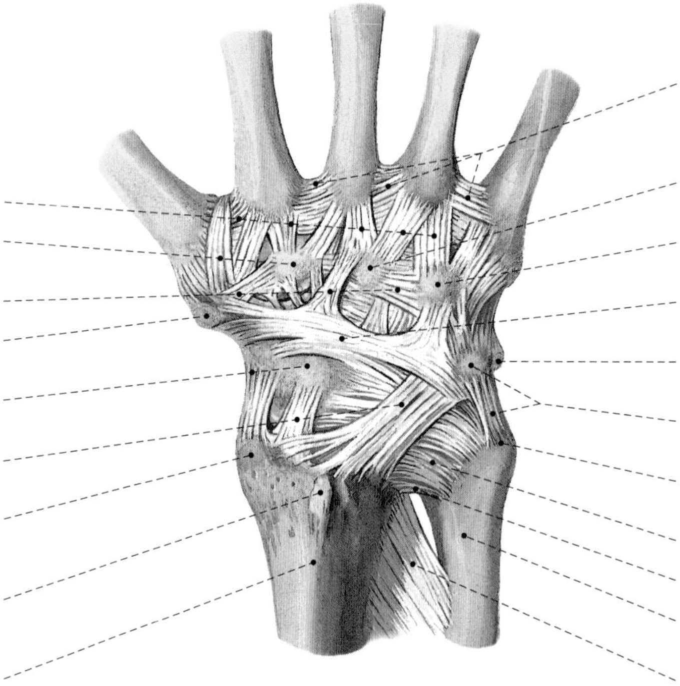
Dorsal carpometacarpal ligaments
1st carpometacarpal joint,
Trapezoid
Dorsal intercarpal ligaments
Trapezium
Radial collateral ligament of wrist joint,
Scaphoid
Dorsal radiocarpal ligament
Radial styloid process
Dorsal tubercle
(LISTER)
Radius
Dorsal metacarpal ligaments
Capitate
Hamate
⟨Dorsal arcuate ligament⟩
Pisiform
Triquetrum,
Ulnar collateral ligament of wrist joint
Ulnar styloid process
Distal radio-ulnar joint
Sacciform recess
Ulna
Interosseous membrane of forearm

108 Joints of the right hand (75%)

a Palmar aspect

b Dorsal aspect

a

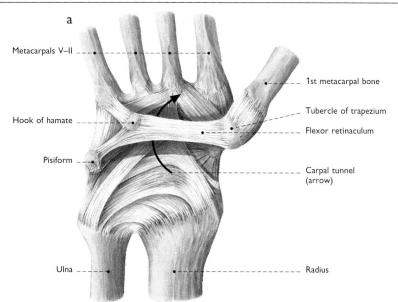

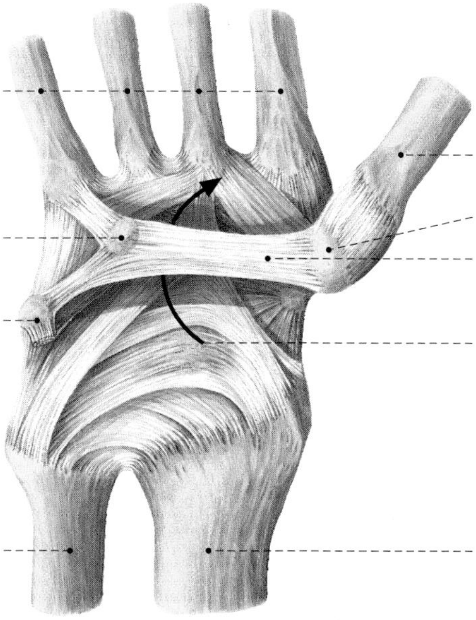
Metacarpals V–II
1st metacarpal bone
Tubercle of trapezium
Hook of hamate
Flexor retinaculum
Pisiform
Carpal tunnel
(arrow)
Ulna
Radius

b

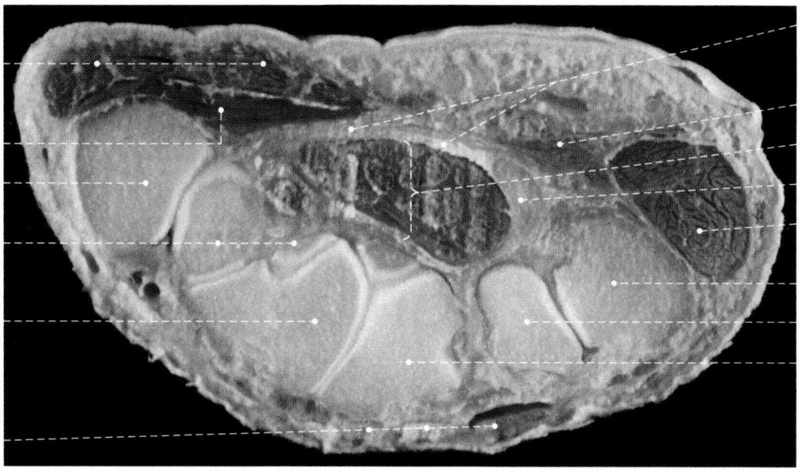
Flexor retinaculum
Abductor pollicis brevis muscle,
Superficial head of flexor pollicis
brevis muscle
Opponens digiti minimi muscle
Opponens pollicis muscle
Carpal tunnel
Base of 1st metacarpal bone
Hook of hamate
Abductor digiti minimi muscle
Trapezium,
Trapezoid
Base of 5th metacarpal bone
Base of 2nd metacarpal bone
Hamate
Capitate
Tendons
of extensor digitorum muscle

c

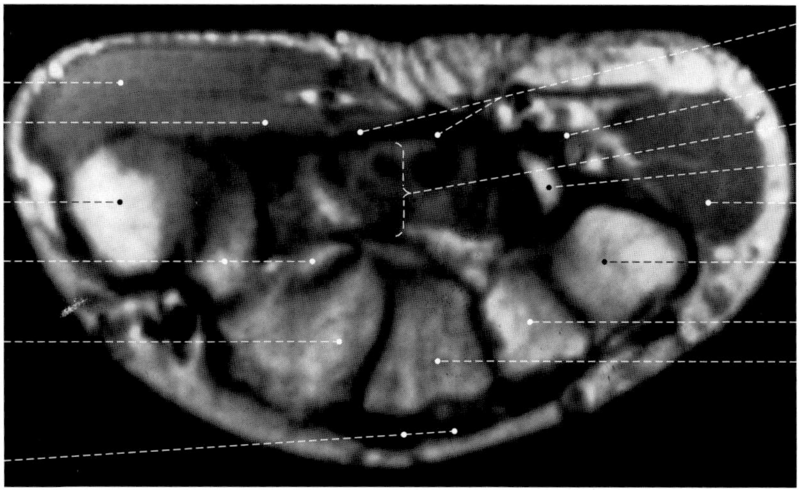
Flexor retinaculum
Abductor pollicis brevis muscle
Opponens digiti minimi muscle
Opponens pollicis muscle
Carpal tunnel
Hook of hamate
Base of 1st metacarpal bone
Abductor digiti minimi muscle
Trapezium,
Trapezoid
Base of 5th metacarpal bone
Hamate
Base of 2nd metacarpal bone
Capitate
Tendons
of extensor digitorum muscle

109 Carpal tunnel of the right hand

a Palmar aspect (80%)
b Anatomical axial section through the wrist and the carpal tunnel (130%), distal aspect
c Axial (transverse) magnetic resonance image (MRI, T_1-weighted) of the wrist and the carpal tunnel (140%), distal aspect
b, c Hand in full supination

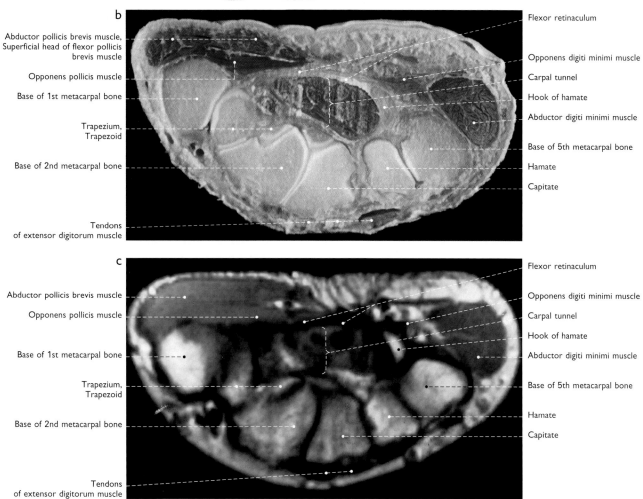

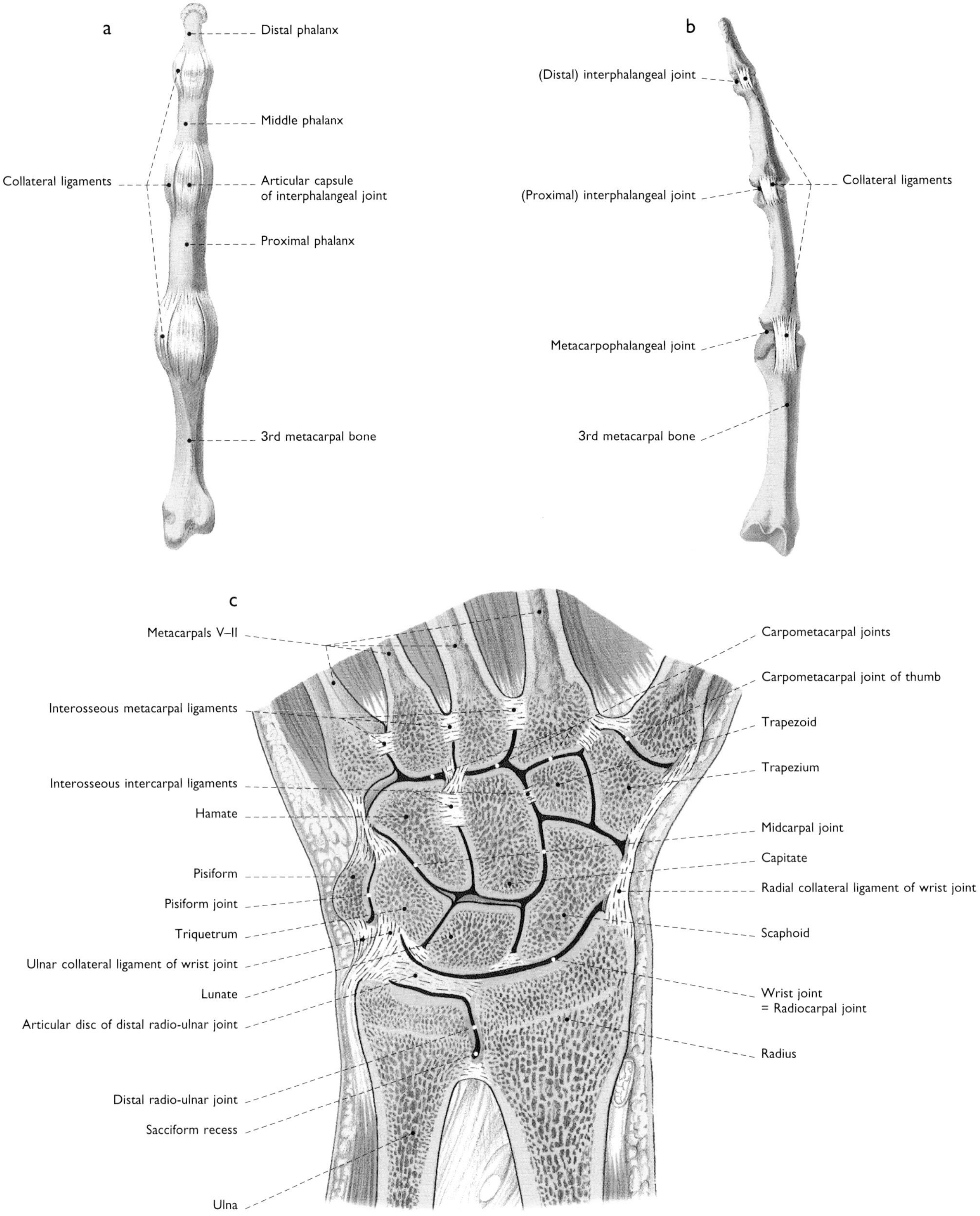
a
Distal phalanx
Middle phalanx
Collateral ligaments
Articular capsule
of interphalangeal joint
Proximal phalanx
3rd metacarpal bone
b
(Distal) interphalangeal joint
Collateral ligaments
(Proximal) interphalangeal joint
Metacarpophalangeal joint
3rd metacarpal bone
c
Metacarpals V–II
Interosseous metacarpal ligaments
Interosseous intercarpal ligaments
Hamate
Pisiform
Pisiform joint
Triquetrum
Ulnar collateral ligament of wrist joint
Lunate
Articular disc of distal radio-ulnar joint
Distal radio-ulnar joint
Sacciform recess
Ulna
Carpometacarpal joints
Carpometacarpal joint of thumb
Trapezoid
Trapezium
Midcarpal joint
Capitate
Radial collateral ligament of wrist joint
Scaphoid
Wrist joint
= Radiocarpal joint
Radius

110 Joints of the right hand

a, b Middle finger (60%)
a Dorsal aspect
b Lateral aspect
c Radio-ulnar (coronal) cut through the wrist (100%), palmar aspect

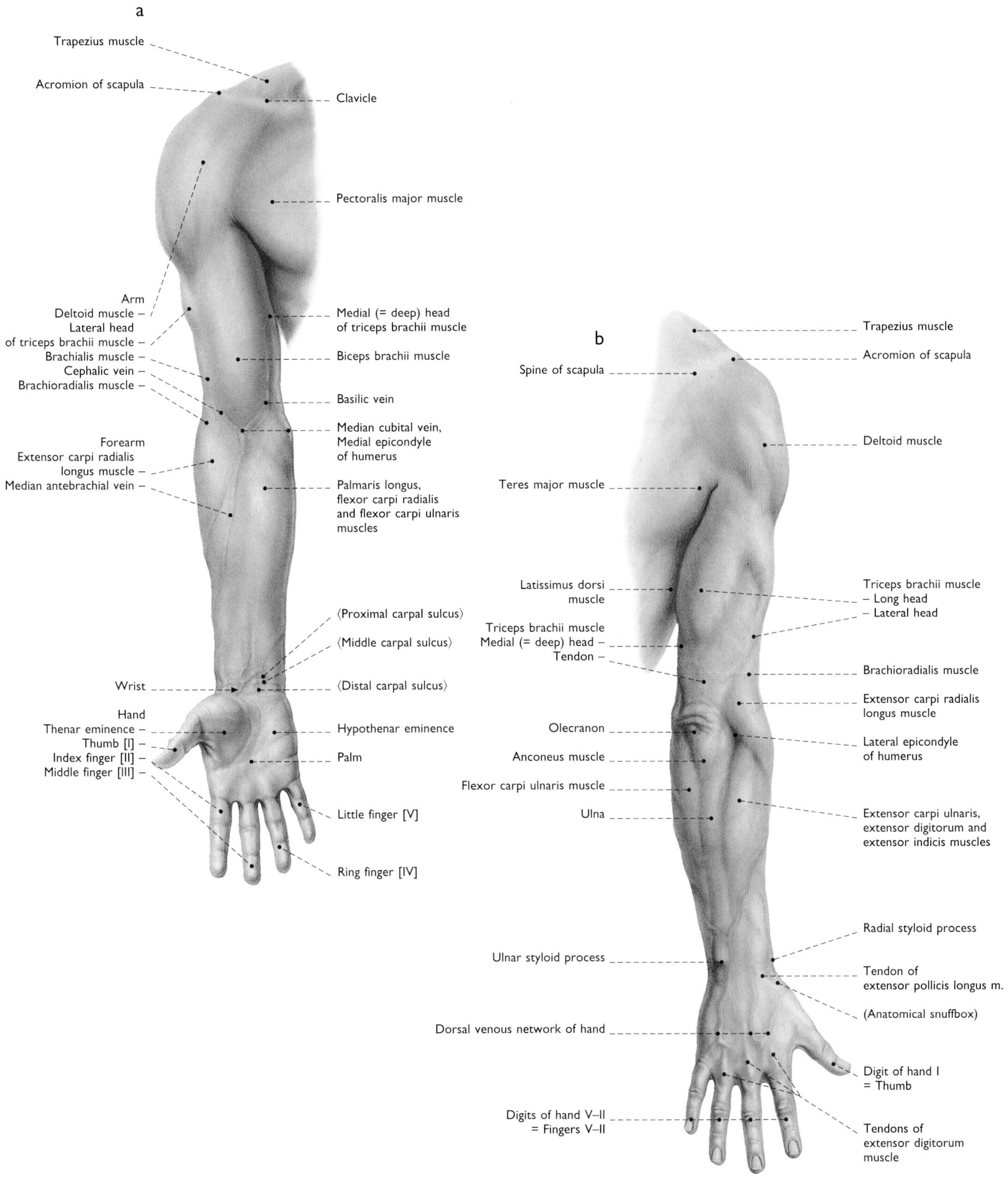
a
Trapezius muscle
Acromion of scapula
Clavicle
Pectoralis major muscle
Arm
Deltoid muscle –
Lateral head
of triceps brachii muscle –
Brachialis muscle –
Cephalic vein –
Brachioradialis muscle –
Medial (= deep) head
of triceps brachii muscle
Biceps brachii muscle
Basilic vein
Median cubital vein,
Medial epicondyle
of humerus
Forearm
Extensor carpi radialis
longus muscle –
Median antebrachial vein –
Palmaris longus,
flexor carpi radialis
and flexor carpi ulnaris
muscles
⟨Proximal carpal sulcus⟩
⟨Middle carpal sulcus⟩
Wrist
⟨Distal carpal sulcus⟩
Hand
Thenar eminence –
Thumb [I] –
Index finger [II] –
Middle finger [III] –
Hypothenar eminence
Palm
Little finger [V]
Ring finger [IV]
b
Trapezius muscle
Acromion of scapula
Spine of scapula
Deltoid muscle
Teres major muscle
Latissimus dorsi
muscle
Triceps brachii muscle
– Long head
– Lateral head
Triceps brachii muscle
Medial (= deep) head –
Tendon –
Brachioradialis muscle
Extensor carpi radialis
longus muscle
Olecranon
Lateral epicondyle
of humerus
Anconeus muscle
Flexor carpi ulnaris muscle
Ulna
Extensor carpi ulnaris,
extensor digitorum and
extensor indicis muscles
Radial styloid process
Ulnar styloid process
Tendon of
extensor pollicis longus m.
(Anatomical snuffbox)
Dorsal venous network of hand
Digit of hand I
= Thumb
Digits of hand V–II
= Fingers V–II
Tendons of
extensor digitorum
muscle

111 Surface anatomy of the right upper limb (20%)

a Ventral aspect
b Dorsal aspect

a

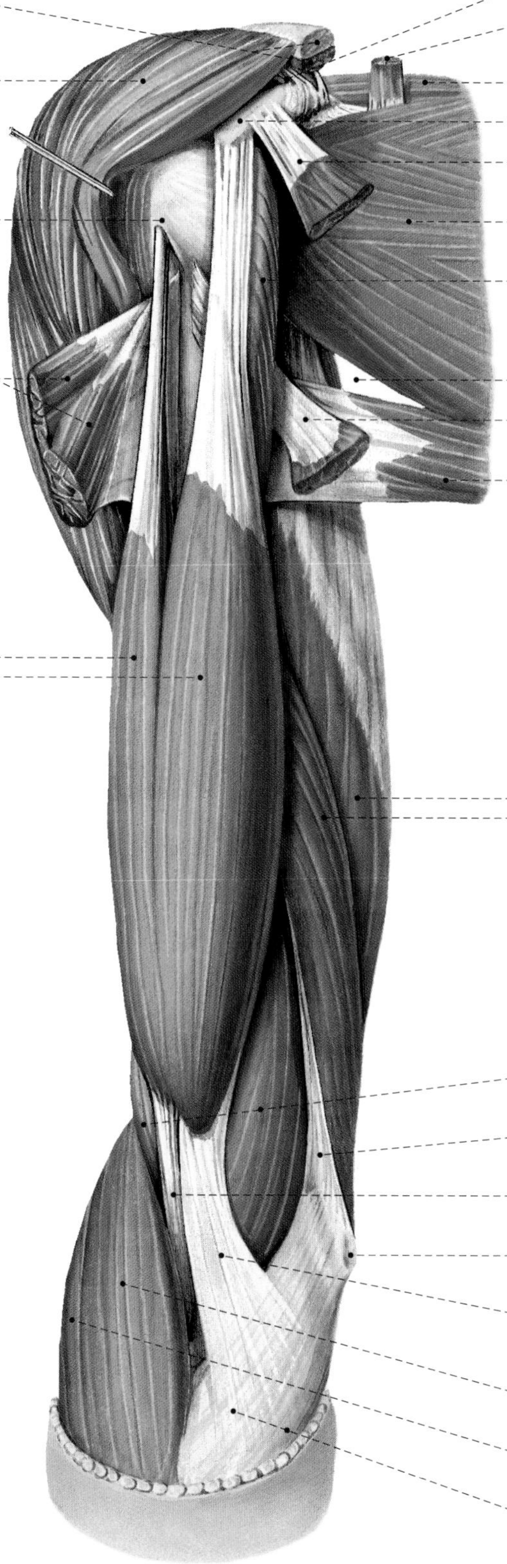
Clavicle,
Subclavius muscle
Deltoid muscle
Intertubercular tendon sheath
Pectoralis major muscle
Biceps brachii muscle
Long head –
Short head –
Coracoclavicular ligament
Inferior belly
of omohyoid muscle
Supraspinatus muscle
Coracoid process
Pectoralis minor muscle
Subscapularis muscle
Coracobrachialis muscle
⟨Triangular space⟩
Latissimus dorsi muscle
Teres major muscle
Triceps brachii muscle
– Long head
– Medial head
= Deep head
Brachialis muscle
Medial intermuscular
septum of arm
Tendon
of biceps brachii muscle
Medial epicondyle
of humerus
Bicipital aponeurosis
Brachioradialis muscle
Extensor carpi radialis
longus muscle
Antebrachial fascia

b

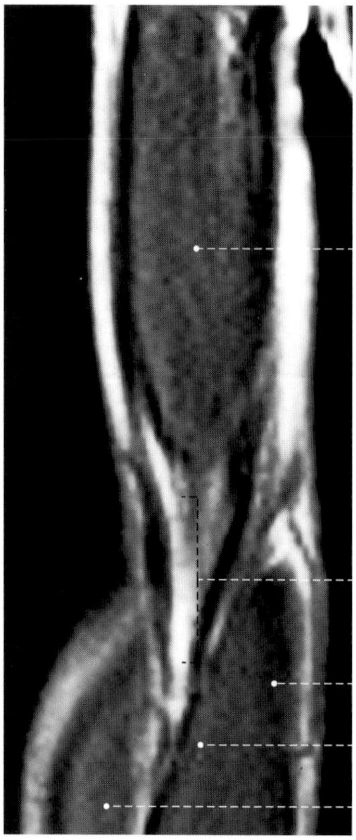
Biceps brachii muscle
Cubital fossa
Flexor carpi radialis muscle
Pronator teres muscle
Brachioradialis muscle

112 Muscles of the right shoulder and the right arm (50%)

a Ventral aspect

b Coronal magnetic resonance image of the anterior region of elbow (MRI, T_1-weighted)

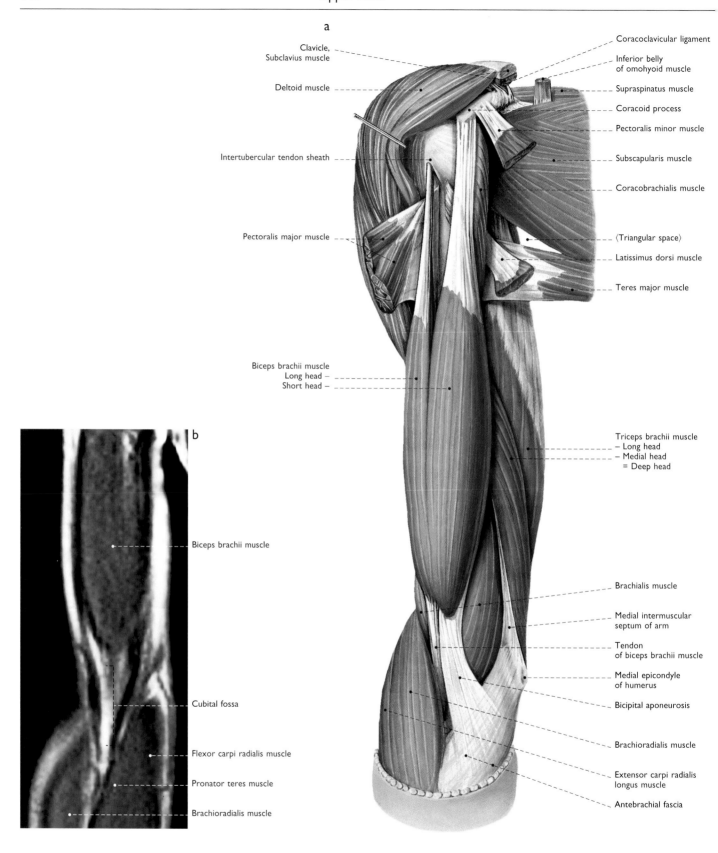

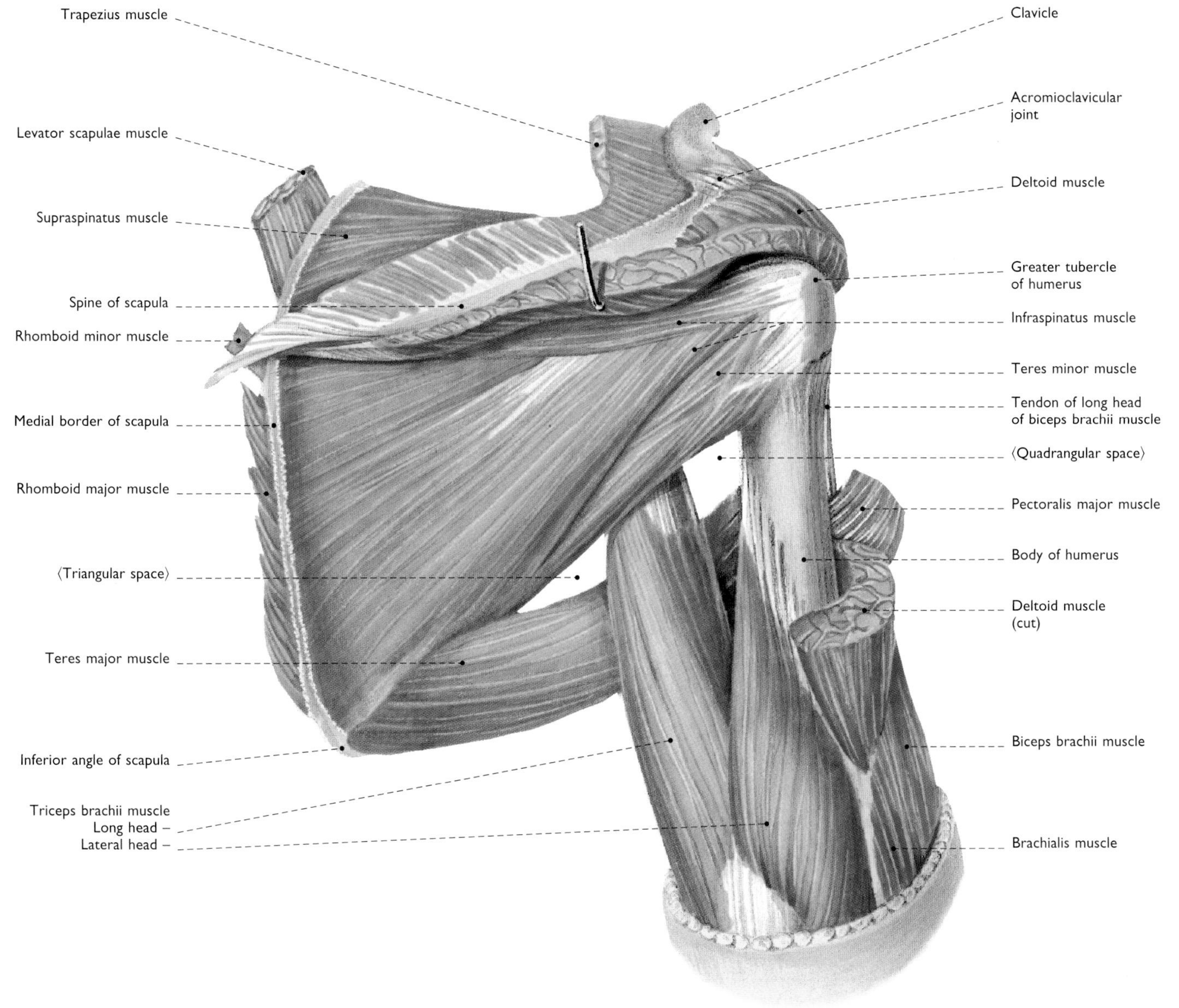

Trapezius muscle
Levator scapulae muscle
Supraspinatus muscle
Spine of scapula
Rhomboid minor muscle
Medial border of scapula
Rhomboid major muscle
⟨Triangular space⟩
Teres major muscle
Inferior angle of scapula
Triceps brachii muscle
Long head –
Lateral head –
Clavicle
Acromioclavicular joint
Deltoid muscle
Greater tubercle of humerus
Infraspinatus muscle
Teres minor muscle
Tendon of long head of biceps brachii muscle
⟨Quadrangular space⟩
Pectoralis major muscle
Body of humerus
Deltoid muscle (cut)
Biceps brachii muscle
Brachialis muscle

117 Muscles of the right shoulder and the right arm (60%)

The deltoid muscle was partially removed.
Dorsal aspect

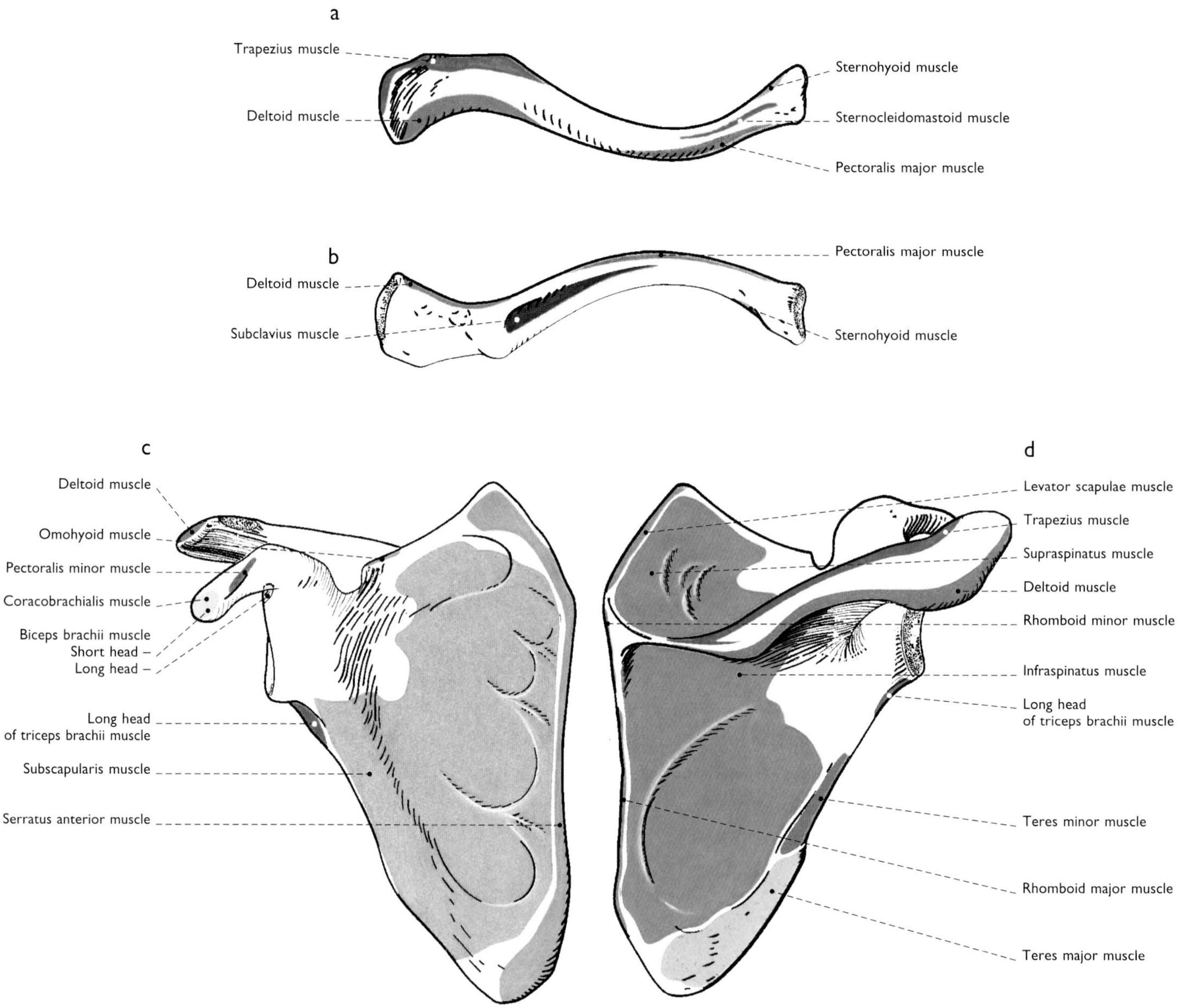
a
Trapezius muscle
Deltoid muscle
Sternohyoid muscle
Sternocleidomastoid muscle
Pectoralis major muscle
b
Deltoid muscle
Subclavius muscle
Pectoralis major muscle
Sternohyoid muscle
c
Deltoid muscle
Omohyoid muscle
Pectoralis minor muscle
Coracobrachialis muscle
Biceps brachii muscle
Short head
Long head
Long head
of triceps brachii muscle
Subscapularis muscle
Serratus anterior muscle
d
Levator scapulae muscle
Trapezius muscle
Supraspinatus muscle
Deltoid muscle
Rhomboid minor muscle
Infraspinatus muscle
Long head
of triceps brachii muscle
Teres minor muscle
Rhomboid major muscle
Teres major muscle

- Ansa cervicalis
- Accessory nerve [XI]
- Axillary nerve
- Medial and lateral pectoral nerves
- Subclavian nerve
- Subscapular nerves
- Long thoracic nerve
- Dorsal scapular nerve
- Suprascapular nerve
- Thoracodorsal nerve
- Radial nerve
- Musculocutaneous nerve

118 Muscle attachments to the right pectoral girdle

The colors indicate the innervation of the muscles attaching to the

a superior surface of the clavicle
b inferior surface of the clavicle
c costal surface of the scapula
d posterior surface of the scapula.

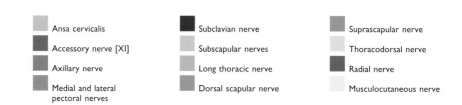

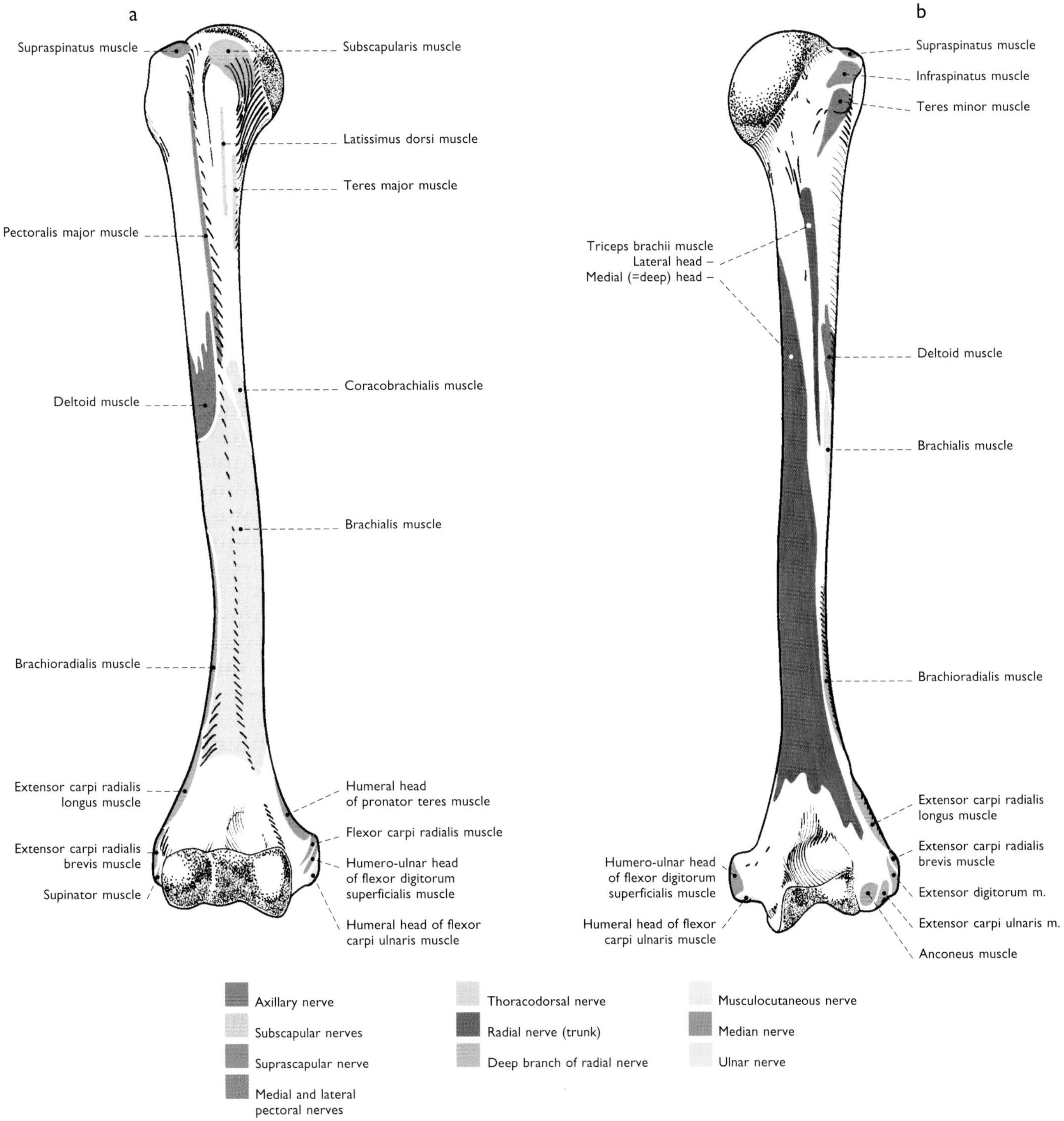
a
Supraspinatus muscle
Subscapularis muscle
Latissimus dorsi muscle
Teres major muscle
Pectoralis major muscle
Coracobrachialis muscle
Deltoid muscle
Brachialis muscle
Brachioradialis muscle
Extensor carpi radialis longus muscle
Humeral head of pronator teres muscle
Flexor carpi radialis muscle
Extensor carpi radialis brevis muscle
Humero-ulnar head of flexor digitorum superficialis muscle
Supinator muscle
Humeral head of flexor carpi ulnaris muscle
b
Supraspinatus muscle
Infraspinatus muscle
Teres minor muscle
Triceps brachii muscle
Lateral head –
Medial (=deep) head –
Deltoid muscle
Brachialis muscle
Brachioradialis muscle
Extensor carpi radialis longus muscle
Extensor carpi radialis brevis muscle
Humero-ulnar head of flexor digitorum superficialis muscle
Extensor digitorum m.
Humeral head of flexor carpi ulnaris muscle
Extensor carpi ulnaris m.
Anconeus muscle
Axillary nerve
Subscapular nerves
Suprascapular nerve
Medial and lateral pectoral nerves
Thoracodorsal nerve
Radial nerve (trunk)
Deep branch of radial nerve
Musculocutaneous nerve
Median nerve
Ulnar nerve

119 Muscle attachments to the right humerus

The colors indicate the innervation of the muscles attaching to the

a ventral surface
b dorsal surface.

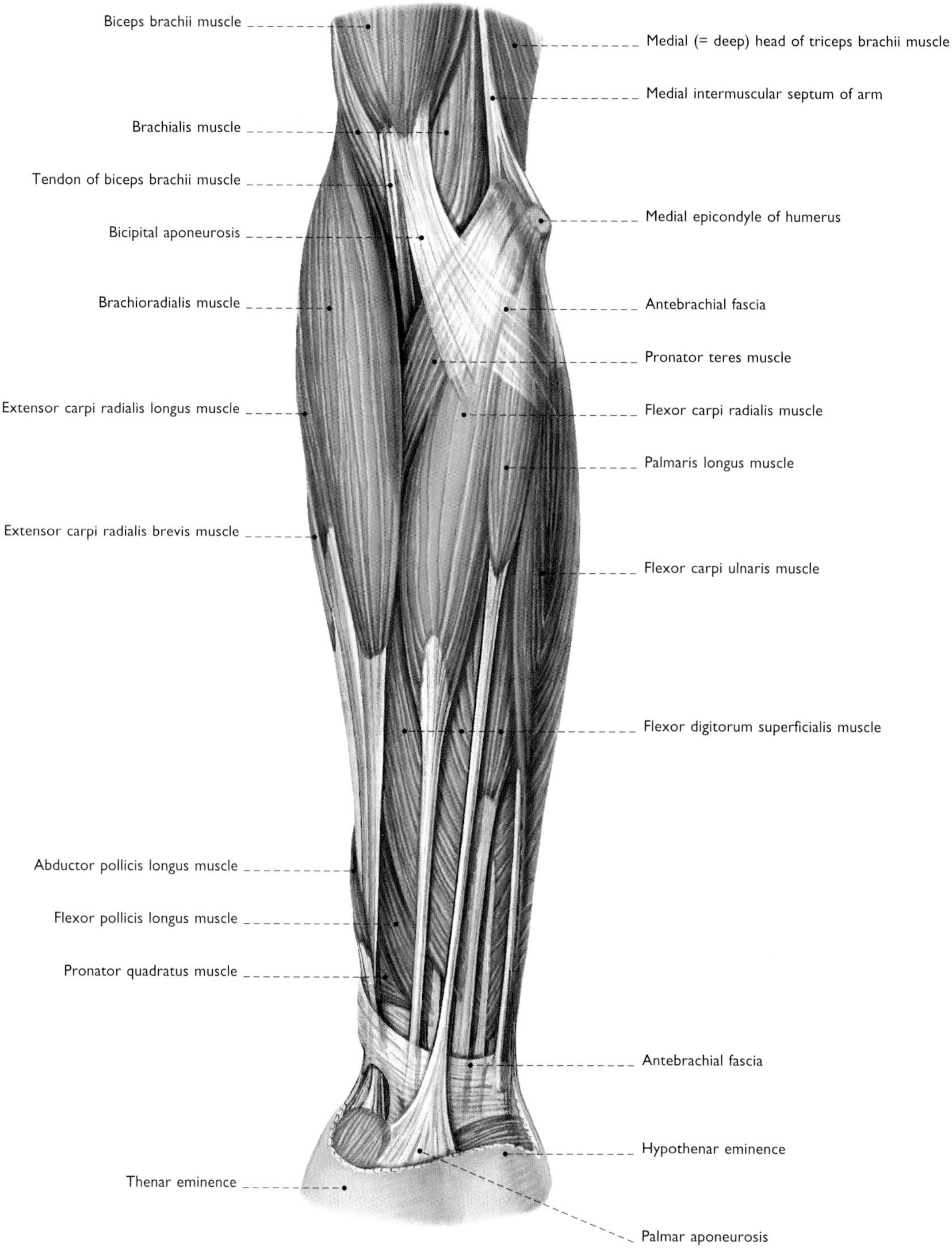
Biceps brachii muscle
Brachialis muscle
Tendon of biceps brachii muscle
Bicipital aponeurosis
Brachioradialis muscle
Extensor carpi radialis longus muscle
Extensor carpi radialis brevis muscle
Abductor pollicis longus muscle
Flexor pollicis longus muscle
Pronator quadratus muscle
Thenar eminence
Medial (= deep) head of triceps brachii muscle
Medial intermuscular septum of arm
Medial epicondyle of humerus
Antebrachial fascia
Pronator teres muscle
Flexor carpi radialis muscle
Palmaris longus muscle
Flexor carpi ulnaris muscle
Flexor digitorum superficialis muscle
Antebrachial fascia
Hypothenar eminence
Palmar aponeurosis

120 Muscles of the right forearm (50%)

Superficial layer, ventral aspect

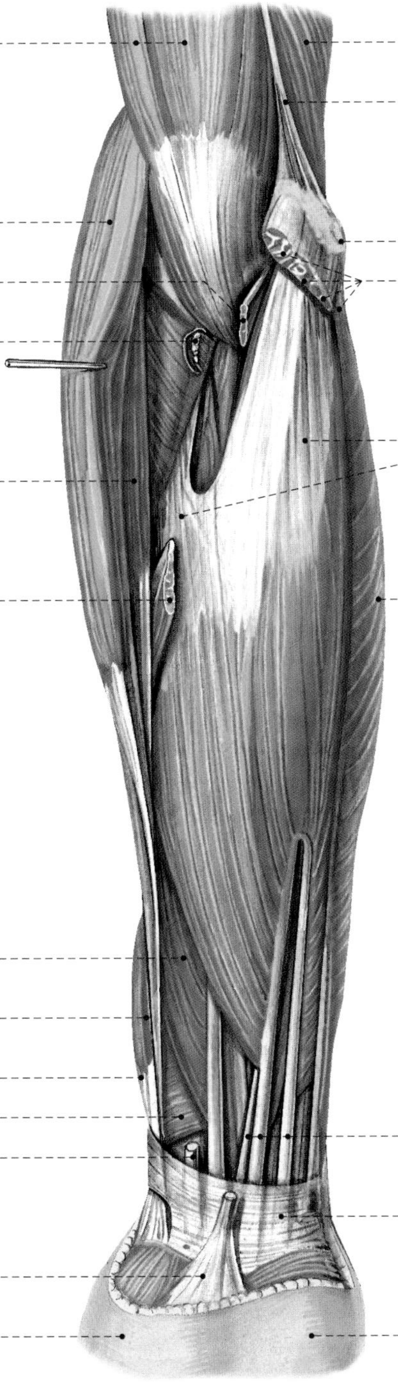
Brachialis muscle
Medial (= deep) head of triceps brachii muscle
Medial intermuscular septum of arm
Brachioradialis muscle
Medial epicondyle of humerus
Ulnar head of pronator teres muscle
⟨Common flexor tendon⟩
– Humeral head
of pronator teres muscle
– Flexor carpi radialis muscle
– Palmaris longus muscle
– Flexor carpi ulnaris muscle
Tendon of biceps brachii muscle
Flexor digitorum superficialis muscle
– Humero-ulnar head
– Radial head
Extensor carpi radialis longus muscle
Pronator teres muscle
Flexor carpi ulnaris muscle
Flexor pollicis longus muscle
Abductor pollicis longus muscle
Extensor pollicis brevis muscle
Pronator quadratus muscle
Tendons of flexor
digitorum superficialis muscle
Tendon of flexor carpi radialis muscle
Antebrachial fascia
Palmar aponeurosis
Thenar eminence
Hypothenar eminence

121 Muscles of the right forearm (50%)

Superficial layer. Some superficial forearm flexors were removed.
Ventral aspect

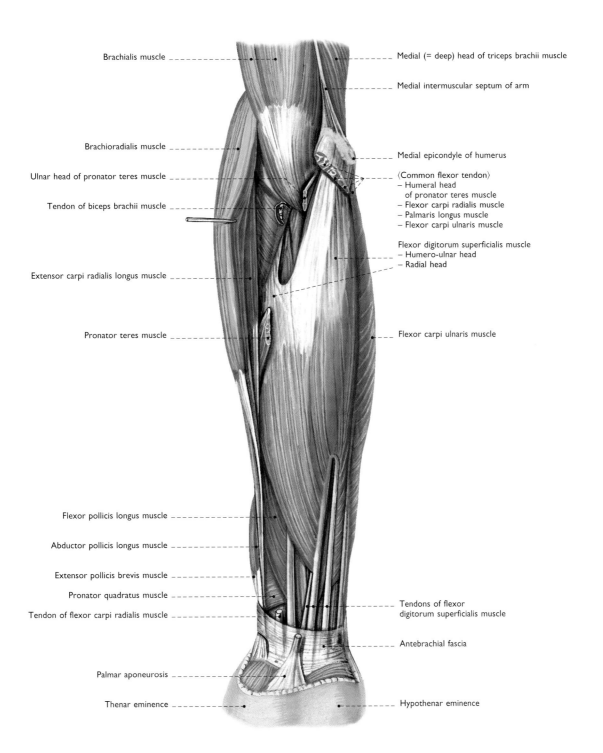

a

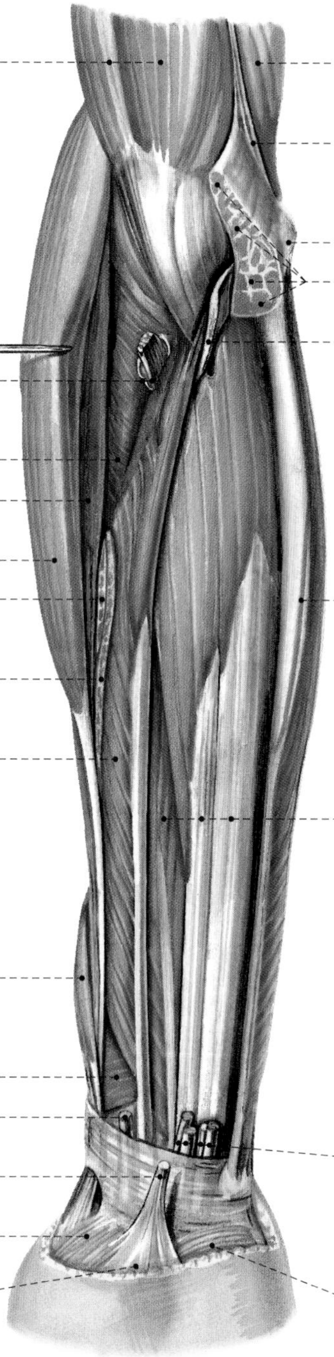
Brachialis muscle
Medial (= deep) head of triceps brachii muscle
Medial intermuscular septum of arm
Medial epicondyle of humerus
⟨Common flexor tendon⟩
Ulnar head of pronator teres muscle
Bicipitoradial bursa, Tendon of biceps brachii muscle
Supinator muscle
Extensor carpi radialis longus muscle
Brachioradialis muscle
Pronator teres muscle
Flexor carpi ulnaris muscle
Flexor digitorum superficialis muscle
Flexor pollicis longus muscle
Flexor digitorum profundus muscle
Abductor pollicis longus muscle
Pronator quadratus muscle
Tendon of flexor carpi radialis muscle
Tendons of flexor digitorum superficialis muscle
Tendon of palmaris longus muscle
Abductor pollicis brevis muscle
Palmar aponeurosis
Palmaris brevis muscle

b

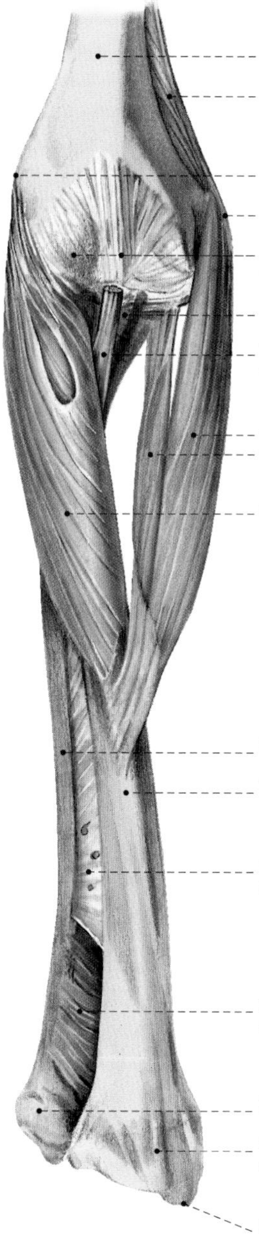
Humerus
Medial intermuscular septum of arm
Lateral epicondyle
Medial epicondyle
Articular capsule of elbow joint
Coronoid process
Tendon of biceps brachii muscle
Pronator teres muscle
– Humeral head
– Ulnar head
Supinator muscle
Ulna
Radius
Interosseous membrane of forearm
Pronator quadratus muscle
Head of ulna
Dorsal tubercle of radius (LISTER)
Radial styloid process

122 Muscles of the right forearm (50%)

Ventral aspect
a Deep layer
b Supinator and pronator muscles in pronated position of the forearm

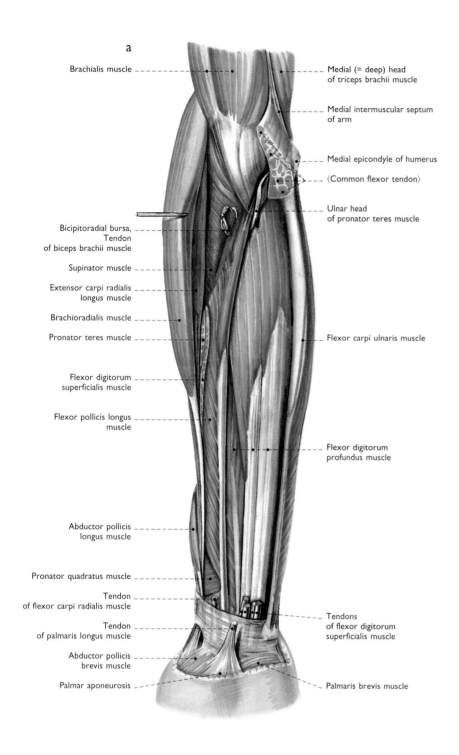

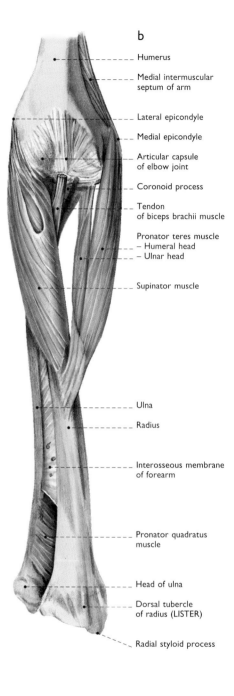

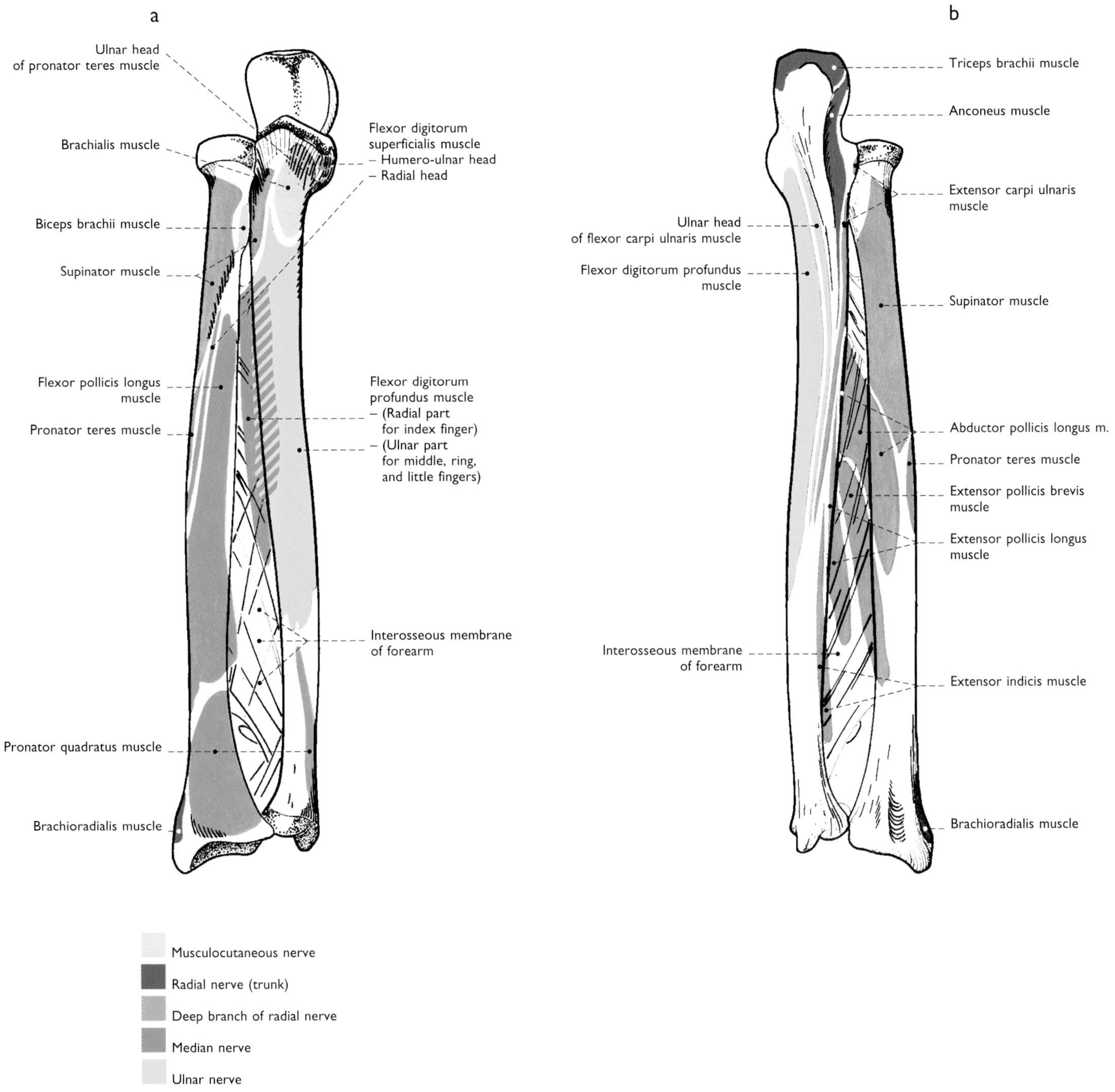
a
Ulnar head of pronator teres muscle
Brachialis muscle
Biceps brachii muscle
Supinator muscle
Flexor pollicis longus muscle
Pronator teres muscle
Pronator quadratus muscle
Brachioradialis muscle
Flexor digitorum superficialis muscle
– Humero-ulnar head
– Radial head
Flexor digitorum profundus muscle
– (Radial part for index finger)
– (Ulnar part for middle, ring, and little fingers)
Interosseous membrane of forearm
b
Triceps brachii muscle
Anconeus muscle
Extensor carpi ulnaris muscle
Ulnar head of flexor carpi ulnaris muscle
Flexor digitorum profundus muscle
Supinator muscle
Abductor pollicis longus m.
Pronator teres muscle
Extensor pollicis brevis muscle
Extensor pollicis longus muscle
Interosseous membrane of forearm
Extensor indicis muscle
Brachioradialis muscle
Musculocutaneous nerve
Radial nerve (trunk)
Deep branch of radial nerve
Median nerve
Ulnar nerve

123 Muscle attachments to the radius, ulna, and interosseous membrane of the right forearm

The colors indicate the innervation of the muscles attaching to the

a ventral surface
b dorsal surface.

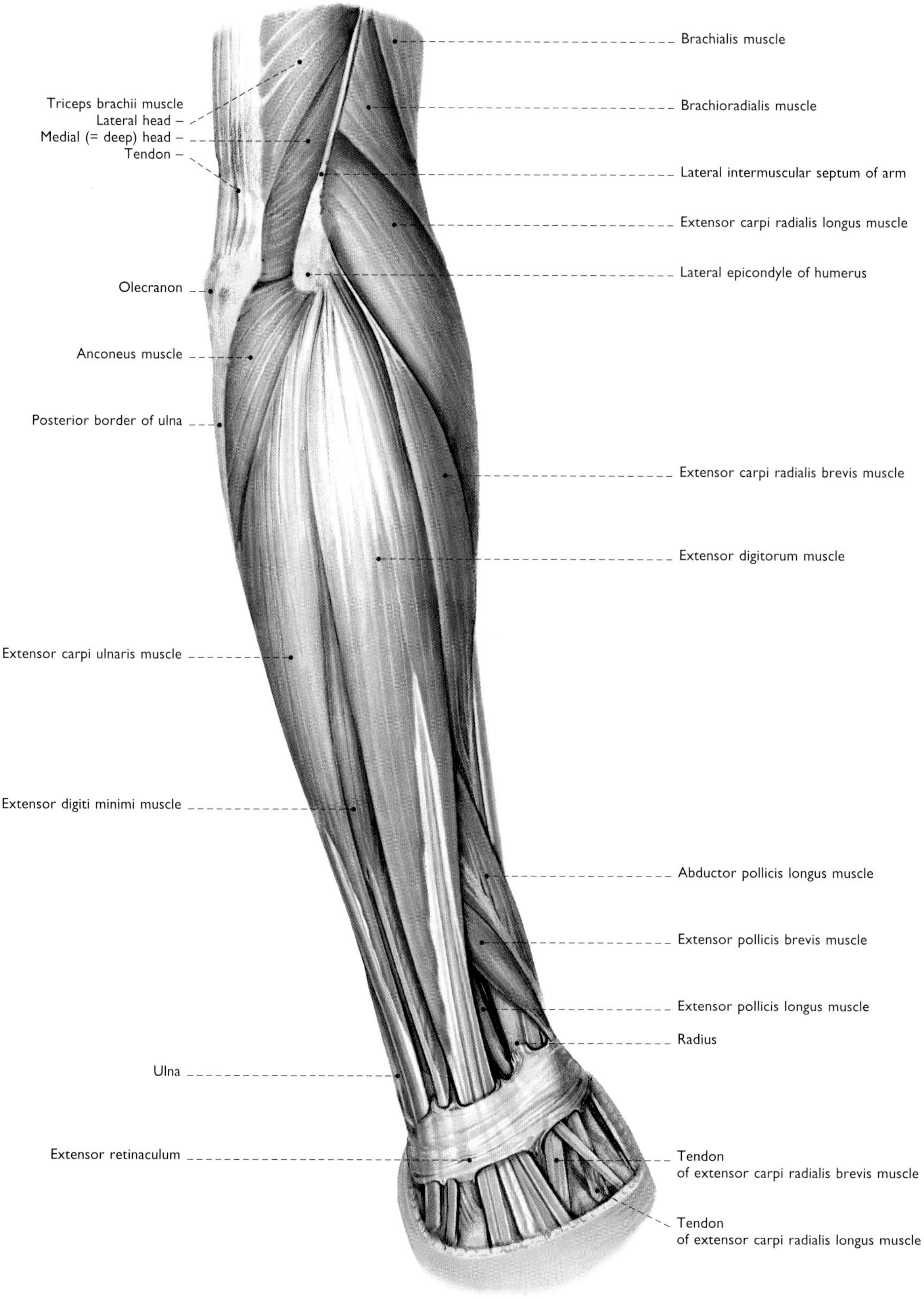

Brachialis muscle
Brachioradialis muscle
Lateral intermuscular septum of arm
Extensor carpi radialis longus muscle
Lateral epicondyle of humerus
Triceps brachii muscle
Lateral head
Medial (= deep) head
Tendon
Olecranon
Anconeus muscle
Posterior border of ulna
Extensor carpi radialis brevis muscle
Extensor digitorum muscle
Extensor carpi ulnaris muscle
Extensor digiti minimi muscle
Abductor pollicis longus muscle
Extensor pollicis brevis muscle
Extensor pollicis longus muscle
Radius
Ulna
Extensor retinaculum
Tendon of extensor carpi radialis brevis muscle
Tendon of extensor carpi radialis longus muscle

124 Muscles of the right forearm (50%)

Superficial layer. The forearm is slightly pronated.
Dorsolateral aspect

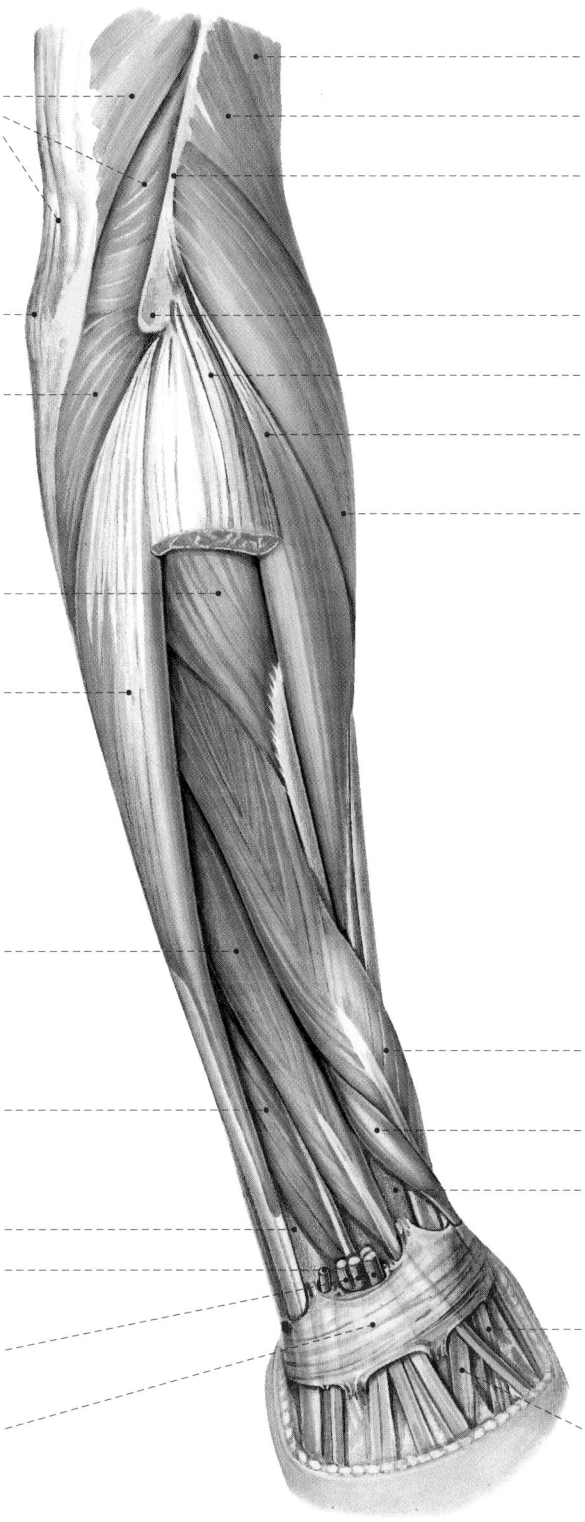
Triceps brachii muscle
Lateral head
Medial (= deep) head
Tendon
Olecranon
Anconeus muscle
Supinator muscle
Extensor carpi ulnaris muscle
Extensor pollicis longus muscle
Extensor indicis muscle
Ulna
Tendon of extensor digiti minimi muscle
Tendons of extensor digitorum muscle
Extensor retinaculum
Brachialis muscle
Brachioradialis muscle
Lateral intermuscular septum of arm
Lateral epicondyle of humerus
Antebrachial fascia,
Extensor digitorum muscle
Extensor carpi radialis brevis muscle
Extensor carpi radialis longus muscle
Abductor pollicis longus muscle
Extensor pollicis brevis muscle
Radius
Tendon of extensor carpi radialis longus muscle
Tendon of extensor carpi radialis brevis muscle

125 Muscles of the right forearm (50%)

Deep layer. The forearm is slightly pronated.
Dorsolateral aspect

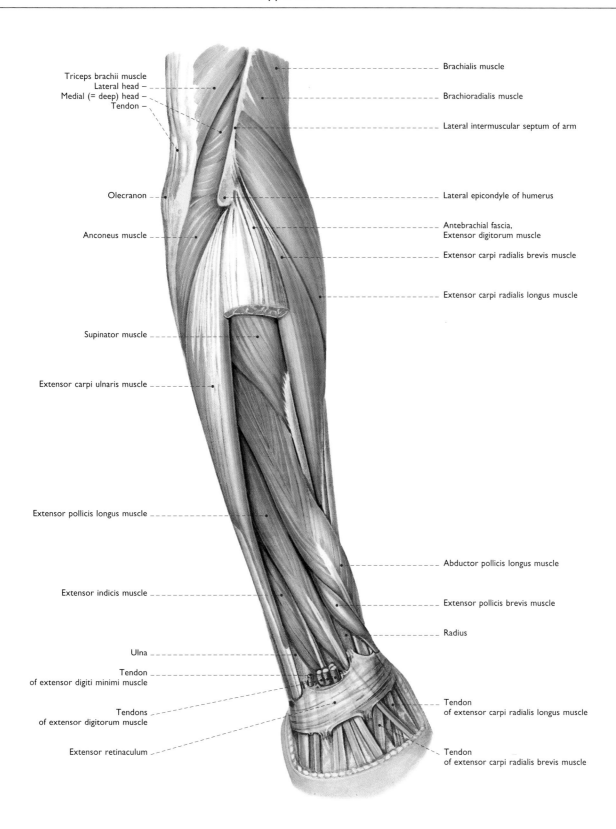

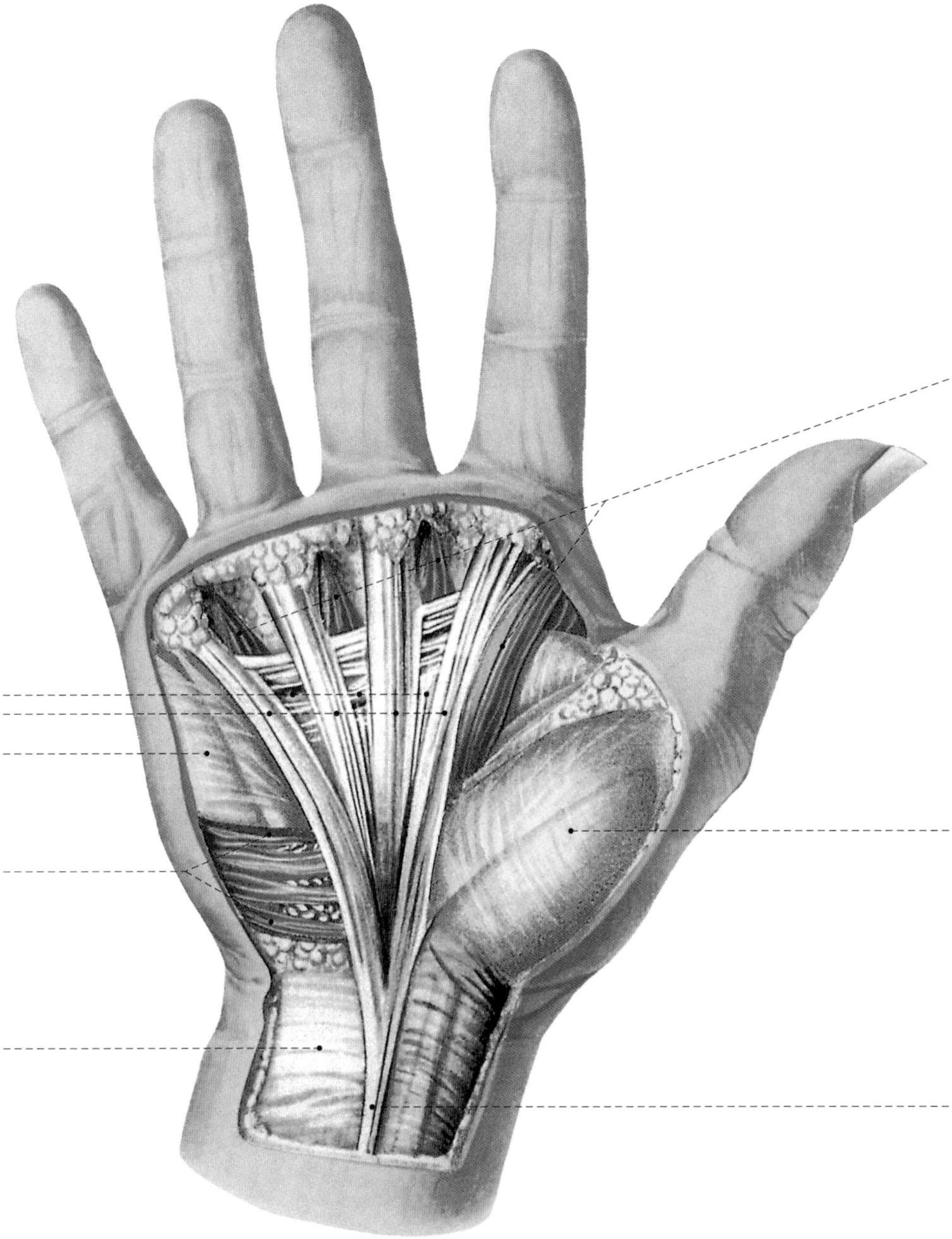
Lumbrical muscles IV–I
Palmar aponeurosis
⟨Transverse fascicles⟩
⟨Longitudinal fascicles⟩
Hypothenar eminence
Thenar eminence
Palmaris brevis muscle
Antebrachial fascia
Tendon
of palmaris longus muscle

126 Palmar aponeurosis of the right hand (75%)

Palmar aspect

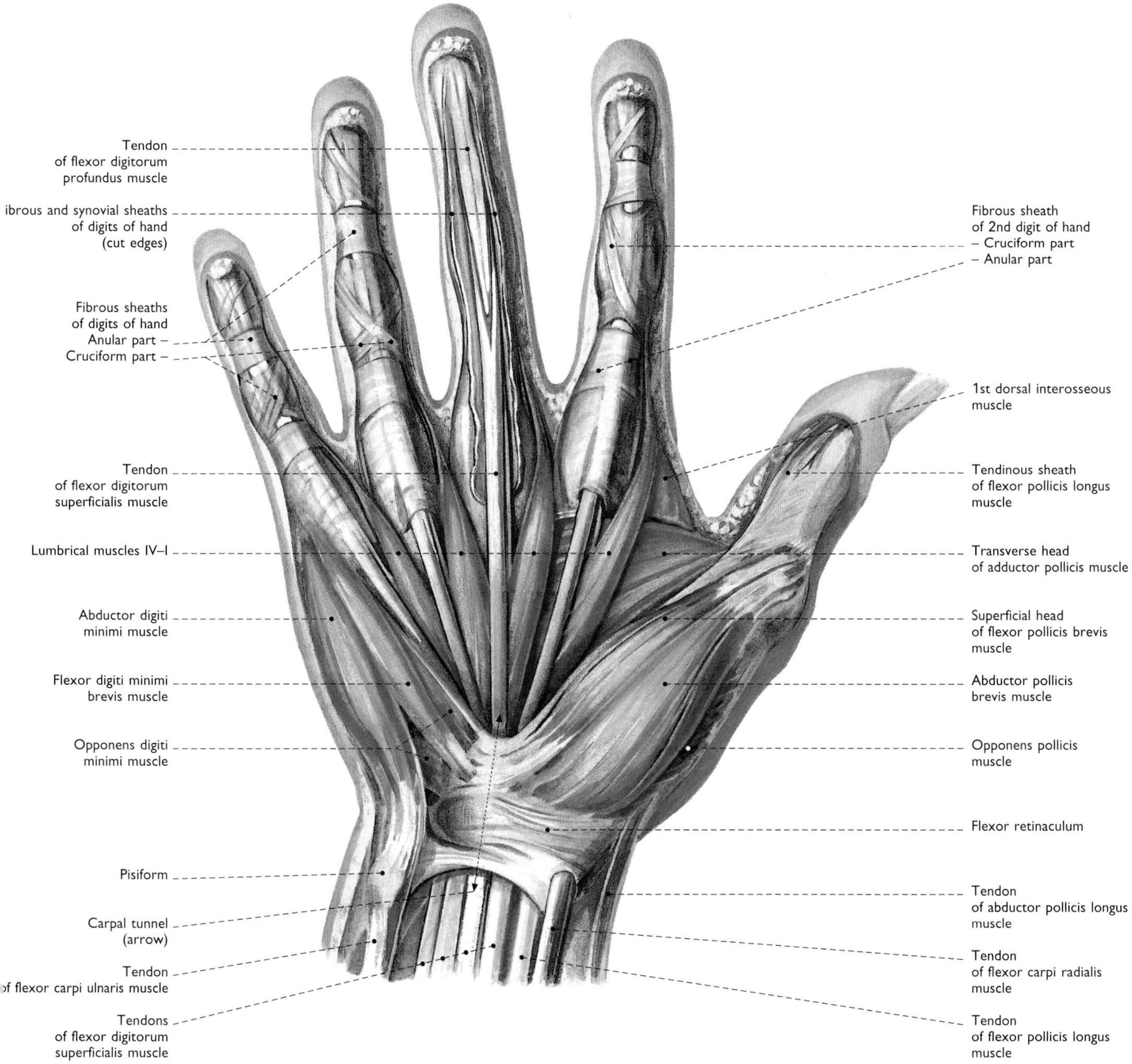
Tendon
of flexor digitorum
profundus muscle
ibrous and synovial sheaths
of digits of hand
(cut edges)
Fibrous sheaths
of digits of hand
Anular part –
Cruciform part –
Tendon
of flexor digitorum
superficialis muscle
Lumbrical muscles IV–I
Abductor digiti
minimi muscle
Flexor digiti minimi
brevis muscle
Opponens digiti
minimi muscle
Pisiform
Carpal tunnel
(arrow)
Tendon
of flexor carpi ulnaris muscle
Tendons
of flexor digitorum
superficialis muscle
Fibrous sheath
of 2nd digit of hand
– Cruciform part
– Anular part
1st dorsal interosseous
muscle
Tendinous sheath
of flexor pollicis longus
muscle
Transverse head
of adductor pollicis muscle
Superficial head
of flexor pollicis brevis
muscle
Abductor pollicis
brevis muscle
Opponens pollicis
muscle
Flexor retinaculum
Tendon
of abductor pollicis longus
muscle
Tendon
of flexor carpi radialis
muscle
Tendon
of flexor pollicis longus
muscle

127 Muscles of the right hand (75%)

Superficial layer. The palmar aponeurosis was removed.
Palmar aspect

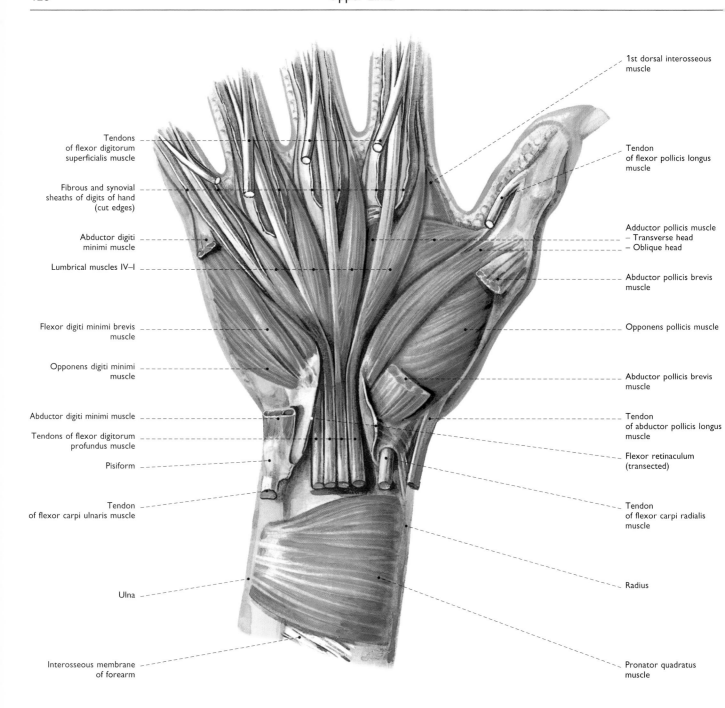

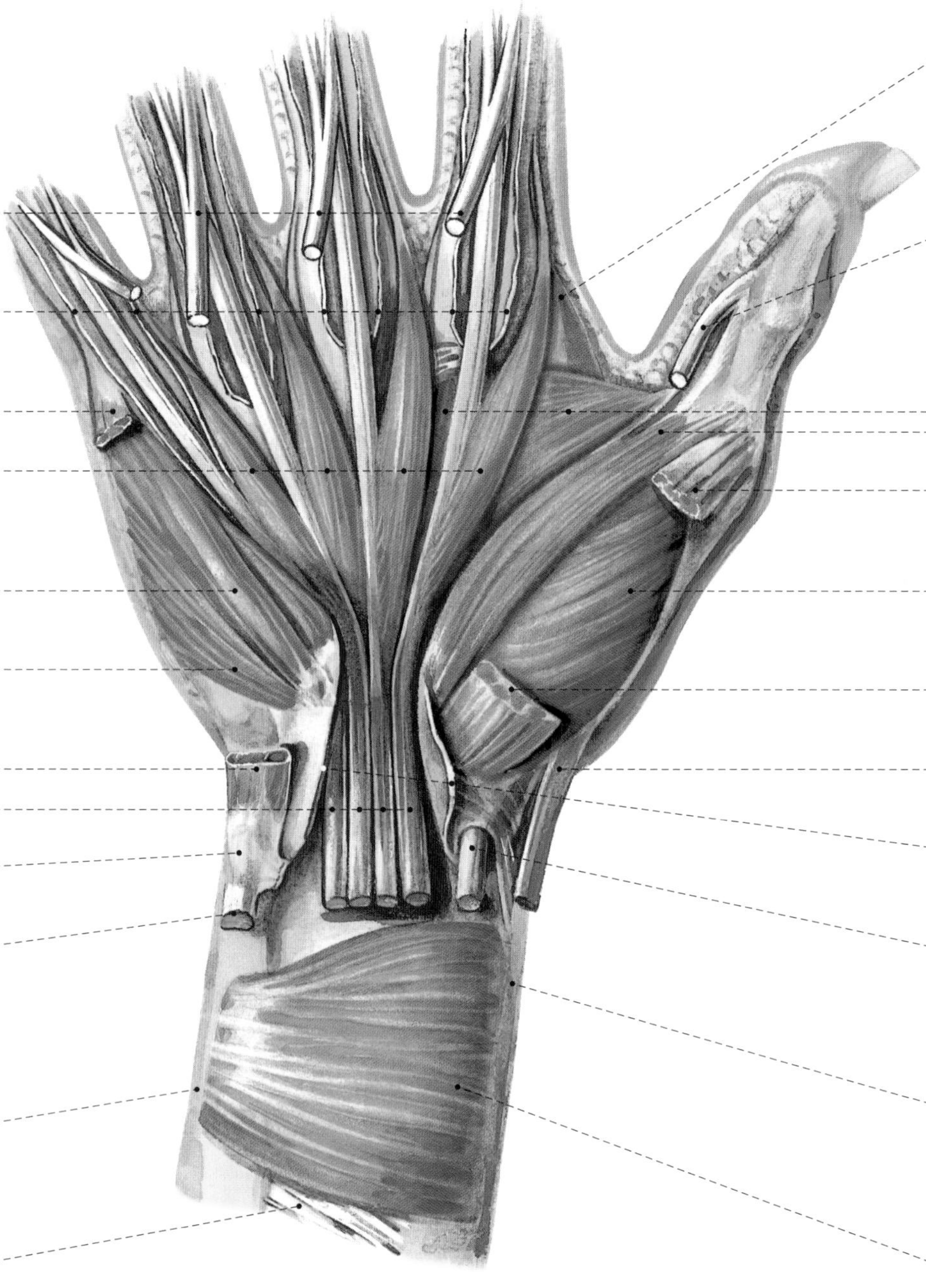
1st dorsal interosseous muscle
Tendons of flexor digitorum superficialis muscle
Tendon of flexor pollicis longus muscle
Fibrous and synovial sheaths of digits of hand (cut edges)
Adductor pollicis muscle
– Transverse head
– Oblique head
Abductor digiti minimi muscle
Lumbrical muscles IV–I
Abductor pollicis brevis muscle
Flexor digiti minimi brevis muscle
Opponens pollicis muscle
Opponens digiti minimi muscle
Abductor pollicis brevis muscle
Abductor digiti minimi muscle
Tendon of abductor pollicis longus muscle
Tendons of flexor digitorum profundus muscle
Flexor retinaculum (transected)
Pisiform
Tendon of flexor carpi ulnaris muscle
Tendon of flexor carpi radialis muscle
Radius
Ulna
Interosseous membrane of forearm
Pronator quadratus muscle

128 Muscles of the right hand (75%)

Superficial layer. The flexor digitorum superficialis muscle was removed and the carpal tunnel opened.
Palmar aspect

a

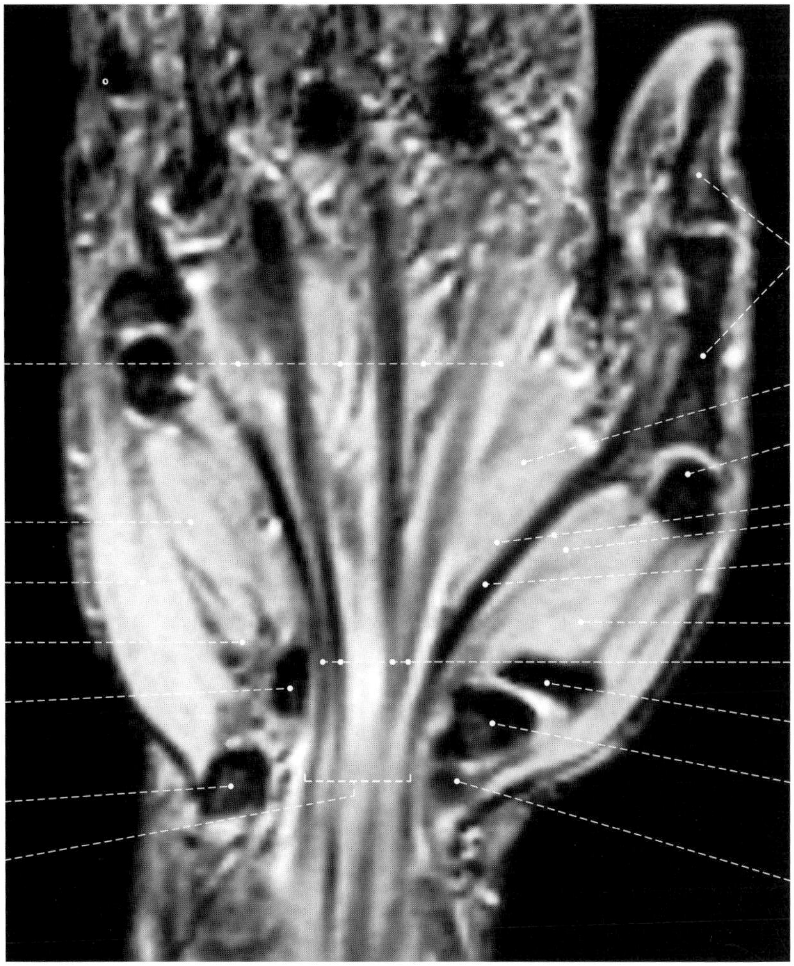

Lumbrical muscles IV–I
Opponens digiti minimi muscle
Abductor digiti minimi muscle
Flexor digiti minimi brevis muscle
Hook of hamate
Pisiform
Carpal tunnel
Thumb
– Distal phalanx
– Proximal phalanx
Adductor pollicis muscle
Head of 1st metacarpal bone
Flexor pollicis brevis muscle
– Deep head
– Superficial head
Tendon of flexor pollicis longus muscle
Opponens pollicis muscle
Tendons of flexor digitorum profundus muscle
Base of 1st metacarpal bone
Trapezium
Tubercle of scaphoid

b

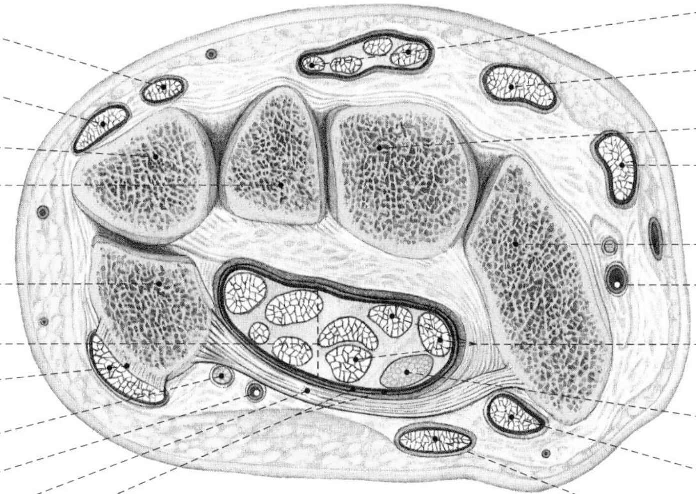

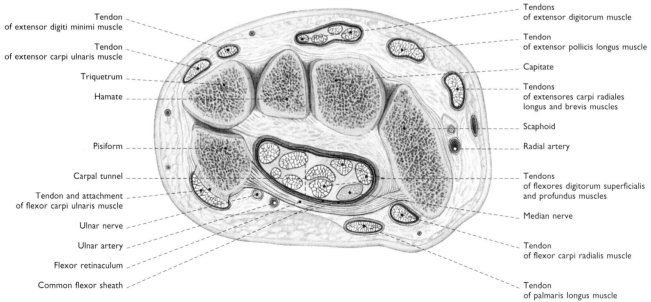

Tendon of extensor digiti minimi muscle
Tendon of extensor carpi ulnaris muscle
Triquetrum
Hamate
Pisiform
Carpal tunnel
Tendon and attachment of flexor carpi ulnaris muscle
Ulnar nerve
Ulnar artery
Flexor retinaculum
Common flexor sheath
Tendons of extensor digitorum muscle
Tendon of extensor pollicis longus muscle
Capitate
Tendons of extensores carpi radiales longus and brevis muscles
Scaphoid
Radial artery
Tendons of flexores digitorum superficialis and profundus muscles
Median nerve
Tendon of flexor carpi radialis muscle
Tendon of palmaris longus muscle

129 Muscles of the right hand

a Radio-ulnar (coronal) magnetic resonance image (MRI, T_2-weighted) (100%)

b Axial (transverse) section through the wrist and the carpal tunnel (140%), hand in pronated position, distal aspect

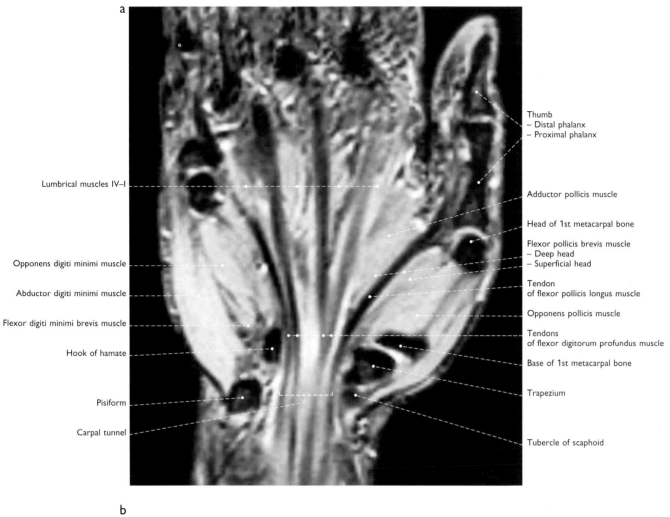

a

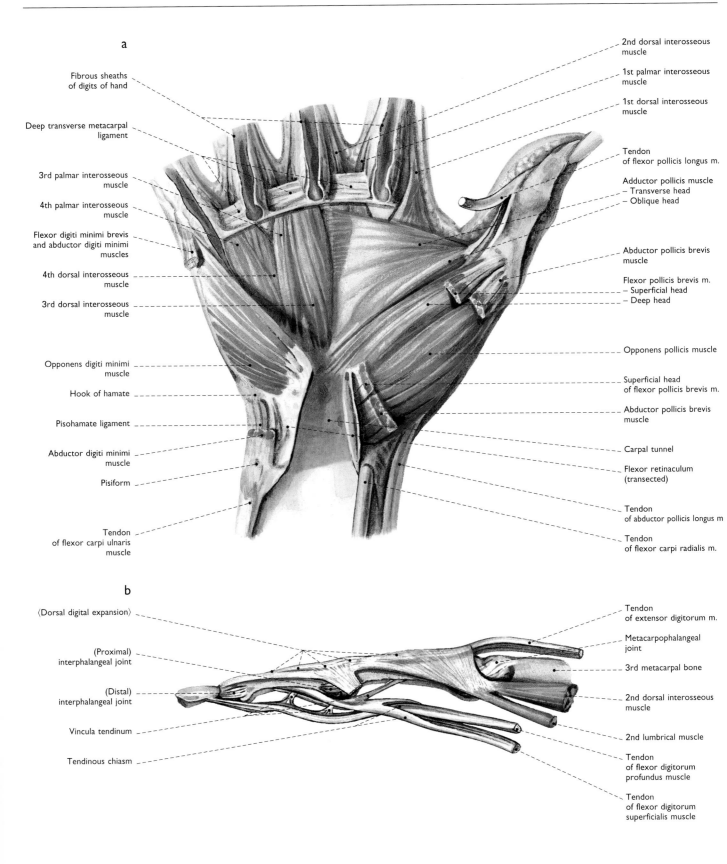

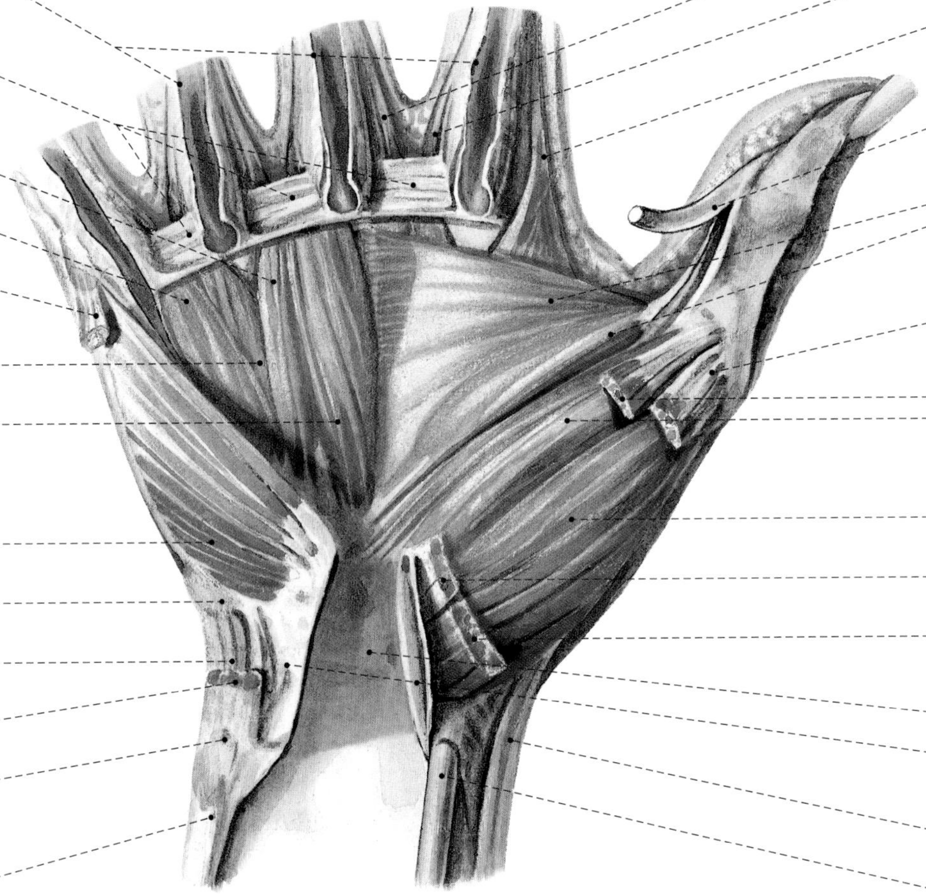
Fibrous sheaths of digits of hand
Deep transverse metacarpal ligament
3rd palmar interosseous muscle
4th palmar interosseous muscle
Flexor digiti minimi brevis and abductor digiti minimi muscles
4th dorsal interosseous muscle
3rd dorsal interosseous muscle
Opponens digiti minimi muscle
Hook of hamate
Pisohamate ligament
Abductor digiti minimi muscle
Pisiform
Tendon of flexor carpi ulnaris muscle
2nd dorsal interosseous muscle
1st palmar interosseous muscle
1st dorsal interosseous muscle
Tendon of flexor pollicis longus m.
Adductor pollicis muscle
– Transverse head
– Oblique head
Abductor pollicis brevis muscle
Flexor pollicis brevis m.
– Superficial head
– Deep head
Opponens pollicis muscle
Superficial head of flexor pollicis brevis m.
Abductor pollicis brevis muscle
Carpal tunnel
Flexor retinaculum (transected)
Tendon of abductor pollicis longus m
Tendon of flexor carpi radialis m.

b

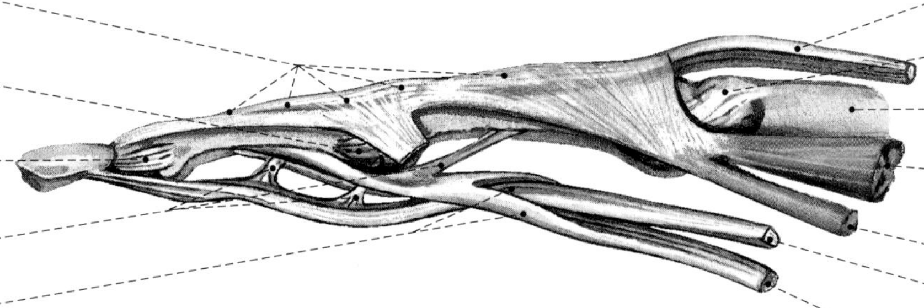
⟨Dorsal digital expansion⟩
(Proximal) interphalangeal joint
(Distal) interphalangeal joint
Vincula tendinum
Tendinous chiasm
Tendon of extensor digitorum m.
Metacarpophalangeal joint
3rd metacarpal bone
2nd dorsal interosseous muscle
2nd lumbrical muscle
Tendon of flexor digitorum profundus muscle
Tendon of flexor digitorum superficialis muscle

130 Muscles of the right hand (75%)

a Deep layer, palmar aspect
b Middle finger with the dorsal digital expansion, radial aspect

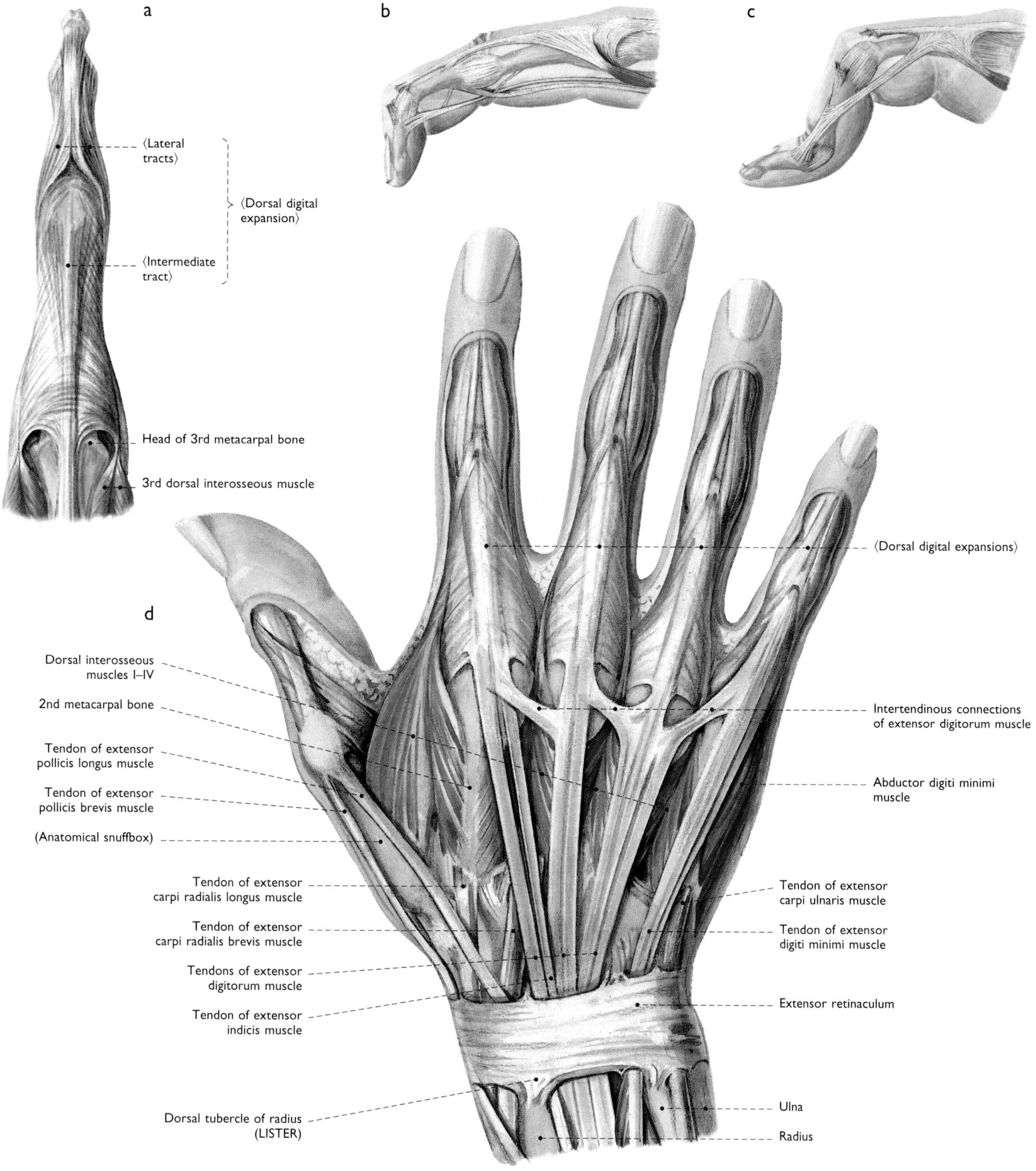
a
b
c
⟨Lateral tracts⟩
⟨Dorsal digital expansion⟩
⟨Intermediate tract⟩
Head of 3rd metacarpal bone
3rd dorsal interosseous muscle
d
⟨Dorsal digital expansions⟩
Dorsal interosseous muscles I–IV
2nd metacarpal bone
Tendon of extensor pollicis longus muscle
Tendon of extensor pollicis brevis muscle
(Anatomical snuffbox)
Intertendinous connections of extensor digitorum muscle
Abductor digiti minimi muscle
Tendon of extensor carpi radialis longus muscle
Tendon of extensor carpi radialis brevis muscle
Tendons of extensor digitorum muscle
Tendon of extensor indicis muscle
Tendon of extensor carpi ulnaris muscle
Tendon of extensor digiti minimi muscle
Extensor retinaculum
Dorsal tubercle of radius (LISTER)
Ulna
Radius

131 Muscles of the right hand

a Muscles of the dorsum and dorsal digital expansion of the middle finger (75%), dorsal aspect

b, c Ruptures of the dorsal digital expansion above the distal (b) and proximal (c) interphalangeal joints (50%)

d Muscles of the dorsum of hand (75%), dorsal aspect

a

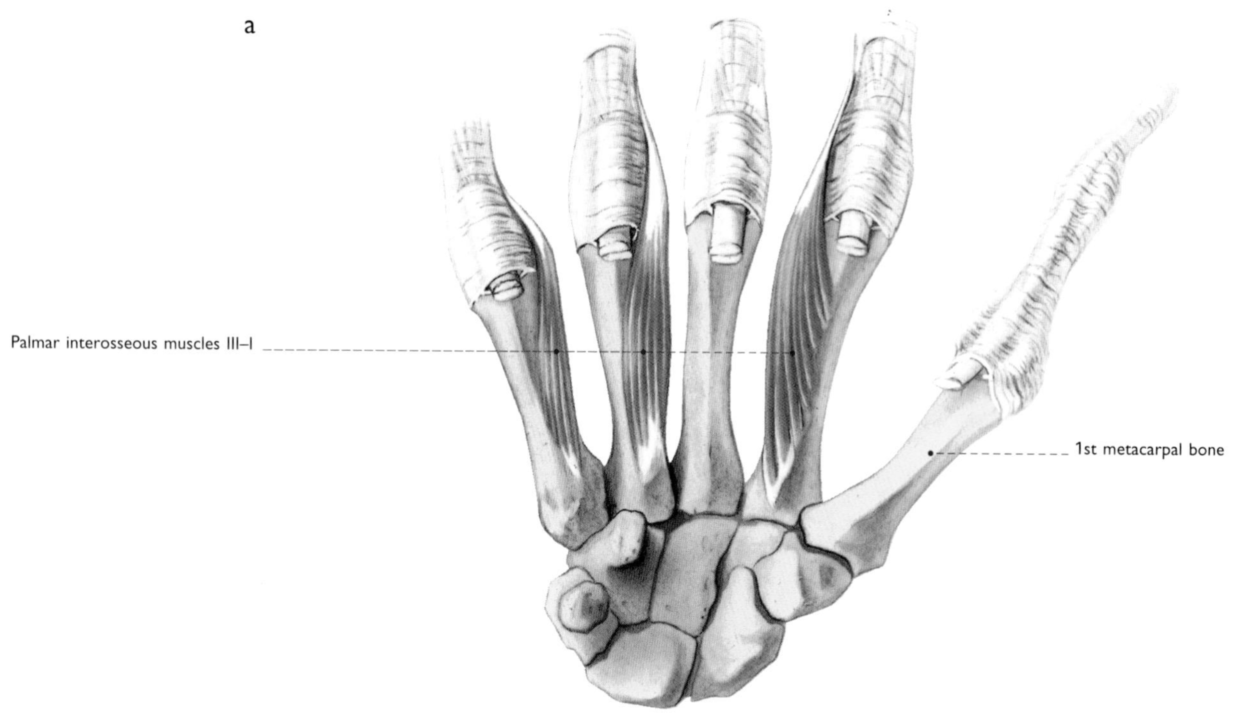
Palmar interosseous muscles III–I
1st metacarpal bone

b

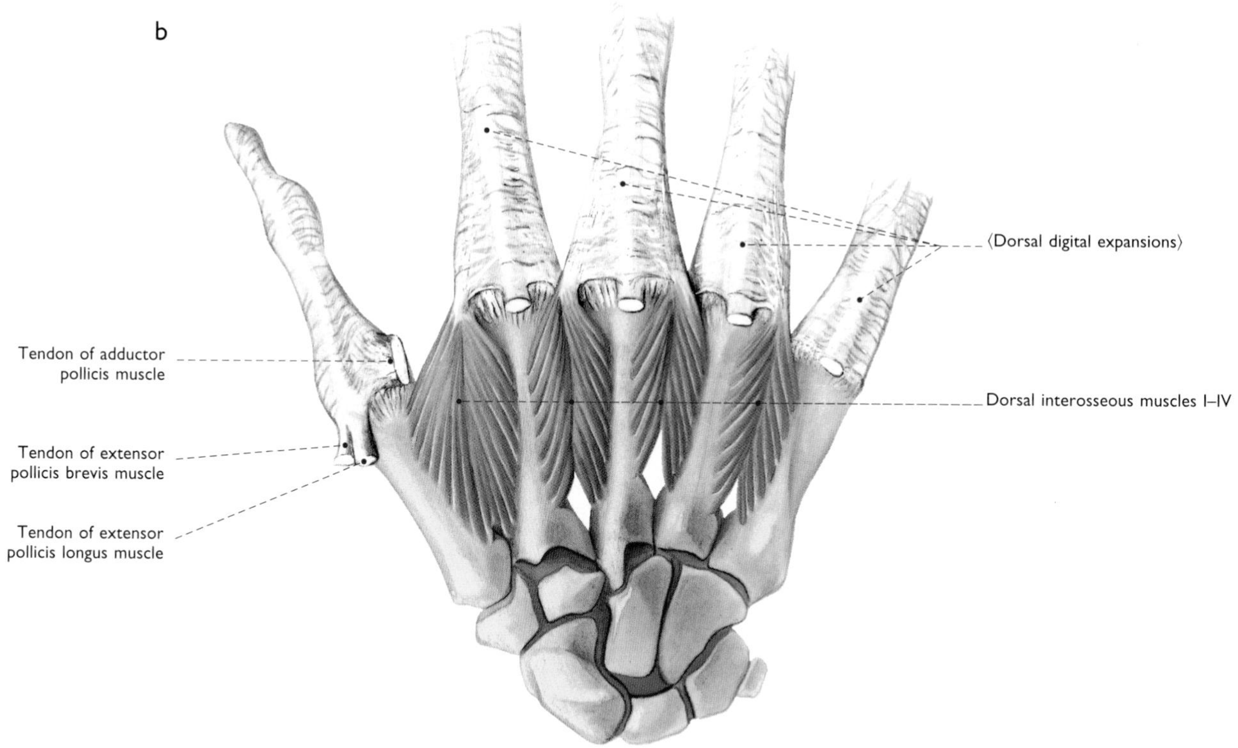
⟨Dorsal digital expansions⟩
Tendon of adductor pollicis muscle
Dorsal interosseous muscles I–IV
Tendon of extensor pollicis brevis muscle
Tendon of extensor pollicis longus muscle

132 Interosseous muscles of the right hand (75%)

a Palmar interosseous muscles, palmar aspect
b Dorsal interosseous muscles, dorsal aspect

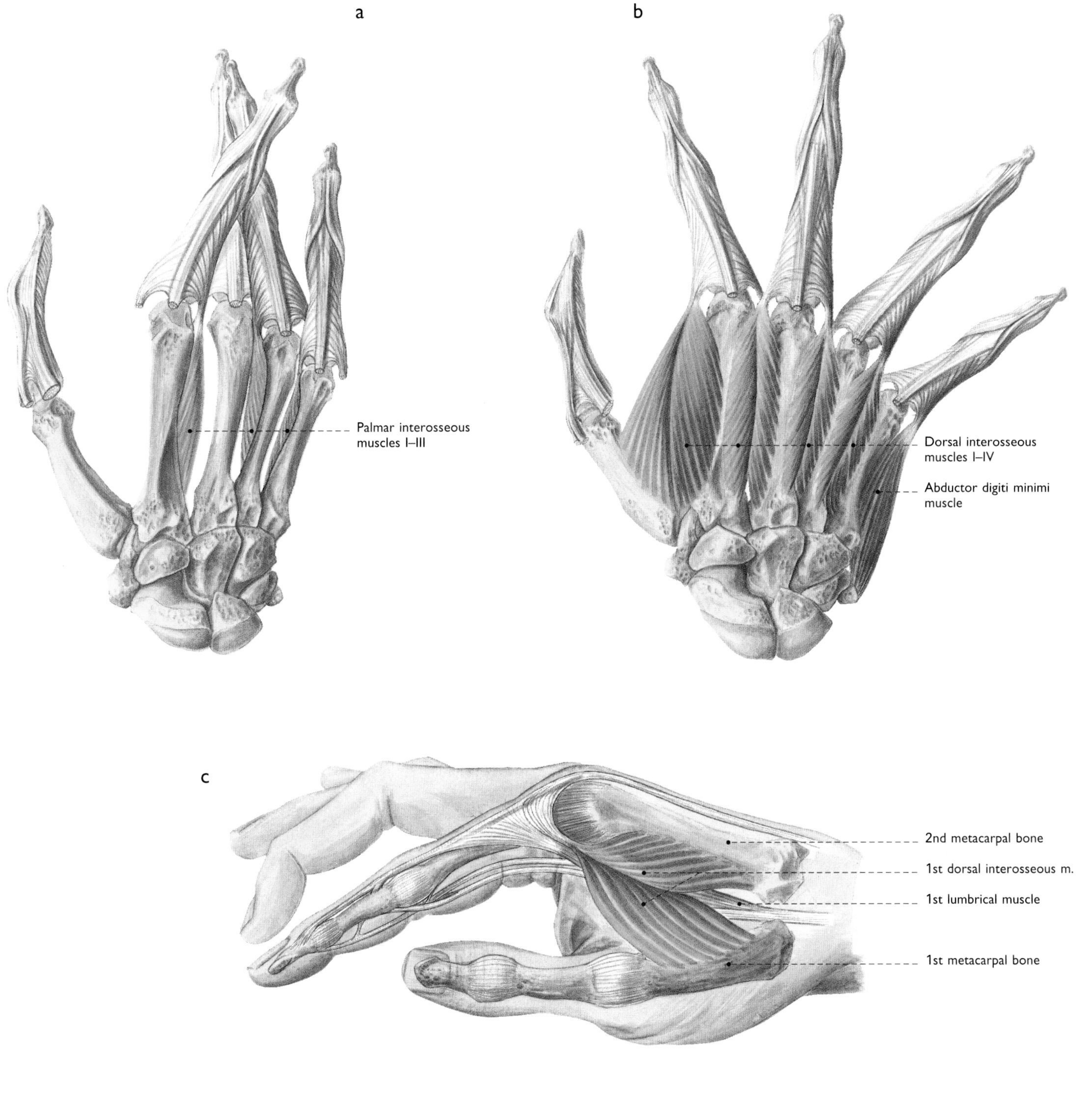
a
Palmar interosseous muscles I–III
b
Dorsal interosseous muscles I–IV
Abductor digiti minimi muscle
c
2nd metacarpal bone
1st dorsal interosseous m.
1st lumbrical muscle
1st metacarpal bone

133 Interosseous and lumbrical muscles of the right hand (60%)

a Function of the palmar interosseous muscles, dorsal aspect
b Function of the dorsal interosseous muscles, dorsal aspect
c Function of the first lumbrical and first dorsal interosseous muscles, radial aspect

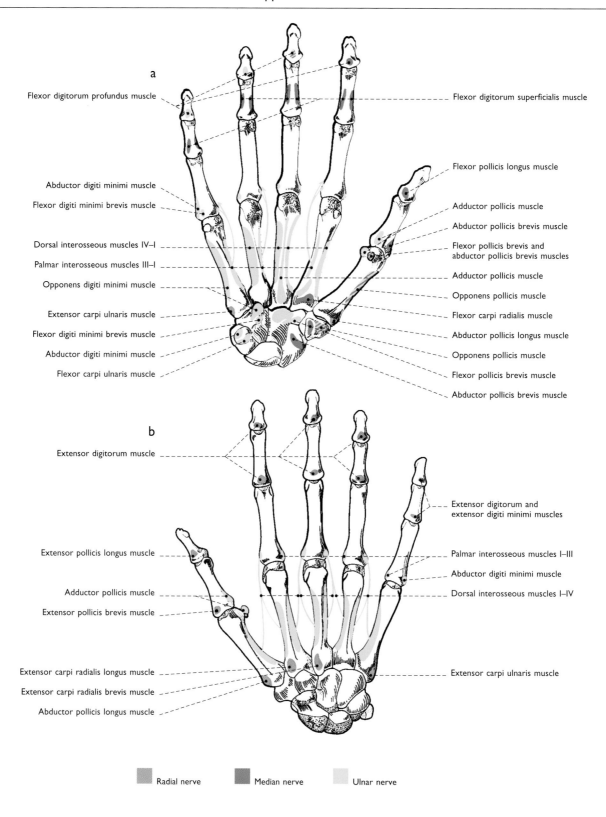

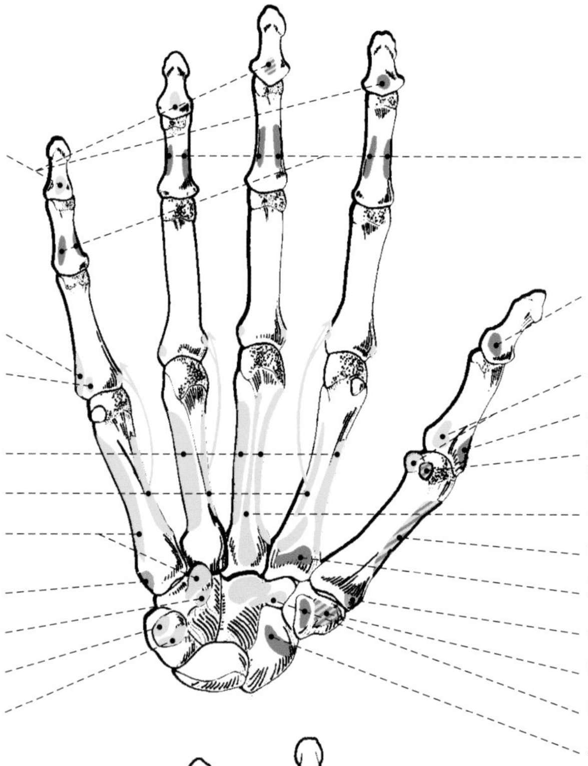
a
Flexor digitorum profundus muscle
Abductor digiti minimi muscle
Flexor digiti minimi brevis muscle
Dorsal interosseous muscles IV–I
Palmar interosseous muscles III–I
Opponens digiti minimi muscle
Extensor carpi ulnaris muscle
Flexor digiti minimi brevis muscle
Abductor digiti minimi muscle
Flexor carpi ulnaris muscle
Flexor digitorum superficialis muscle
Flexor pollicis longus muscle
Adductor pollicis muscle
Abductor pollicis brevis muscle
Flexor pollicis brevis and abductor pollicis brevis muscles
Adductor pollicis muscle
Opponens pollicis muscle
Flexor carpi radialis muscle
Abductor pollicis longus muscle
Opponens pollicis muscle
Flexor pollicis brevis muscle
Abductor pollicis brevis muscle

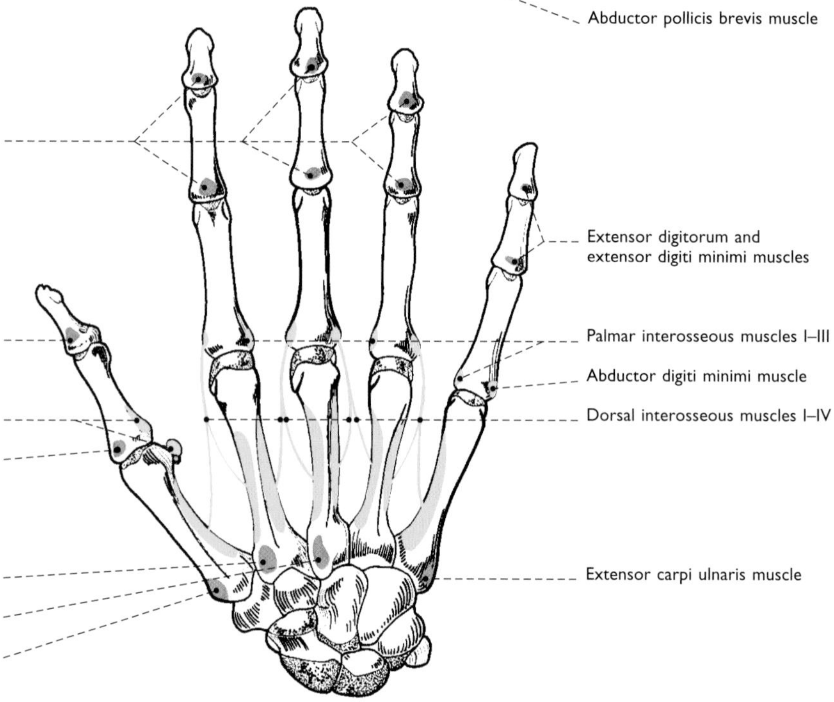
b
Extensor digitorum muscle
Extensor pollicis longus muscle
Adductor pollicis muscle
Extensor pollicis brevis muscle
Extensor carpi radialis longus muscle
Extensor carpi radialis brevis muscle
Abductor pollicis longus muscle
Extensor digitorum and extensor digiti minimi muscles
Palmar interosseous muscles I–III
Abductor digiti minimi muscle
Dorsal interosseous muscles I–IV
Extensor carpi ulnaris muscle

Radial nerve Median nerve Ulnar nerve

134 Muscle attachments to the bones of the right hand

The colors indicate the innervation of the muscles attaching to the

a palmar surface

b dorsal surface.

a

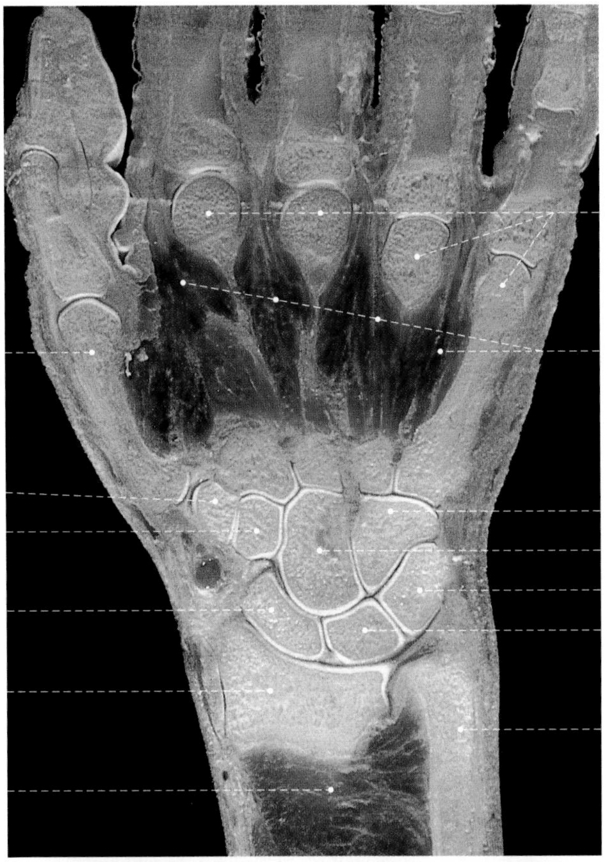
Heads of metacarpals II–V
1st metacarpal bone
Dorsal interosseous muscles I–IV
Trapezium
Trapezoid
Hamate
Capitate
Triquetrum
Scaphoid
Lunate
Radius
Ulna
Pronator quadratus muscle

b

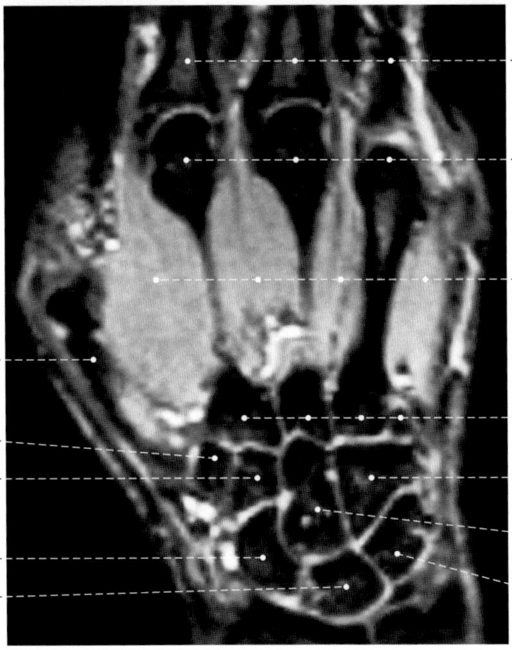
Proximal phalanges of digits II–IV
Heads of metacarpals II–IV
Dorsal interosseous muscles I–IV
1st metacarpal bone
Bases of metacarpals II–V
Trapezium
Trapezoid
Hamate
Capitate
Scaphoid
Triquetrum
Lunate

135 Dorsal interosseous muscles of the right hand (75%)

a Anatomical radio-ulnar (coronal) section, dorsal aspect
b Radio-ulnar (coronal) magnetic resonance image (MRI, T_2-weighted) of the wrist and the metacarpus

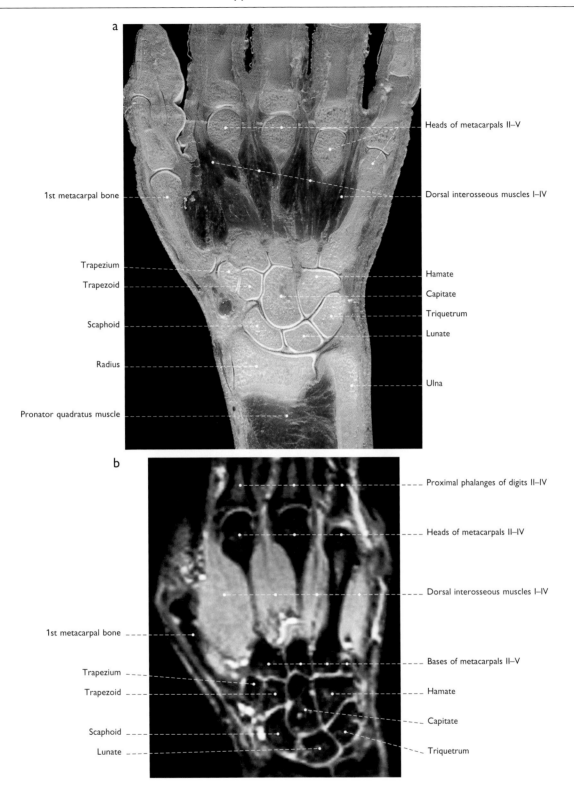

a

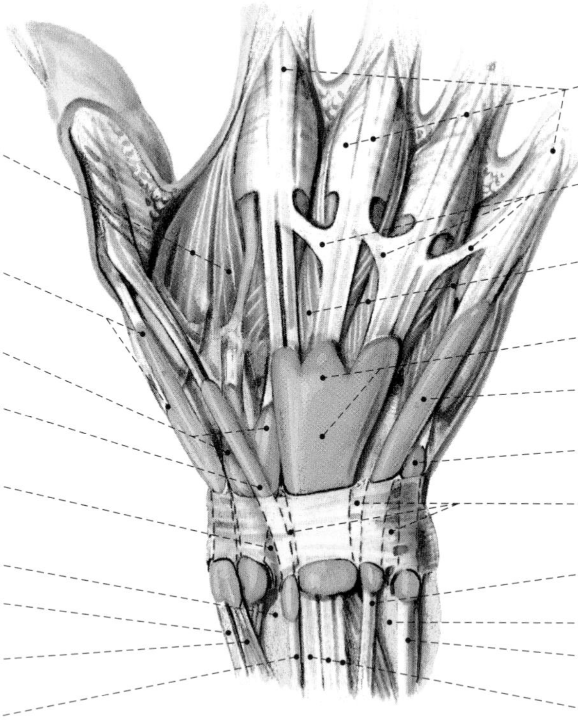
1st dorsal interosseous muscle
Tendinous sheath of abductor longus and extensor pollicis brevis muscles
Tendinous sheath of extensores carpi radiales muscles
Tendinous sheath of extensor pollicis longus muscle
Dorsal tubercle of radius (LISTER)
Radius
Tendon of abductor pollicis longus muscle
Tendon of extensor pollicis brevis muscle
Tendon of extensor pollicis longus muscle
⟨Dorsal digital expansions⟩
Intertendinous connections of extensor digitorum muscle
Dorsal interosseous muscles II–IV
Tendinous sheath of extensor digitorum and extensor indicis muscles
Tendinous sheath of extensor digiti minimi muscle
Tendinous sheath of extensor carpi ulnaris muscle
Extensor retinaculum
Tendon of extensor digiti minimi muscle
Ulna
Tendon of extensor carpi ulnaris muscle
Tendons of extensor digitorum muscle

b

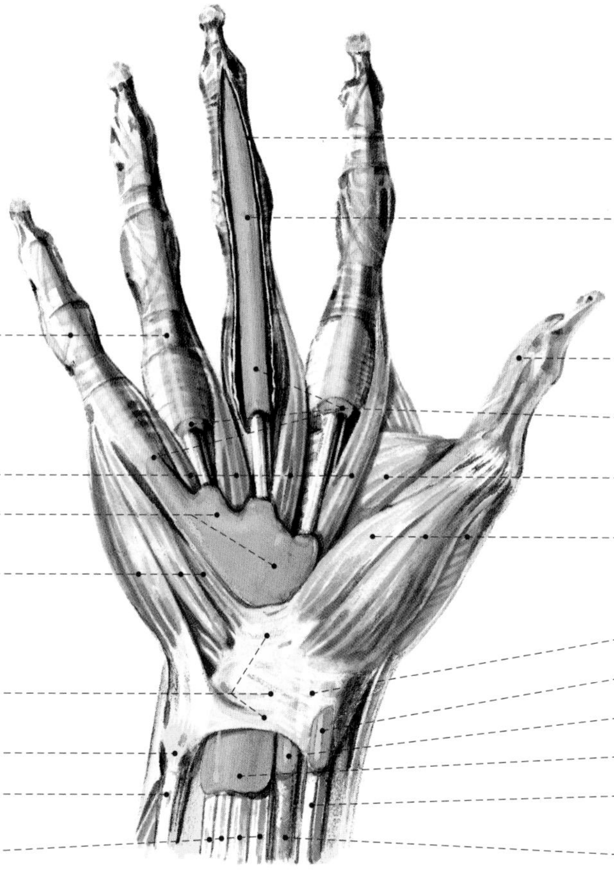
Fibrous sheaths of digits of hand
Lumbrical muscles IV–I
Common flexor sheath
Abductor digiti minimi muscle, Flexor digiti minimi brevis muscle, Opponens digiti minimi muscle
Flexor retinaculum
Pisiform
Tendon of flexor carpi ulnaris muscle
Tendons of flexor digitorum superficialis muscle
Fibrous sheath of 3rd digit of hand (cut edge)
Synovial sheath of 3rd digit of hand
Tendinous sheath of flexor pollicis longus muscle
Synovial sheaths of digits of hand
Adductor pollicis muscle
Flexor pollicis brevis muscle, Abductor pollicis brevis muscle, Opponens pollicis muscle
Tubercle of scaphoid
Tendinous sheath of flexor carpi radialis m.
Tendinous sheath of flexor pollicis longus m.
Common flexor sheath
Tendon of flexor carpi radialis muscle
Tendon of flexor pollicis longus muscle

136 Tendinous sheaths on the wrist and the fingers of the right hand (50%)

a Dorsal aspect
b Palmar aspect

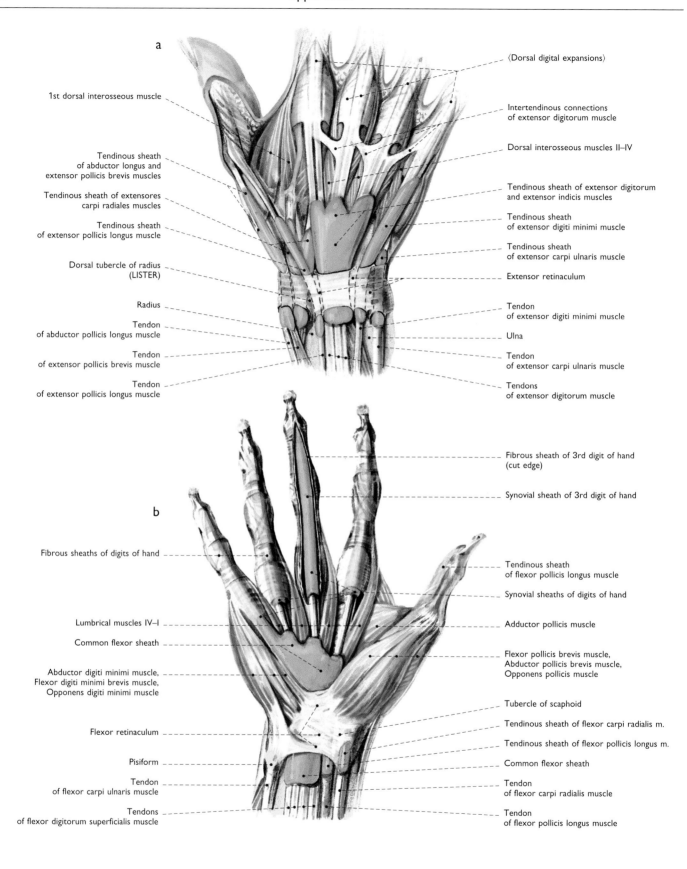

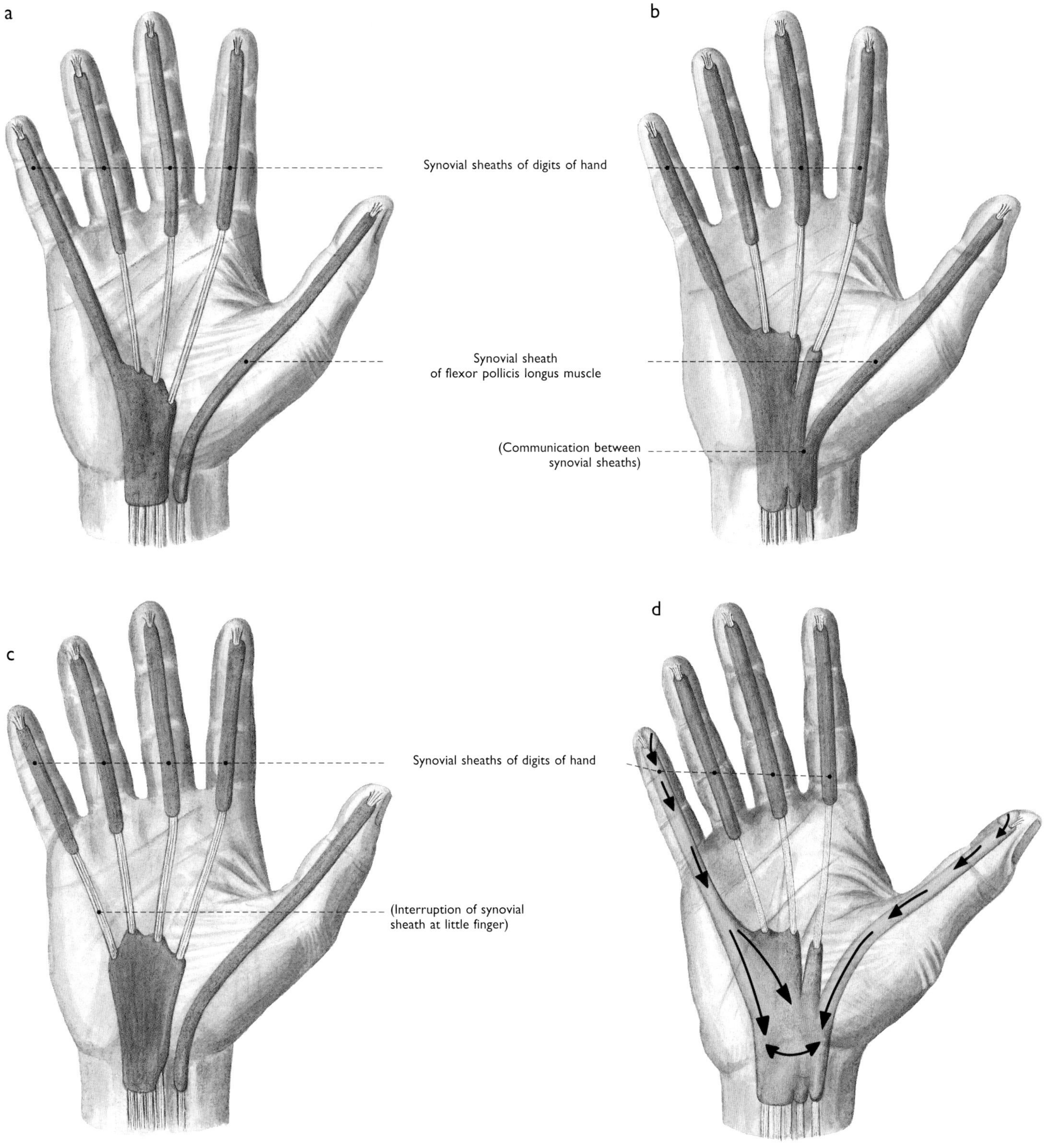
a
b
Synovial sheaths of digits of hand
Synovial sheath
of flexor pollicis longus muscle
(Communication between
synovial sheaths)
c
d
Synovial sheaths of digits of hand
(Interruption of synovial
sheath at little finger)

137 Tendinous sheaths on the wrist and the fingers of the right hand (40%)

Palmar aspect

- a Usual arrangement
- b Most common variation
- c Other common variation
- d V-phlegmona following an abscess at the distal phalanx of the thumb or the little finger

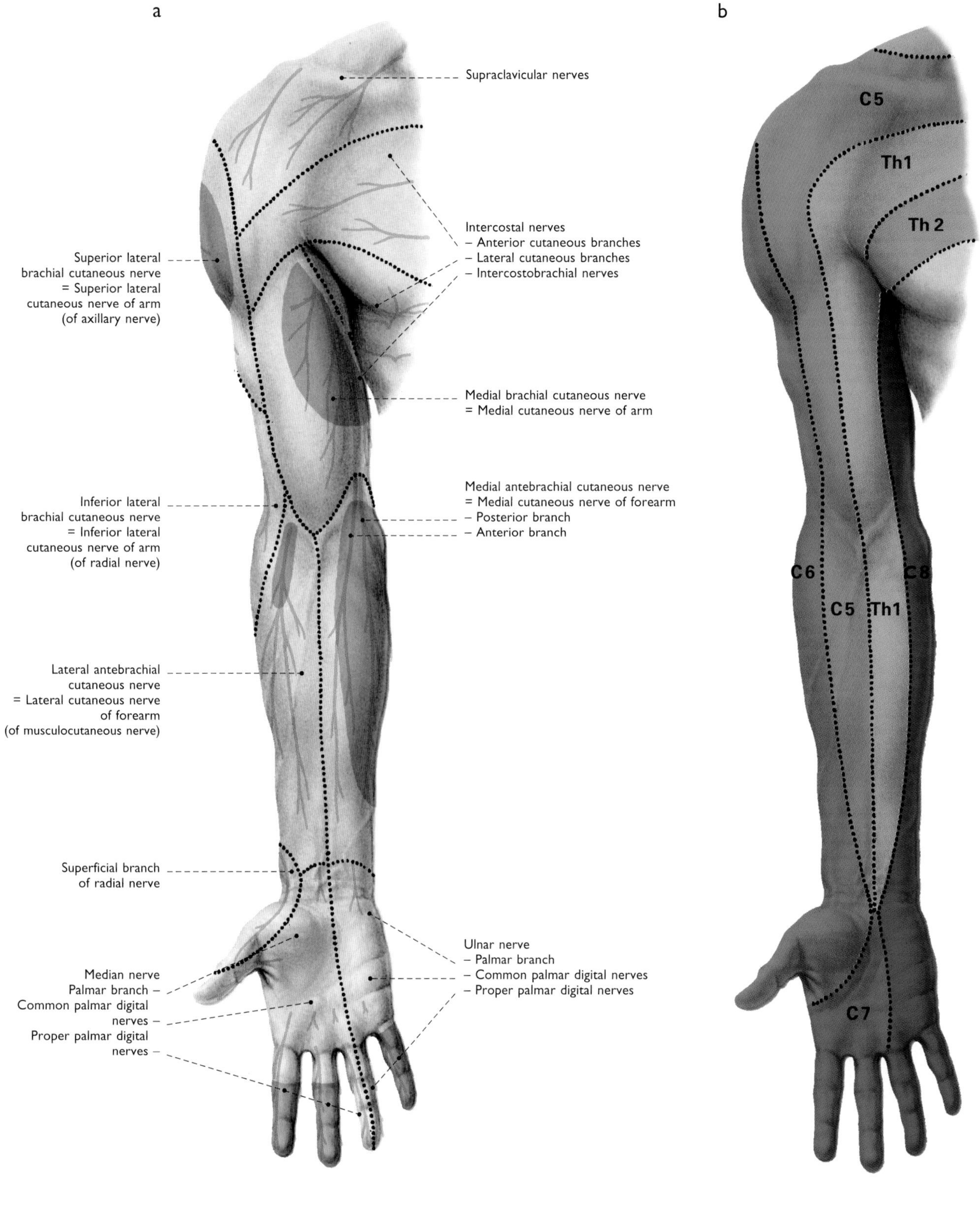
a
Supraclavicular nerves
Intercostal nerves
– Anterior cutaneous branches
– Lateral cutaneous branches
– Intercostobrachial nerves
Superior lateral brachial cutaneous nerve = Superior lateral cutaneous nerve of arm (of axillary nerve)
Medial brachial cutaneous nerve = Medial cutaneous nerve of arm
Medial antebrachial cutaneous nerve = Medial cutaneous nerve of forearm
– Posterior branch
– Anterior branch
Inferior lateral brachial cutaneous nerve = Inferior lateral cutaneous nerve of arm (of radial nerve)
Lateral antebrachial cutaneous nerve = Lateral cutaneous nerve of forearm (of musculocutaneous nerve)
Superficial branch of radial nerve
Ulnar nerve
– Palmar branch
– Common palmar digital nerves
– Proper palmar digital nerves
Median nerve
Palmar branch –
Common palmar digital nerves –
Proper palmar digital nerves –
b
C5
Th1
Th 2
C6
C8
C5
Th1
C7

138 Cutaneous and segmental innervation of the right upper limb (25%)

Schematic representations, ventral aspect

a Cutaneous nerves and areas of distribution, the autonomic areas of the different nerves are given in a darker gray.

b Segmental innervation (dermatomes)

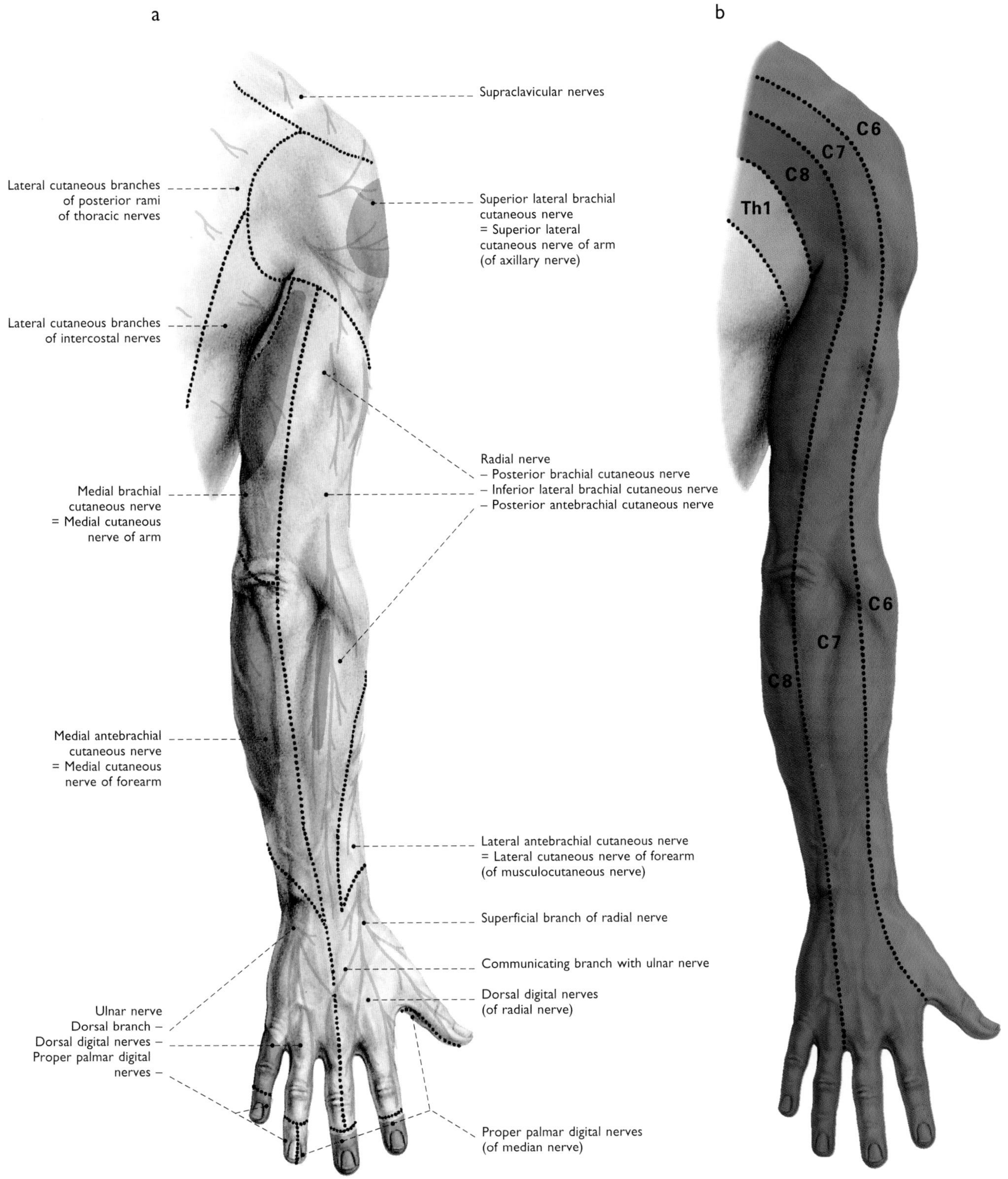
a
b
Supraclavicular nerves
Lateral cutaneous branches of posterior rami of thoracic nerves
Superior lateral brachial cutaneous nerve = Superior lateral cutaneous nerve of arm (of axillary nerve)
Lateral cutaneous branches of intercostal nerves
Radial nerve
– Posterior brachial cutaneous nerve
– Inferior lateral brachial cutaneous nerve
– Posterior antebrachial cutaneous nerve
Medial brachial cutaneous nerve = Medial cutaneous nerve of arm
Medial antebrachial cutaneous nerve = Medial cutaneous nerve of forearm
Lateral antebrachial cutaneous nerve = Lateral cutaneous nerve of forearm (of musculocutaneous nerve)
Superficial branch of radial nerve
Communicating branch with ulnar nerve
Dorsal digital nerves (of radial nerve)
Ulnar nerve
Dorsal branch –
Dorsal digital nerves –
Proper palmar digital nerves –
Proper palmar digital nerves (of median nerve)
C6
C7
C8
Th1
C6
C7
C8

139 Cutaneous and segmental innervation of the right upper limb (25%)

Schematic representations, dorsal aspect

a Cutaneous nerves and areas of distribution, the autonomic areas of the different nerves are given in a darker gray.

b Segmental innervation (dermatomes)

a

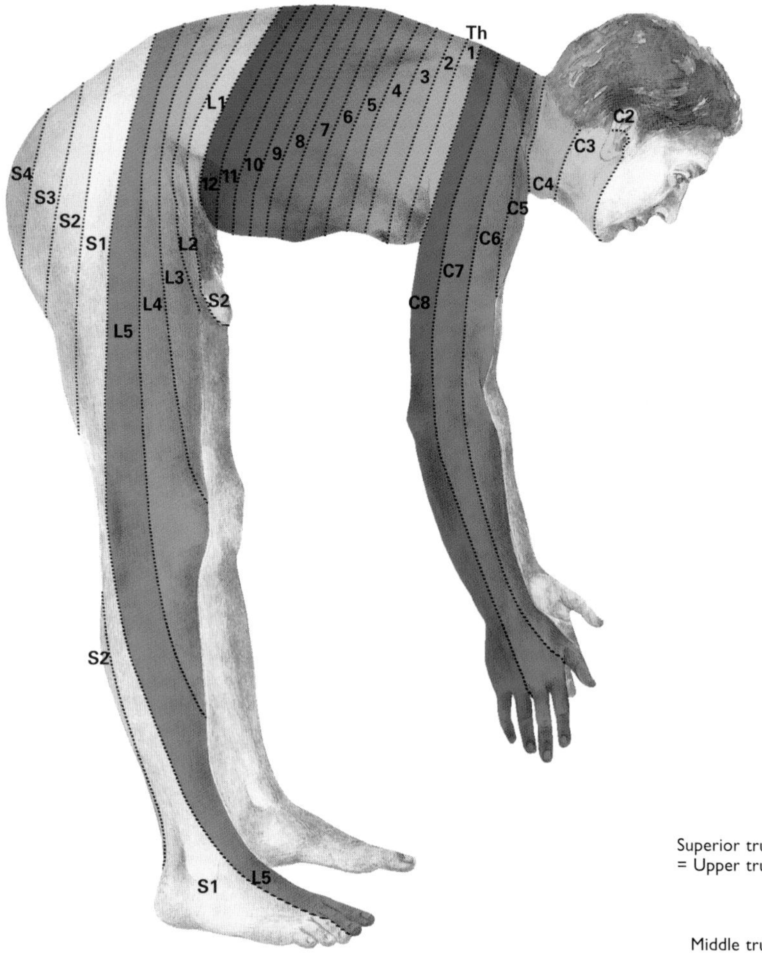

b

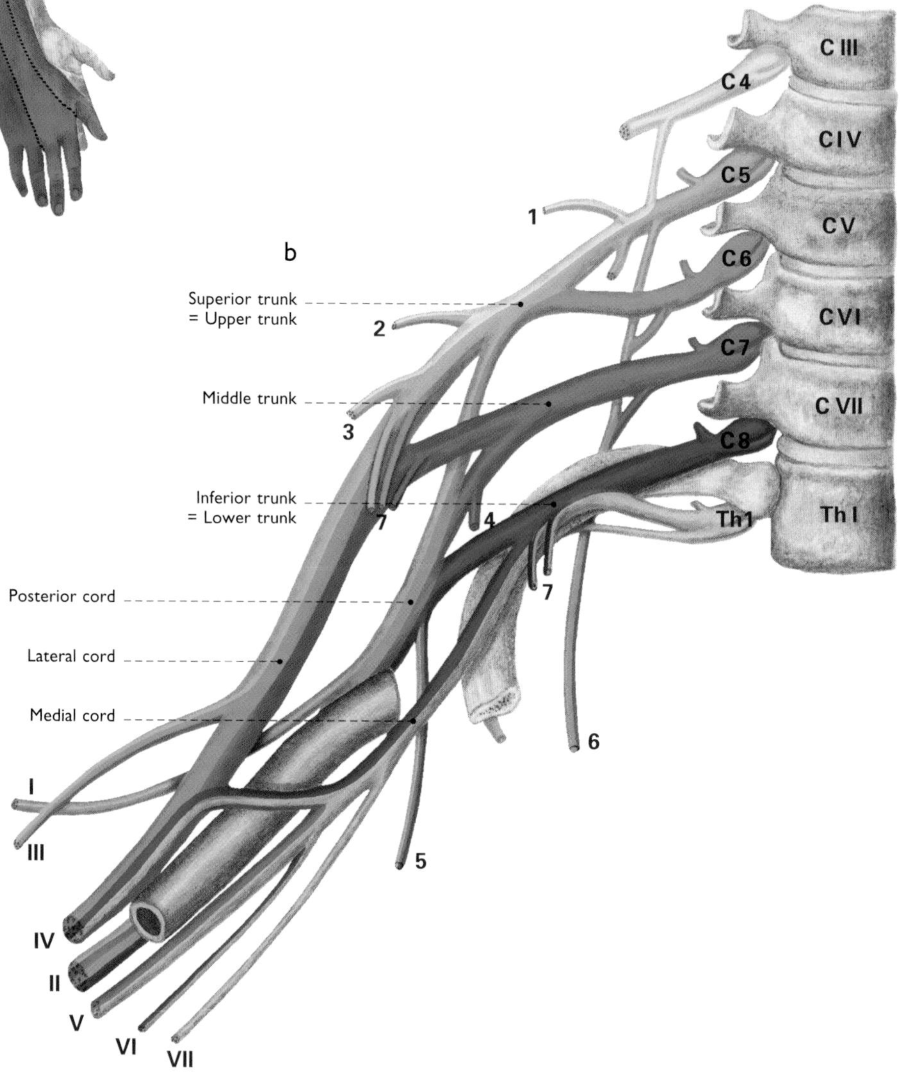

Supraclavicular part
1 Dorsal scapular nerve
2 Suprascapular nerve
3 Subclavian nerve
4 Subscapular nerves
5 Thoracodorsal nerve
6 Long thoracic nerve (BELL)
7 Medial and lateral pectoral nerves

Infraclavicular part

Posterior cord	→ I	Axillary nerve
	→ II	Radial nerve
Lateral cord	→ III	Musculocutaneous nerve
	→ IV	Median nerve
Medial cord	→ IV	Median nerve
	→ V	Ulnar nerve
	→ VI	Medial antebrachial cutaneous nerve
	→ VII	Medial brachial cutaneous nerve

140 Segmental innervation and brachial plexus

a Segmental innervation (dermatomes) of the upper limb, trunk, and lower limb (according to von LANZ and WACHSMUTH, 1959)
b Plan of the brachial plexus

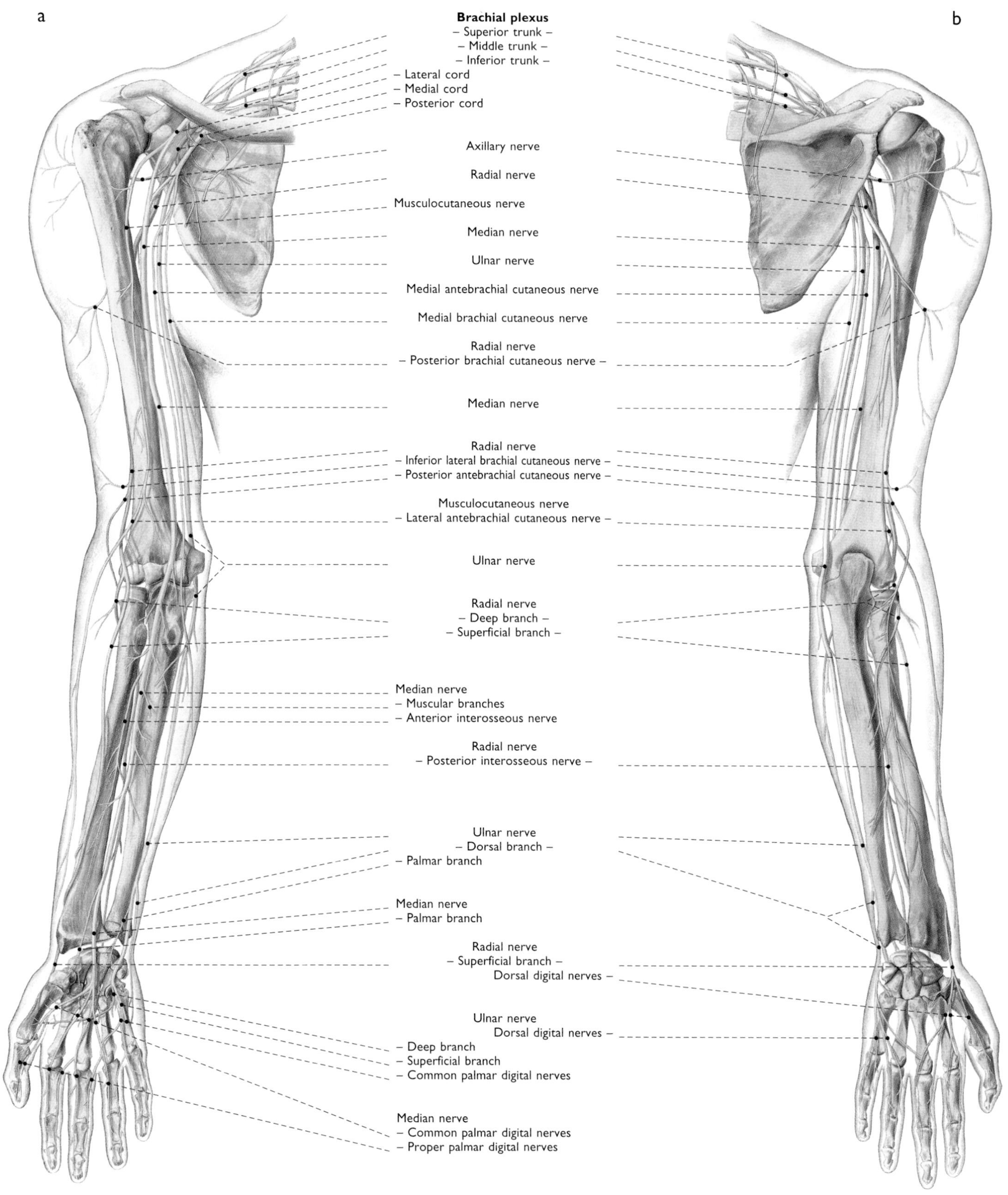
a
b
Brachial plexus
– Superior trunk –
– Middle trunk –
– Inferior trunk –
– Lateral cord
– Medial cord
– Posterior cord
Axillary nerve
Radial nerve
Musculocutaneous nerve
Median nerve
Ulnar nerve
Medial antebrachial cutaneous nerve
Medial brachial cutaneous nerve
Radial nerve
– Posterior brachial cutaneous nerve –
Median nerve
Radial nerve
– Inferior lateral brachial cutaneous nerve –
– Posterior antebrachial cutaneous nerve –
Musculocutaneous nerve
– Lateral antebrachial cutaneous nerve –
Ulnar nerve
Radial nerve
– Deep branch –
– Superficial branch –
Median nerve
– Muscular branches
– Anterior interosseous nerve
Radial nerve
– Posterior interosseous nerve –
Ulnar nerve
– Dorsal branch –
– Palmar branch
Median nerve
– Palmar branch
Radial nerve
– Superficial branch –
Dorsal digital nerves –
Ulnar nerve
Dorsal digital nerves –
– Deep branch
– Superficial branch
– Common palmar digital nerves
Median nerve
– Common palmar digital nerves
– Proper palmar digital nerves

141 Nerves of the right upper limb (30%)

Schematic representations

a Ventral aspect

b Dorsal aspect

b

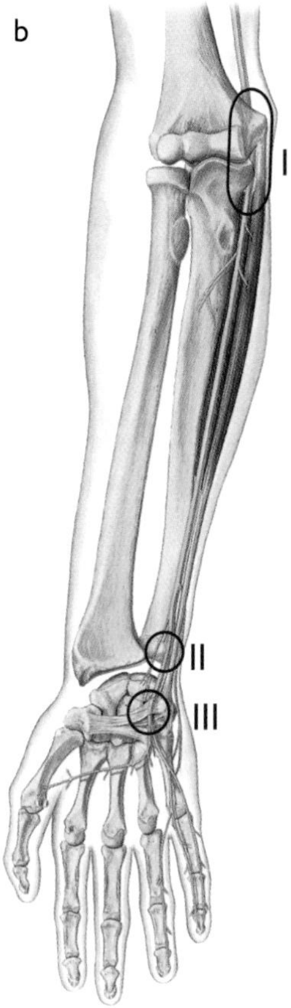

Ulnar nerve (b)

I Pressure in the ulnar groove, fracture of the medial epicondyle of humerus or compression along the passage through the flexor carpi ulnaris muscle
II Pressure or cuts at the distal ulna
III Compression in the ulnar canal ('GUYON's canal syndrome')

c

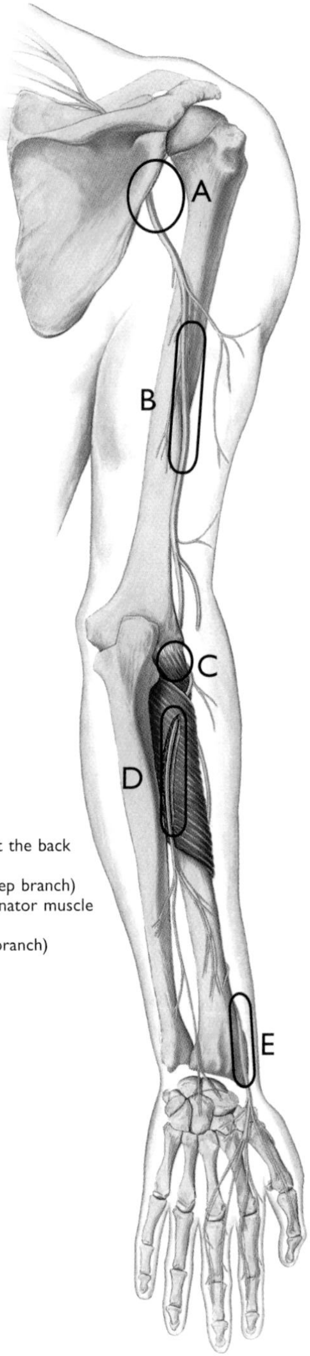

Median nerve (a)

1 Pressure against the humerus ('paralysie des amants')
2 Supracondylar fracture of humerus
3 Compression along the passage through the pronator teres muscle ('pronator syndrome')
4 Cuts or fracture at the distal forearm
5 Compression within the carpal tunnel ('carpal tunnel syndrome')

a

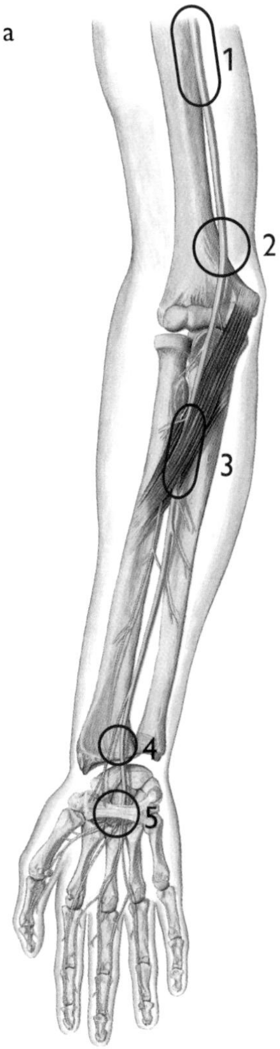

Radial nerve (c)

A Pressure in the axilla ('crutch palsy')
B Fracture of the humeral shaft or pressure against the back of humerus ('Saturday night palsy')
C Fracture or dislocation of the head of radius (deep branch)
D Compression along the passage through the supinator muscle (deep branch, 'supinator syndrome')
E Pressure or cuts at the distal radius (superficial branch)

142 Nerves of the right upper limb (25%)

Typical sites of injury of the three main nerves of the upper limb
a Median nerve
b Ulnar nerve
c Radial nerve

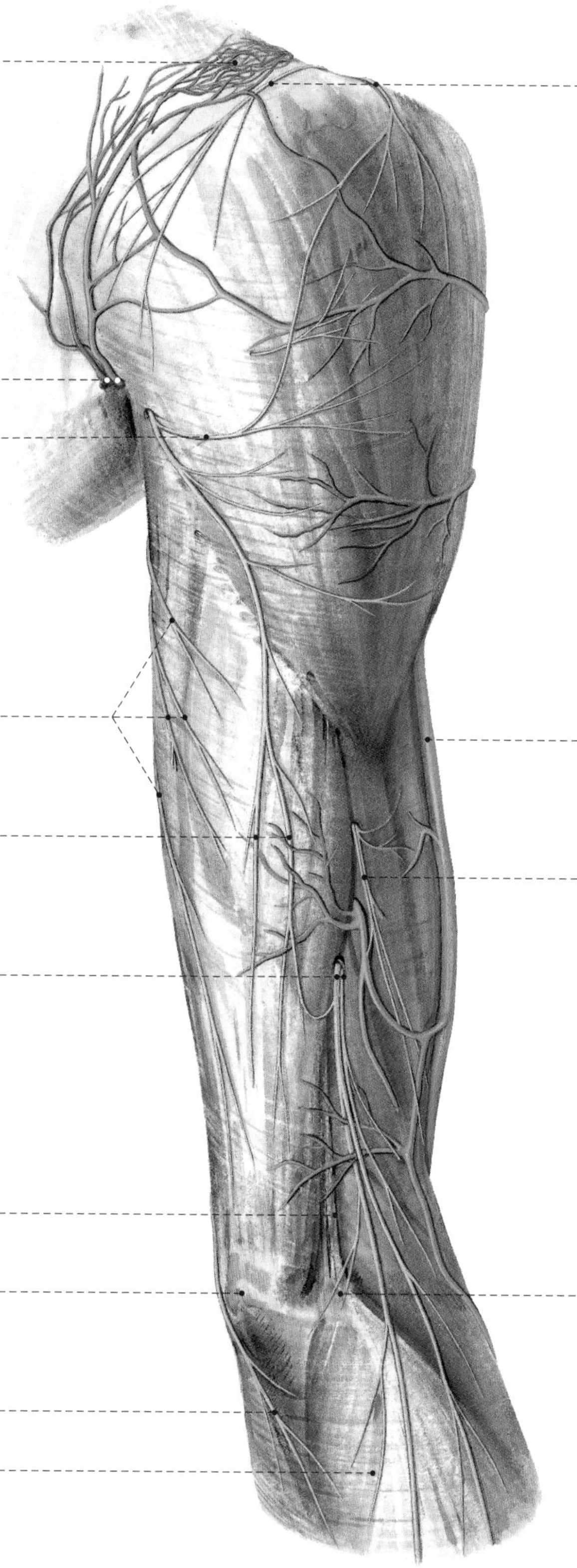
Acromial anastomosis
Lateral supraclavicular nerves
Branches of circumflex scapular artery and vein
Superior lateral brachial cutaneous nerve = Superior lateral cutaneous nerve of arm
Medial brachial cutaneous nerve = Medial cutaneous nerve of arm
Cephalic vein
Posterior brachial cutaneous nerve = Posterior cutaneous nerve of arm
Inferior lateral brachial cutaneous nerve = Inferior lateral cutaneous nerve of arm
Posterior antebrachial cutaneous nerve = Posterior cutaneous nerve of forearm
Lateral intermuscular septum of arm
Olecranon of ulna
Lateral epicondyle of humerus
Posterior branch of medial antebrachial cutaneous nerve
Antebrachial fascia

143 Subcutaneous veins and nerves of the right shoulder and the right arm (50%)

In this case the inferior lateral brachial cutaneous nerve originates from the axillary nerve. Dorsolateral aspect

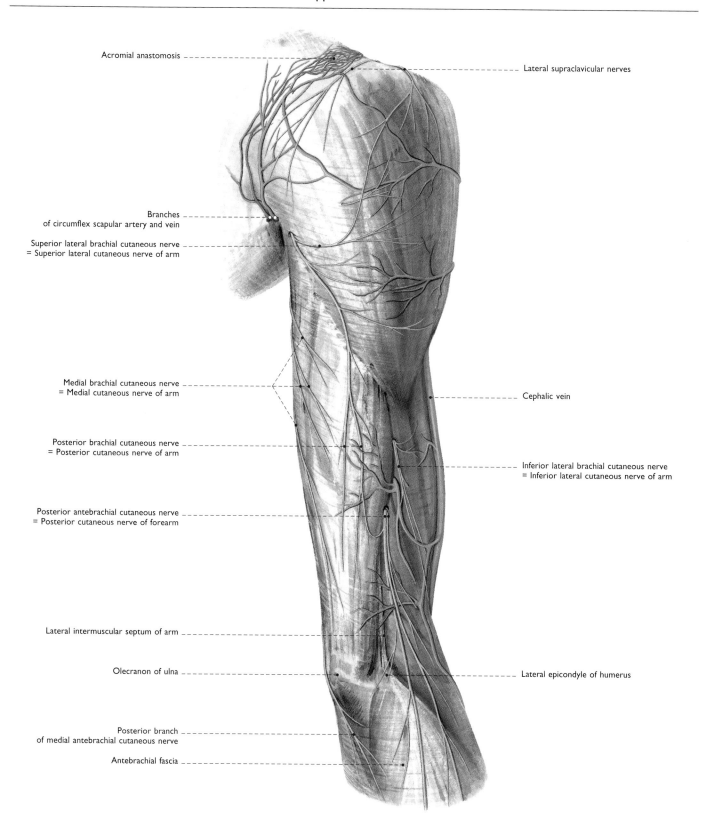

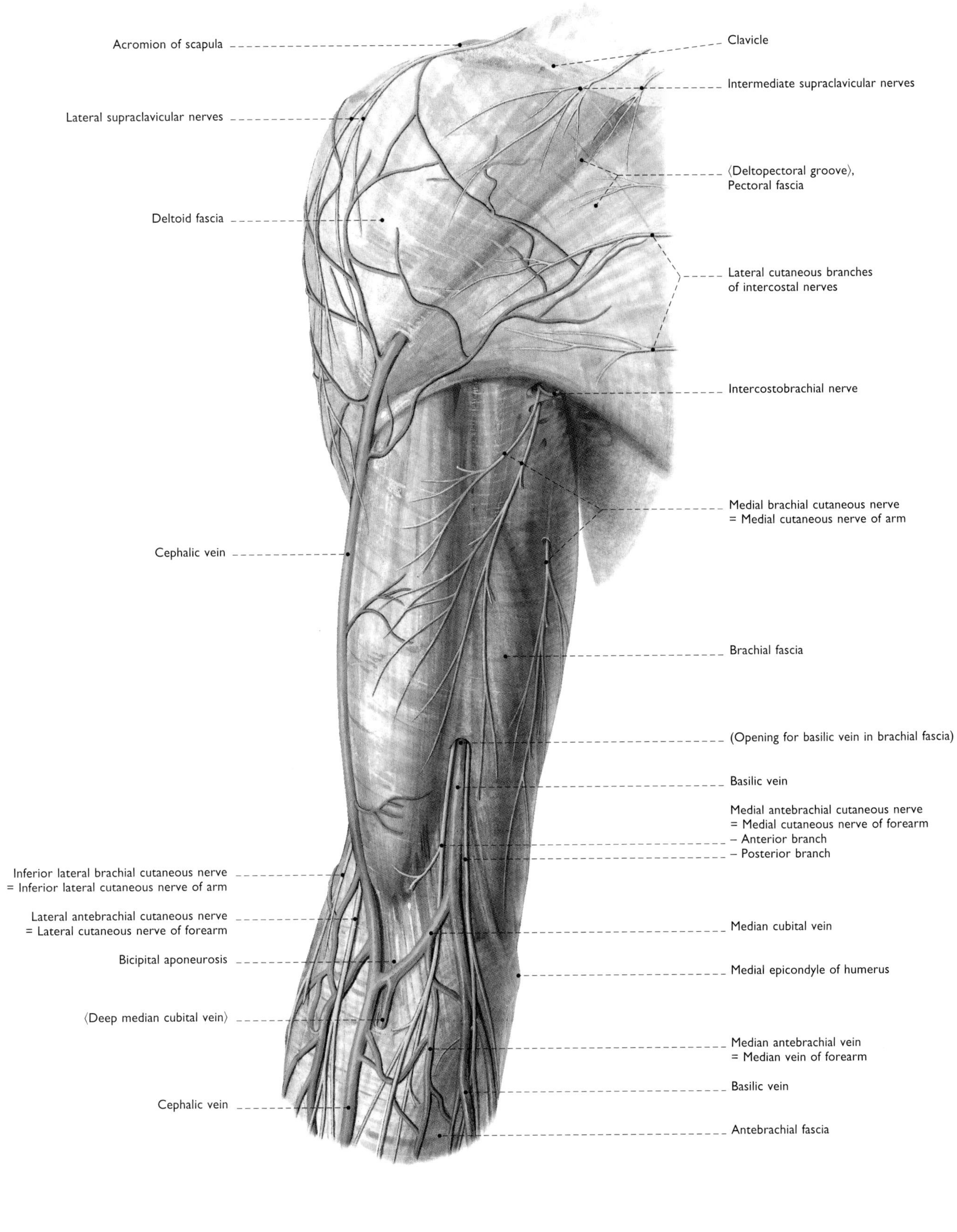
Acromion of scapula
Clavicle
Intermediate supraclavicular nerves
Lateral supraclavicular nerves
⟨Deltopectoral groove⟩,
Pectoral fascia
Deltoid fascia
Lateral cutaneous branches
of intercostal nerves
Intercostobrachial nerve
Medial brachial cutaneous nerve
= Medial cutaneous nerve of arm
Cephalic vein
Brachial fascia
(Opening for basilic vein in brachial fascia)
Basilic vein
Medial antebrachial cutaneous nerve
= Medial cutaneous nerve of forearm
– Anterior branch
– Posterior branch
Inferior lateral brachial cutaneous nerve
= Inferior lateral cutaneous nerve of arm
Lateral antebrachial cutaneous nerve
= Lateral cutaneous nerve of forearm
Median cubital vein
Bicipital aponeurosis
Medial epicondyle of humerus
⟨Deep median cubital vein⟩
Median antebrachial vein
= Median vein of forearm
Basilic vein
Cephalic vein
Antebrachial fascia

144 Subcutaneous veins and nerves of the right shoulder and the right arm (50%)

Ventral aspect

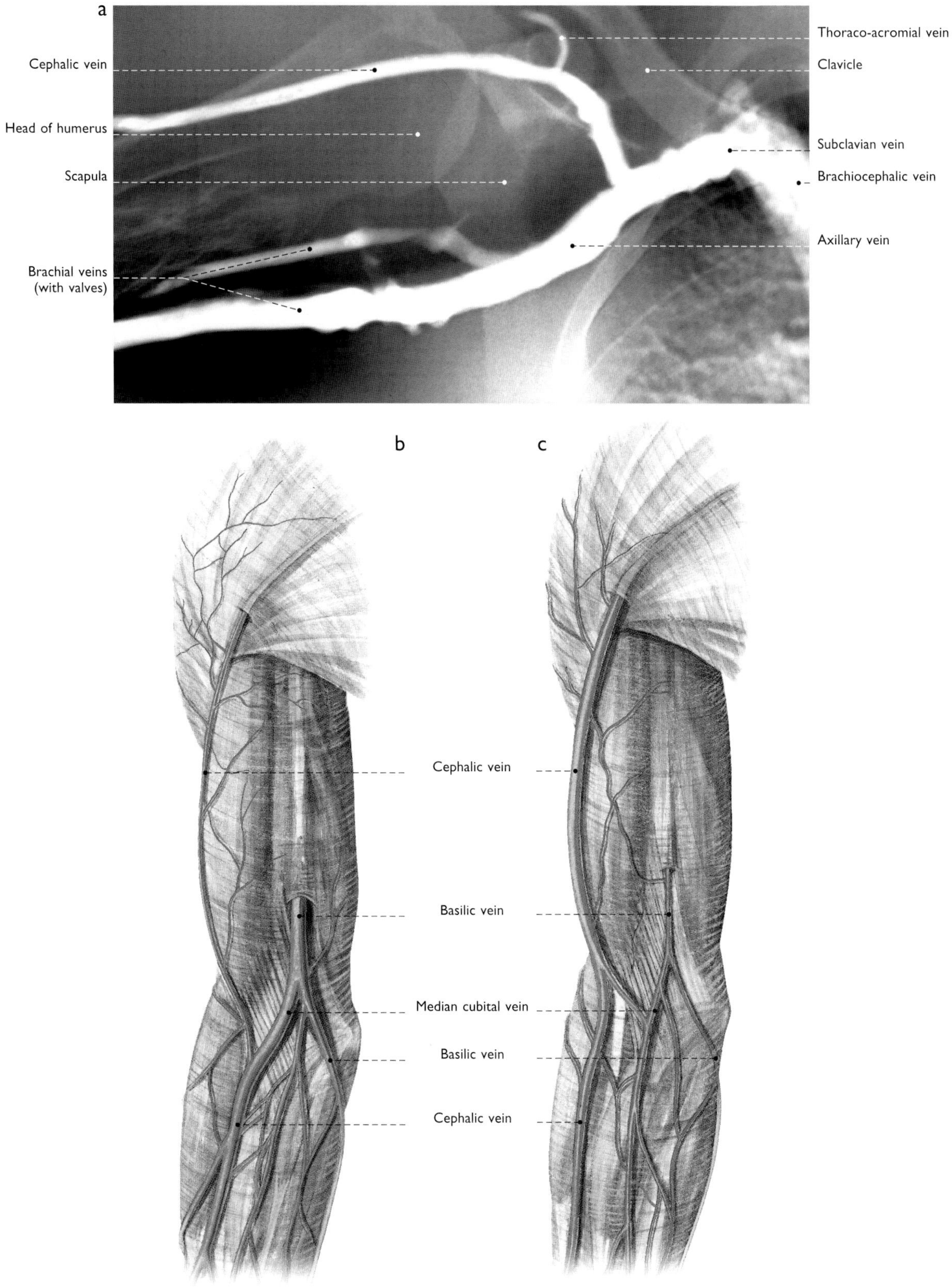
a
Cephalic vein
Head of humerus
Scapula
Brachial veins
(with valves)
Thoraco-acromial vein
Clavicle
Subclavian vein
Brachiocephalic vein
Axillary vein
b
c
Cephalic vein
Basilic vein
Median cubital vein
Basilic vein
Cephalic vein

145 Subcutaneous veins of the right shoulder, the right arm and forearm

a Phlebogram of the veins of the arm and the axilla (50%)

b, c Common variations of the subcutaneous veins of the arm and the anterior region of elbow (30%), ventral aspect

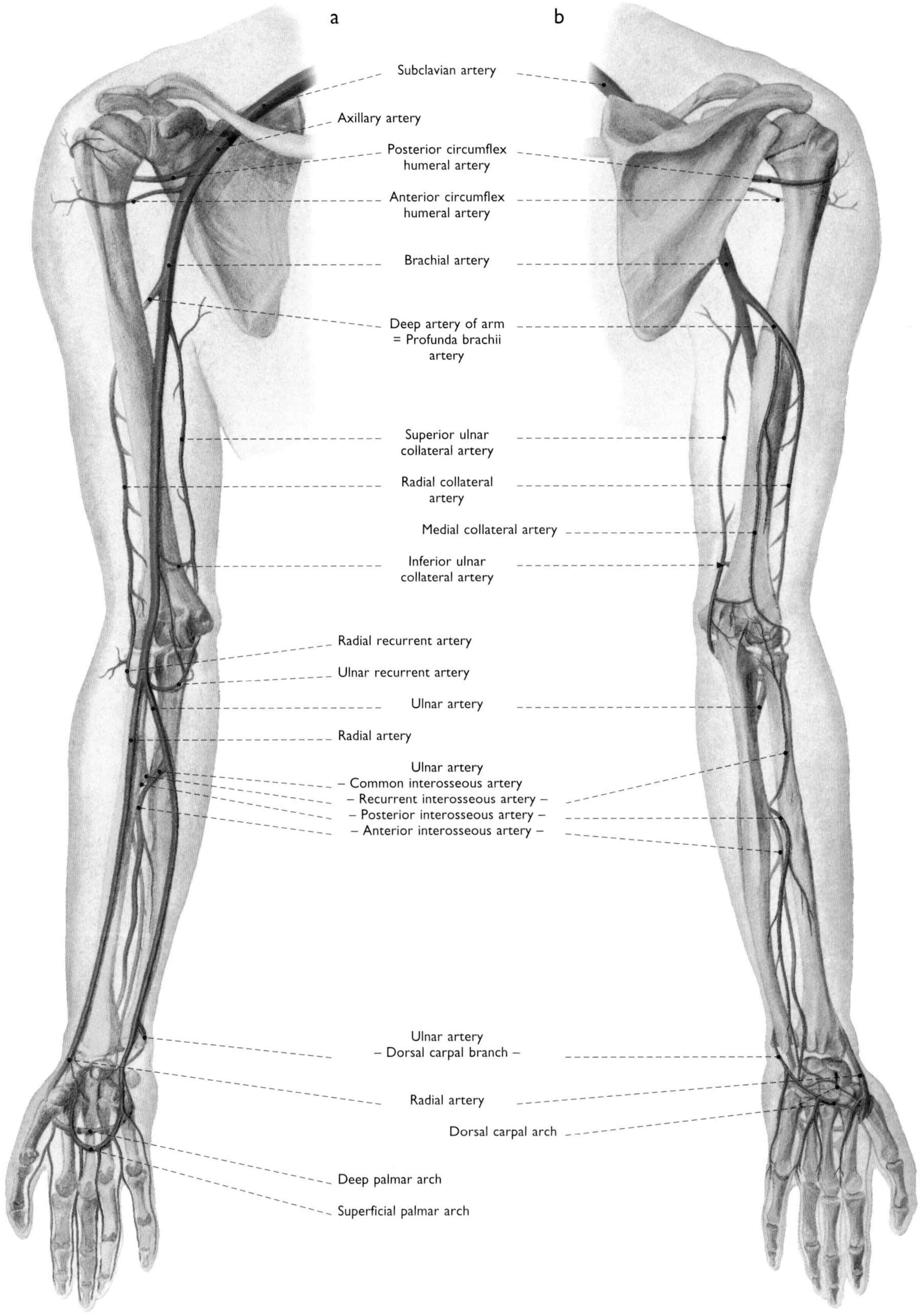
a
b
Subclavian artery
Axillary artery
Posterior circumflex humeral artery
Anterior circumflex humeral artery
Brachial artery
Deep artery of arm = Profunda brachii artery
Superior ulnar collateral artery
Radial collateral artery
Medial collateral artery
Inferior ulnar collateral artery
Radial recurrent artery
Ulnar recurrent artery
Ulnar artery
Radial artery
Ulnar artery
– Common interosseous artery
– Recurrent interosseous artery –
– Posterior interosseous artery –
– Anterior interosseous artery –
Ulnar artery
– Dorsal carpal branch –
Radial artery
Dorsal carpal arch
Deep palmar arch
Superficial palmar arch

146 Arteries of the right upper limb (30%)

Schematic representations
a Ventral aspect
b Dorsal aspect

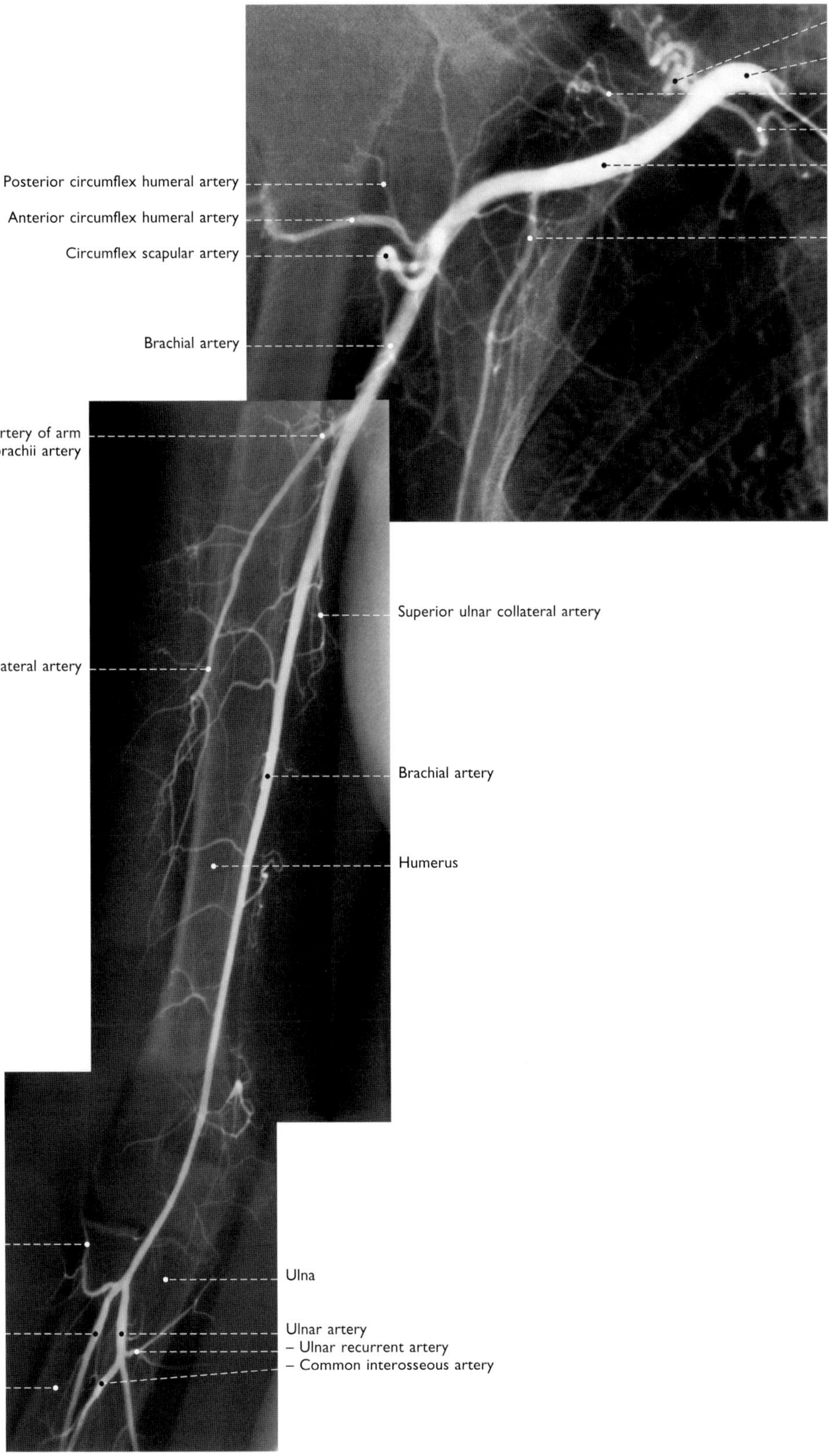
Thyrocervical trunk
Subclavian artery
Costocervical trunk
Internal thoracic artery
Axillary artery
Lateral thoracic artery
Posterior circumflex humeral artery
Anterior circumflex humeral artery
Circumflex scapular artery
Brachial artery
Deep artery of arm
= Profunda brachii artery
Superior ulnar collateral artery
Radial collateral artery
Brachial artery
Humerus
Radial recurrent artery
Ulna
Radial artery
Ulnar artery
– Ulnar recurrent artery
– Common interosseous artery
Radius

147 Arteries of the right upper limb (50%)

Arteriogram of the arteries of the upper limb (subclavian, axillary, brachial, radial, and ulnar arteries)

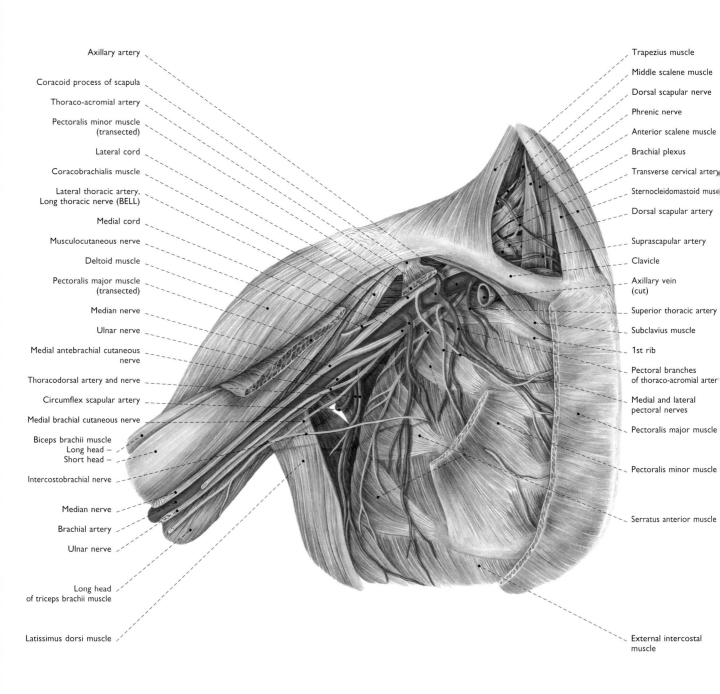

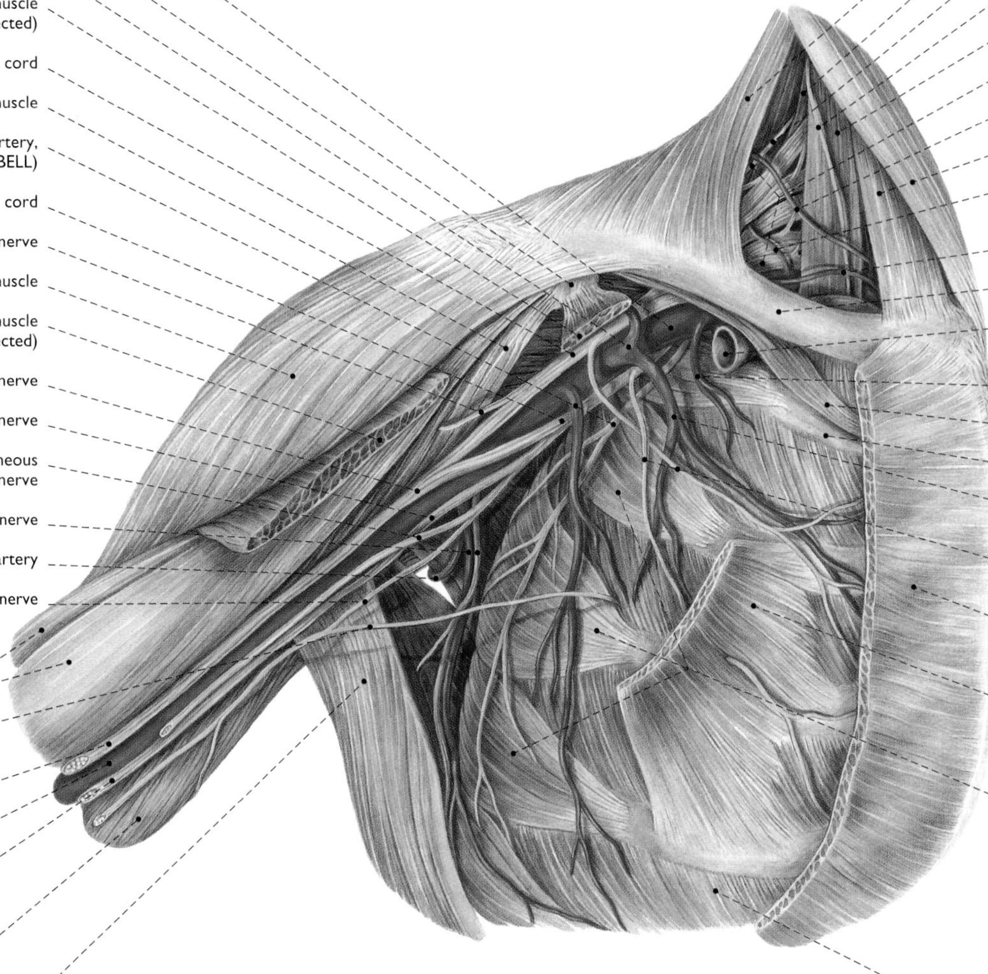
Axillary artery
Coracoid process of scapula
Thoraco-acromial artery
Pectoralis minor muscle (transected)
Lateral cord
Coracobrachialis muscle
Lateral thoracic artery, Long thoracic nerve (BELL)
Medial cord
Musculocutaneous nerve
Deltoid muscle
Pectoralis major muscle (transected)
Median nerve
Ulnar nerve
Medial antebrachial cutaneous nerve
Thoracodorsal artery and nerve
Circumflex scapular artery
Medial brachial cutaneous nerve
Biceps brachii muscle
Long head –
Short head –
Intercostobrachial nerve
Median nerve
Brachial artery
Ulnar nerve
Long head of triceps brachii muscle
Latissimus dorsi muscle
Trapezius muscle
Middle scalene muscle
Dorsal scapular nerve
Phrenic nerve
Anterior scalene muscle
Brachial plexus
Transverse cervical artery
Sternocleidomastoid muscle
Dorsal scapular artery
Suprascapular artery
Clavicle
Axillary vein (cut)
Superior thoracic artery
Subclavius muscle
1st rib
Pectoral branches of thoraco-acromial artery
Medial and lateral pectoral nerves
Pectoralis major muscle
Pectoralis minor muscle
Serratus anterior muscle
External intercostal muscle

148 Axilla (50%)

Axilla with axillary artery and brachial plexus.
The axillary vein was transected beneath the clavicle, the omohyoid muscle is omitted.
Ventral aspect

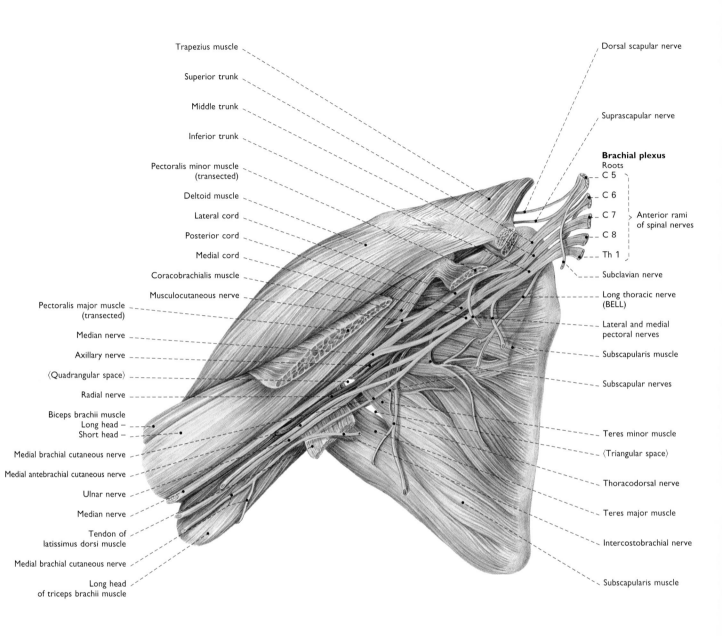

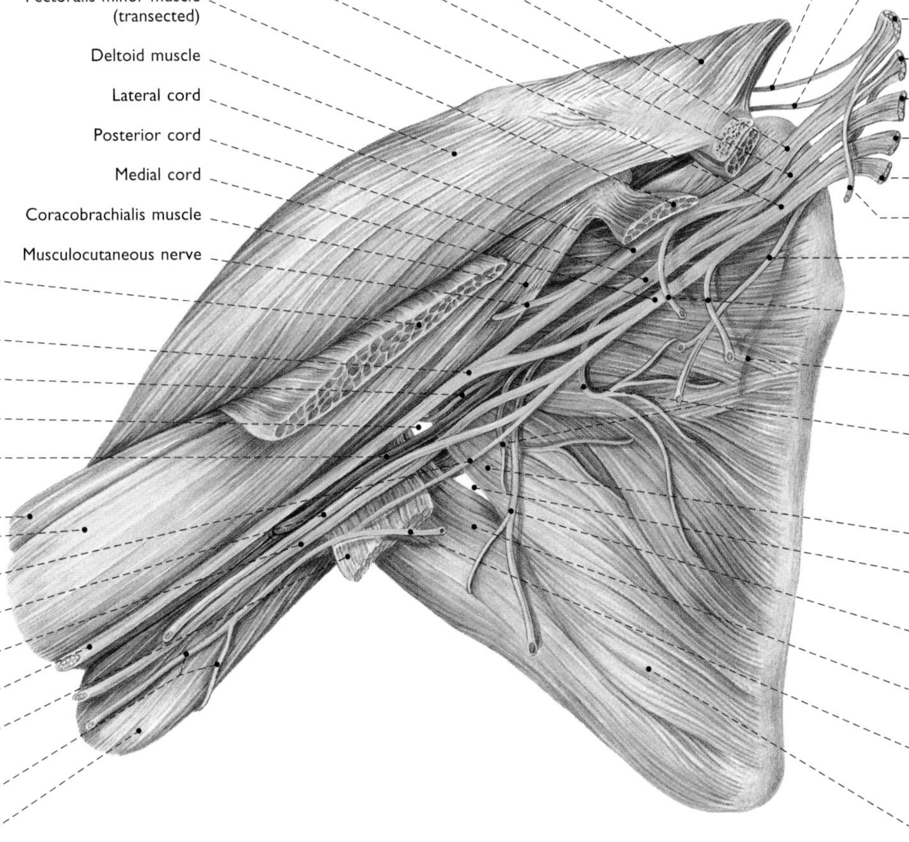
Trapezius muscle
Superior trunk
Middle trunk
Inferior trunk
Pectoralis minor muscle (transected)
Deltoid muscle
Lateral cord
Posterior cord
Medial cord
Coracobrachialis muscle
Musculocutaneous nerve
Pectoralis major muscle (transected)
Median nerve
Axillary nerve
⟨Quadrangular space⟩
Radial nerve
Biceps brachii muscle
Long head
Short head
Medial brachial cutaneous nerve
Medial antebrachial cutaneous nerve
Ulnar nerve
Median nerve
Tendon of latissimus dorsi muscle
Medial brachial cutaneous nerve
Long head of triceps brachii muscle
Dorsal scapular nerve
Suprascapular nerve
Brachial plexus
Roots
C 5
C 6
C 7
C 8
Th 1
Anterior rami of spinal nerves
Subclavian nerve
Long thoracic nerve (BELL)
Lateral and medial pectoral nerves
Subscapularis muscle
Subscapular nerves
Teres minor muscle
⟨Triangular space⟩
Thoracodorsal nerve
Teres major muscle
Intercostobrachial nerve
Subscapularis muscle

149 Brachial plexus (50%)

Brachial plexus in the axilla and in the proximal arm, ventral aspect

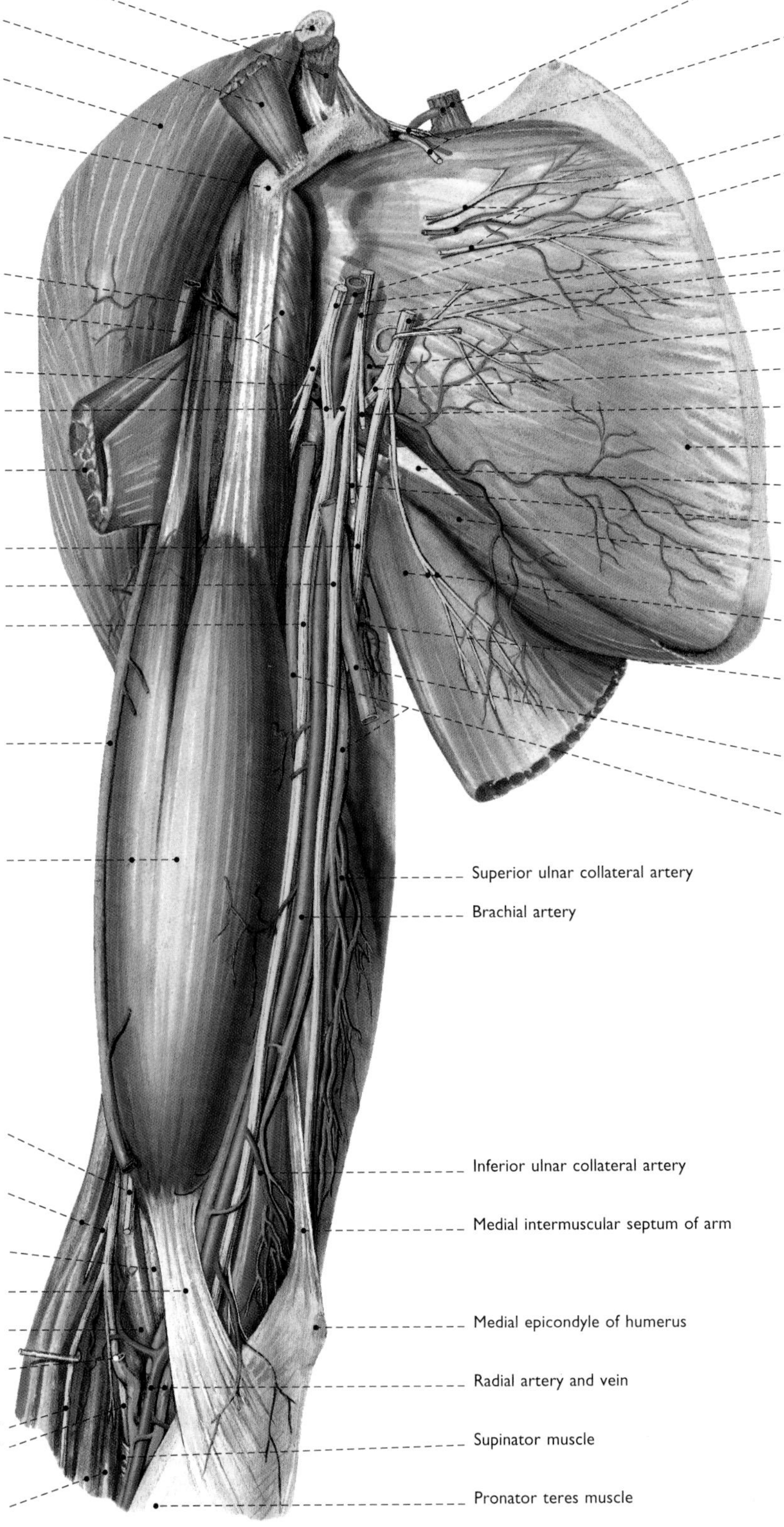

Clavicle,
Subclavius muscle
Pectoralis minor muscle
(turned upwards)
Deltoid muscle
Coracoid process of scapula
Anterior circumflex humeral artery
Coracobrachialis muscle,
Musculocutaneous nerve
Posterior circumflex humeral artery
Lateral and medial roots
of median nerve
Pectoralis major muscle
Radial nerve
Ulnar nerve
Median nerve
Cephalic vein
Biceps brachii muscle
Lateral antebrachial
cutaneous nerve
Brachioradialis muscle,
Muscular branch of radial nerve
Tendon of biceps brachii muscle
Bicipital aponeurosis
Brachialis muscle
⟨Deep median cubital vein⟩
Radial nerve
Superficial branch –
Deep branch –
Extensores carpi radiales muscles
Suprascapular artery,
Inferior belly
of omohyoid muscle
Superior transverse scapular ligament,
Suprascapular nerve
Subscapular nerves and artery
Axillary artery
Infraclavicular part
of brachial plexus
– Lateral cord
– Medial cord
– Posterior cord
Subscapular artery
Axillary nerve
Medial brachial cutaneous nerve
Subscapularis muscle
⟨Triangular space⟩
Medial antebrachial cutaneous nerve
Teres major muscle
Latissimus dorsi muscle,
Thoracodorsal nerve
Deep artery of arm
= Profunda brachii artery
Basilic vein
Brachial veins
Superior ulnar collateral artery
Brachial artery
Inferior ulnar collateral artery
Medial intermuscular septum of arm
Medial epicondyle of humerus
Radial artery and vein
Supinator muscle
Pronator teres muscle

150 Blood vessels and nerves of the right shoulder, the right arm, and the anterior region of elbow (50%)

Ventral aspect

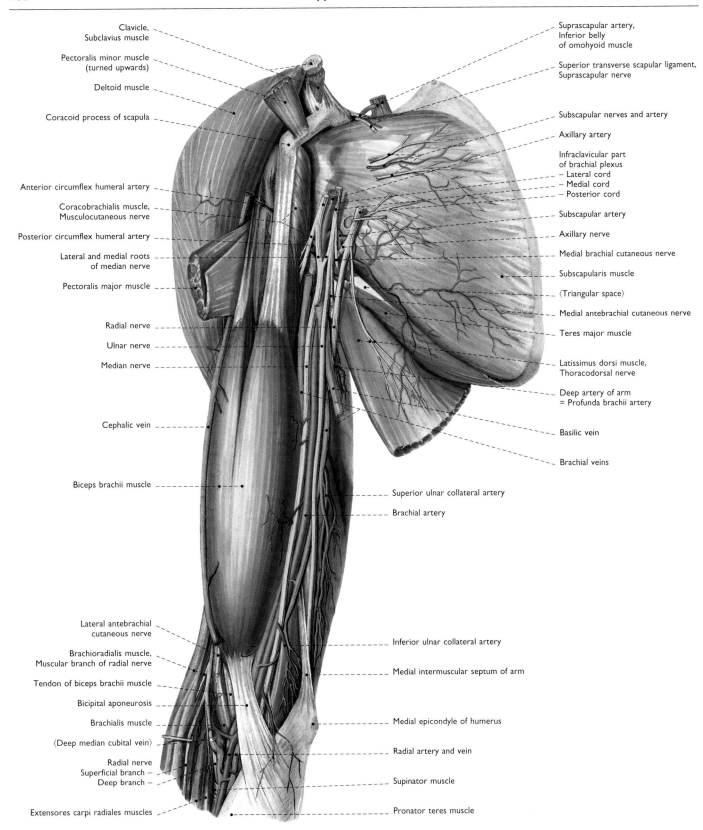

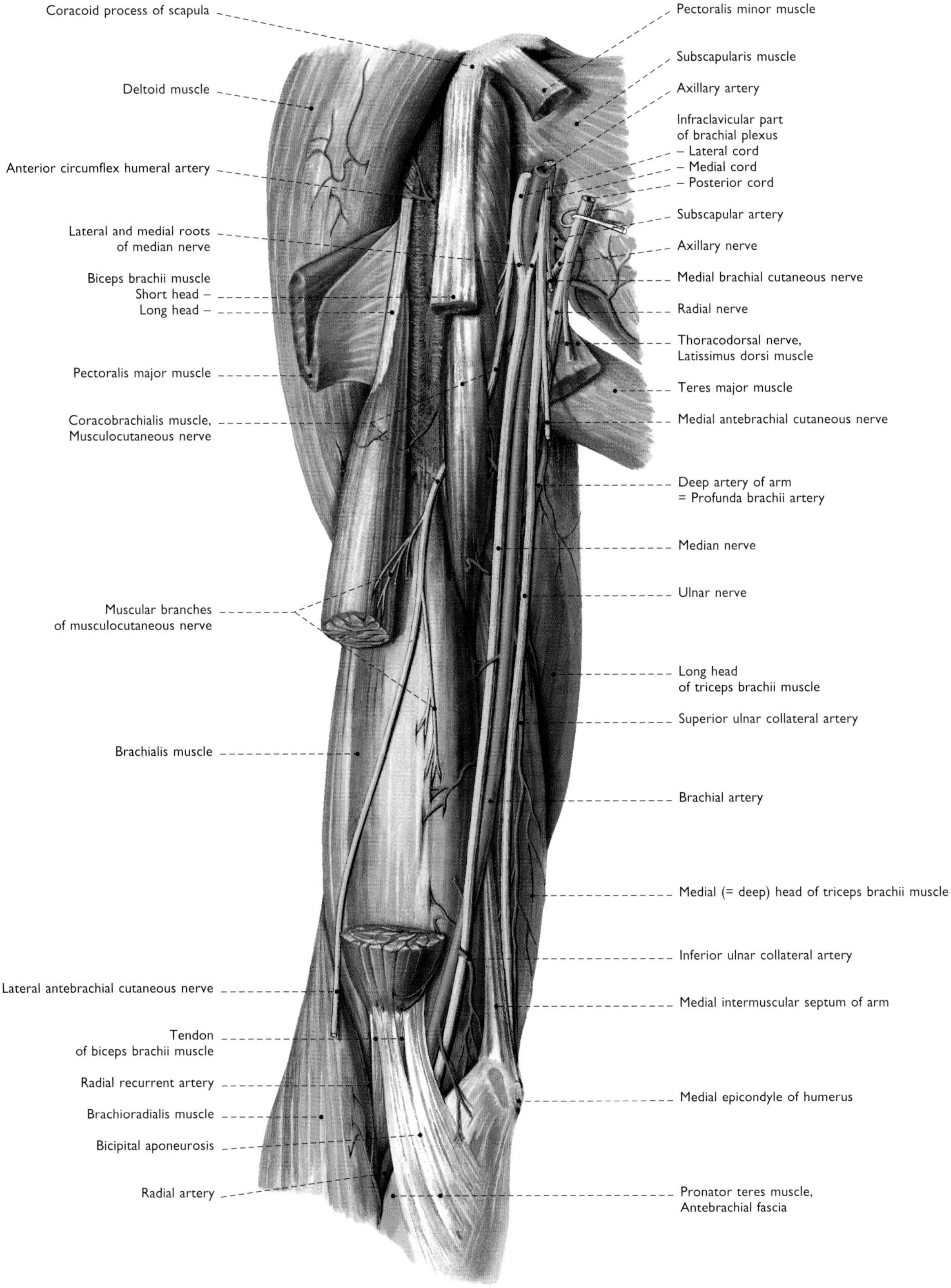

Coracoid process of scapula
Deltoid muscle
Anterior circumflex humeral artery
Lateral and medial roots of median nerve
Biceps brachii muscle
Short head –
Long head –
Pectoralis major muscle
Coracobrachialis muscle, Musculocutaneous nerve
Muscular branches of musculocutaneous nerve
Brachialis muscle
Lateral antebrachial cutaneous nerve
Tendon of biceps brachii muscle
Radial recurrent artery
Brachioradialis muscle
Bicipital aponeurosis
Radial artery
Pectoralis minor muscle
Subscapularis muscle
Axillary artery
Infraclavicular part of brachial plexus
– Lateral cord
– Medial cord
– Posterior cord
Subscapular artery
Axillary nerve
Medial brachial cutaneous nerve
Radial nerve
Thoracodorsal nerve, Latissimus dorsi muscle
Teres major muscle
Medial antebrachial cutaneous nerve
Deep artery of arm = Profunda brachii artery
Median nerve
Ulnar nerve
Long head of triceps brachii muscle
Superior ulnar collateral artery
Brachial artery
Medial (= deep) head of triceps brachii muscle
Inferior ulnar collateral artery
Medial intermuscular septum of arm
Medial epicondyle of humerus
Pronator teres muscle, Antebrachial fascia

151 Arteries and nerves of the right arm and the anterior region of elbow (50%)

The biceps brachii muscle was partially removed.
Ventral aspect

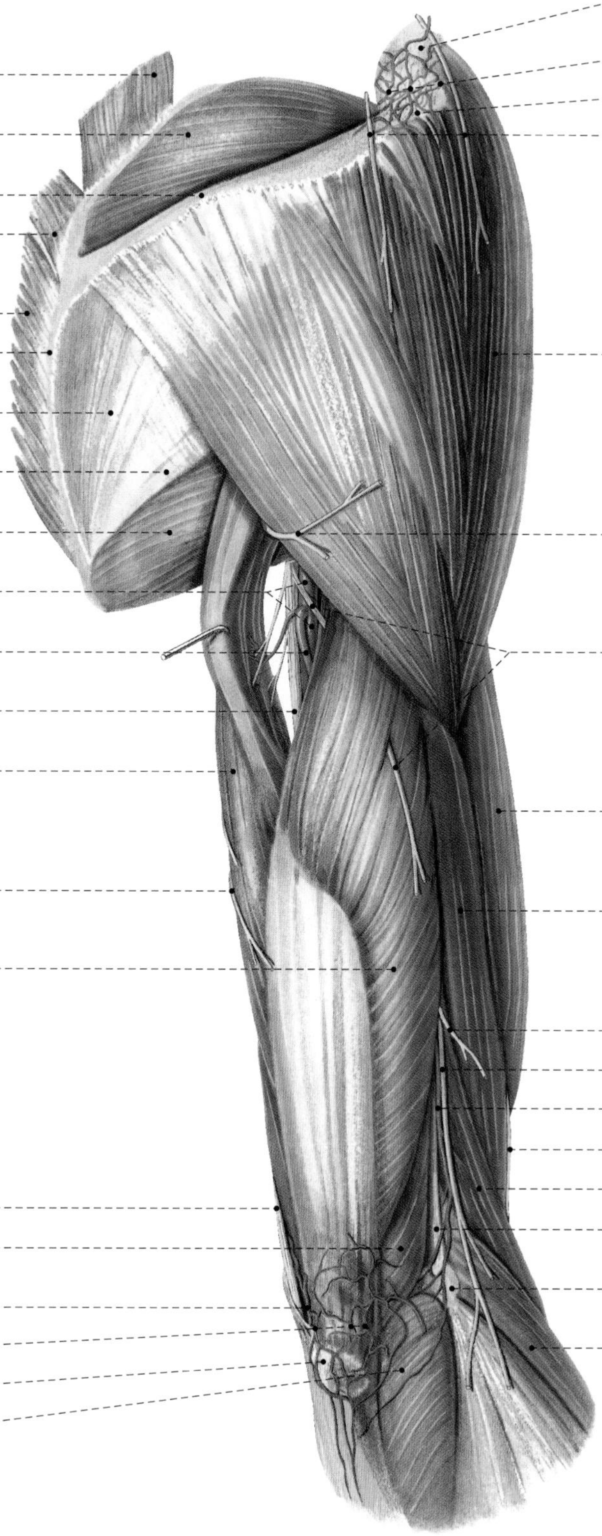
Acromial end of clavicle
Acromial anastomosis
Acromion of scapula
Lateral supraclavicular nerves
Levator scapulae muscle
Supraspinatus muscle
Spine of scapula
Rhomboid minor muscle
Rhomboid major muscle
Medial border of scapula
Infraspinatus muscle
Teres minor muscle
Teres major muscle
Brachial artery
Deep artery of arm
= Profunda brachii artery
Radial nerve
Long head
of triceps brachii muscle
Medial brachial cutaneous nerve
Lateral head
of triceps brachii muscle
Ulnar nerve
Medial (= deep) head
of triceps brachii muscle
Superior ulnar collateral artery
Cubital anastomosis
Olecranon of ulna
Anconeus muscle
Deltoid muscle
Superior lateral brachial cutaneous nerve
Posterior brachial cutaneous nerve
Biceps brachii muscle
Brachialis muscle
Inferior lateral brachial cutaneous nerve
Posterior antebrachial cutaneous nerve
Radial collateral artery
Lateral antebrachial cutaneous nerve
Brachioradialis muscle
Lateral intermuscular septum of arm
Lateral epicondyle of humerus
Extensor carpi radialis longus muscle

152 Arteries and nerves of the right shoulder, the right arm, and the posterior region of elbow (50%)

Dorsolateral aspect

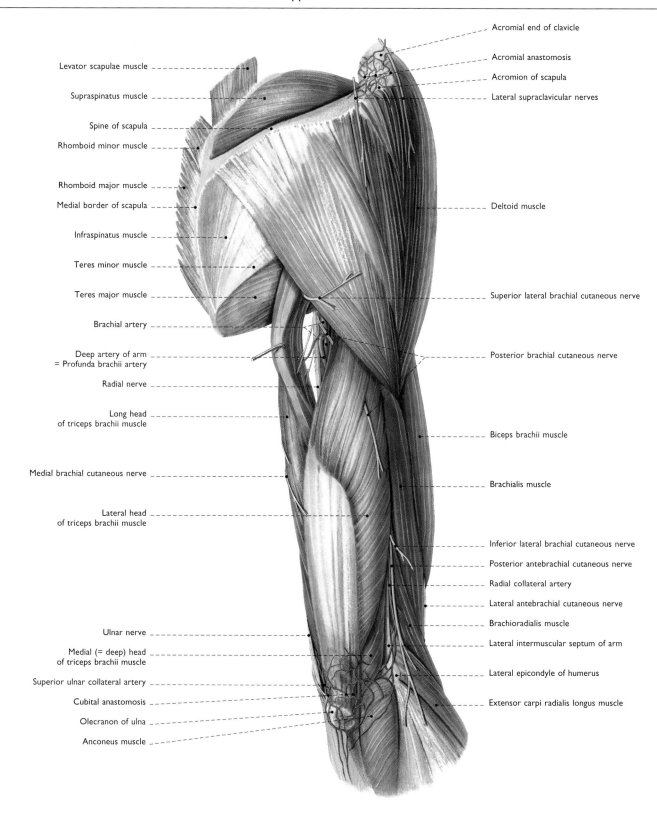

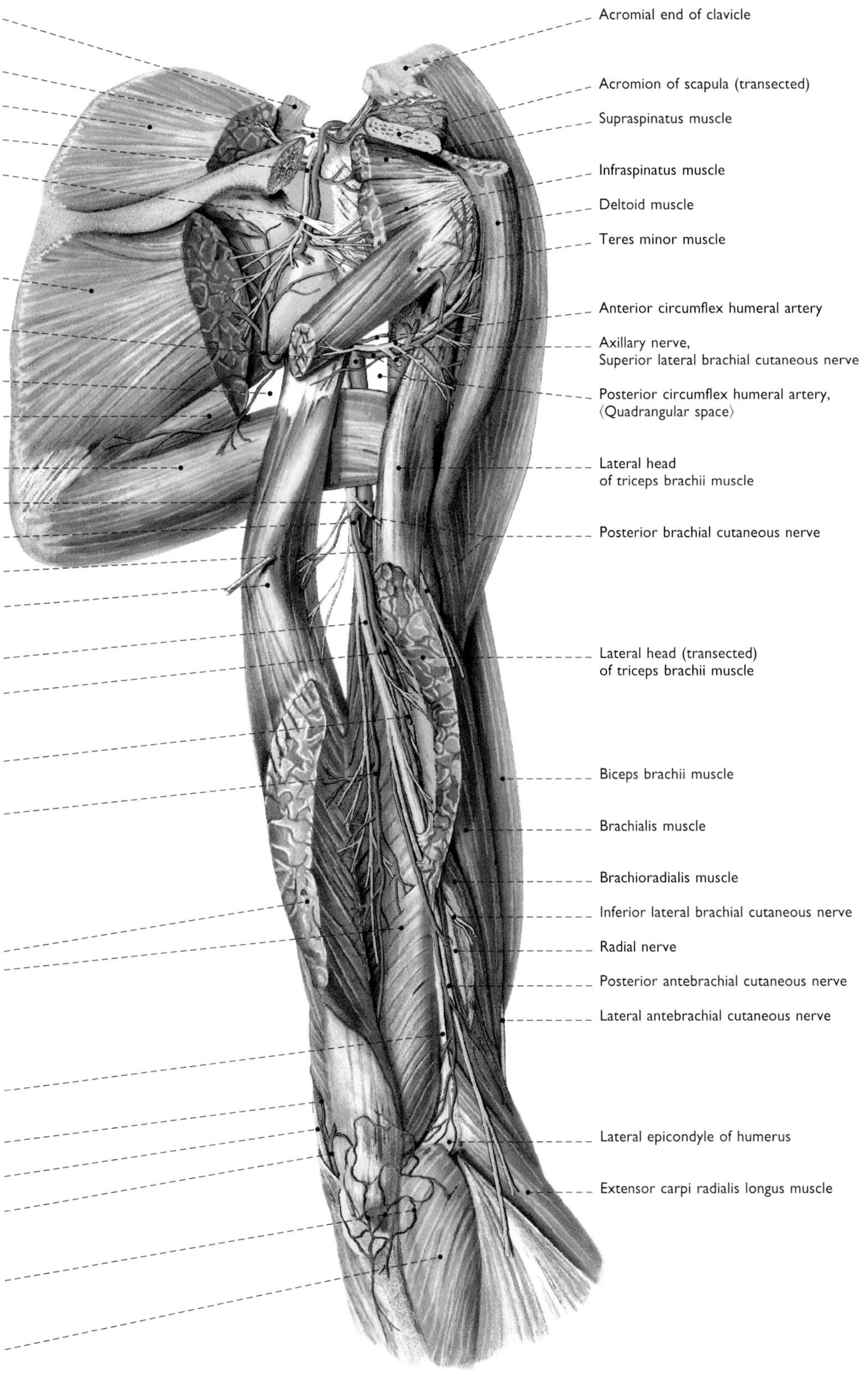
Inferior belly of omohyoid muscle
Superior transverse scapular ligament
Supraspinatus muscle
Suprascapular nerve
(Inferior transverse scapular ligament)
Infraspinatus muscle
Circumflex scapular artery, Axillary artery
⟨Triangular space⟩
Teres minor muscle
Teres major muscle
Brachial artery
Deep artery of arm
Deltoid branch
Long head of triceps brachii muscle
Radial nerve
Radial collateral artery
Nutrient artery of humerus
Medial collateral artery
Triceps brachii muscle
Lateral head (transected) –
Medial (= deep) head –
Lateral intermuscular septum of arm
Superior ulnar collateral artery
Ulnar nerve
Ulnar recurrent artery
Cubital anastomosis
Anconeus muscle
Acromial end of clavicle
Acromion of scapula (transected)
Supraspinatus muscle
Infraspinatus muscle
Deltoid muscle
Teres minor muscle
Anterior circumflex humeral artery
Axillary nerve,
Superior lateral brachial cutaneous nerve
Posterior circumflex humeral artery,
⟨Quadrangular space⟩
Lateral head of triceps brachii muscle
Posterior brachial cutaneous nerve
Lateral head (transected) of triceps brachii muscle
Biceps brachii muscle
Brachialis muscle
Brachioradialis muscle
Inferior lateral brachial cutaneous nerve
Radial nerve
Posterior antebrachial cutaneous nerve
Lateral antebrachial cutaneous nerve
Lateral epicondyle of humerus
Extensor carpi radialis longus muscle

153 Arteries and nerves of the right shoulder, the right arm, and the posterior region of elbow (50%)

The lateral head of the triceps brachii muscle was divided, the radial nerve channel opened. Dorsolateral aspect

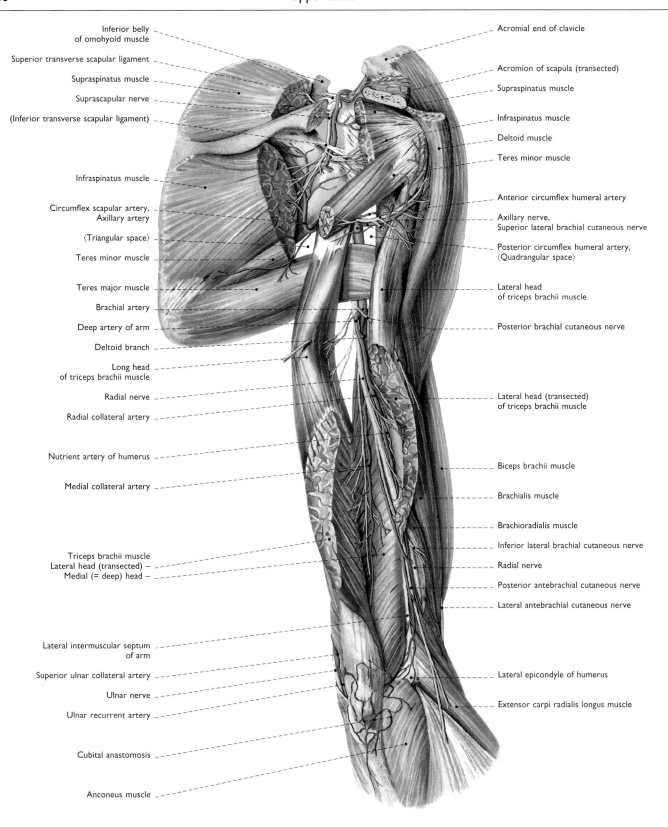

a

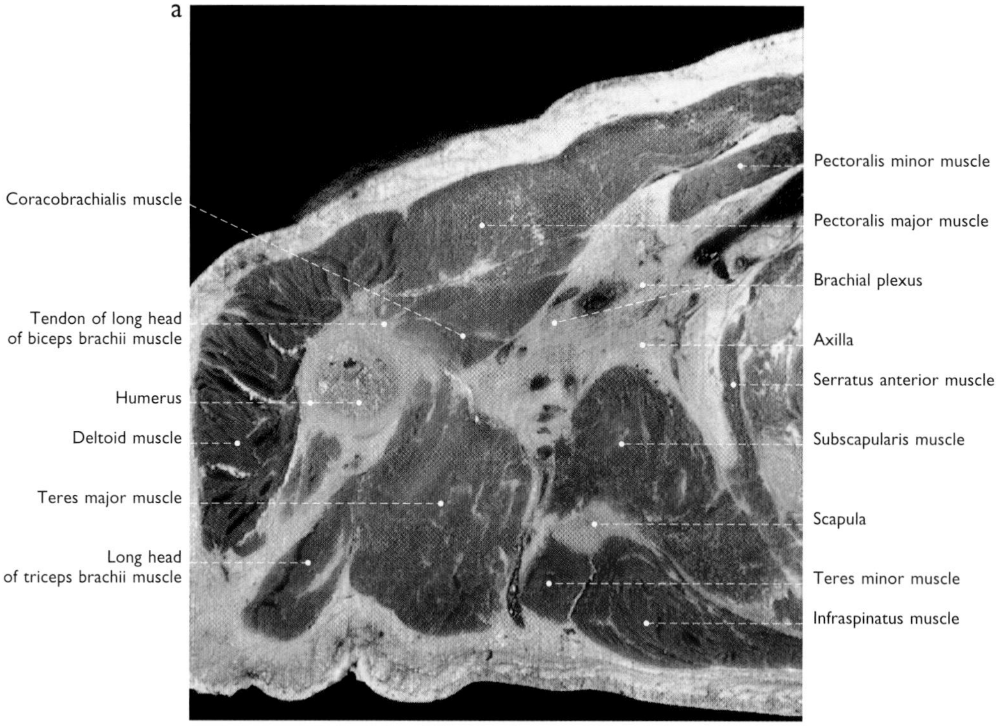
Coracobrachialis muscle
Tendon of long head of biceps brachii muscle
Humerus
Deltoid muscle
Teres major muscle
Long head of triceps brachii muscle
Pectoralis minor muscle
Pectoralis major muscle
Brachial plexus
Axilla
Serratus anterior muscle
Subscapularis muscle
Scapula
Teres minor muscle
Infraspinatus muscle

b

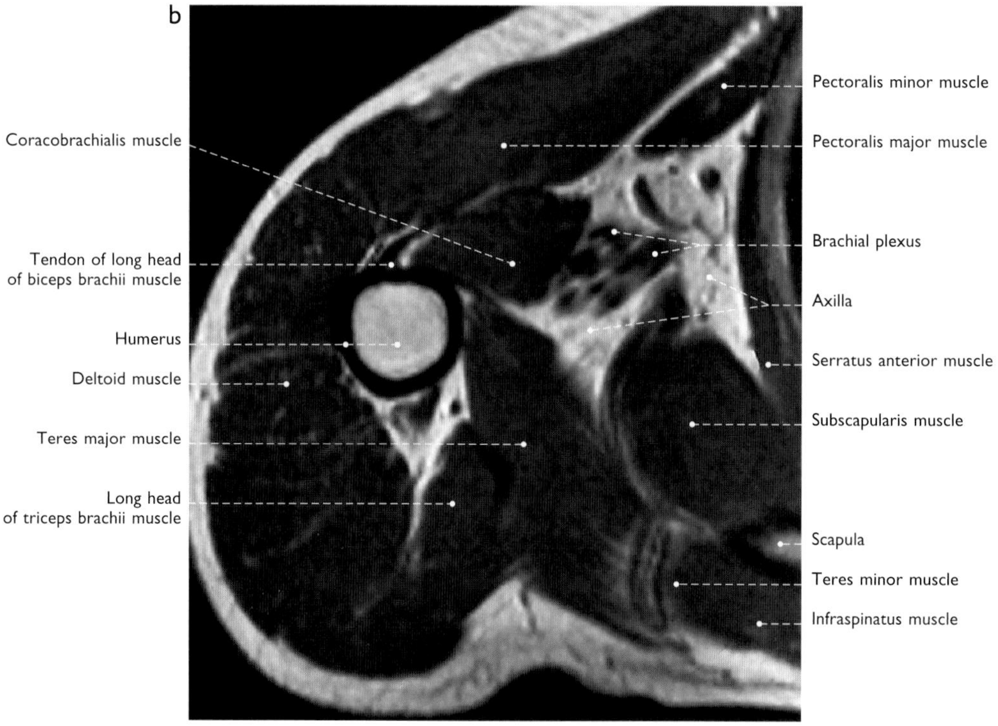
Coracobrachialis muscle
Tendon of long head of biceps brachii muscle
Humerus
Deltoid muscle
Teres major muscle
Long head of triceps brachii muscle
Pectoralis minor muscle
Pectoralis major muscle
Brachial plexus
Axilla
Serratus anterior muscle
Subscapularis muscle
Scapula
Teres minor muscle
Infraspinatus muscle

154 Right arm (80%)

Axial (transverse) sections through the proximal arm at the level of the shoulder and the axilla, distal aspect

a Anatomical section

b Magnetic resonance image (MRI, T_1-weighted)

a

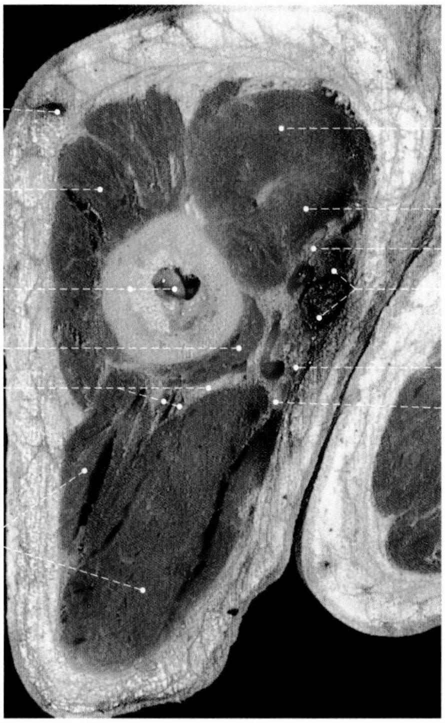
Cephalic vein
Deltoid muscle
Body of humerus
Triceps brachii muscle
Medial (= deep) head –
Radial nerve,
Deep artery and vein of arm
Triceps brachii muscle
Lateral head –
Long head –
Biceps brachii muscle
Coracobrachialis muscle
Musculocutaneous nerve
Brachial artery and vein
Median nerve
Ulnar nerve

b

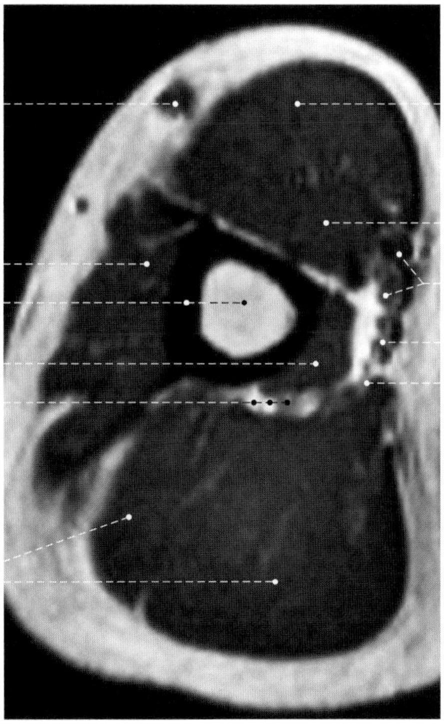
Cephalic vein
Deltoid muscle
Body of humerus
Triceps brachii muscle
Medial (= deep) head –
Deep artery and vein of arm,
Radial nerve
Triceps brachii muscle
Lateral head –
Long head –
Biceps brachii muscle
Coracobrachialis muscle
Brachial artery and vein
Median nerve
Ulnar nerve

155 Right arm (80%)

Axial (transverse) sections through the proximal third of the arm, distal aspect

a Anatomical section

b Magnetic resonance image (MRI, T_1-weighted)

a

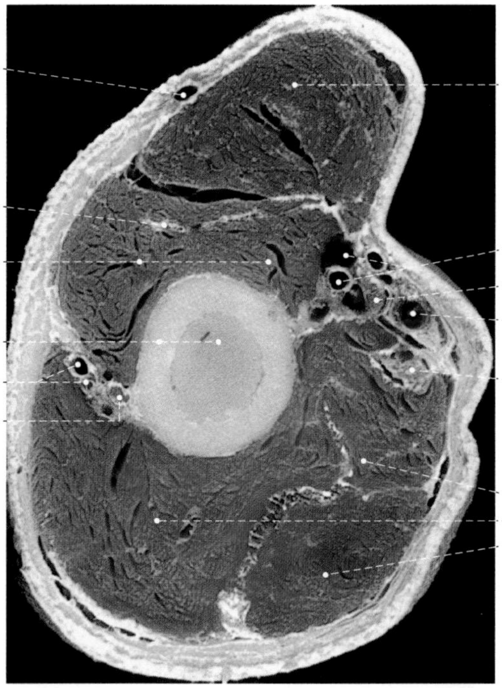
Cephalic vein
Musculocutaneous nerve
Brachialis muscle
Body of humerus
Deep artery and vein of arm
Radial nerve
Biceps brachii muscle
Brachial vein and artery
Median nerve
Basilic vein
Ulnar nerve
Triceps brachii muscle
– Medial (= deep) head
– Lateral head
– Long head

b

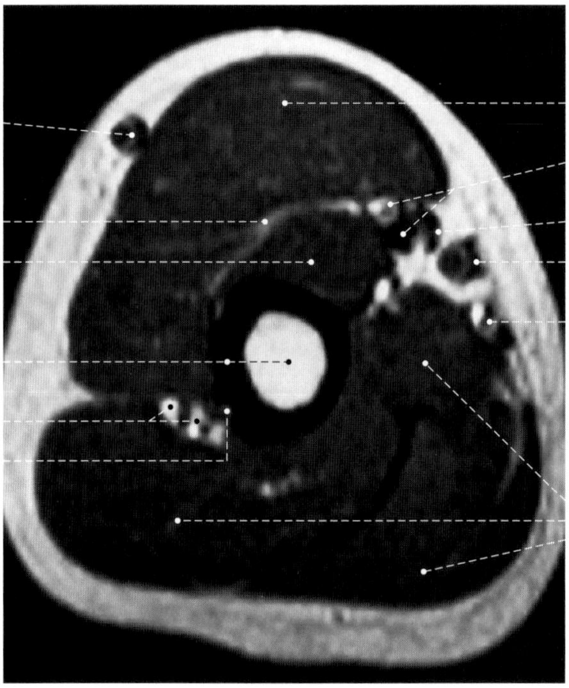
Cephalic vein
Musculocutaneous nerve
Brachialis muscle
Body of humerus
Deep artery and vein of arm
Radial nerve
Biceps brachii muscle
Brachial vein and artery
Median nerve
Basilic vein
Ulnar nerve
Triceps brachii muscle
– Medial (= deep) head
– Lateral head
– Long head

156 Right arm (100%)

Axial (transverse) sections through the middle third of the arm, distal aspect

a Anatomical section

b Magnetic resonance image (MRI, T_1-weighted)

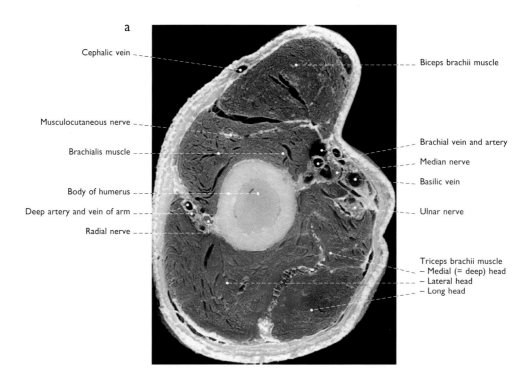

a

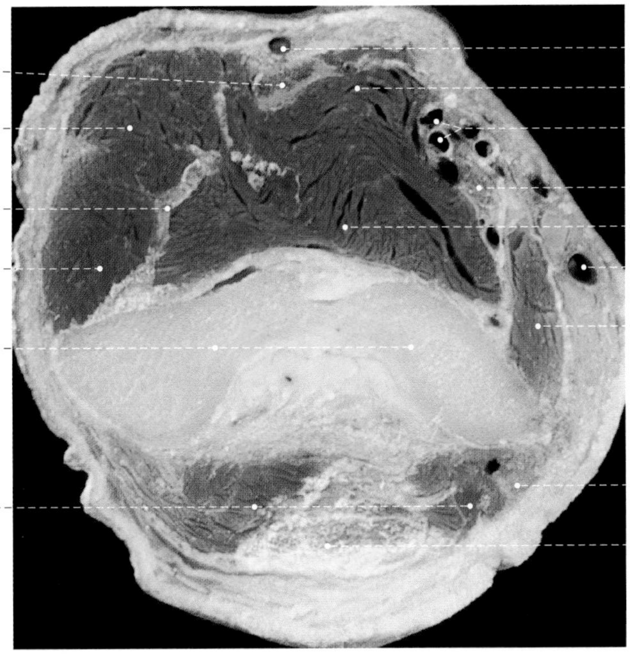
Tendon of biceps brachii muscle
Brachioradialis muscle
Radial nerve
Extensor carpi radialis longus muscle
Humerus
Triceps brachii muscle
Cephalic vein
Biceps brachii muscle
Brachial vein and artery
Median nerve
Brachialis muscle
Basilic vein
Pronator teres muscle
Ulnar nerve
Tendon of triceps brachii muscle

b

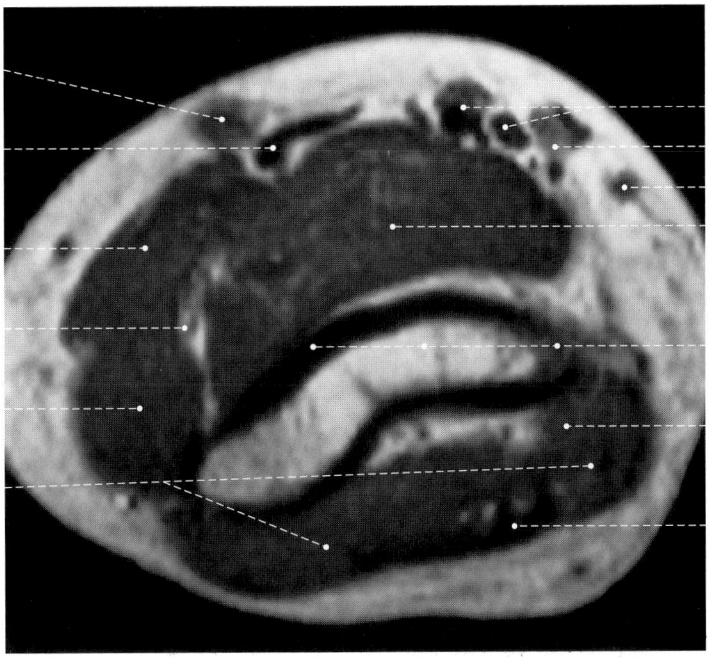
Cephalic vein
Tendon of biceps brachii muscle
Brachioradialis muscle
Radial nerve
Extensor carpi radialis longus muscle
Triceps brachii muscle
Brachial vein and artery
Median nerve
Basilic vein
Brachialis muscle
Humerus
Ulnar nerve
Tendon of triceps brachii muscle

157 Right arm (100%)

Axial (transverse) sections through the distal third of the arm just above the elbow joint, distal aspect

a Anatomical section

b Magnetic resonance image (MRI, T_1-weighted)

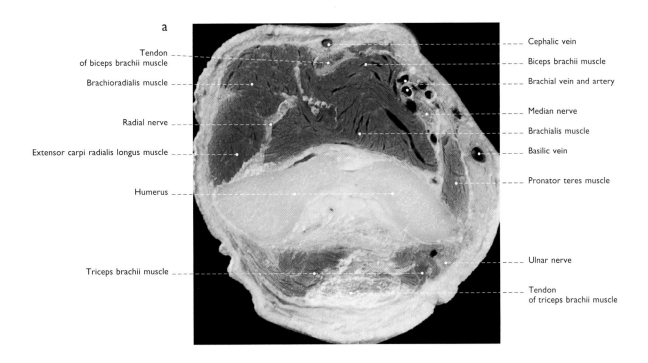

a

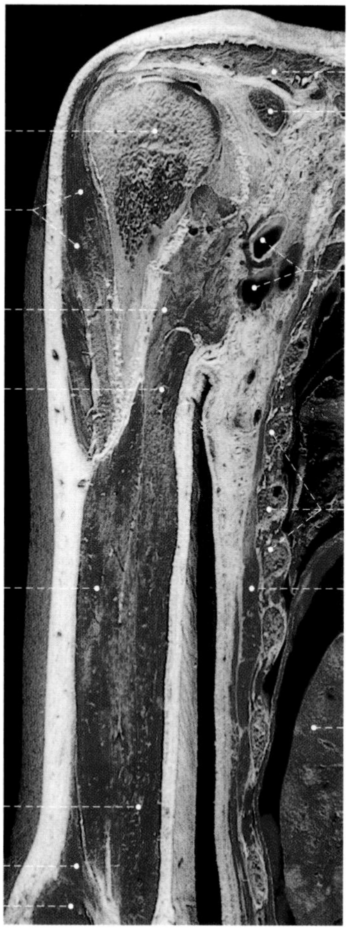
Supraspinatus muscle
Coracoid process of scapula
Head of humerus
Deltoid muscle
Axillary artery and vein
Coracobrachialis muscle
Biceps brachii muscle
Ribs
Brachialis muscle
Serratus anterior muscle
Liver
Biceps brachii muscle
Brachioradialis muscle
Extensor carpi radialis longus muscle

b

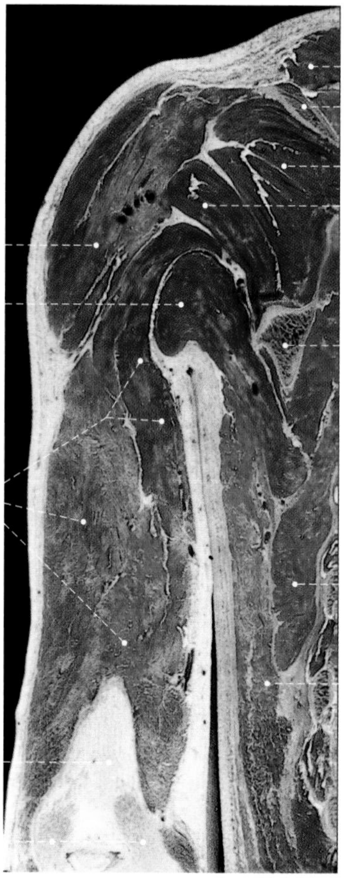
Trapezius muscle
Spine of scapula
Infraspinatus muscle
Teres minor muscle
Deltoid muscle
Teres major muscle
Scapula
Triceps brachii muscle
Long head –
Lateral head –
Medial (= deep) head –
Serratus anterior muscle
Latissimus dorsi muscle
Olecranon fossa
Lateral and medial epicondyles of humerus

158 Right arm (35%)

Coronal anatomical sections

a through the ventral part (flexor compartment)

b through the dorsal part (extensor compartment) of the arm, ventral aspect

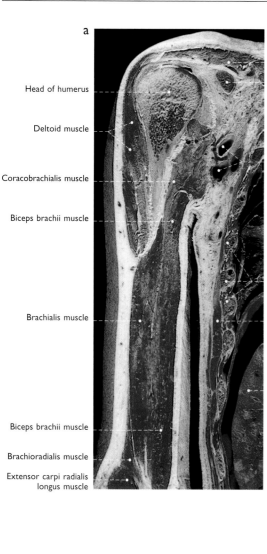

a

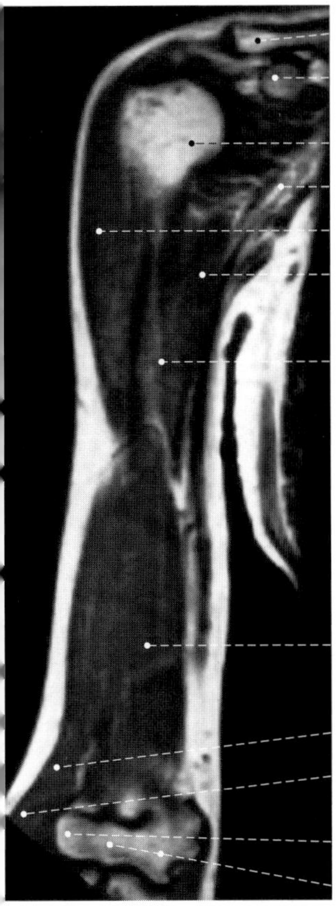
Clavicle
Coracoid process of scapula
Head of humerus
Axillary fossa
Deltoid muscle
Coracobrachialis muscle
Biceps brachii muscle
Brachialis muscle
Brachioradialis muscle
Extensor carpi radialis longus muscle
Capitulum of humerus
Trochlea of humerus

b

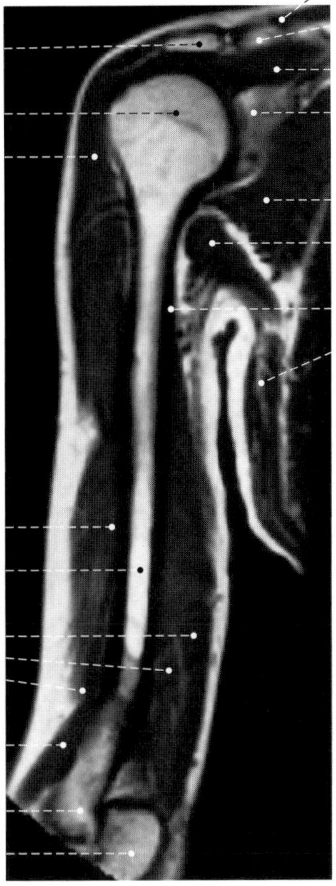
Acromion of scapula
Head of humerus
Deltoid muscle
Brachialis muscle
Body of humerus
Triceps brachii muscle
Long head –
Medial (= deep) head –
Lateral head –
Brachioradialis muscle
Capitulum of humerus
Olecranon of ulna
Trapezius muscle
Clavicle
Supraspinatus muscle
Scapula
Subscapularis muscle
Teres major muscle
Coracobrachialis muscle
Latissimus dorsi muscle

c

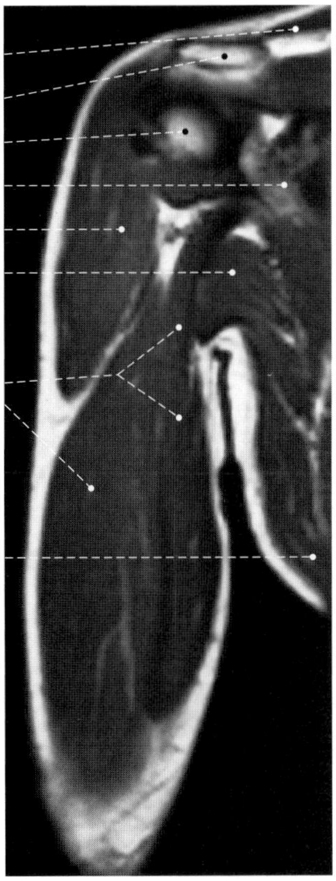
Trapezius muscle
Acromion of scapula
Head of humerus
Scapula
Deltoid muscle
Teres major muscle
Triceps brachii muscle
Long head –
Lateral head –
Latissimus dorsi muscle

159 Right arm (30%)

Coronal magnetic resonance images (MRI, T_1-weighted)
a through the ventral part (flexor compartment)
b through the middle part
c through the dorsal part (extensor compartment) of the arm, ventral aspect

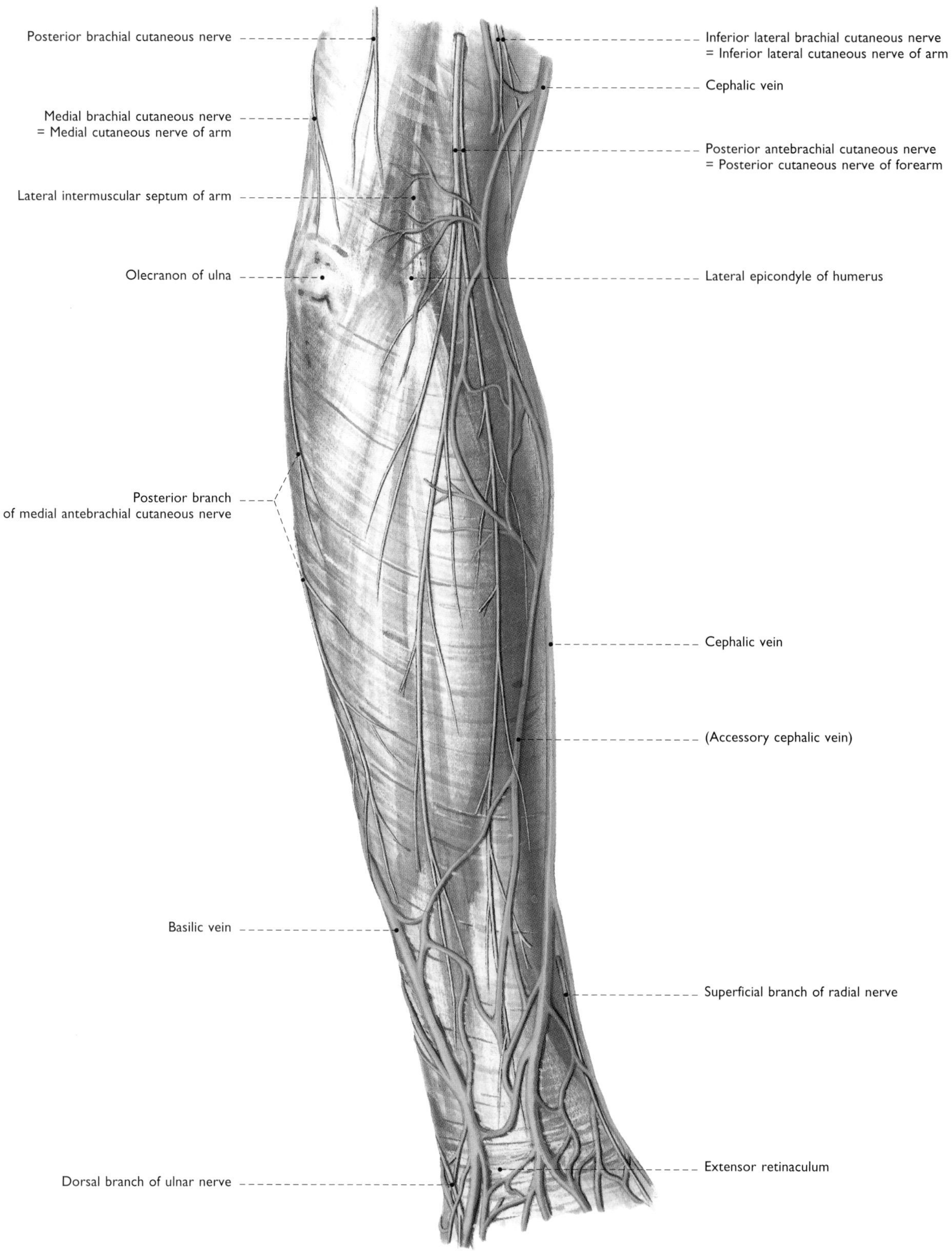
Posterior brachial cutaneous nerve
Medial brachial cutaneous nerve = Medial cutaneous nerve of arm
Lateral intermuscular septum of arm
Olecranon of ulna
Posterior branch of medial antebrachial cutaneous nerve
Basilic vein
Dorsal branch of ulnar nerve
Inferior lateral brachial cutaneous nerve = Inferior lateral cutaneous nerve of arm
Cephalic vein
Posterior antebrachial cutaneous nerve = Posterior cutaneous nerve of forearm
Lateral epicondyle of humerus
Cephalic vein
(Accessory cephalic vein)
Superficial branch of radial nerve
Extensor retinaculum

160 Subcutaneous veins and nerves of the posterior (extensor) region of the right forearm (50%)

Dorsolateral aspect

a

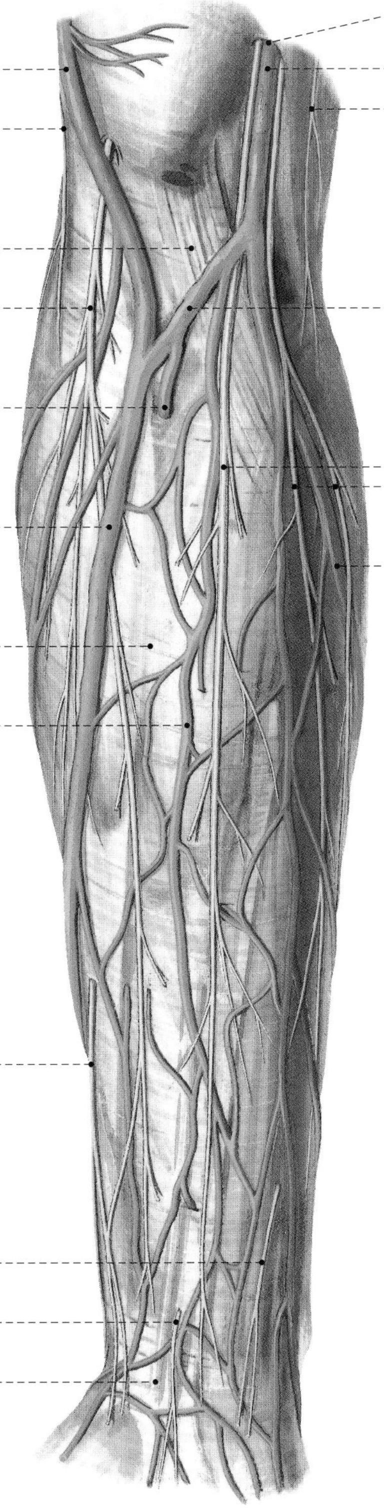
(Opening for basilic vein in brachial fascia)
Cephalic vein
Basilic vein
Posterior brachial cutaneous nerve
= Posterior cutaneous nerve of arm
Medial brachial cutaneous nerve
= Medial cutaneous nerve of arm
Bicipital aponeurosis
Lateral antebrachial cutaneous nerve
= Lateral cutaneous nerve of forearm
Median cubital vein
⟨Deep median cubital vein⟩
Medial antebrachial cutaneous nerve
= Medial cutaneous nerve of forearm
– Anterior branch
– Posterior branch
Cephalic vein
Basilic vein
Antebrachial fascia
Median antebrachial vein
= Median vein of forearm
Superficial branch
of radial nerve
Palmar branch of ulnar nerve
Palmar branch of median nerve
Tendon
of palmaris longus muscle

b

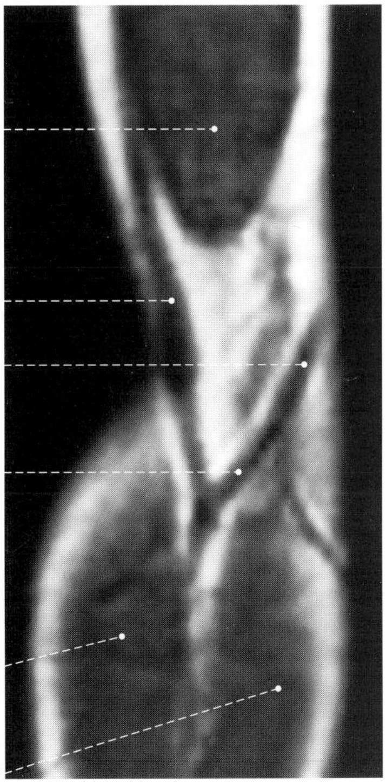
Biceps brachii muscle
Cephalic vein
Basilic vein
Median cubital vein
Brachioradialis muscle
Flexor carpi radialis muscle

161 Subcutaneous veins and nerves of the anterior region of elbow and the anterior (flexor) region of the right forearm (50%)

a Ventral aspect
b Coronal magnetic resonance image (MRI, T_1-weighted)

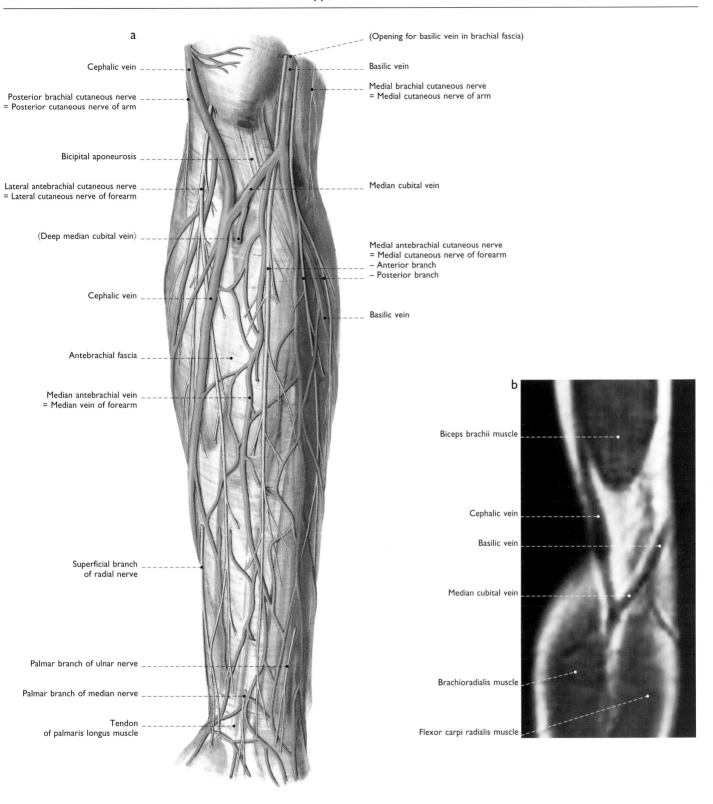

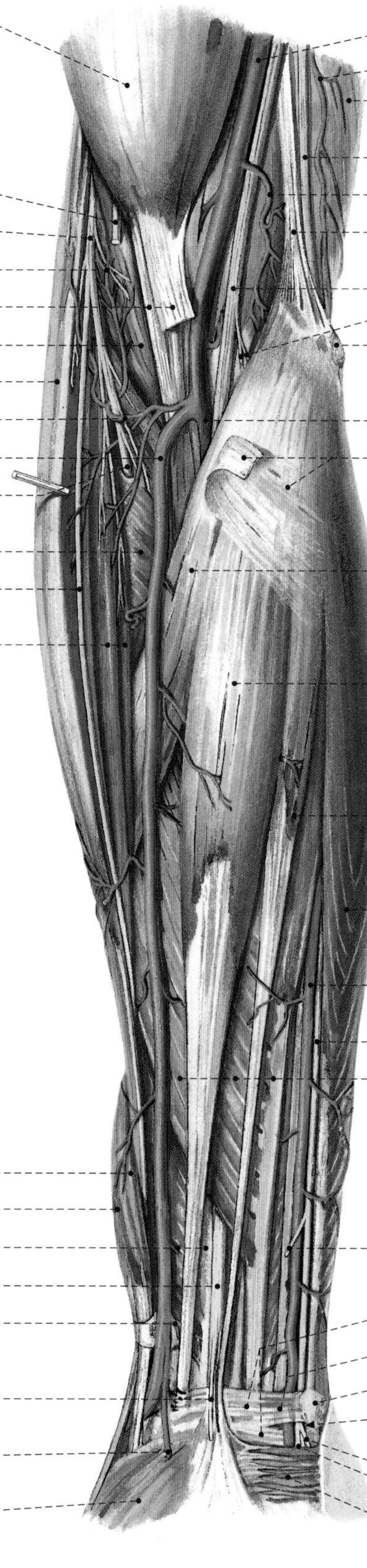
Biceps brachii muscle
Lateral antebrachial cutaneous nerve
Radial nerve
Radial collateral artery
Tendon and aponeurosis of biceps brachii muscle
Brachialis muscle
Brachioradialis muscle
Radial recurrent artery
Radial artery
Deep branch of radial nerve
Supinator muscle
Superficial branch of radial nerve
Extensor carpi radialis longus muscle,
Extensor carpi radialis brevis muscle
Abductor pollicis longus muscle
Extensor pollicis brevis muscle
Flexor pollicis longus muscle
Median nerve
Palmar carpal branch of radial artery
Palmar branch of median nerve
Superficial palmar branch of radial artery
Abductor pollicis brevis muscle
Brachial artery
Superior ulnar collateral artery
Medial (= deep) head of triceps brachii muscle
Ulnar nerve
Inferior ulnar collateral artery
Medial intermuscular septum of arm
Median nerve
– Muscular branches
Medial epicondyle of humerus
Ulnar artery
Bicipital aponeurosis,
Antebrachial fascia
Pronator teres muscle
Flexor carpi radialis muscle
Palmaris longus muscle
Flexor carpi ulnaris muscle
Ulnar artery
Ulnar nerve
Flexor digitorum superficialis muscle
Palmar branch of ulnar nerve
Flexor retinaculum
⟨Palmar carpal ligament⟩
Pisiform
Ulnar canal (Loge of GUYON)
Ulnar nerve
– Deep branch
– Superficial branch
Palmaris brevis muscle

162 Arteries and nerves of the right forearm (50%)
Ventral aspect

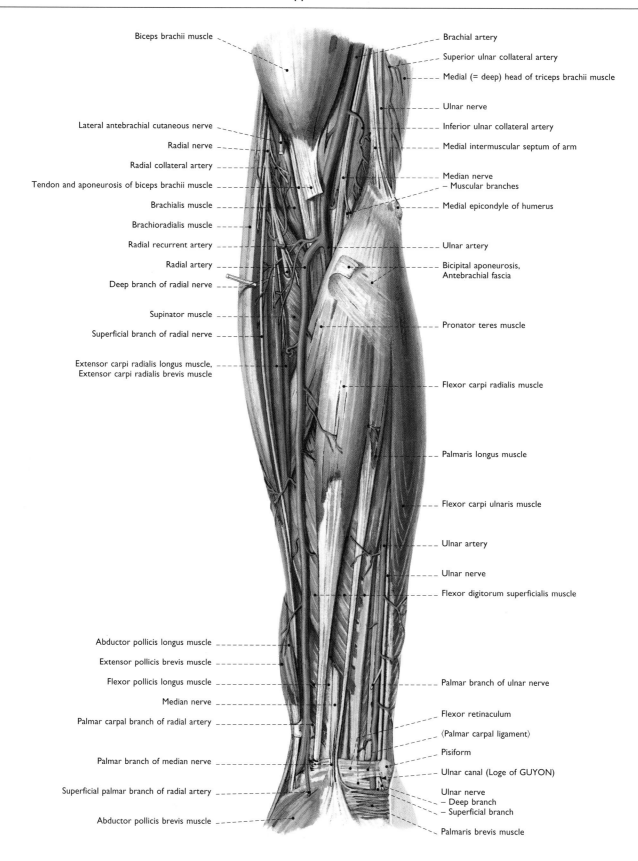

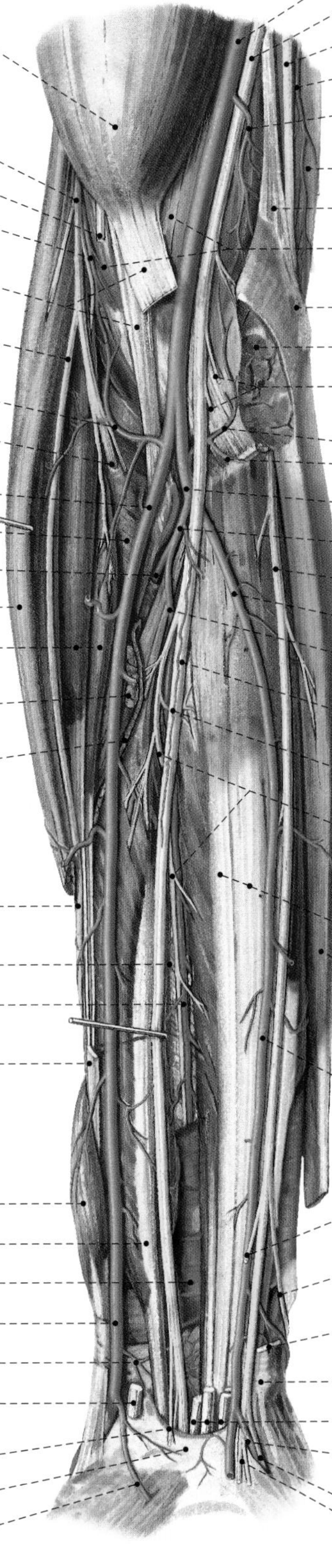
Brachial artery
Median nerve
Ulnar nerve
Superior ulnar collateral artery
Inferior ulnar collateral artery
Triceps brachii muscle
Medial intermuscular septum of arm
Brachialis muscle
Medial epicondyle of humerus
⟨Common flexor tendon⟩
Muscular branches of median nerve
Ulnar recurrent artery
– Anterior branch
– Posterior branch
Ulnar artery
Common interosseous artery
Ulnar nerve
Ulnar artery
Anterior interosseous artery
Median nerve
Median artery
Anterior interosseous nerve
(of median nerve)
Flexor digitorum profundus muscle
Flexor carpi ulnaris muscle
Ulnar artery
Palmar branch of ulnar nerve
Dorsal branch of ulnar nerve
Tendon of flexor carpi ulnaris muscle
Pisiform
Tendons of flexor digitorum superficialis muscle
Deep palmar branch of ulnar artery
Ulnar nerve
– Deep branch
– Superficial branch
Biceps brachii muscle
Radial nerve
Lateral antebrachial cutaneous nerve
Radial collateral artery
Aponeurosis and tendon
of biceps brachii muscle
Superficial branch of radial nerve
Radial recurrent artery
Deep branch of radial nerve
Radial artery
Supinator muscle
Posterior interosseous artery
Brachioradialis muscle
Extensor carpi radialis longus muscle,
Extensor carpi radialis brevis muscle
Pronator teres muscle
(cut edge)
Flexor digitorum superficialis muscle
(cut edge)
Superficial branch of radial nerve
Interosseous membrane of forearm
Anterior interosseous artery
Tendon of brachioradialis muscle
Abductor pollicis longus muscle
Flexor pollicis longus muscle
Pronator quadratus muscle
Radial artery
Palmar carpal branch of radial artery
Tendon of flexor carpi radialis muscle
Palmar branch of median nerve
Flexor retinaculum
Superficial palmar branch of radial artery

163 Arteries and nerves of the right forearm (50%)

The superficial muscles were removed.
Ventral aspect

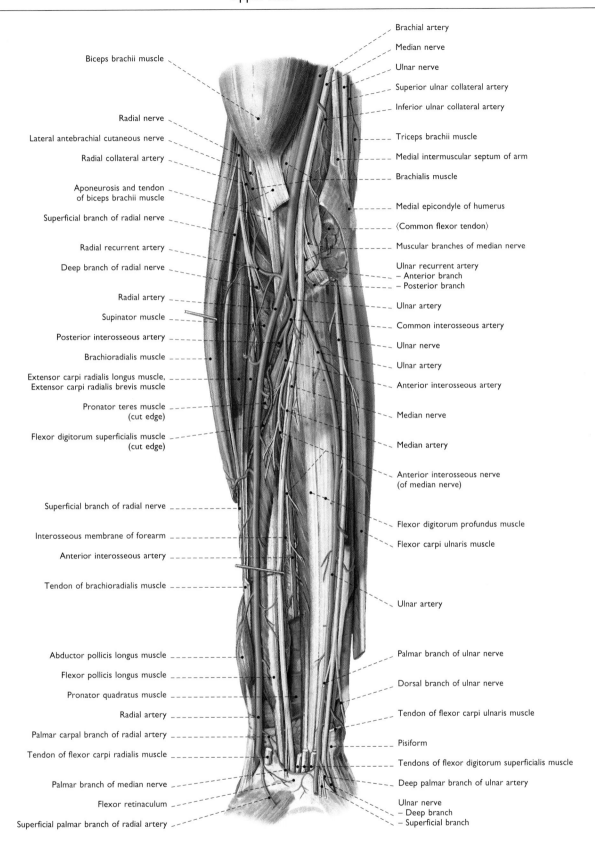

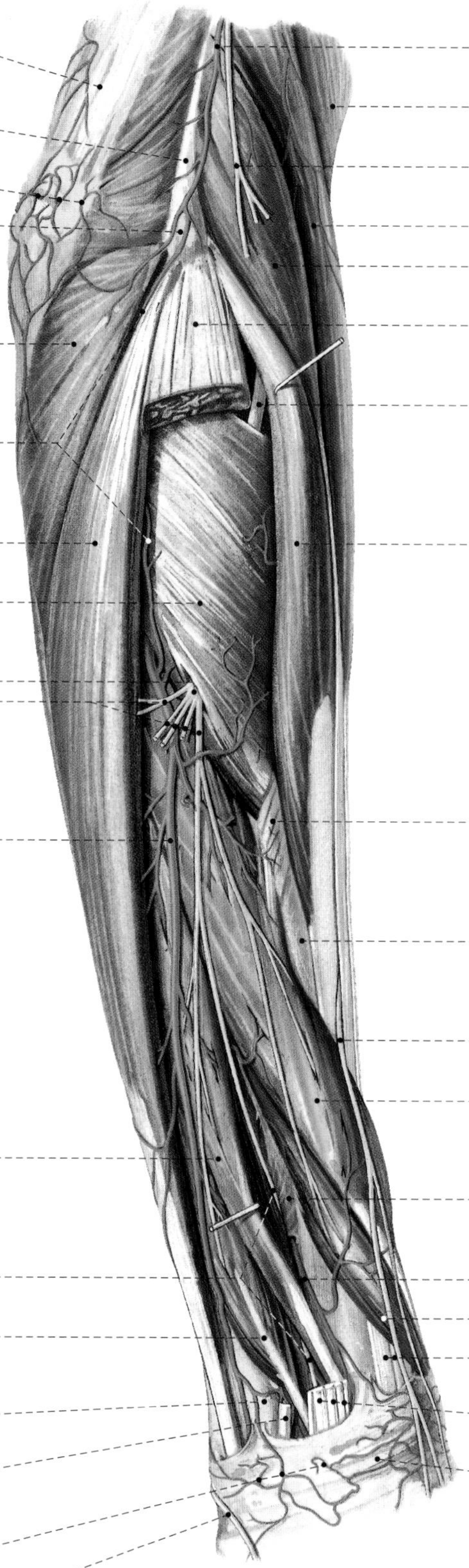
Tendon of triceps brachii muscle
Lateral intermuscular septum of arm
Cubital anastomosis
Lateral epicondyle of humerus
Anconeus muscle
Recurrent interosseous artery
Extensor carpi ulnaris muscle
Supinator muscle
Radial nerve
Deep branch –
Muscular branches –
Posterior interosseous artery
Extensor pollicis longus muscle
Posterior interosseous nerve (of radial nerve)
Extensor indicis muscle
Ulna
Tendon of extensor digiti minimi muscle
Dorsal carpal arch
Dorsal branch of ulnar nerve
Radial collateral artery
Brachialis muscle
Posterior antebrachial cutaneous nerve
Brachioradialis muscle
Extensor carpi radialis longus muscle
Extensor digitorum muscle
Deep branch of radial nerve
Extensor carpi radialis brevis muscle
Pronator teres muscle
Radius
Superficial branch of radial nerve
Abductor pollicis longus muscle
Interosseous membrane of forearm
Anterior interosseous artery
Extensor pollicis brevis muscle
Tendons of extensores carpi radiales longus and brevis muscles
Tendons of extensor digitorum muscle
Extensor retinaculum

164 **Arteries and nerves of the right forearm** (50%)

The superficial muscles were partially removed.
Dorsolateral aspect

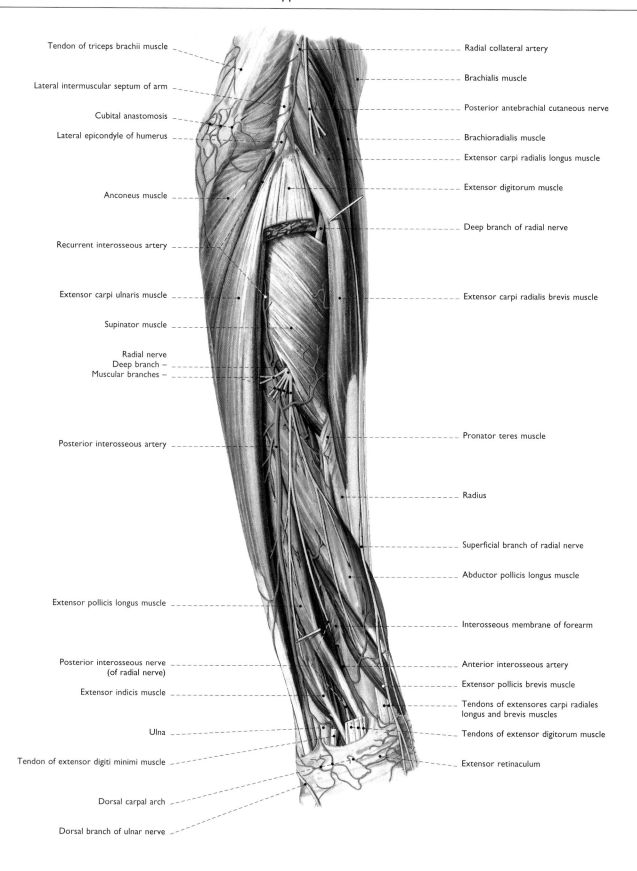

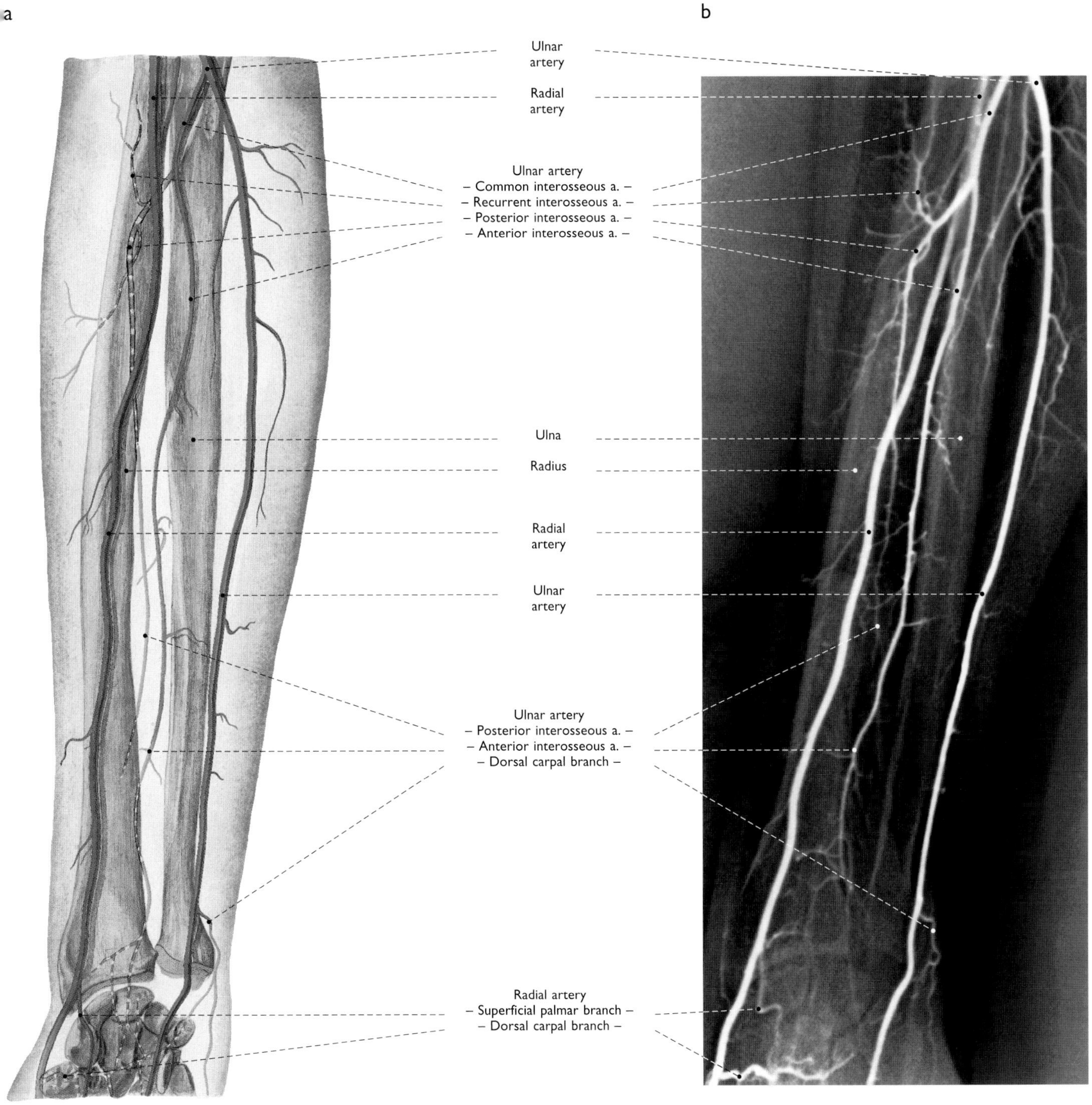
a
b
Ulnar artery
Radial artery
Ulnar artery
– Common interosseous a. –
– Recurrent interosseous a. –
– Posterior interosseous a. –
– Anterior interosseous a. –
Ulna
Radius
Radial artery
Ulnar artery
Ulnar artery
– Posterior interosseous a. –
– Anterior interosseous a. –
– Dorsal carpal branch –
Radial artery
– Superficial palmar branch –
– Dorsal carpal branch –

165 Arteries of the right forearm (60%)

Ventral aspect
a Schematic representation
b Arteriogram

a

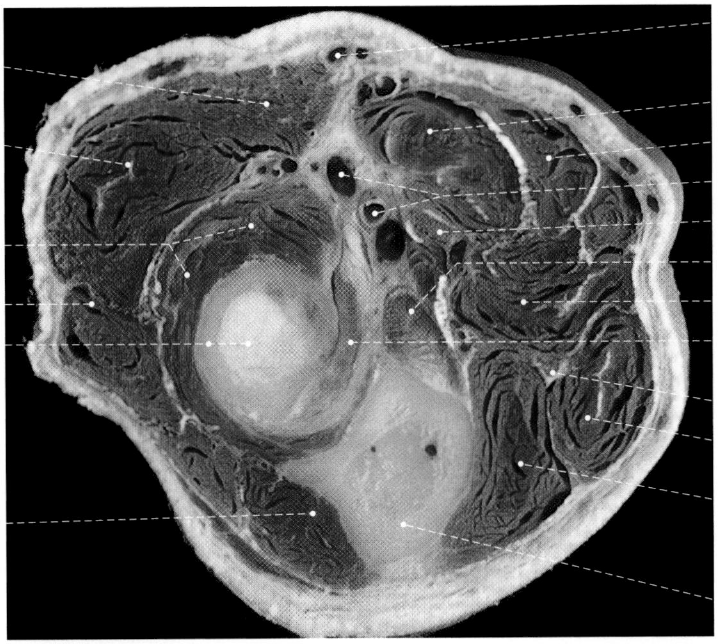
Cephalic vein
Brachioradialis muscle
Pronator teres muscle
Flexor carpi radialis muscle
Extensor carpi radialis longus muscle
Brachial vein and artery
Median nerve
Supinator muscle
Brachialis muscle
Extensor carpi radialis brevis muscle
Flexor digitorum superficialis muscle
Radius
Tendon of biceps brachii muscle
Ulnar nerve
Flexor carpi ulnaris muscle
Flexor digitorum profundus muscle
Anconeus muscle
Ulna

b

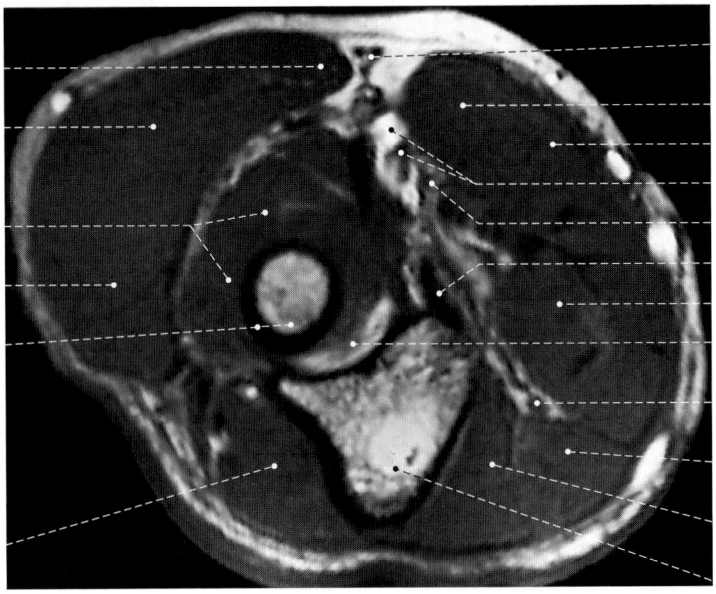
Cephalic vein
Brachioradialis muscle
Pronator teres muscle
Extensor carpi radialis longus muscle
Flexor carpi radialis muscle
Brachial vein and artery
Supinator muscle
Median nerve
Brachialis muscle
Extensor carpi radialis brevis muscle
Flexor digitorum superficialis muscle
Radius
Tendon of biceps brachii muscle
Ulnar nerve
Flexor carpi ulnaris muscle
Flexor digitorum profundus muscle
Anconeus muscle
Ulna

166 Right forearm (110%)

Axial (transverse) sections through the proximal forearm just below the elbow joint, distal aspect

a Anatomical section

b Magnetic resonance image (MRI, T_1-weighted)

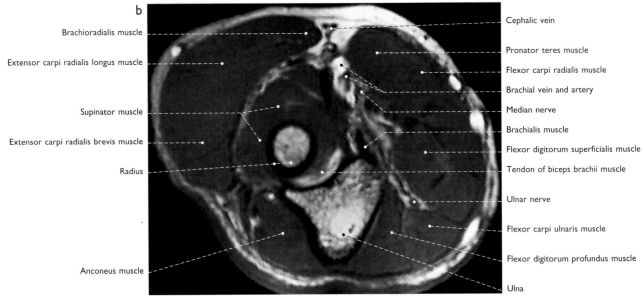

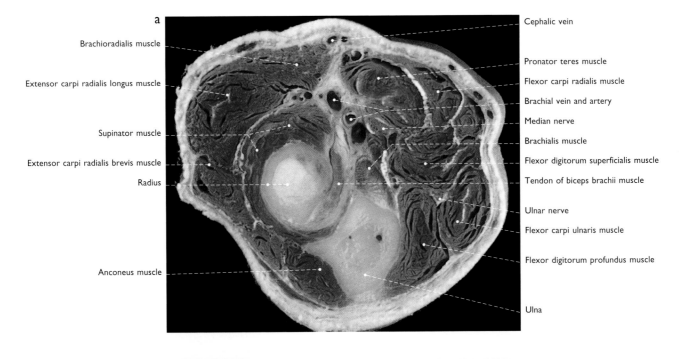

a

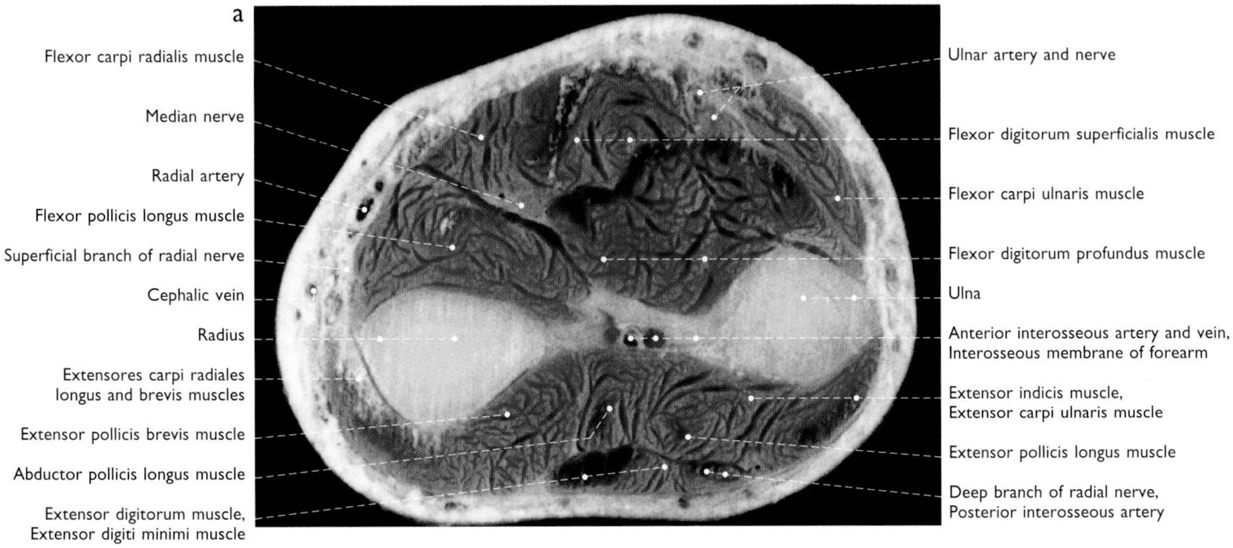
Flexor carpi radialis muscle
Median nerve
Radial artery
Flexor pollicis longus muscle
Superficial branch of radial nerve
Cephalic vein
Radius
Extensores carpi radiales longus and brevis muscles
Extensor pollicis brevis muscle
Abductor pollicis longus muscle
Extensor digitorum muscle, Extensor digiti minimi muscle
Ulnar artery and nerve
Flexor digitorum superficialis muscle
Flexor carpi ulnaris muscle
Flexor digitorum profundus muscle
Ulna
Anterior interosseous artery and vein, Interosseous membrane of forearm
Extensor indicis muscle, Extensor carpi ulnaris muscle
Extensor pollicis longus muscle
Deep branch of radial nerve, Posterior interosseous artery

b

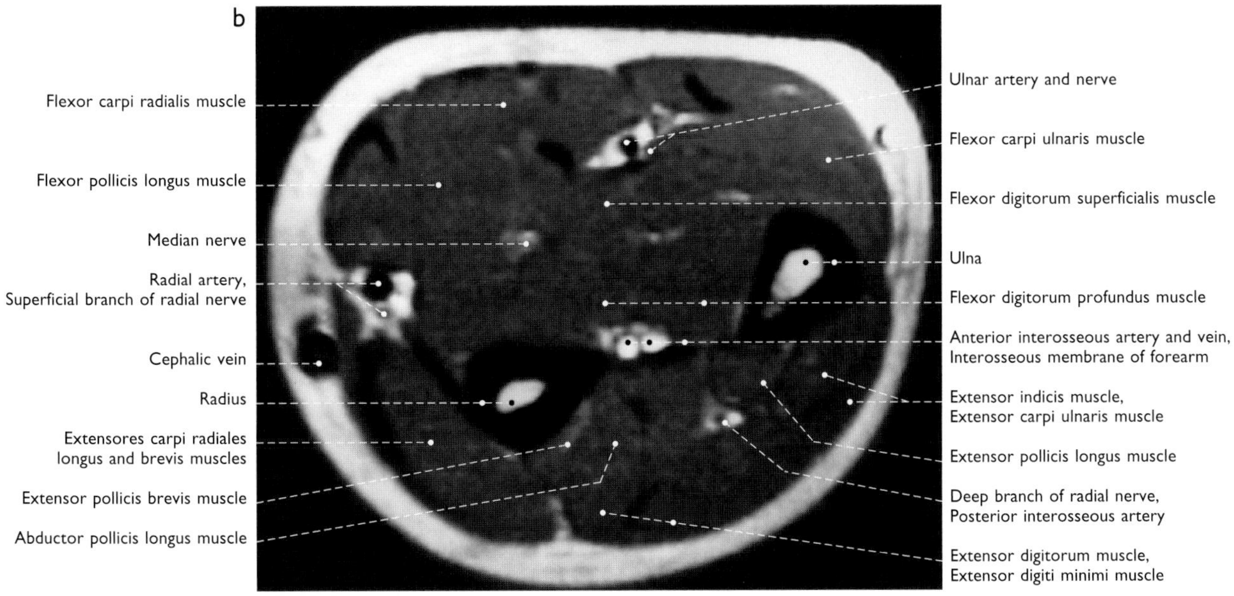
Flexor carpi radialis muscle
Flexor pollicis longus muscle
Median nerve
Radial artery, Superficial branch of radial nerve
Cephalic vein
Radius
Extensores carpi radiales longus and brevis muscles
Extensor pollicis brevis muscle
Abductor pollicis longus muscle
Ulnar artery and nerve
Flexor carpi ulnaris muscle
Flexor digitorum superficialis muscle
Ulna
Flexor digitorum profundus muscle
Anterior interosseous artery and vein, Interosseous membrane of forearm
Extensor indicis muscle, Extensor carpi ulnaris muscle
Extensor pollicis longus muscle
Deep branch of radial nerve, Posterior interosseous artery
Extensor digitorum muscle, Extensor digiti minimi muscle

167 Right forearm (110%)

Axial (transverse) sections through the proximal third of the forearm in supinated position, distal aspect

a Anatomical section

b Magnetic resonance image (MRI, T_1-weighted)

a

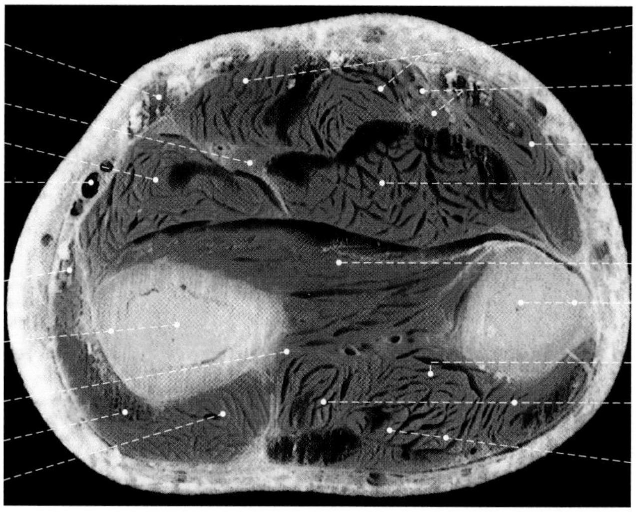
Tendon of flexor carpi radialis muscle
Median nerve
Flexor pollicis longus muscle
Radial artery
Tendon of extensor carpi radialis longus muscle
Radius
Interosseous membrane of forearm
Abductor pollicis longus muscle
Extensor pollicis brevis muscle
Flexor digitorum superficialis muscle
Ulnar artery and nerve
Flexor carpi ulnaris muscle
Flexor digitorum profundus muscle
Pronator quadratus muscle
Ulna
Extensor indicis muscle
Extensor pollicis longus muscle,
Extensor carpi ulnaris muscle
Extensor digitorum muscle,
Extensor digiti minimi muscle

b

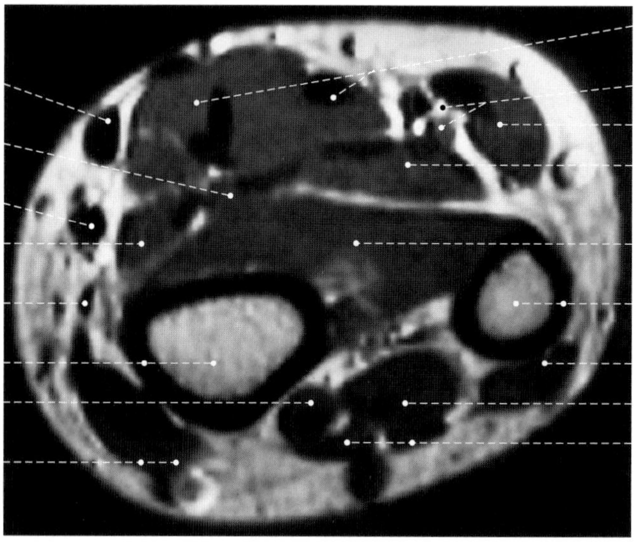
Tendon of flexor carpi radialis muscle
Median nerve
Radial artery
Flexor pollicis longus muscle
Tendon of extensor carpi radialis longus muscle
Radius
Extensor pollicis longus muscle
Abductor pollicis longus muscle,
Extensor pollicis brevis muscle
Flexor digitorum superficialis muscle
Ulnar artery and nerve
Flexor carpi ulnaris muscle
Flexor digitorum profundus muscle
Pronator quadratus muscle
Ulna
Extensor carpi ulnaris muscle
Extensor indicis muscle
Extensor digitorum muscle,
Extensor digiti minimi muscle

168 Right forearm (120%)

Axial (transverse) sections through the distal third of the forearm in supinated position, distal aspect

a Anatomical section

b Magnetic resonance image (MRI, T_1-weighted)

a

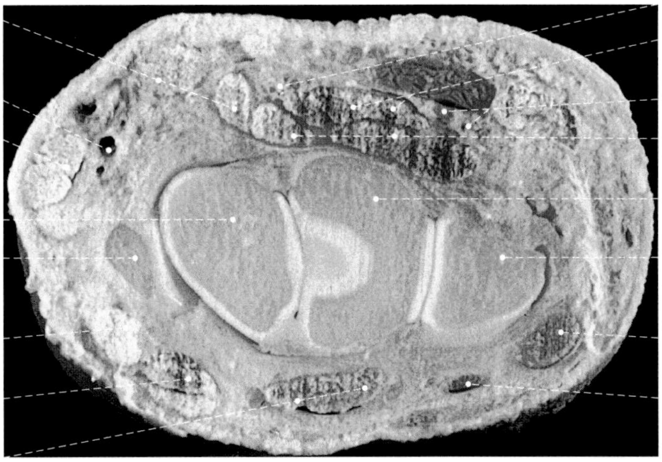
Tendons of flexor carpi radialis and flexor pollicis longus muscles
Radial artery
Tendons of abductor pollicis longus and extensor pollicis brevis muscles
Scaphoid
Radial styloid process
Tendon of extensor carpi radialis longus muscle
Tendon of extensor carpi radialis brevis muscle
Tendons of extensor indicis and extensor digitorum muscles
Median nerve
Tendons of flexor digitorum superficialis muscle
Ulnar nerve and artery
Tendons of flexor digitorum profundus muscle
Lunate
Triquetrum
Tendon of extensor carpi ulnaris muscle
Tendon of extensor digiti minimi muscle

b

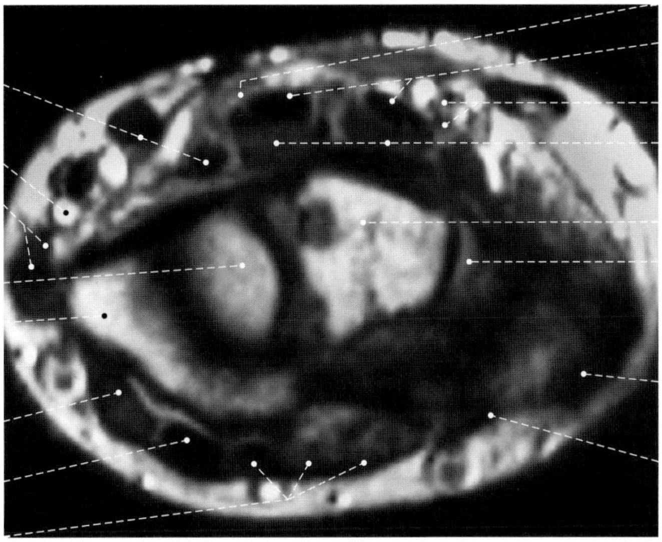
Tendons of flexor carpi radialis and flexor pollicis longus muscles
Radial artery
Tendons of abductor pollicis longus and extensor pollicis brevis muscles
Scaphoid
Radial styloid process
Tendon of extensor carpi radialis longus muscle
Tendon of extensor carpi radialis brevis muscle
Tendons of extensor indicis and extensor digitorum muscles
Median nerve
Tendons of flexor digitorum superficialis muscle
Ulnar nerve and artery
Tendons of flexor digitorum profundus muscle
Lunate
Triquetrum
Tendon of extensor carpi ulnaris muscle
Tendon of extensor digiti minimi muscle

169 Right forearm (120%)

Axial (transverse) sections through the distal forearm at the level of the wrist joint. Forearm and hand in supinated position, distal aspect

a Anatomical section

b Magnetic resonance image (MRI, T_1-weighted)

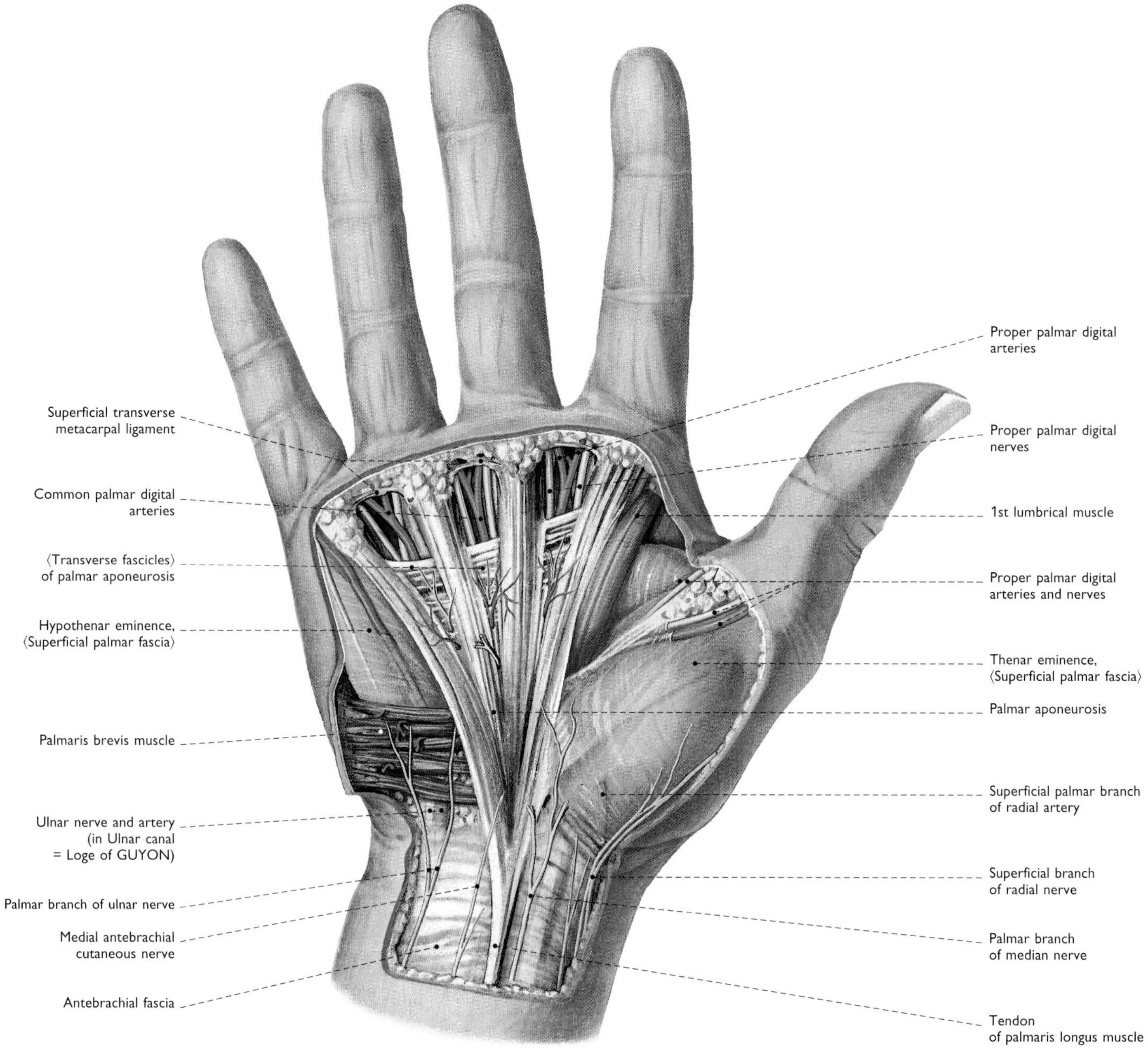
Superficial transverse metacarpal ligament
Common palmar digital arteries
⟨Transverse fascicles⟩ of palmar aponeurosis
Hypothenar eminence, ⟨Superficial palmar fascia⟩
Palmaris brevis muscle
Ulnar nerve and artery (in Ulnar canal = Loge of GUYON)
Palmar branch of ulnar nerve
Medial antebrachial cutaneous nerve
Antebrachial fascia
Proper palmar digital arteries
Proper palmar digital nerves
1st lumbrical muscle
Proper palmar digital arteries and nerves
Thenar eminence, ⟨Superficial palmar fascia⟩
Palmar aponeurosis
Superficial palmar branch of radial artery
Superficial branch of radial nerve
Palmar branch of median nerve
Tendon of palmaris longus muscle

170 Arteries and nerves of the palm of the right hand (75%)

Palmar aspect

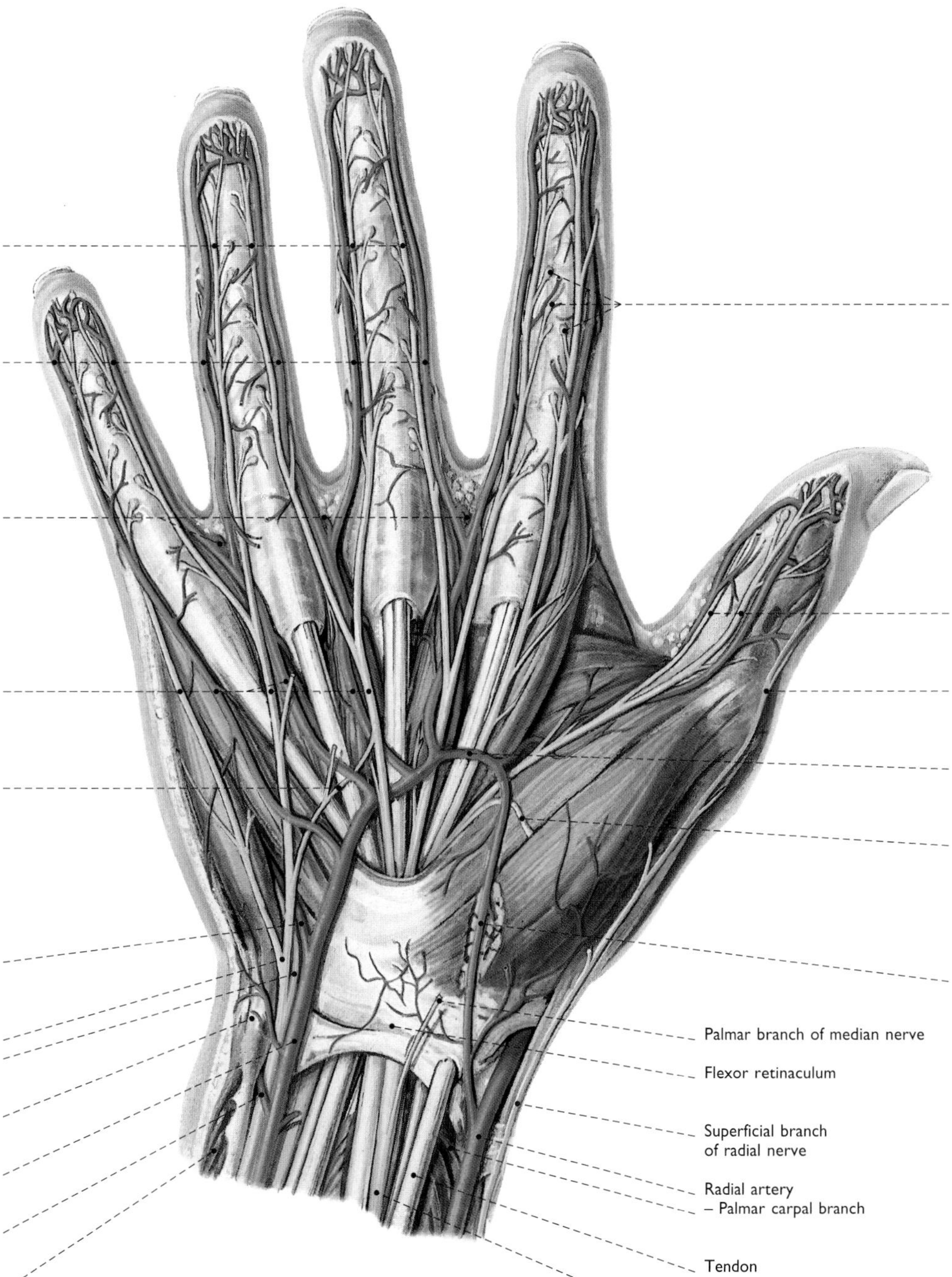

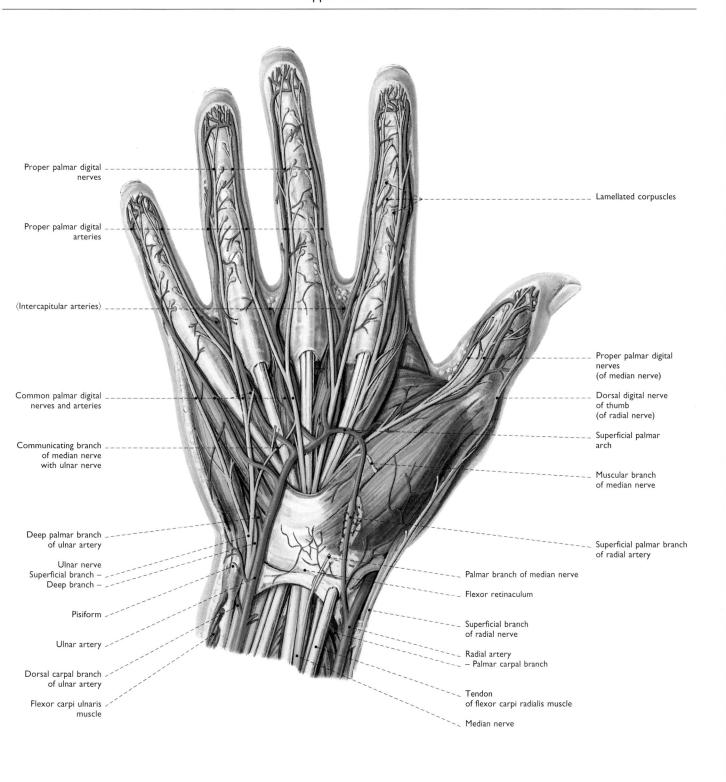

Proper palmar digital nerves
Proper palmar digital arteries
⟨Intercapitular arteries⟩
Common palmar digital nerves and arteries
Communicating branch of median nerve with ulnar nerve
Deep palmar branch of ulnar artery
Ulnar nerve
Superficial branch –
Deep branch –
Pisiform
Ulnar artery
Dorsal carpal branch of ulnar artery
Flexor carpi ulnaris muscle
Lamellated corpuscles
Proper palmar digital nerves (of median nerve)
Dorsal digital nerve of thumb (of radial nerve)
Superficial palmar arch
Muscular branch of median nerve
Superficial palmar branch of radial artery
Palmar branch of median nerve
Flexor retinaculum
Superficial branch of radial nerve
Radial artery
– Palmar carpal branch
Tendon of flexor carpi radialis muscle
Median nerve

171 Arteries and nerves of the palm of the right hand (75%)

The palmar aponeurosis was removed.
Palmar aspect

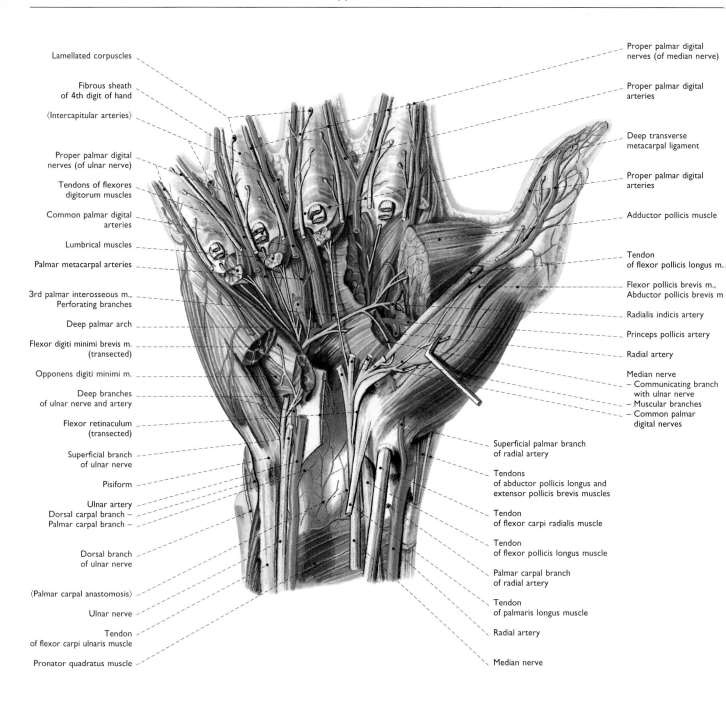

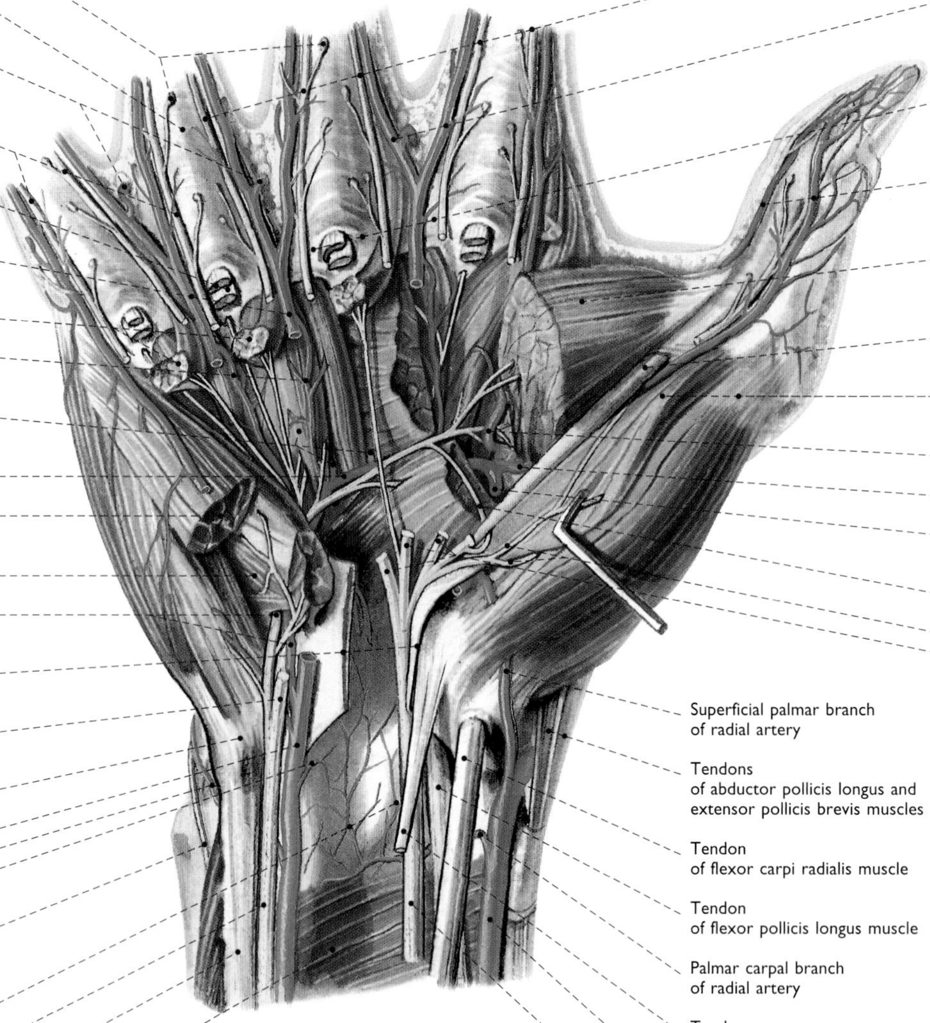
Lamellated corpuscles
Fibrous sheath of 4th digit of hand
⟨Intercapitular arteries⟩
Proper palmar digital nerves (of ulnar nerve)
Tendons of flexores digitorum muscles
Common palmar digital arteries
Lumbrical muscles
Palmar metacarpal arteries
3rd palmar interosseous m., Perforating branches
Deep palmar arch
Flexor digiti minimi brevis m. (transected)
Opponens digiti minimi m.
Deep branches of ulnar nerve and artery
Flexor retinaculum (transected)
Superficial branch of ulnar nerve
Pisiform
Ulnar artery
Dorsal carpal branch –
Palmar carpal branch –
Dorsal branch of ulnar nerve
⟨Palmar carpal anastomosis⟩
Ulnar nerve
Tendon of flexor carpi ulnaris muscle
Pronator quadratus muscle
Proper palmar digital nerves (of median nerve)
Proper palmar digital arteries
Deep transverse metacarpal ligament
Proper palmar digital arteries
Adductor pollicis muscle
Tendon of flexor pollicis longus m.
Flexor pollicis brevis m., Abductor pollicis brevis m
Radialis indicis artery
Princeps pollicis artery
Radial artery
Median nerve
– Communicating branch with ulnar nerve
– Muscular branches
– Common palmar digital nerves
Superficial palmar branch of radial artery
Tendons of abductor pollicis longus and extensor pollicis brevis muscles
Tendon of flexor carpi radialis muscle
Tendon of flexor pollicis longus muscle
Palmar carpal branch of radial artery
Tendon of palmaris longus muscle
Radial artery
Median nerve

172 Arteries and nerves of the palm of the right hand (75%)

The palmar aponeurosis and the flexor muscles of the fingers were removed. Palmar aspect

a

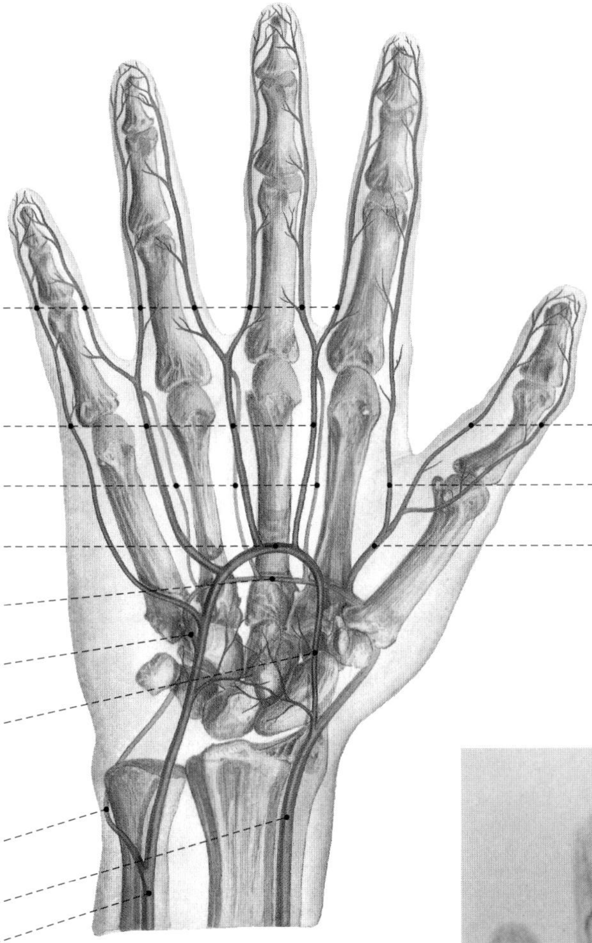
roper palmar digital arteries
mmon palmar digital arteries
Palmar metacarpal arteries
Superficial palmar arch
Deep palmar arch
Deep palmar branch of ulnar artery
Superficial palmar nch of radial artery
orsal carpal branch of ulnar artery
Radial artery
Ulnar artery
Proper palmar digital arteries
Radialis indicis artery
Princeps pollicis artery

b

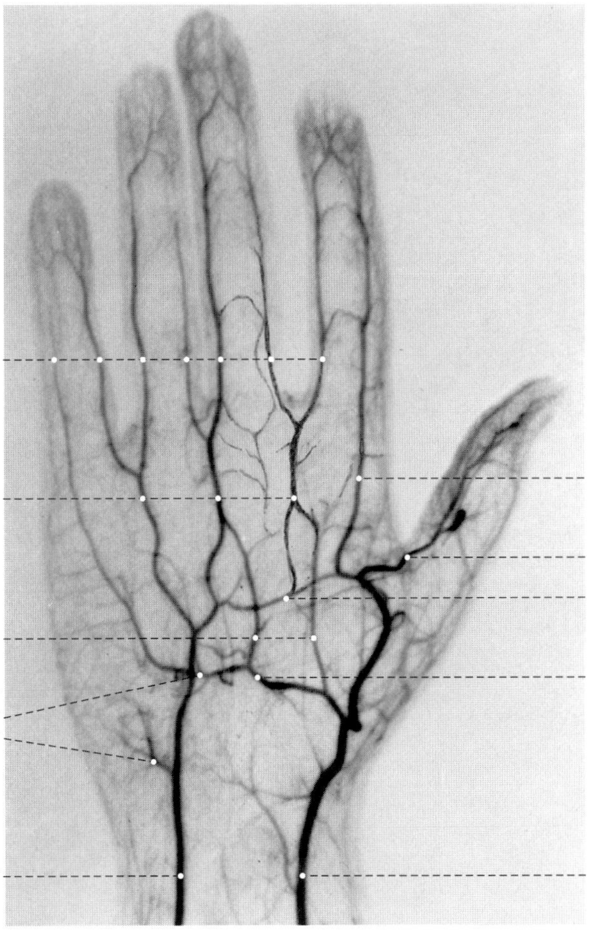
Proper palmar digital arteries
Common palmar digital arteries
Palmar metacarpal arteries
Ulnar artery
Deep palmar branch –
Dorsal carpal branch –
Ulnar artery
Radialis indicis artery
Princeps pollicis artery
Superficial palmar arch
Deep palmar arch
Radial artery

173 Arteries of the right hand (50%)

Palmar aspect

a Schematic representation

b Arteriogram

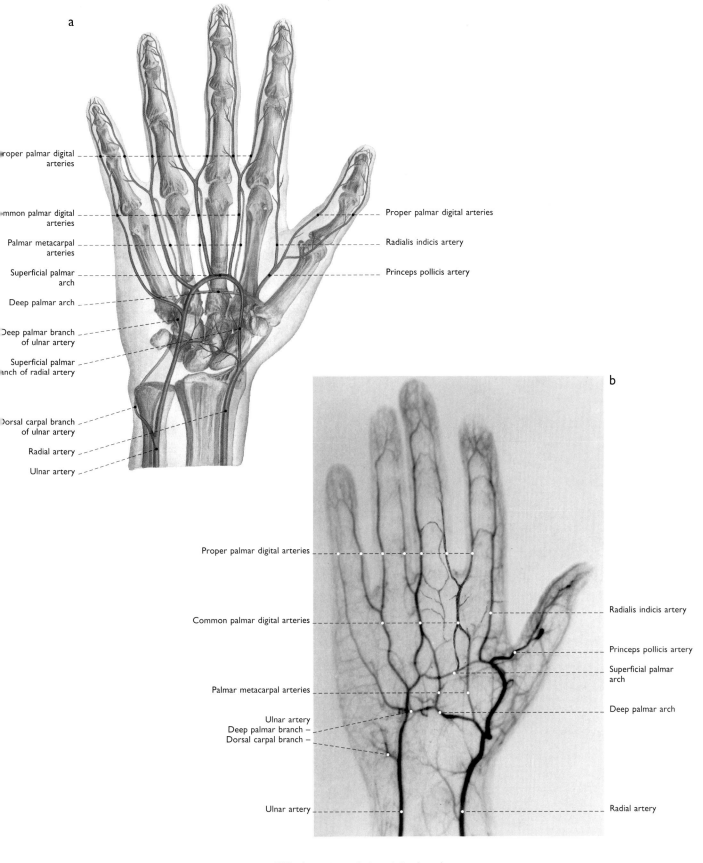

a

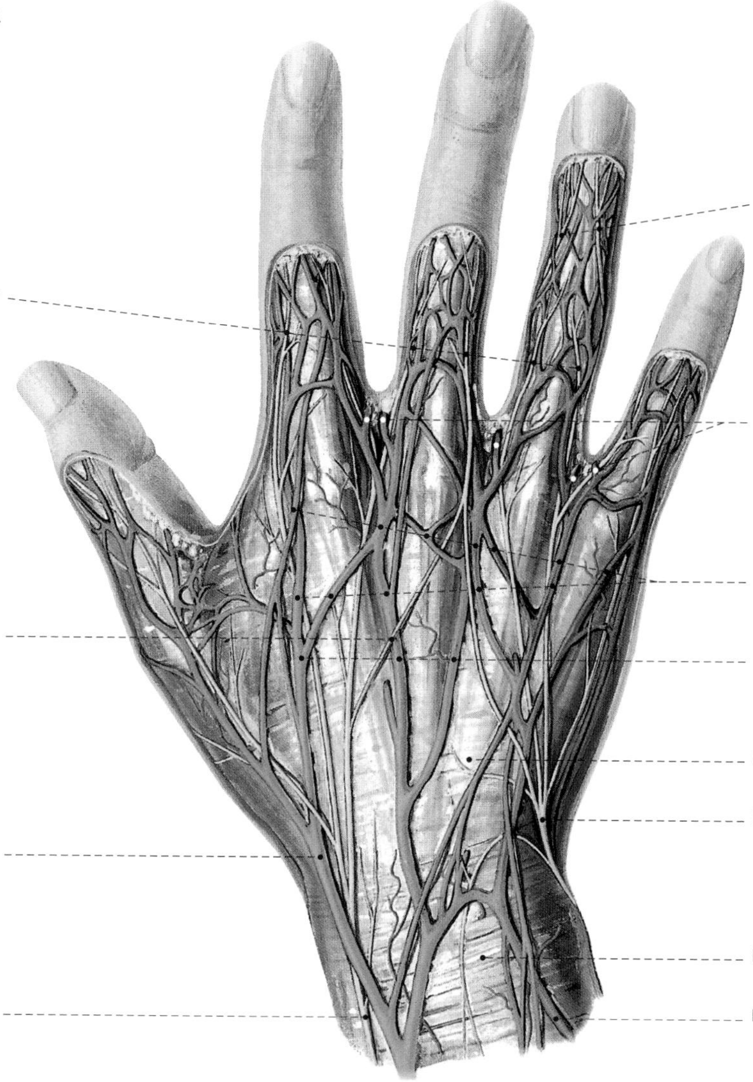
Proper palmar digital nerves
Dorsal digital nerves
Intercapitular veins
Dorsal venous network of hand
Communicating branch of radial nerve with ulnar nerve
Dorsal metacarpal veins
Dorsal fascia of hand
Dorsal branch of ulnar nerve
Cephalic vein
Extensor retinaculum
Superficial branch of radial nerve
Basilic vein

b

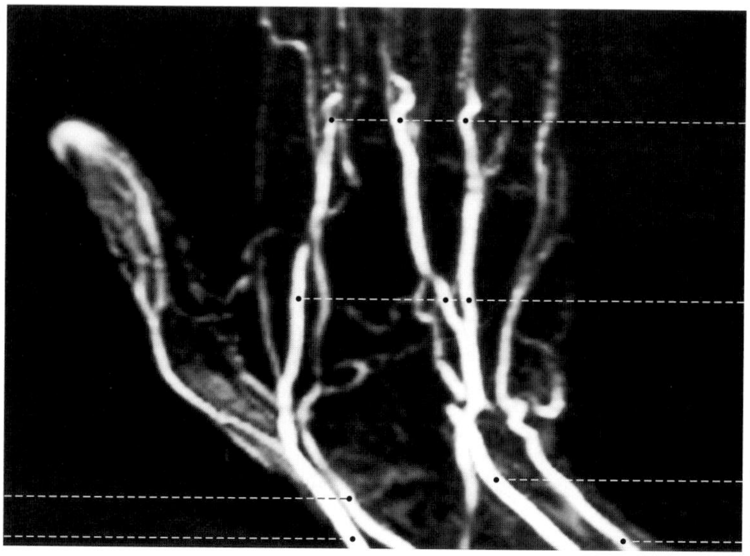
Intercapitular veins
Dorsal venous network of hand
Basilic vein
Radial vein
Cephalic vein
Ulnar vein

174 Subcutaneous veins and nerves of the dorsum of the right hand (60%)

a Dorsal aspect
b Magnetic resonance angiogram (MRA)

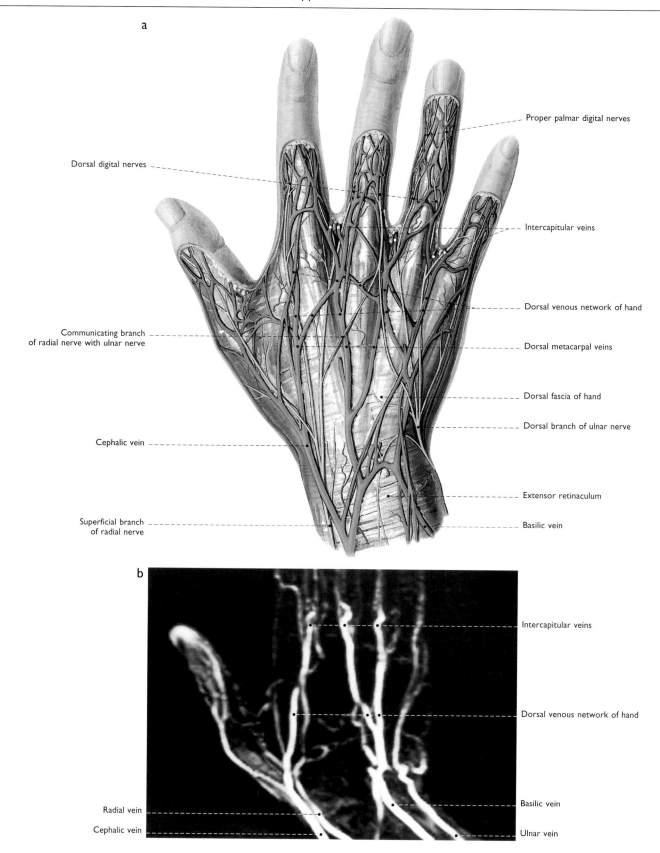

a

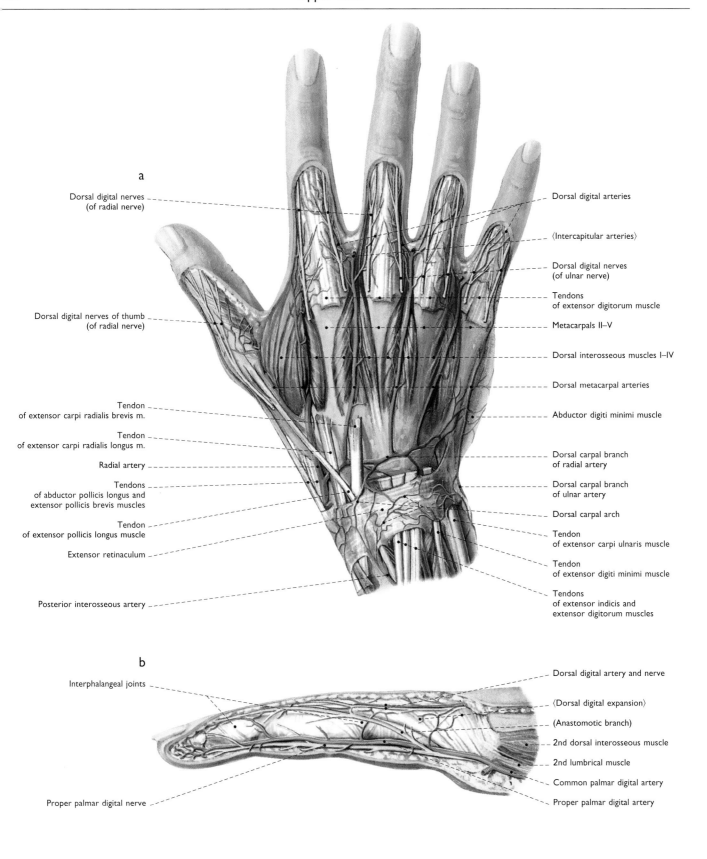

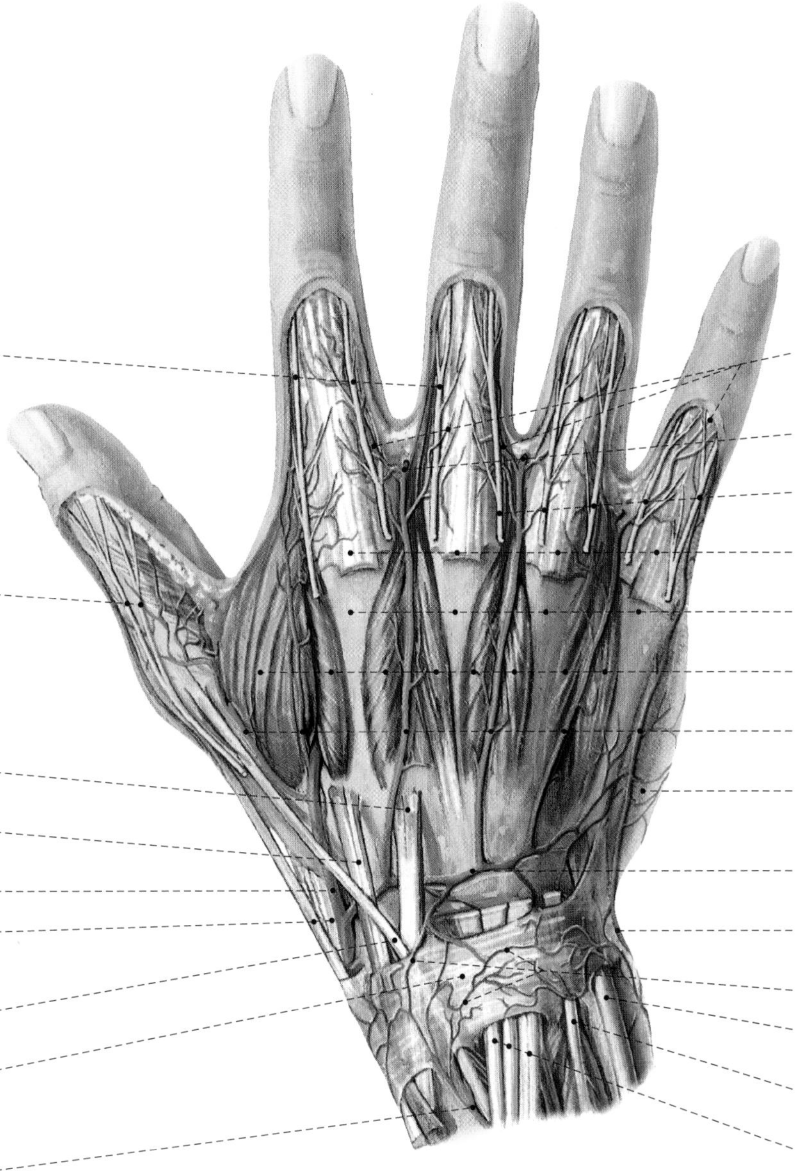
Dorsal digital nerves (of radial nerve)
Dorsal digital nerves of thumb (of radial nerve)
Tendon of extensor carpi radialis brevis m.
Tendon of extensor carpi radialis longus m.
Radial artery
Tendons of abductor pollicis longus and extensor pollicis brevis muscles
Tendon of extensor pollicis longus muscle
Extensor retinaculum
Posterior interosseous artery
Dorsal digital arteries
⟨Intercapitular arteries⟩
Dorsal digital nerves (of ulnar nerve)
Tendons of extensor digitorum muscle
Metacarpals II–V
Dorsal interosseous muscles I–IV
Dorsal metacarpal arteries
Abductor digiti minimi muscle
Dorsal carpal branch of radial artery
Dorsal carpal branch of ulnar artery
Dorsal carpal arch
Tendon of extensor carpi ulnaris muscle
Tendon of extensor digiti minimi muscle
Tendons of extensor indicis and extensor digitorum muscles

b

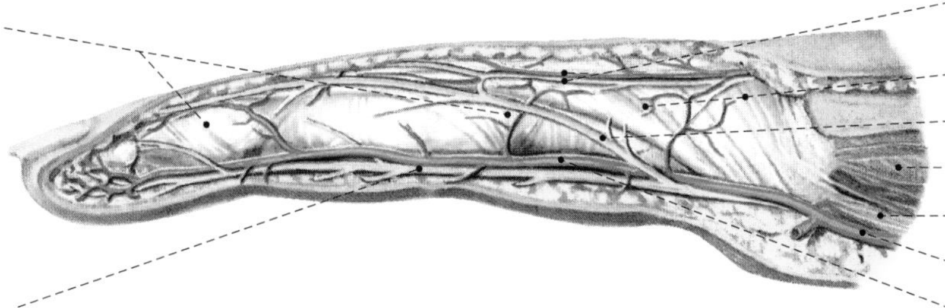
Interphalangeal joints
Proper palmar digital nerve
Dorsal digital artery and nerve
⟨Dorsal digital expansion⟩
(Anastomotic branch)
2nd dorsal interosseous muscle
2nd lumbrical muscle
Common palmar digital artery
Proper palmar digital artery

175 Arteries and nerves of the dorsum of the right hand and the fingers

a The extensor tendons to the fingers were removed. Dorsal aspect of the dorsum of hand (60%)
b Middle finger (90%), radial aspect

a

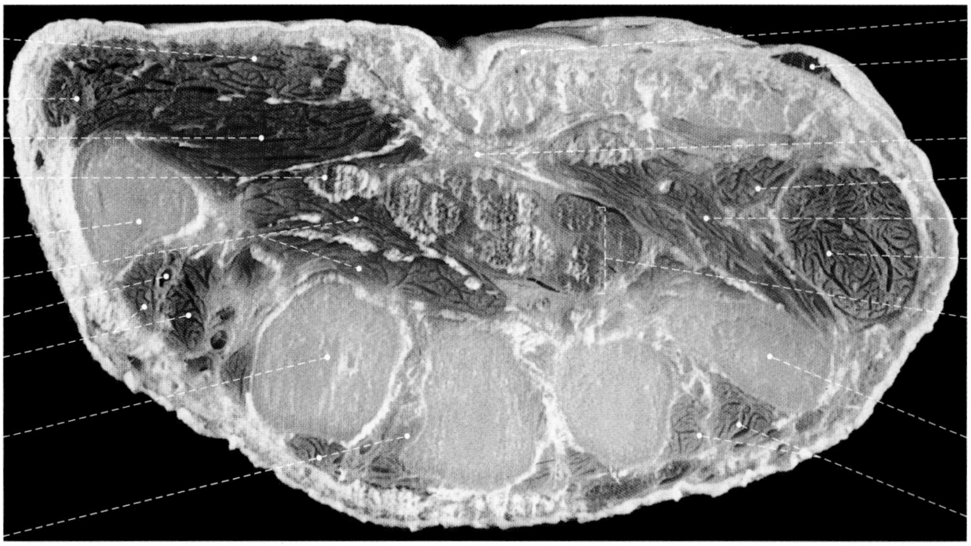
Superficial head of flexor pollicis brevis m.
Abductor pollicis brevis m.
Opponens pollicis muscle
Tendon of flexor pollicis longus m.
1st metacarpal bone
Adductor pollicis muscle
Princeps pollicis artery
1st dorsal interosseous muscle
2nd metacarpal bone
2nd dorsal interosseous muscle
Palmar aponeurosis
Palmaris brevis muscle
Flexor retinaculum
Flexor digiti minimi brevis m.
Opponens digiti minimi m.
Abductor digiti minimi muscle
Carpal tunnel with tendons of flexores digitorum superficialis and profundus muscles
5th metacarpal bone
4th dorsal interosseous muscle

b

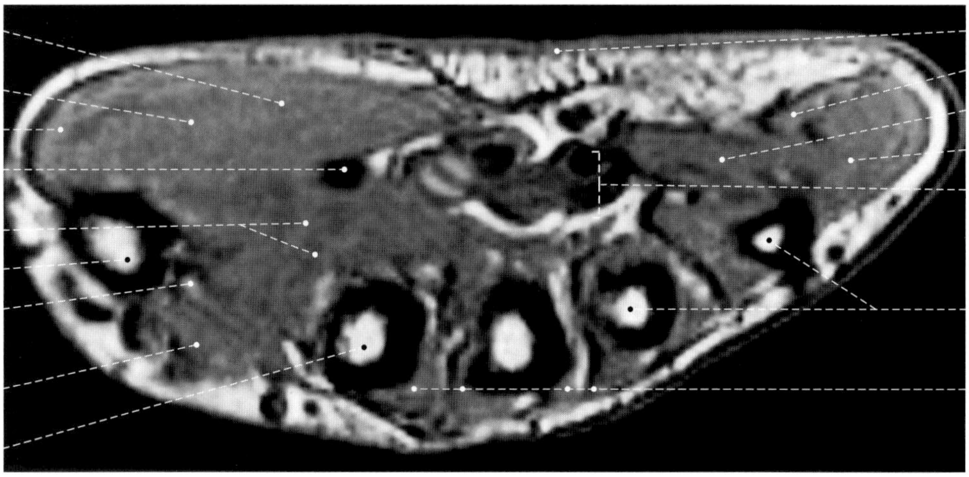
Superficial head of flexor pollicis brevis m.
Opponens pollicis muscle
Abductor pollicis brevis m.
Tendon of flexor pollicis longus m.
Adductor pollicis muscle
1st metacarpal bone
Princeps pollicis artery
1st dorsal interosseous m.
2nd metacarpal bone
Palmar aponeurosis
Flexor digiti minimi brevis m.
Opponens digiti minimi m.
Abductor digiti minimi m.
Carpal tunnel with tendons of flexores digitorum superficialis and profundus muscles
4th and 5th metacarpals
2nd and 3rd dorsal interosseous muscles

176 Right hand (150%)

Axial (transverse) sections through the proximal metacarpus, hand in full supination, distal aspect

a Anatomical section

b Magnetic resonance image (MRI, T_1-weighted)

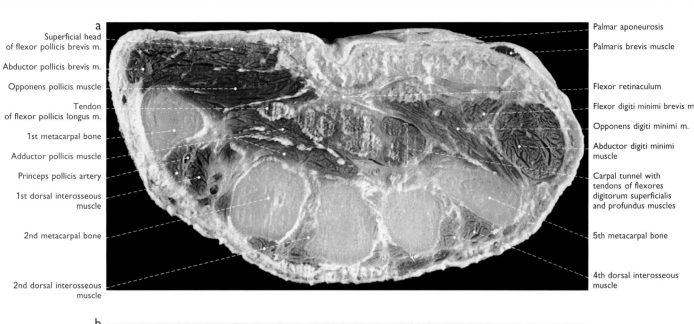

a

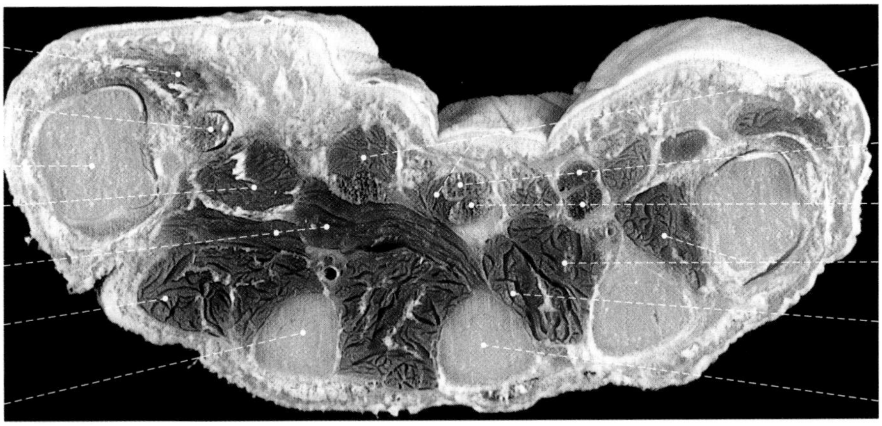
Superficial head of flexor pollicis brevis muscle
Tendon of flexor pollicis longus muscle
1st metacarpal bone
Deep head of flexor pollicis brevis muscle
Adductor pollicis muscle
1st dorsal interosseous muscle
2nd metacarpal bone
1st and 2nd lumbrical muscles
Tendons (II and III) of flexor digitorum superficialis m.
Tendons (II and III) of flexor digitorum profundus m.
2nd and 3rd palmar interosseous muscles
3rd dorsal interosseous muscle
3rd metacarpal bone

b

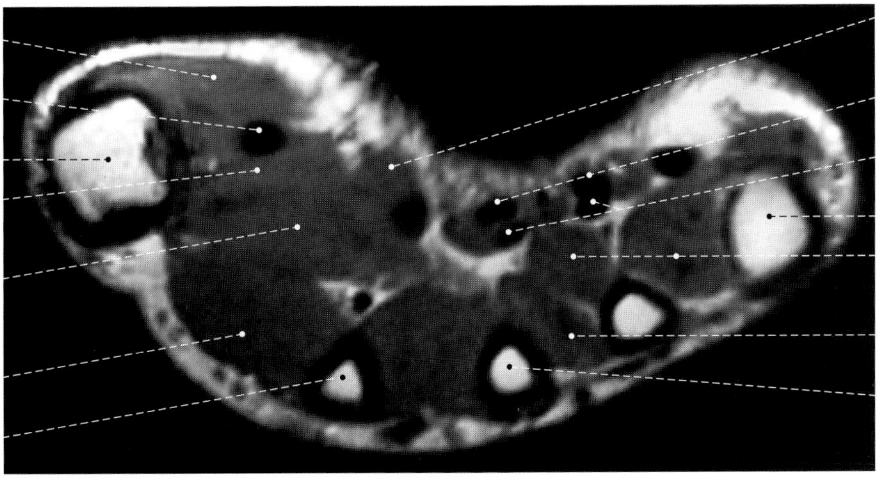
Superficial head of flexor pollicis brevis muscle
Tendon of flexor pollicis longus muscle
1st metacarpal bone
Deep head of flexor pollicis brevis muscle
Adductor pollicis muscle
1st dorsal interosseous muscle
2nd metacarpal bone
1st lumbrical muscle
Tendons (II and III) of flexor digitorum superficialis m.
Tendons (II and III) of flexor digitorum profundus m.
5th metacarpal bone
2nd and 3rd palmar interosseous muscles
3rd dorsal interosseous muscle
3rd metacarpal bone

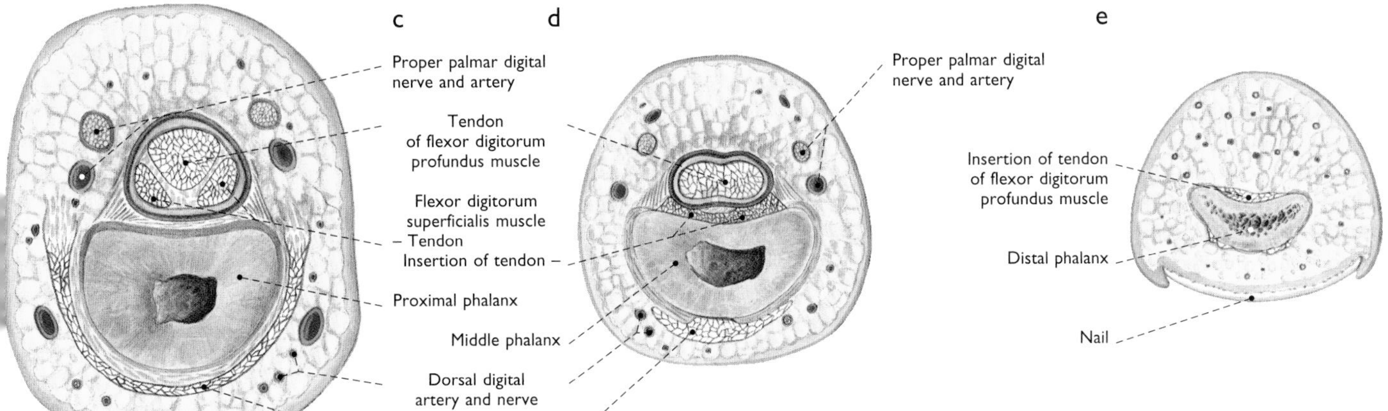
c
d
e
Proper palmar digital nerve and artery
Tendon of flexor digitorum profundus muscle
Flexor digitorum superficialis muscle
– Tendon
Insertion of tendon –
Proximal phalanx
Middle phalanx
Dorsal digital artery and nerve
⟨Dorsal digital expansion⟩
Proper palmar digital nerve and artery
Insertion of tendon of flexor digitorum profundus muscle
Distal phalanx
Nail

177 Right hand

Hand in full supination

a, b Axial (transverse) sections through the middle part of the metacarpus (130%), distal aspect

a Anatomical section

b Magnetic resonance image (MRI, T_1-weighted)

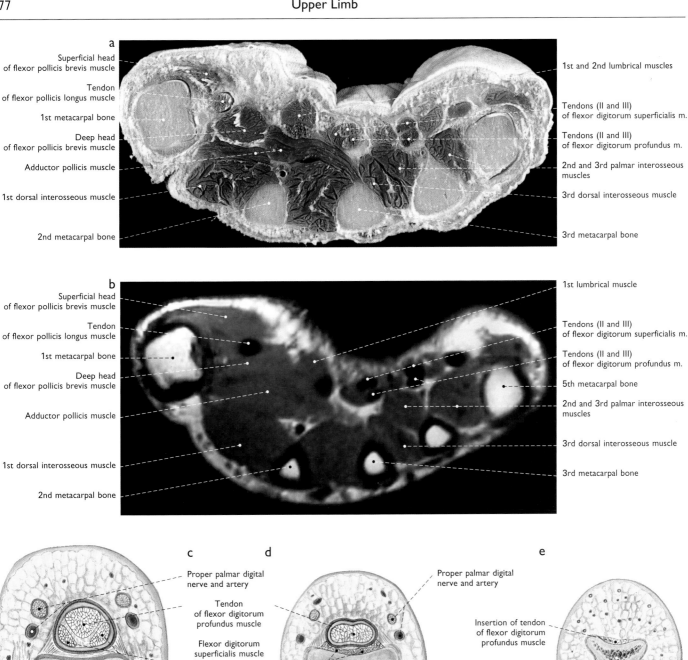

c–e Axial (transverse) sections through

c the proximal phalanx

d the middle phalanx

e the distal phalanx

of the middle finger (230%), distal aspect

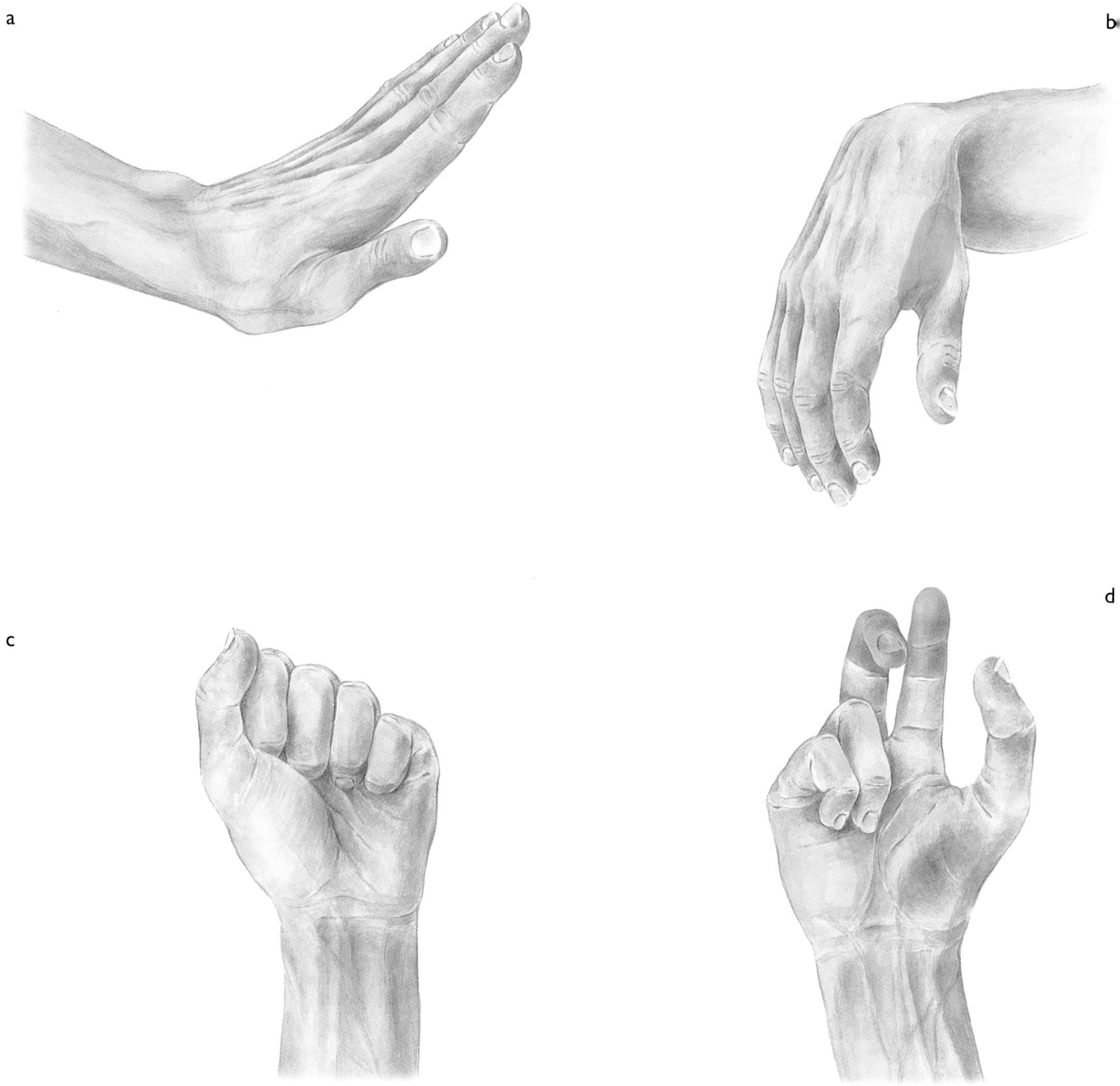

178 Paralysis of nerves of the upper limb (50%)

a, b **Radial nerve palsy,** radial aspect
a Normal extension of the left hand
b 'Wrist drop' due to an injury to the right radial nerve in or above the elbow region

c, d **Median nerve palsy,** palmar aspect
c Normal closure of fist of the left hand
d Incompletely closed fist ('oath hand') due to median nerve palsy at the right upper limb in or above the elbow region, additionally a flattened thenar eminence ('ape hand') because of an atrophy of thenar muscles

The skin regions marked by blue color indicate the autonomic areas of the corresponding nerves.

a

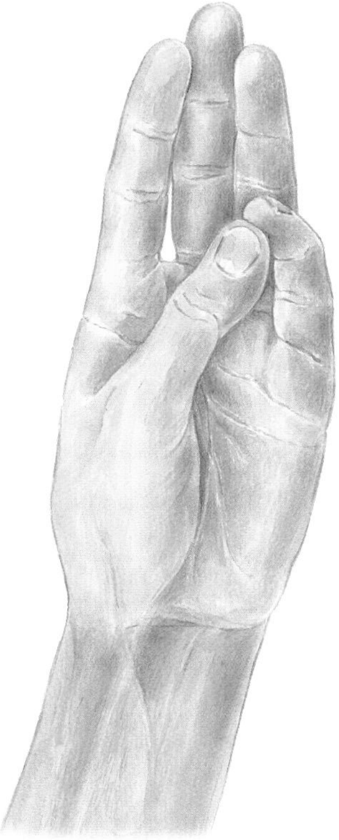

b

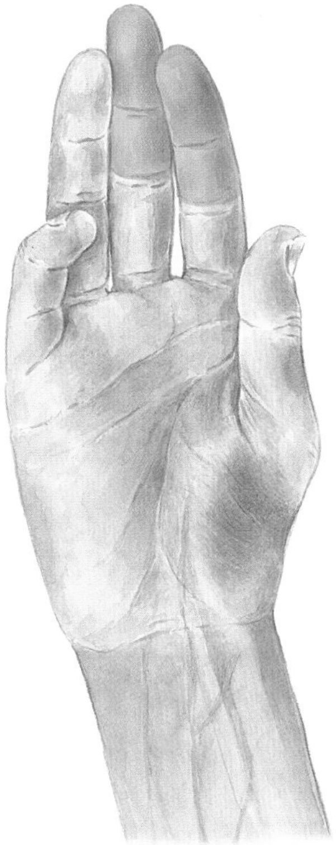

c

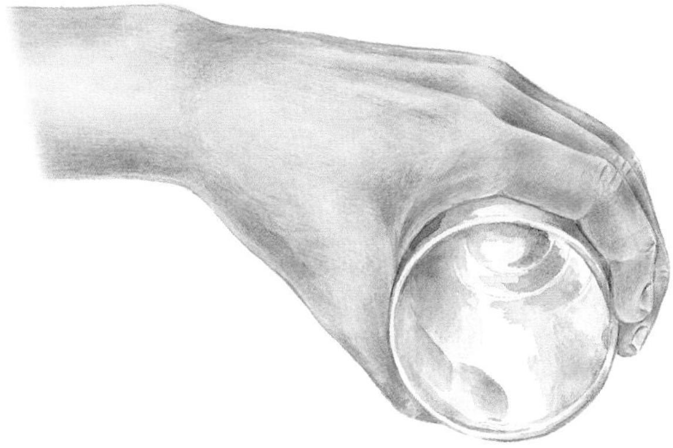

d

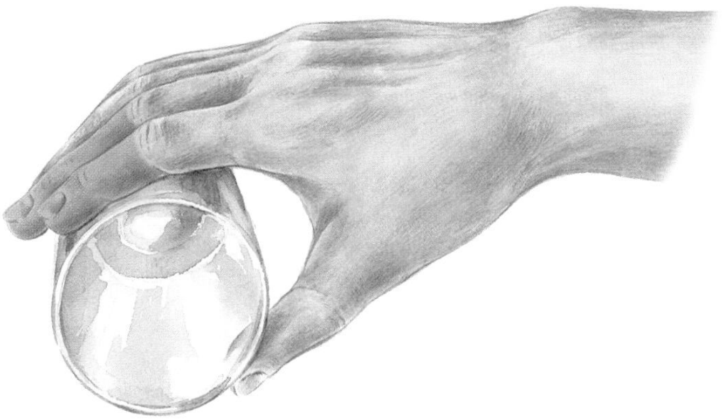

179 Paralysis of nerves of the upper limb (50%)

Median nerve palsy

a, b Opposition of the thumb to the little finger, palmar aspect
a Normal function of the left hand
b Insufficient opposition of the thumb of the right hand due to median nerve palsy, additionally a flattened thenar eminence ('ape hand') because of an atrophy of thenar muscles
c, d Test of the abduction function of the thumb, radial aspect
c Normal function of the left hand
d Insufficient surrounding of a bottle because of an injured abduction function of the thumb due to median nerve palsy

The skin regions marked by blue color indicate the autonomic areas of the median nerve.

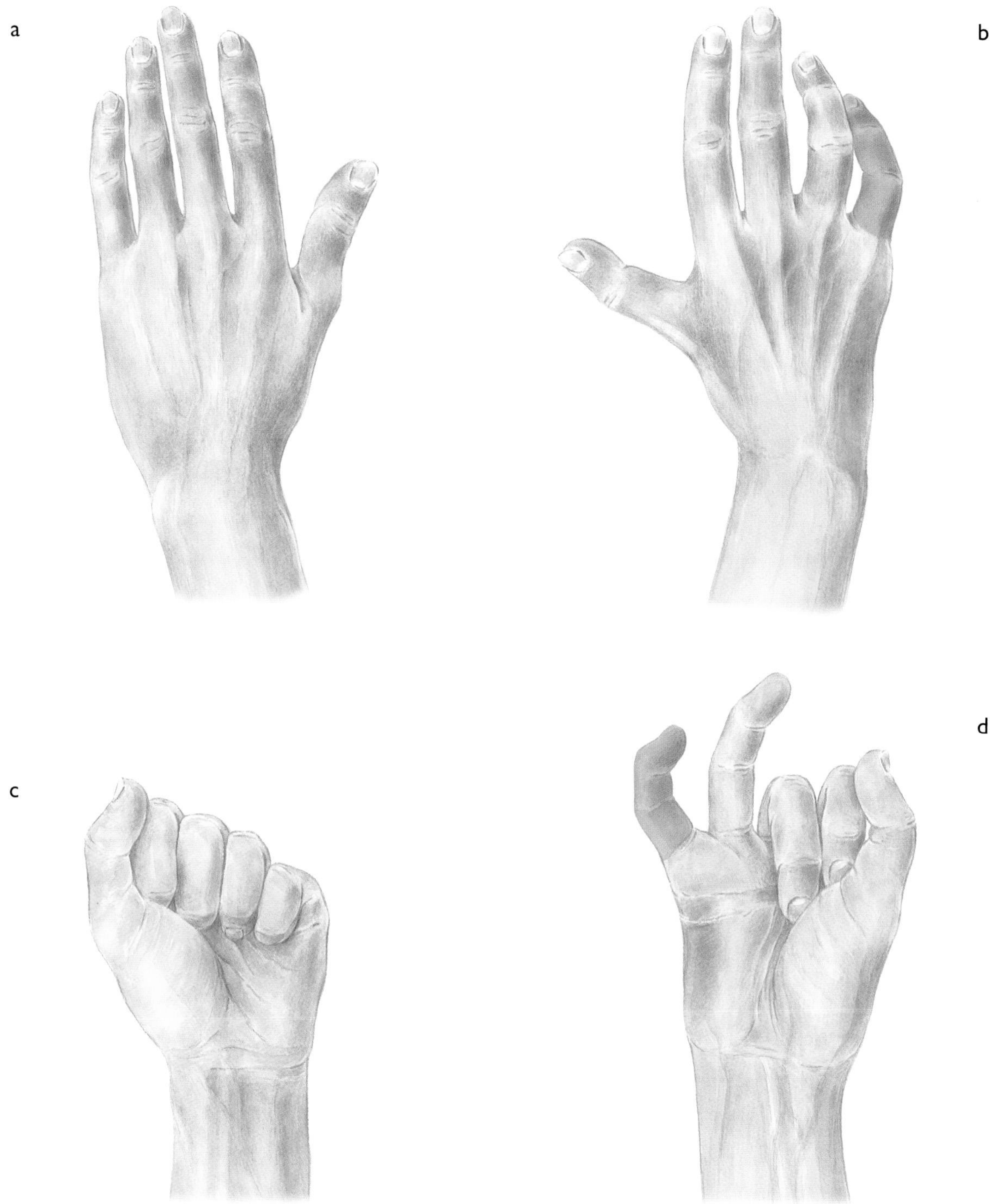

180 Paralysis of nerves of the upper limb (50%)

Ulnar nerve palsy

a, b Dorsal aspect
a Normal state of the left hand
b 'Clawn hand' resulting from a longer lasting ulnar nerve palsy of the right upper limb and atrophy of the hypothenar muscles
c, d Palmar aspect
c Normal closure of fist of the left hand
d Incompletely closed fist of the right hand due to a deficient flexion of the little and ring fingers because of ulnar nerve palsy

The skin area marked by blue color indicates the autonomic area of the ulnar nerve.

a

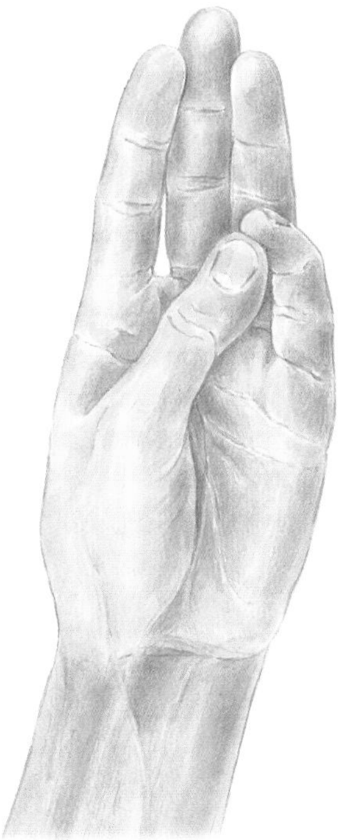

b

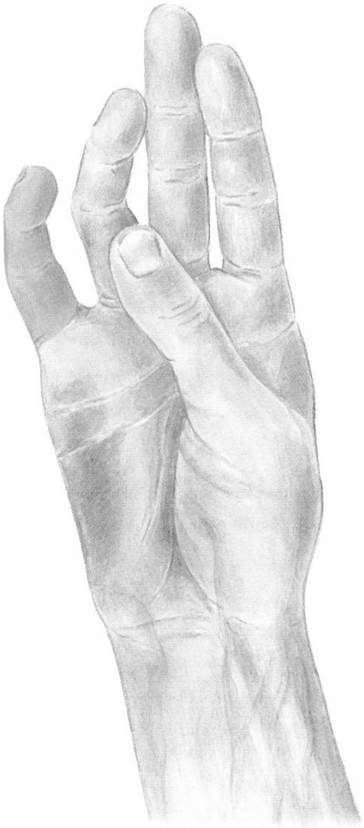

c

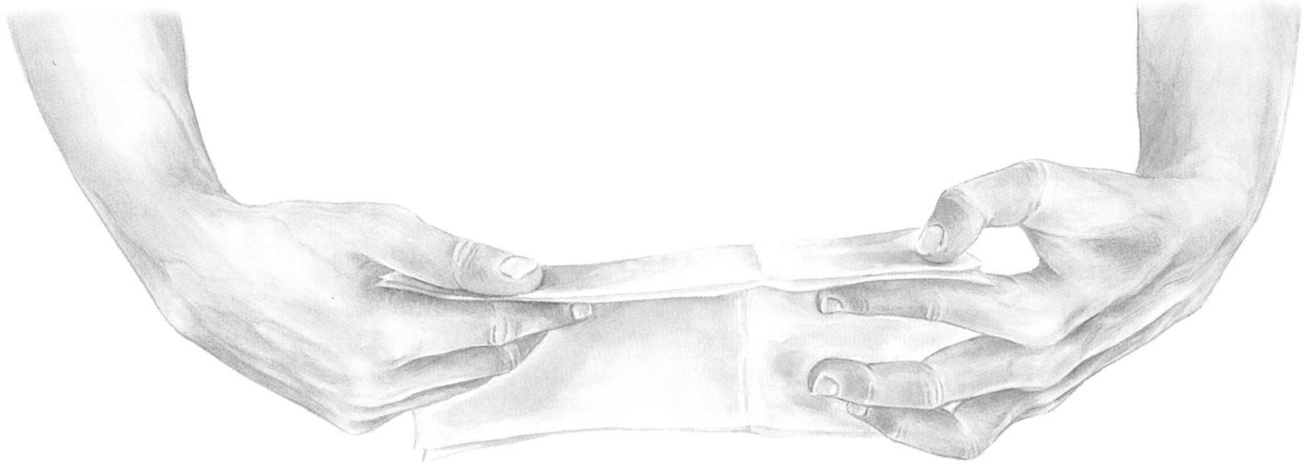

181 Paralysis of nerves of the upper limb (50%)

Ulnar nerve palsy

a, b Opposition of the little finger to the thumb, palmar aspect

a Normal function of the left hand

b Insufficient opposition of the little finger of the right hand due to ulnar nerve palsy, additionally an atrophy of the hypothenar muscles

c Test of the adduction function of the thumb, radial aspect. Normal function of the right hand (on the left side of picture), but insufficient adduction of the thumb ('FROMENT's sign') because of ulnar nerve palsy at the left hand (on the right side of picture)

The skin area marked by blue color indicates the autonomic area of the ulnar nerve.

Lower Limb

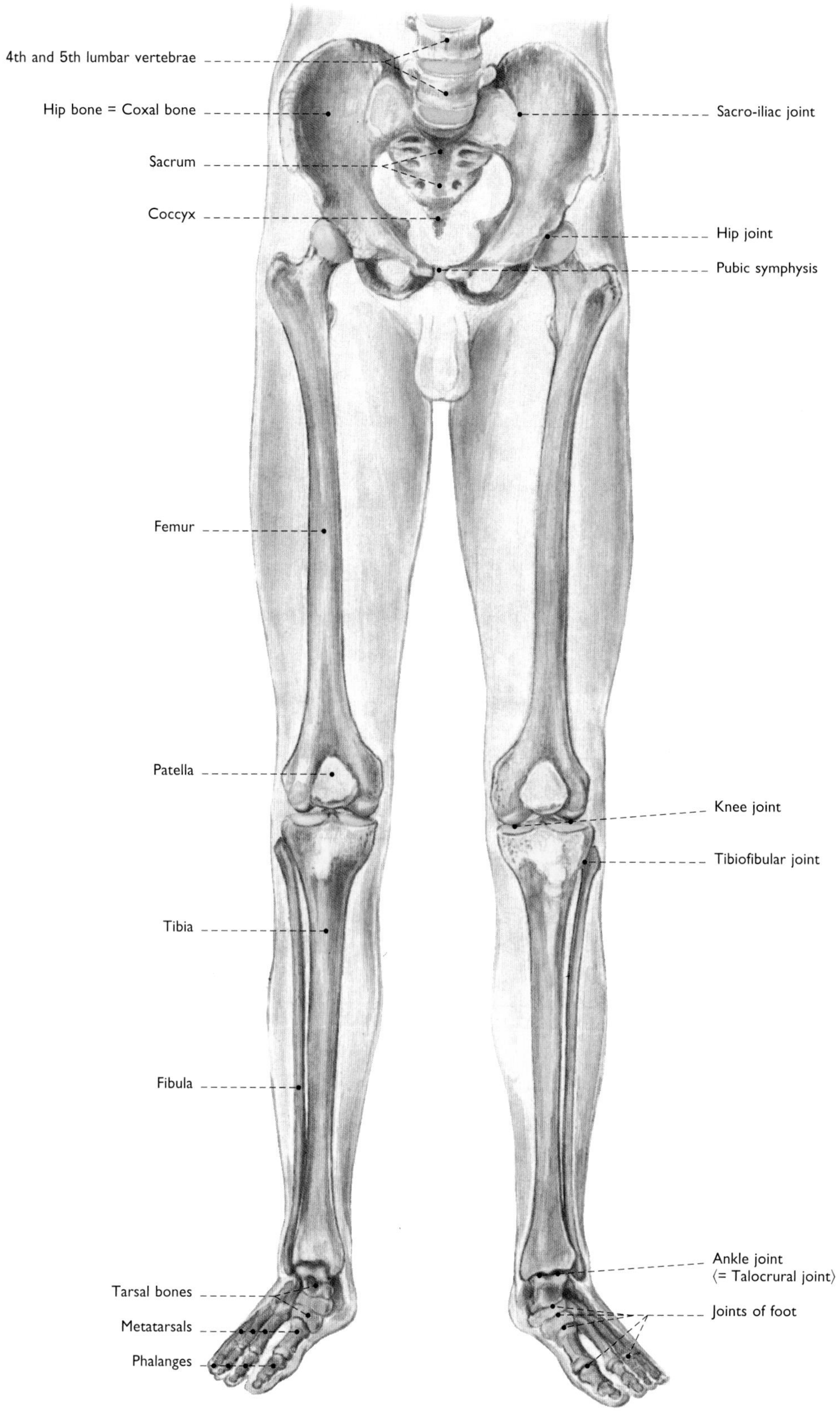
4th and 5th lumbar vertebrae
Hip bone = Coxal bone
Sacrum
Coccyx
Femur
Patella
Tibia
Fibula
Tarsal bones
Metatarsals
Phalanges
Sacro-iliac joint
Hip joint
Pubic symphysis
Knee joint
Tibiofibular joint
Ankle joint
(= Talocrural joint)
Joints of foot

184 Lower limb (20%)

Ventral aspect

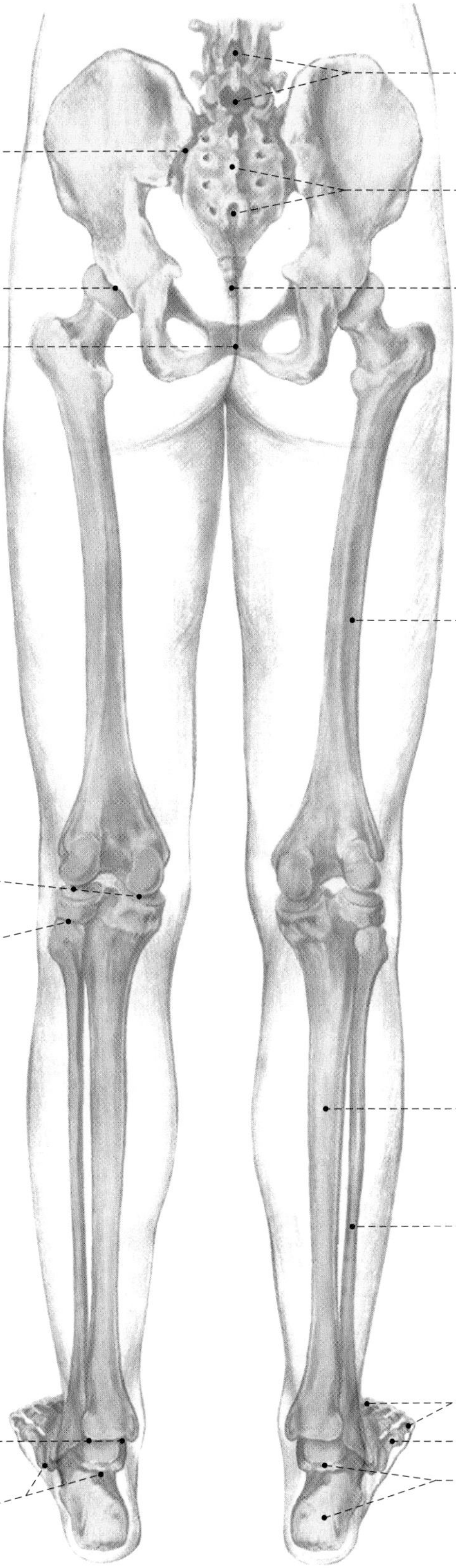
4th and 5th lumbar vertebrae
Sacro-iliac joint
Sacrum
Hip joint
Coccyx
Pubic symphysis
Femur
Knee joint
Tibiofibular joint
Tibia
Fibula
Phalanges
Ankle joint
⟨= Talocrural joint⟩
Metatarsals
Tarsal bones
Joints of foot

185 Lower limb (20%)

Dorsal aspect

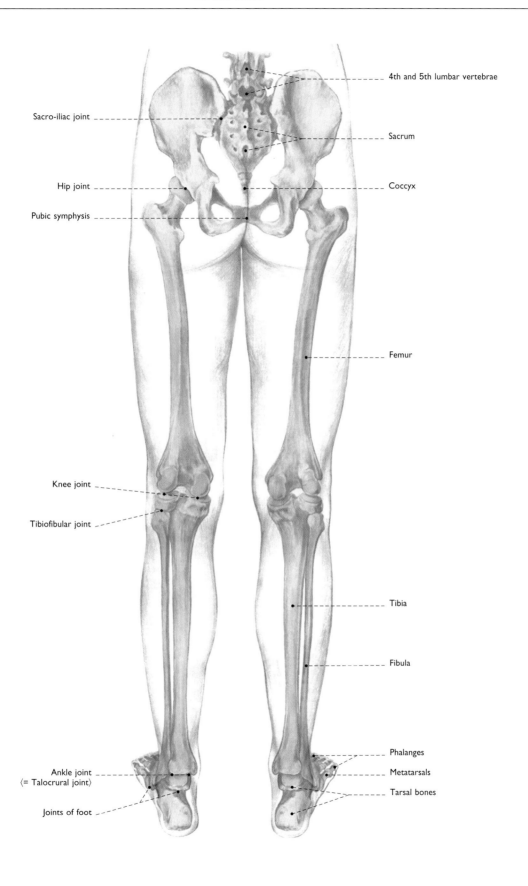

a

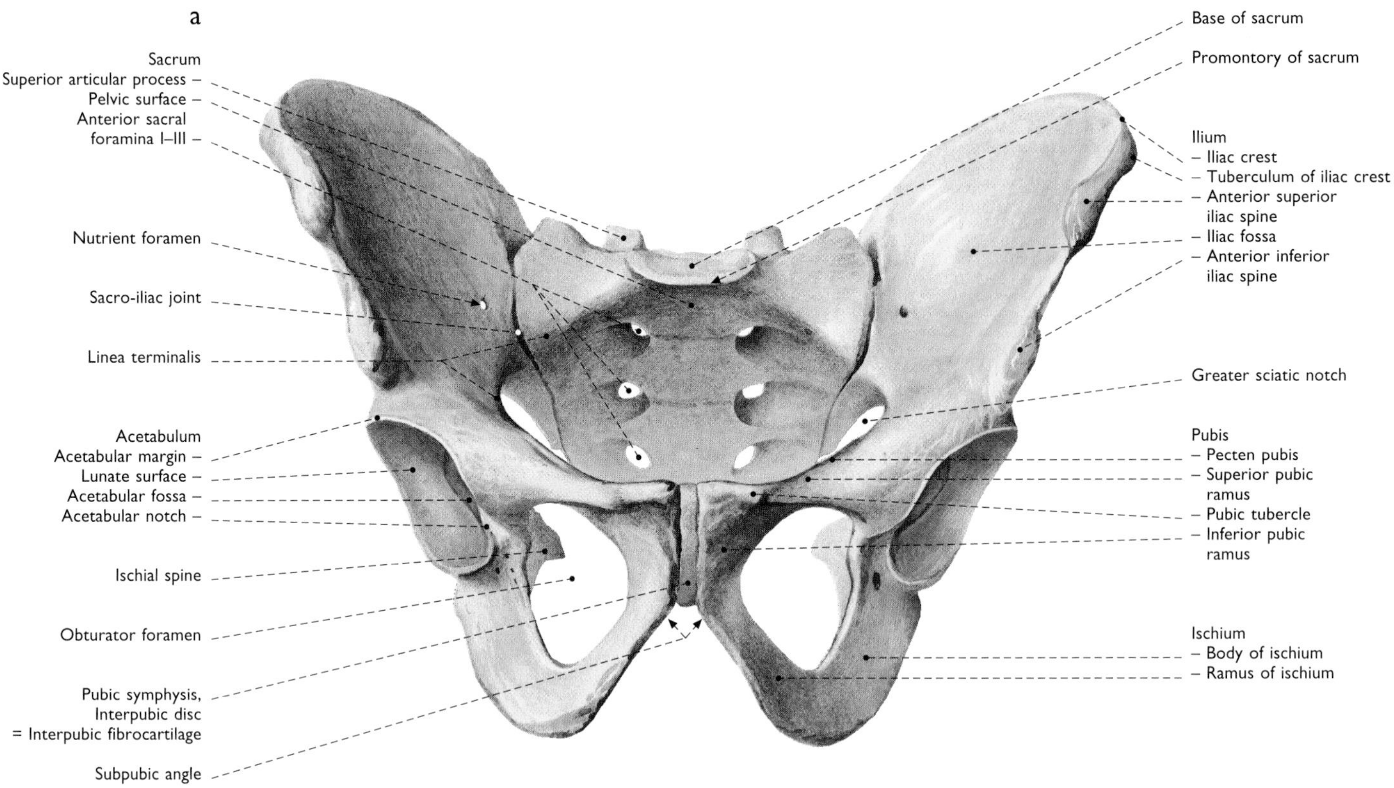
Sacrum
Superior articular process –
Pelvic surface –
Anterior sacral foramina I–III –
Nutrient foramen
Sacro-iliac joint
Linea terminalis
Acetabulum
Acetabular margin –
Lunate surface –
Acetabular fossa –
Acetabular notch –
Ischial spine
Obturator foramen
Pubic symphysis, Interpubic disc = Interpubic fibrocartilage
Subpubic angle
Base of sacrum
Promontory of sacrum
Ilium
– Iliac crest
– Tuberculum of iliac crest
– Anterior superior iliac spine
– Iliac fossa
– Anterior inferior iliac spine
Greater sciatic notch
Pubis
– Pecten pubis
– Superior pubic ramus
– Pubic tubercle
– Inferior pubic ramus
Ischium
– Body of ischium
– Ramus of ischium

b

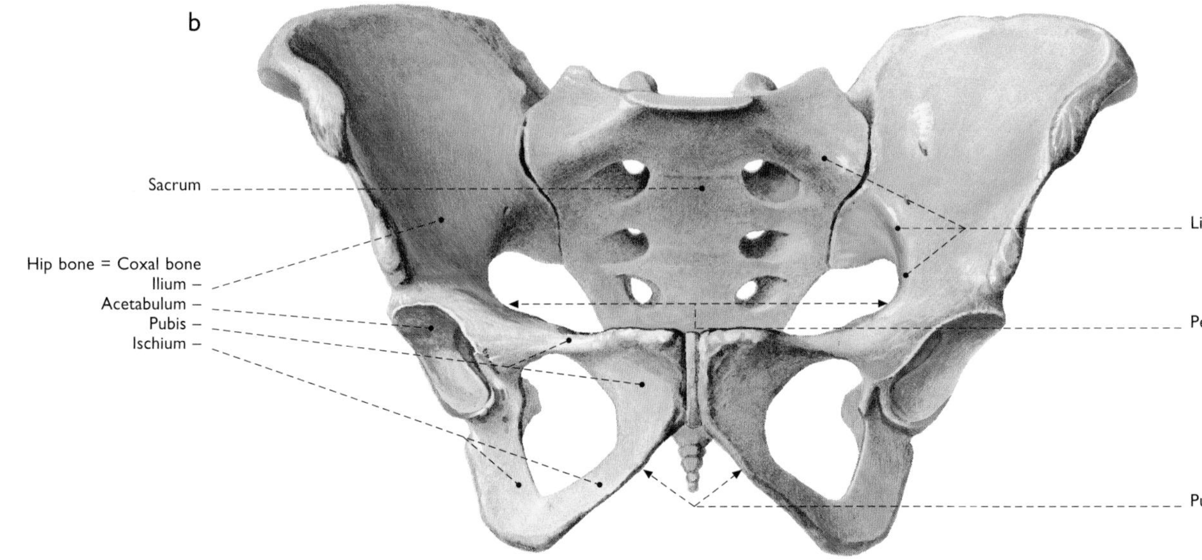
Sacrum
Hip bone = Coxal bone
Ilium –
Acetabulum –
Pubis –
Ischium –
Linea terminalis
Pelvic inlet
Pubic arch

186 Pelvic girdle (40%)

Ventral aspect
a Male pelvis
b Female pelvis

a

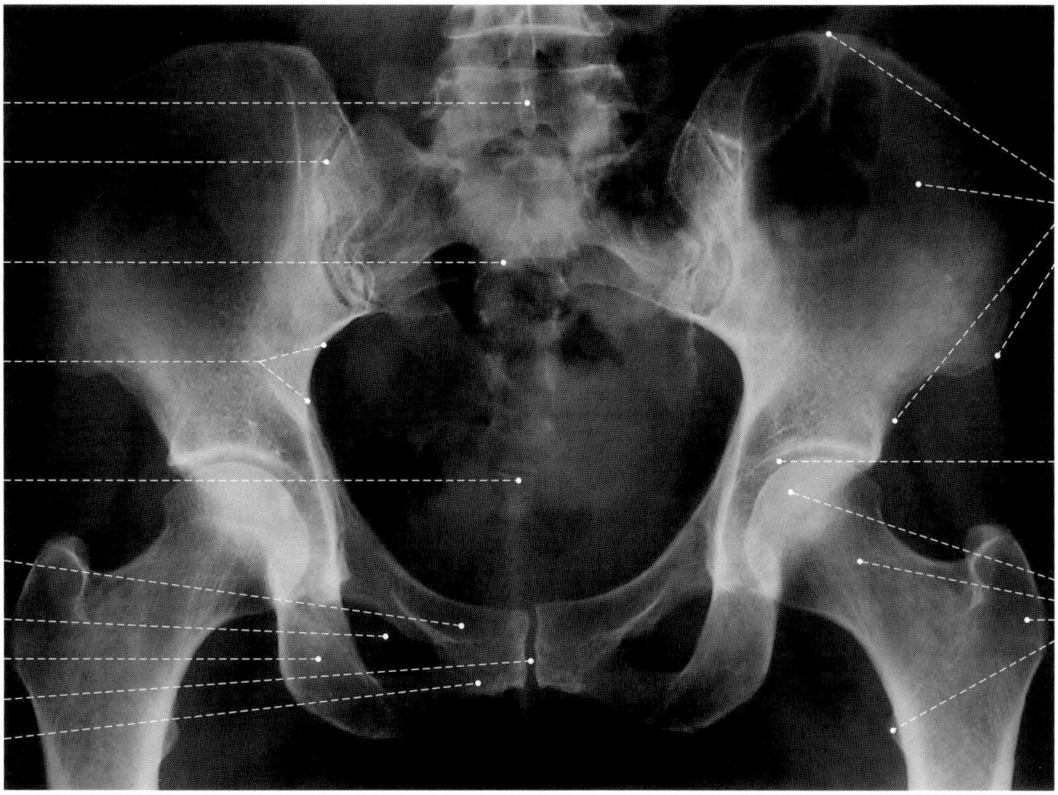
5th lumbar vertebra
Sacro-iliac joint
Sacrum
Linea terminalis
Coccyx
Superior pubic ramus
Obturator foramen
Ischium
Pubic symphysis
Inferior pubic ramus
Ilium
– Iliac crest
– Ala of ilium
– Anterior inferior iliac spine
– Anterior superior iliac spine
Hip joint
Femur
– Head of femur
– Neck of femur
– Greater trochanter
– Lesser trochanter

b

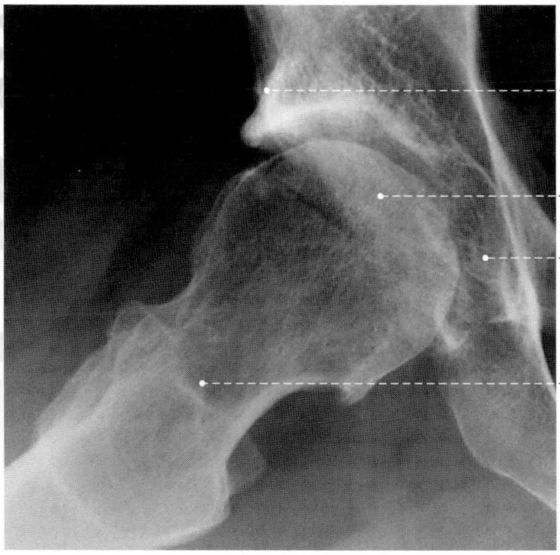
Anterior inferior iliac spine
Head of femur
Acetabular fossa
Neck of femur

c

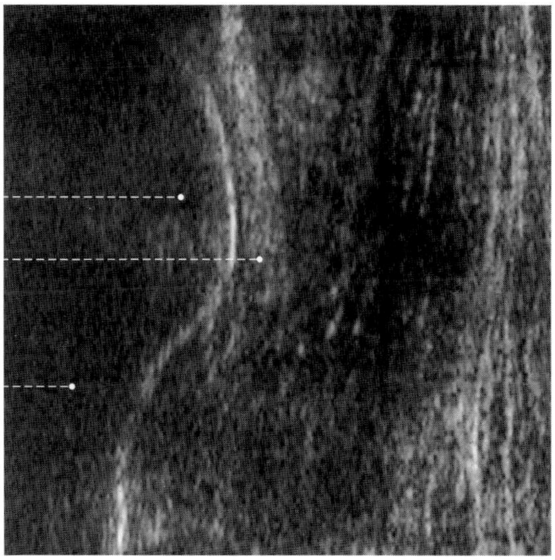

187 Pelvic girdle and proximal thigh bones (= femora)

a Anteroposterior radiograph (50%)
b Anteroposterior radiograph of the right hip joint, the femur in abduction (65%)
c Ultrasonogram of the right hip joint

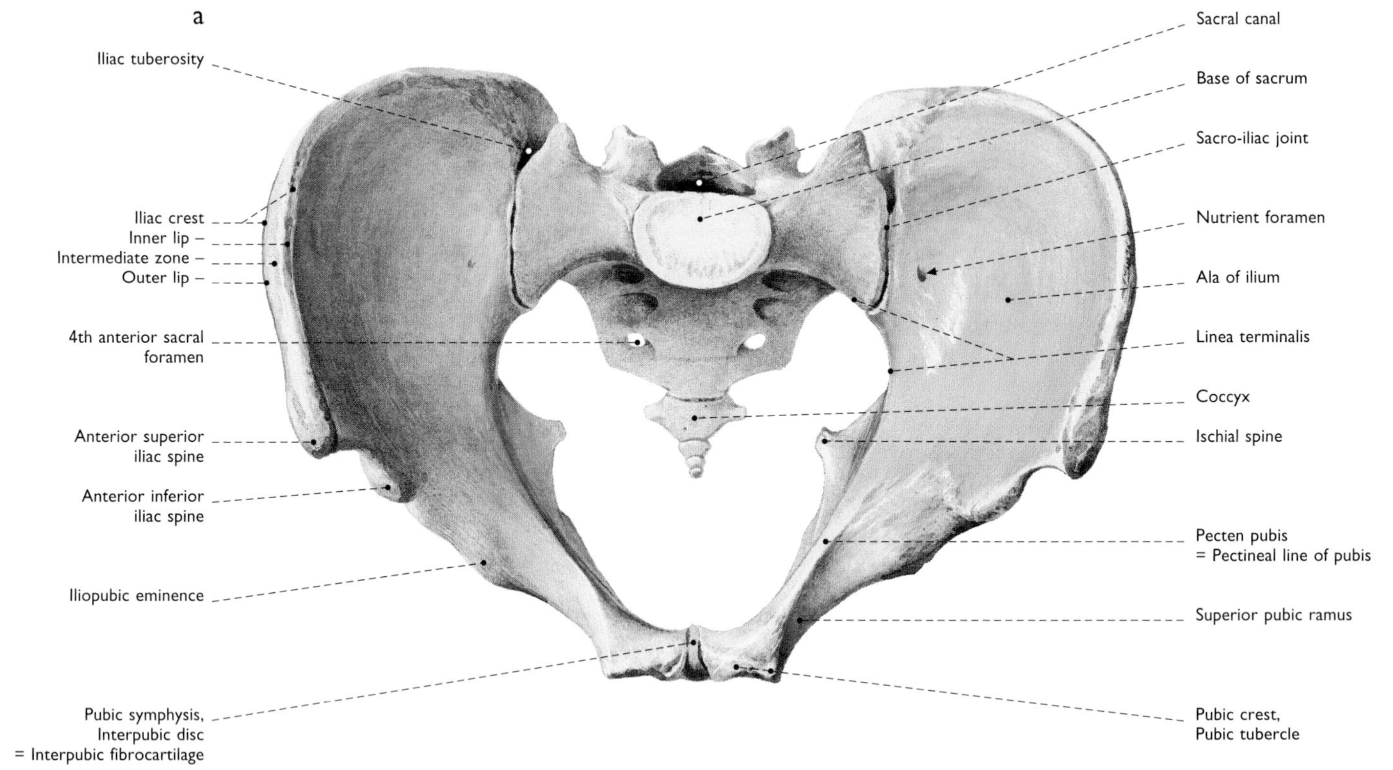
a
Iliac tuberosity
Iliac crest
Inner lip –
Intermediate zone –
Outer lip –
4th anterior sacral foramen
Anterior superior iliac spine
Anterior inferior iliac spine
Iliopubic eminence
Pubic symphysis, Interpubic disc = Interpubic fibrocartilage
Sacral canal
Base of sacrum
Sacro-iliac joint
Nutrient foramen
Ala of ilium
Linea terminalis
Coccyx
Ischial spine
Pecten pubis = Pectineal line of pubis
Superior pubic ramus
Pubic crest, Pubic tubercle

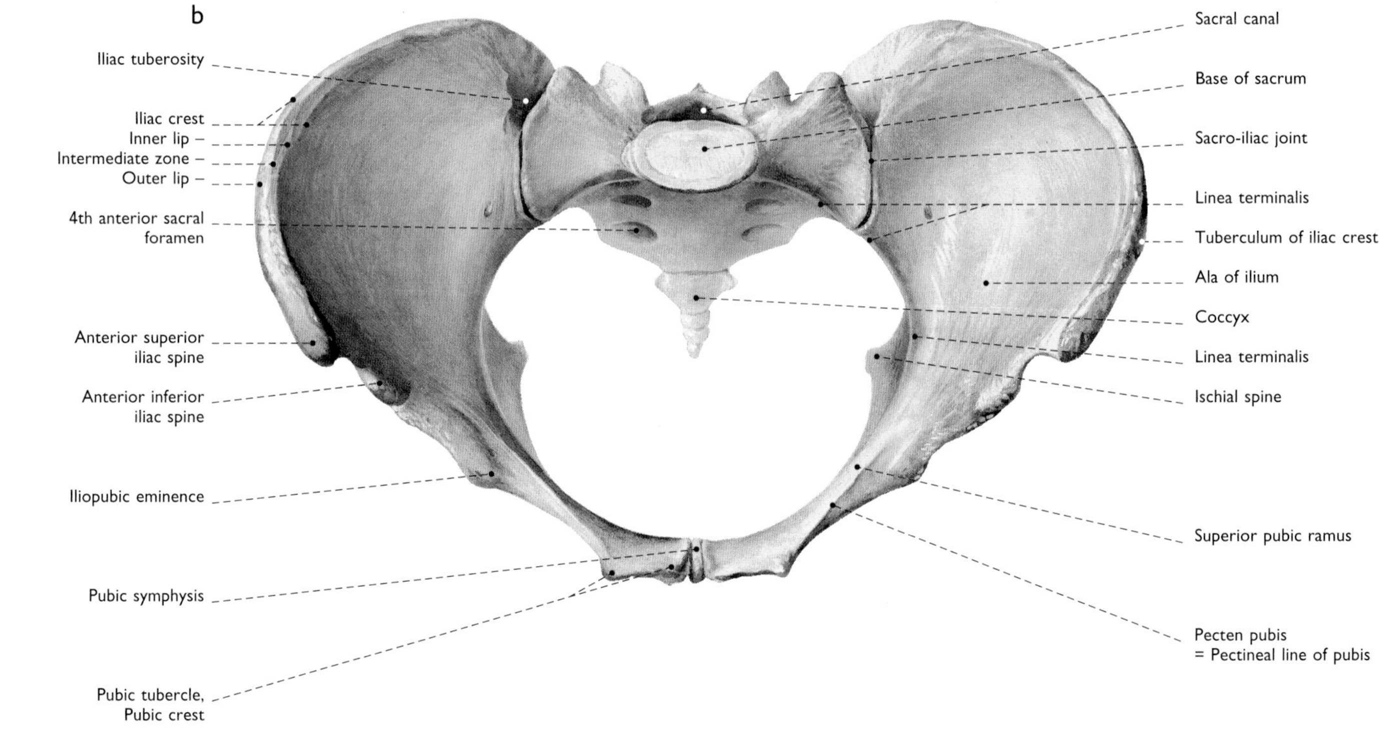
b
Iliac tuberosity
Iliac crest
Inner lip –
Intermediate zone –
Outer lip –
4th anterior sacral foramen
Anterior superior iliac spine
Anterior inferior iliac spine
Iliopubic eminence
Pubic symphysis
Pubic tubercle, Pubic crest
Sacral canal
Base of sacrum
Sacro-iliac joint
Linea terminalis
Tuberculum of iliac crest
Ala of ilium
Coccyx
Linea terminalis
Ischial spine
Superior pubic ramus
Pecten pubis = Pectineal line of pubis

188 Pelvic girdle (40%)

Superior aspect
a Male pelvis
b Female pelvis

a

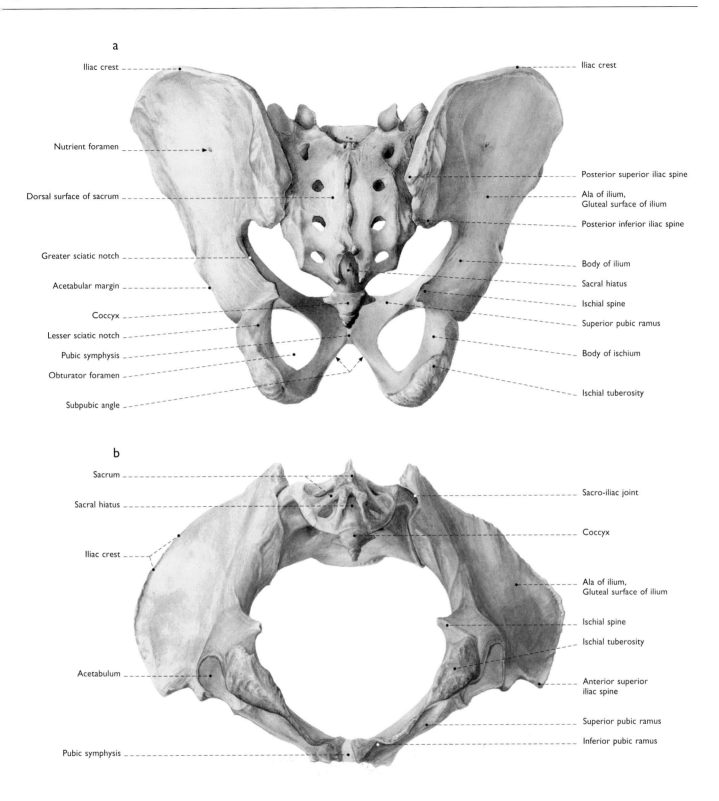

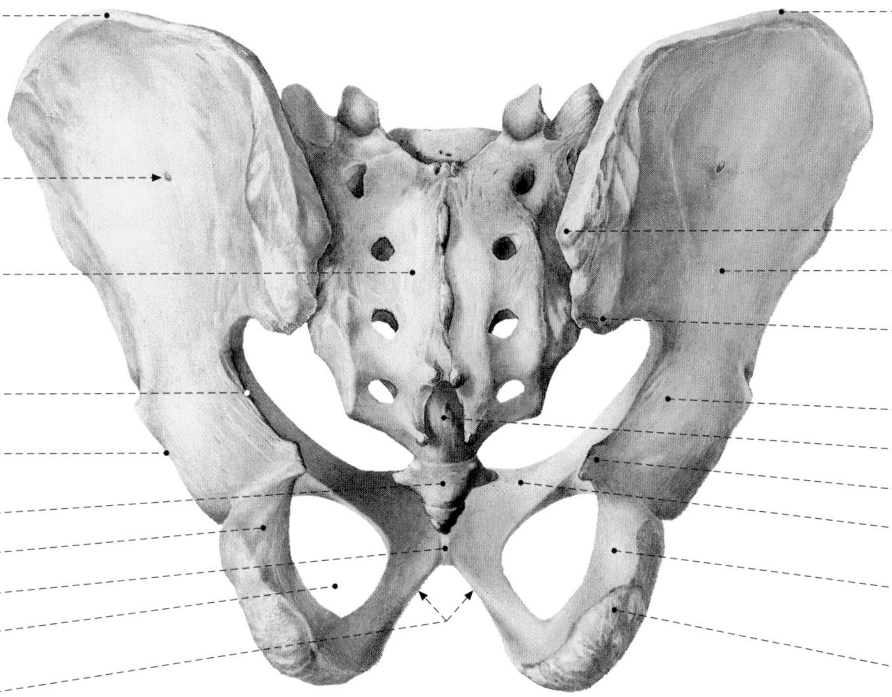
Iliac crest
Nutrient foramen
Dorsal surface of sacrum
Greater sciatic notch
Acetabular margin
Coccyx
Lesser sciatic notch
Pubic symphysis
Obturator foramen
Subpubic angle
Iliac crest
Posterior superior iliac spine
Ala of ilium,
Gluteal surface of ilium
Posterior inferior iliac spine
Body of ilium
Sacral hiatus
Ischial spine
Superior pubic ramus
Body of ischium
Ischial tuberosity

b

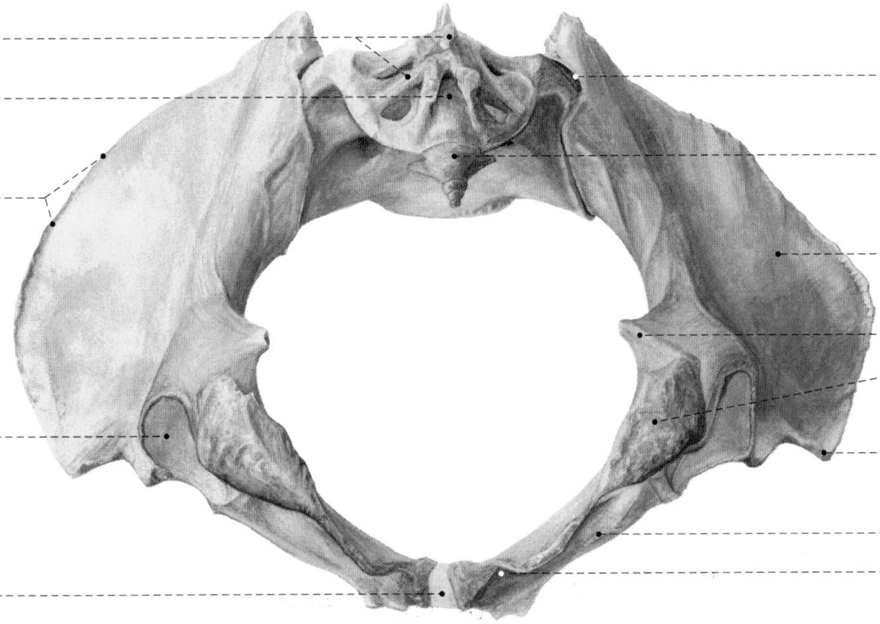
Sacrum
Sacral hiatus
Iliac crest
Acetabulum
Pubic symphysis
Sacro-iliac joint
Coccyx
Ala of ilium,
Gluteal surface of ilium
Ischial spine
Ischial tuberosity
Anterior superior
iliac spine
Superior pubic ramus
Inferior pubic ramus

189 Pelvic girdle of a female (40%)

a Dorsal aspect
b Inferior aspect

a

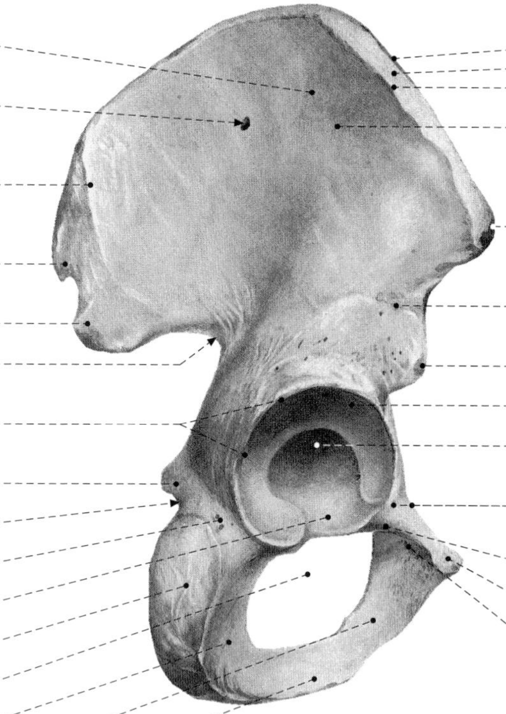
Gluteal surface of ala of ilium
Nutrient foramen
Posterior gluteal line
Posterior superior iliac spine
Posterior inferior iliac spine
Greater sciatic notch
Acetabular margin
Ischial spine
Lesser sciatic notch
Ischium
Acetabular notch
Ischial tuberosity
Obturator foramen
Body of ischium
Inferior pubic ramus
Ramus of ischium
Iliac crest
– Inner lip
– Intermediate zone
– Outer lip
Anterior gluteal line
Anterior superior iliac spine
Inferior gluteal line
Anterior inferior iliac spine
Lunate surface of acetabulum
Acetabular fossa
Superior pubic ramus, Pecten pubis
Obturator crest
Pubic tubercle
Obturator groove

b

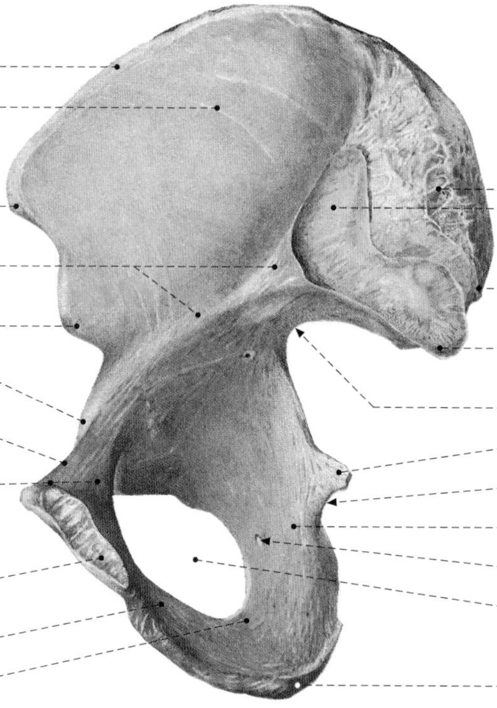
Iliac crest
Iliac fossa of ala of ilium
Anterior superior iliac spine
Arcuate line
Anterior inferior iliac spine
Iliopubic eminence
Pecten pubis = Pectineal line of pubis
Pubic crest, Superior pubic ramus
Symphysial surface
Inferior pubic ramus
Ramus of ischium
Sacropelvic surface
– Iliac tuberosity
– Auricular surface
Posterior superior iliac spine
Posterior inferior iliac spine
Greater sciatic notch
Ischial spine
Lesser sciatic notch
Body of ischium
Nutrient foramen
Obturator foramen
Ischial tuberosity

c

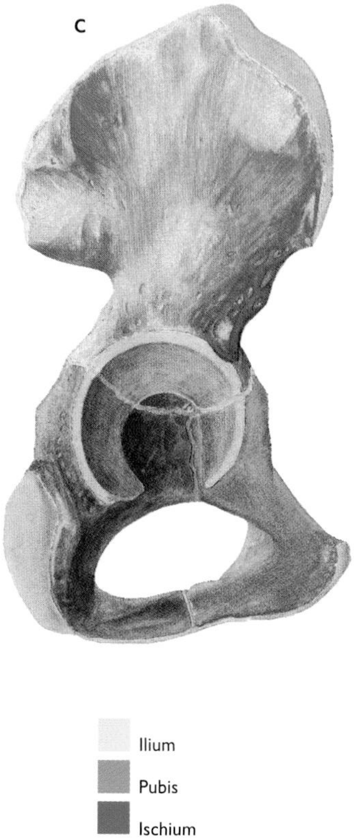
Ilium
Pubis
Ischium

190 Right hip bone (= coxal bone)

a, b Hip bone of an adult (40%)
a Lateral aspect
b Medial aspect
c Hip bone of a 10-year-old child with the typical Y-shaped epiphysial plate (50%), lateral aspect

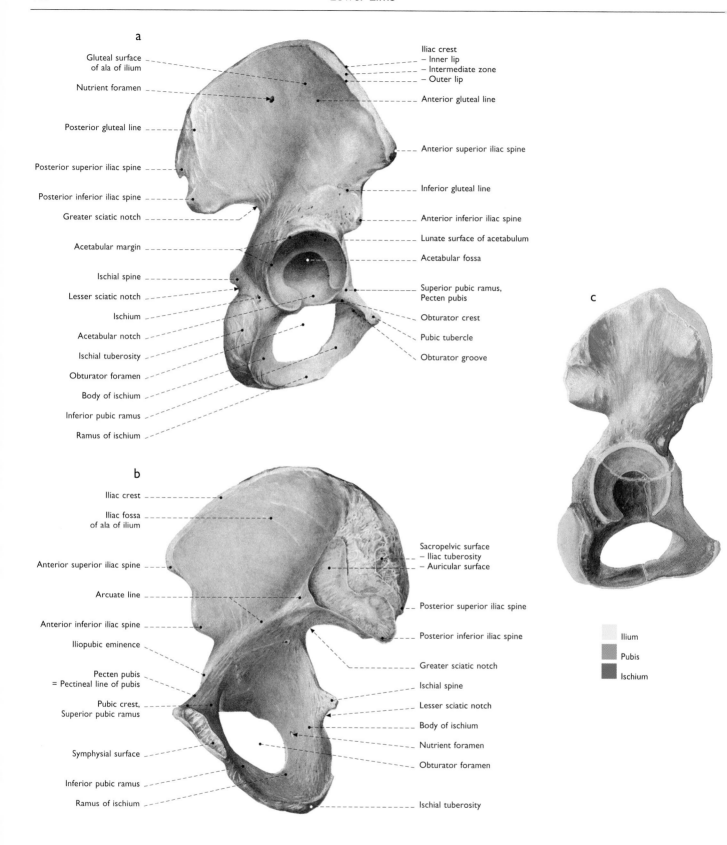

a

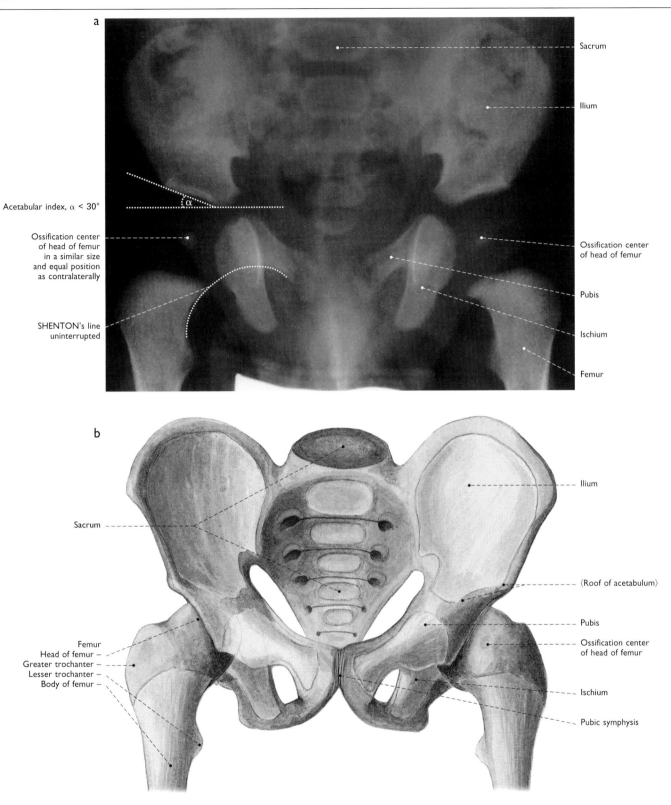

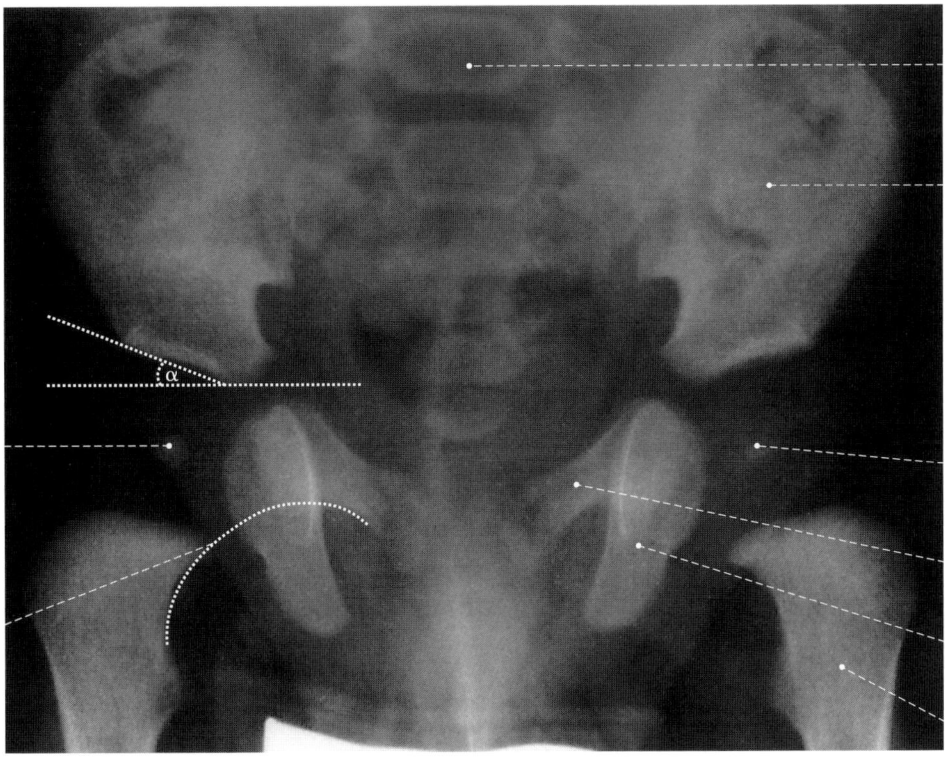
Sacrum
Ilium
Acetabular index, α < 30°
α
Ossification center of head of femur in a similar size and equal position as contralaterally
Ossification center of head of femur
Pubis
SHENTON's line uninterrupted
Ischium
Femur

b

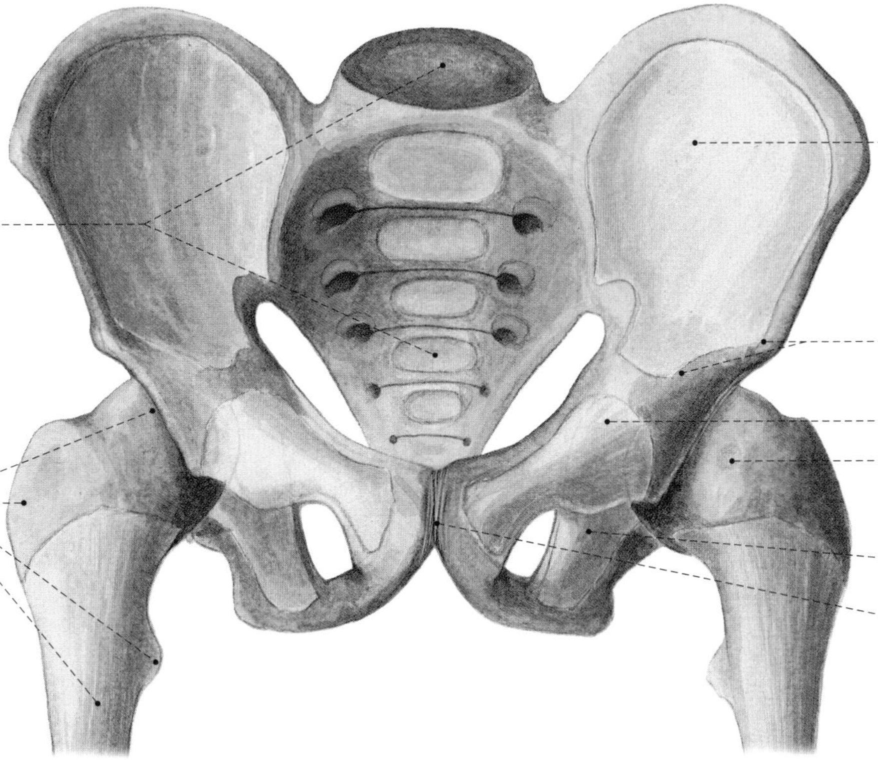
Ilium
Sacrum
⟨Roof of acetabulum⟩
Pubis
Femur
Head of femur
Greater trochanter
Lesser trochanter
Body of femur
Ossification center of head of femur
Ischium
Pubic symphysis

191 Pelvic girdle and proximal thigh bones (= femora) of a 3-month-old child (100%)

a Anteroposterior radiograph. On the left side of the picture, the main radiological criteria for a normal development of the hip joint at this age are indicated.

b Ventral aspect

a

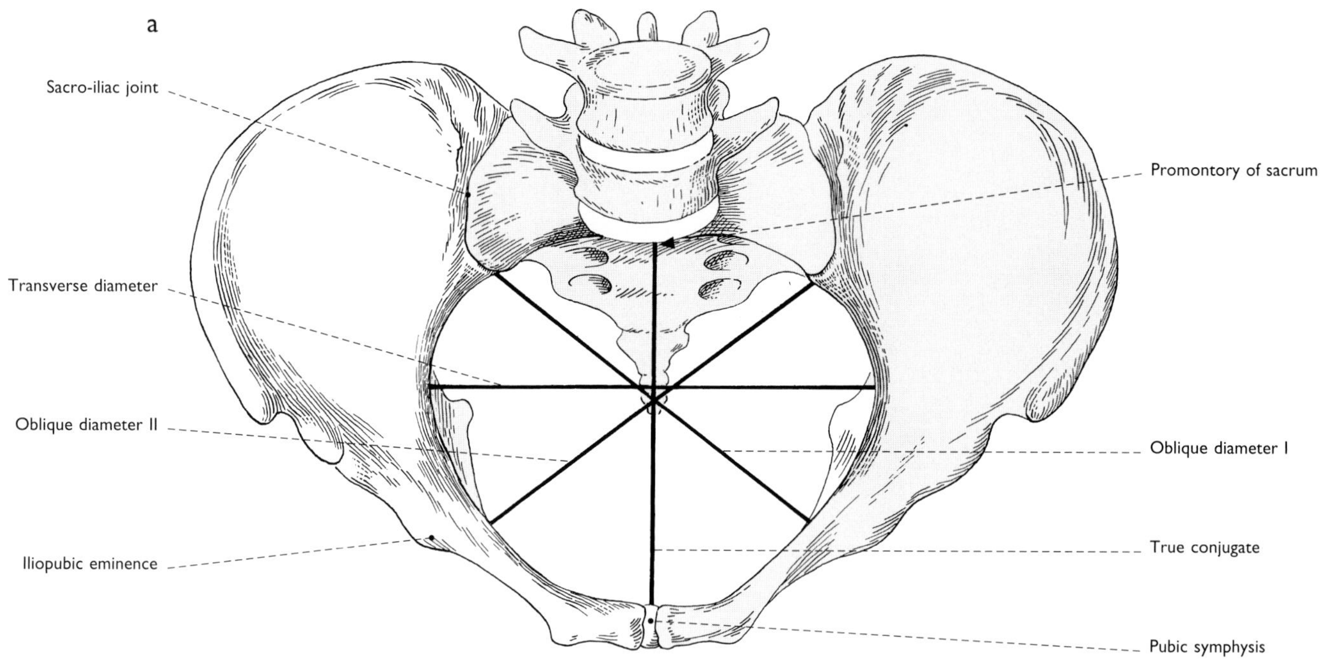
Sacro-iliac joint
Transverse diameter
Oblique diameter II
Iliopubic eminence
Promontory of sacrum
Oblique diameter I
True conjugate
Pubic symphysis

b

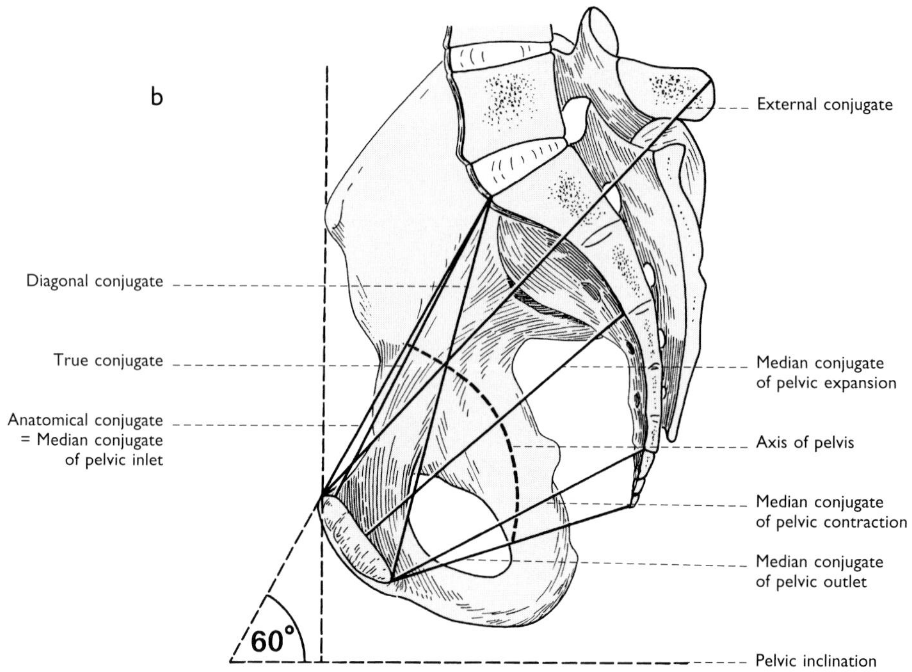
Diagonal conjugate
True conjugate
Anatomical conjugate
= Median conjugate
of pelvic inlet
60°
External conjugate
Median conjugate
of pelvic expansion
Axis of pelvis
Median conjugate
of pelvic contraction
Median conjugate
of pelvic outlet
Pelvic inclination

192 Pelvis of a female (40%)

Schematic representations

a Diameters of the pelvic inlet, cranial aspect

b Inclination of the pelvis and median conjugates, medial aspect of a median section

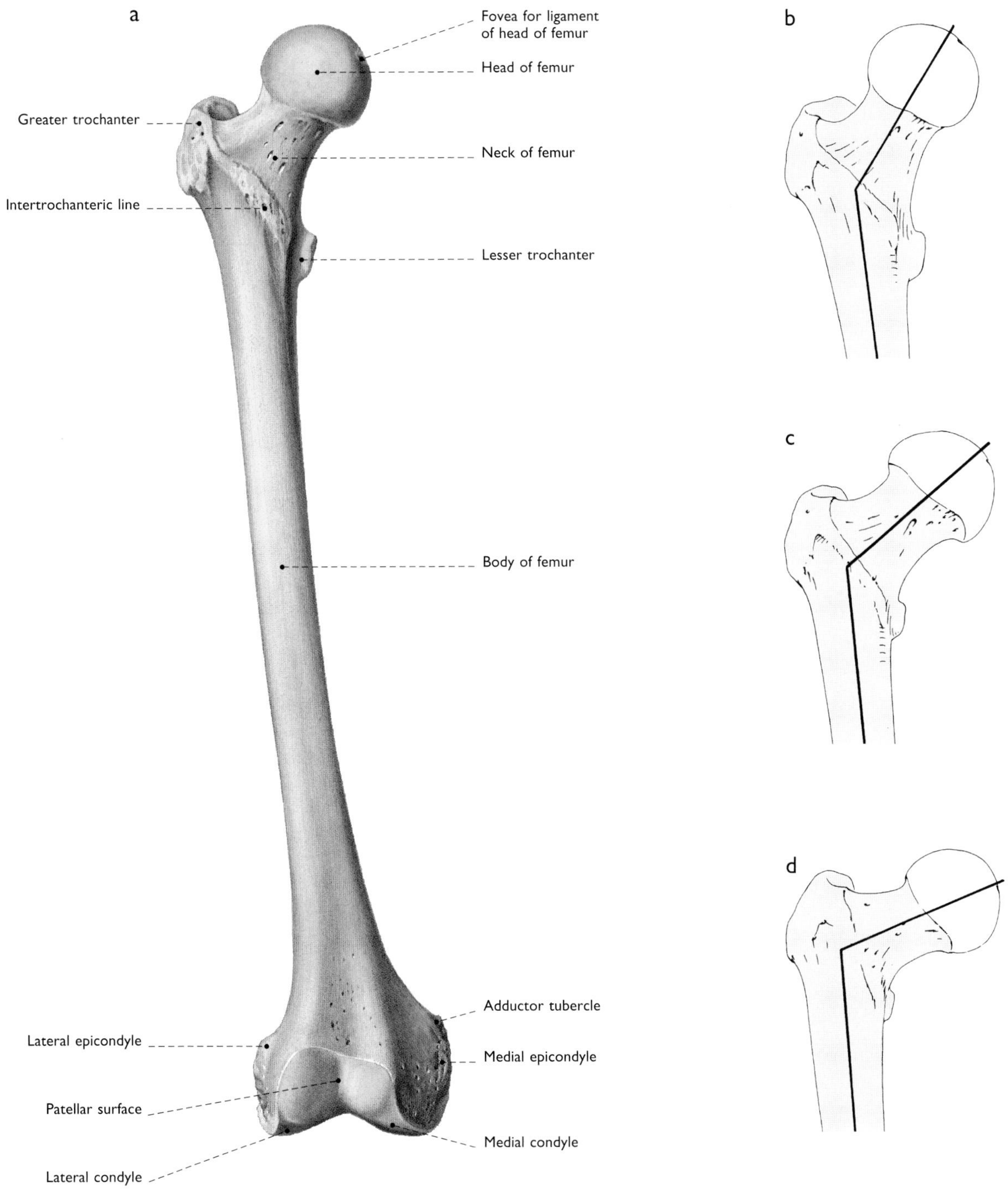
a
Fovea for ligament of head of femur
Head of femur
Greater trochanter
Neck of femur
Intertrochanteric line
Lesser trochanter
Body of femur
Adductor tubercle
Lateral epicondyle
Medial epicondyle
Patellar surface
Medial condyle
Lateral condyle
b
c
d

193 Right thigh bone (= femur) (40%)

a Ventral aspect
b–d Neck-shaft angle
b 140°, coxa valga
c 124°, within the norm of an adult (120–130°)
d 108°, coxa vara

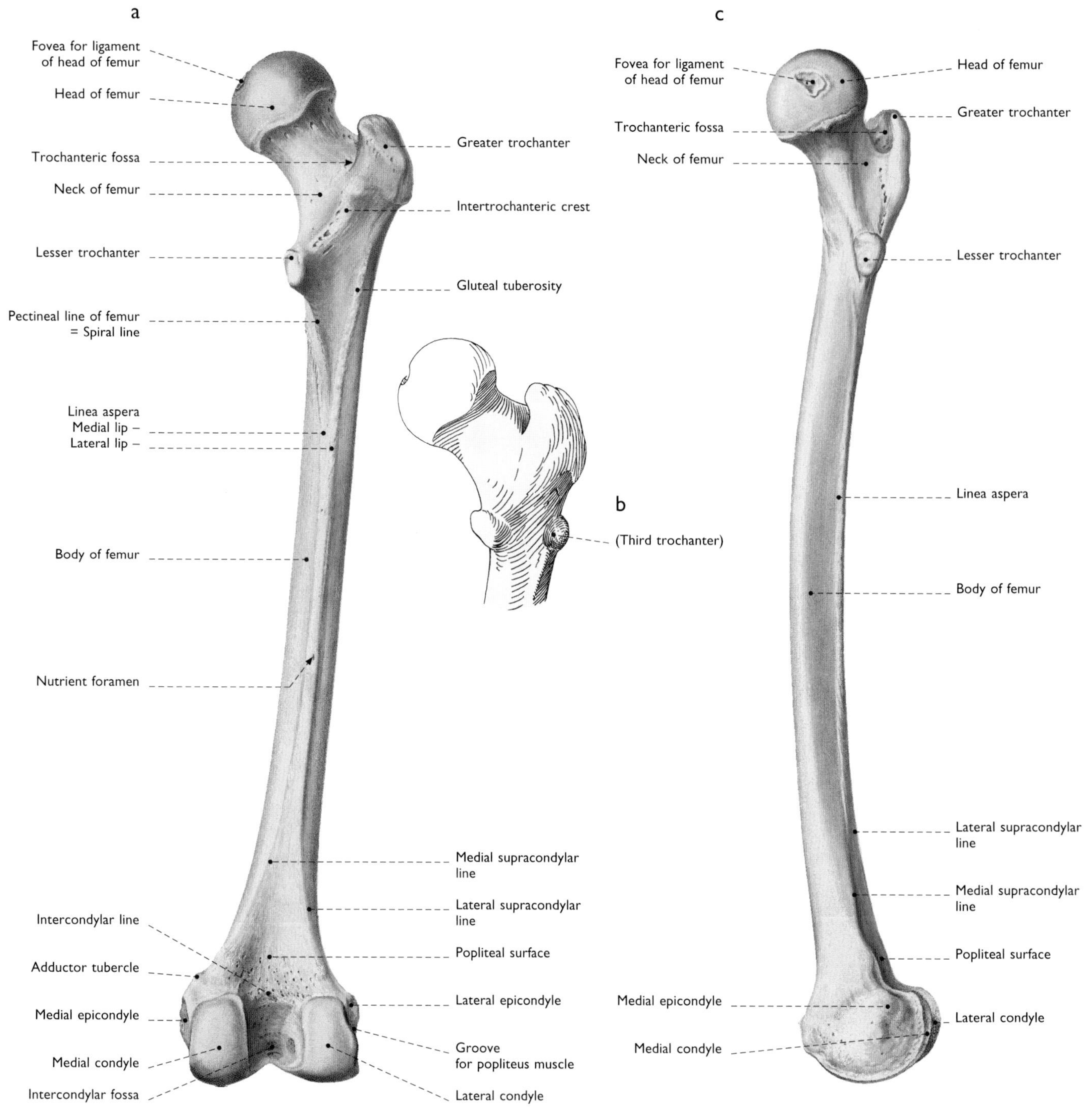

a
Fovea for ligament of head of femur
Head of femur
Trochanteric fossa
Neck of femur
Lesser trochanter
Pectineal line of femur = Spiral line
Linea aspera
Medial lip –
Lateral lip –
Body of femur
Nutrient foramen
Intercondylar line
Adductor tubercle
Medial epicondyle
Medial condyle
Intercondylar fossa
Greater trochanter
Intertrochanteric crest
Gluteal tuberosity
Medial supracondylar line
Lateral supracondylar line
Popliteal surface
Lateral epicondyle
Groove for popliteus muscle
Lateral condyle
b
(Third trochanter)
c
Fovea for ligament of head of femur
Trochanteric fossa
Neck of femur
Head of femur
Greater trochanter
Lesser trochanter
Linea aspera
Body of femur
Lateral supracondylar line
Medial supracondylar line
Popliteal surface
Medial epicondyle
Medial condyle
Lateral condyle

194 Right thigh bone (= femur) (40%)

a Dorsal aspect
b Proximal end of the thigh bone with a third trochanter, dorsal aspect
c Medial aspect

a

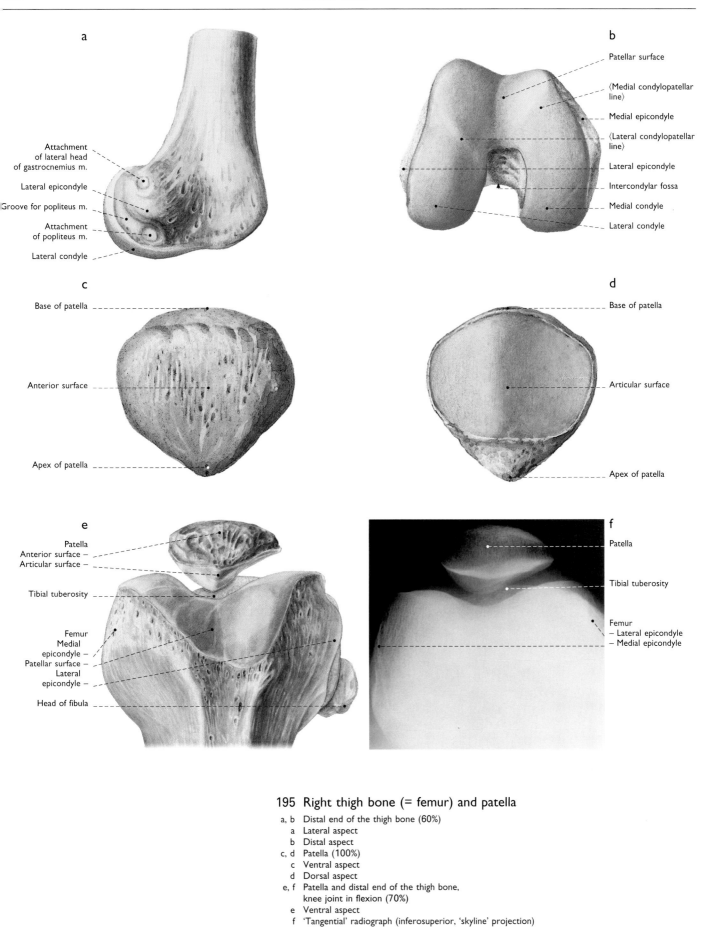

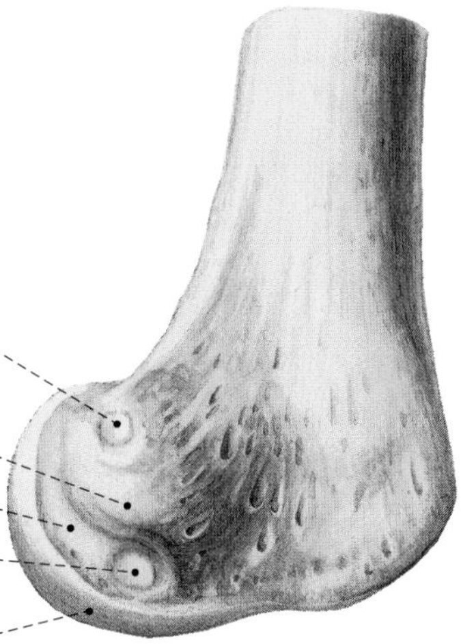
Attachment of lateral head of gastrocnemius m.
Lateral epicondyle
Groove for popliteus m.
Attachment of popliteus m.
Lateral condyle

b

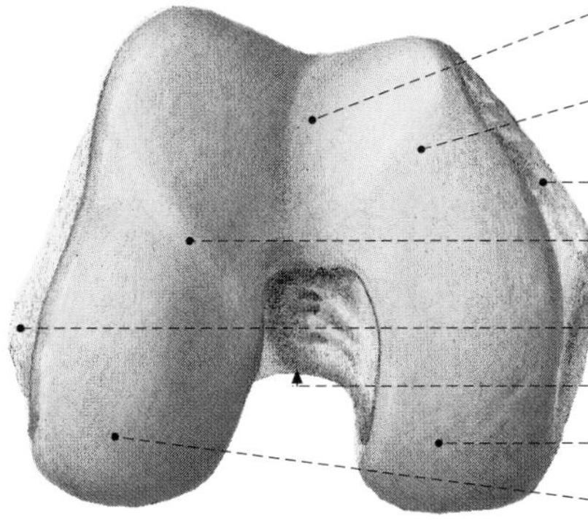
Patellar surface
⟨Medial condylopatellar line⟩
Medial epicondyle
⟨Lateral condylopatellar line⟩
Lateral epicondyle
Intercondylar fossa
Medial condyle
Lateral condyle

c

Base of patella
Anterior surface
Apex of patella

d

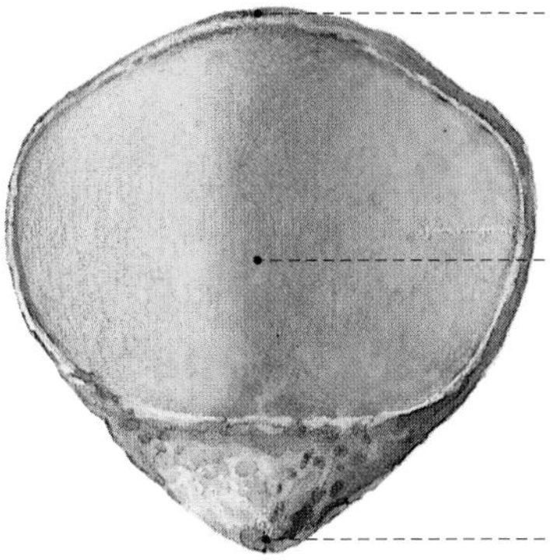
Base of patella
Articular surface
Apex of patella

e

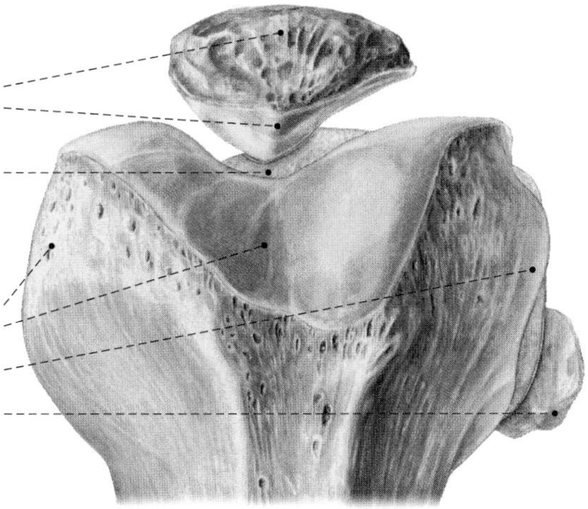
Patella
Anterior surface –
Articular surface –
Tibial tuberosity
Femur
Medial epicondyle –
Patellar surface –
Lateral epicondyle –
Head of fibula

f

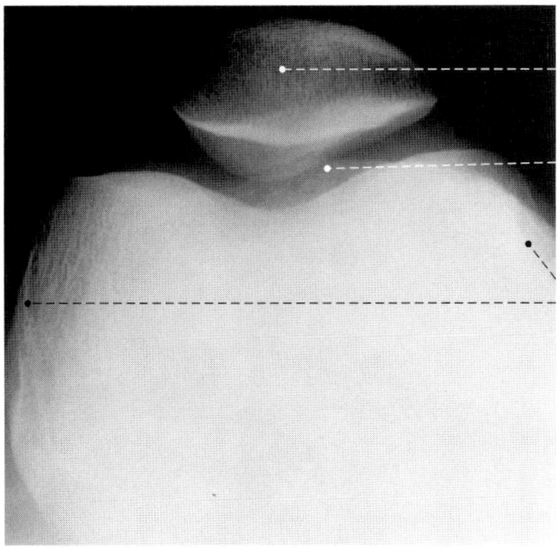
Patella
Tibial tuberosity
Femur
– Lateral epicondyle
– Medial epicondyle

195 Right thigh bone (= femur) and patella

a, b Distal end of the thigh bone (60%)
a Lateral aspect
b Distal aspect
c, d Patella (100%)
c Ventral aspect
d Dorsal aspect
e, f Patella and distal end of the thigh bone, knee joint in flexion (70%)
e Ventral aspect
f 'Tangential' radiograph (inferosuperior, 'skyline' projection)

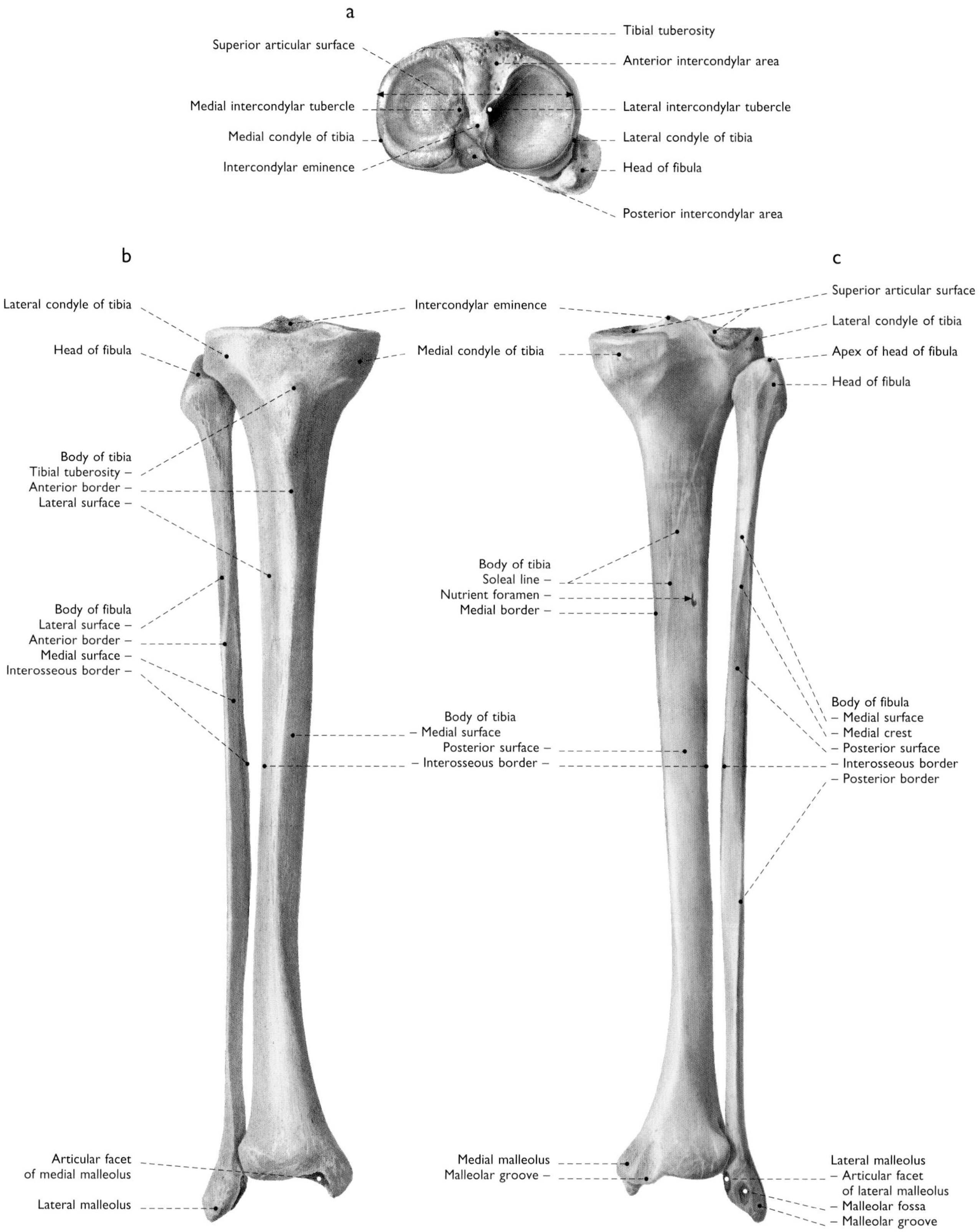
a
Superior articular surface
Medial intercondylar tubercle
Medial condyle of tibia
Intercondylar eminence
Tibial tuberosity
Anterior intercondylar area
Lateral intercondylar tubercle
Lateral condyle of tibia
Head of fibula
Posterior intercondylar area
b
Lateral condyle of tibia
Head of fibula
Body of tibia
Tibial tuberosity –
Anterior border –
Lateral surface –
Body of fibula
Lateral surface –
Anterior border –
Medial surface –
Interosseous border –
Articular facet of medial malleolus
Lateral malleolus
Intercondylar eminence
Medial condyle of tibia
Body of tibia
Soleal line –
Nutrient foramen –
Medial border –
Body of tibia
– Medial surface
Posterior surface –
– Interosseous border –
Medial malleolus
Malleolar groove –
c
Superior articular surface
Lateral condyle of tibia
Apex of head of fibula
Head of fibula
Body of fibula
– Medial surface
– Medial crest
– Posterior surface
– Interosseous border
– Posterior border
Lateral malleolus
– Articular facet of lateral malleolus
– Malleolar fossa
– Malleolar groove

196 Bones of the right leg (40%)

a Proximal aspect
b Ventral aspect
c Dorsal aspect

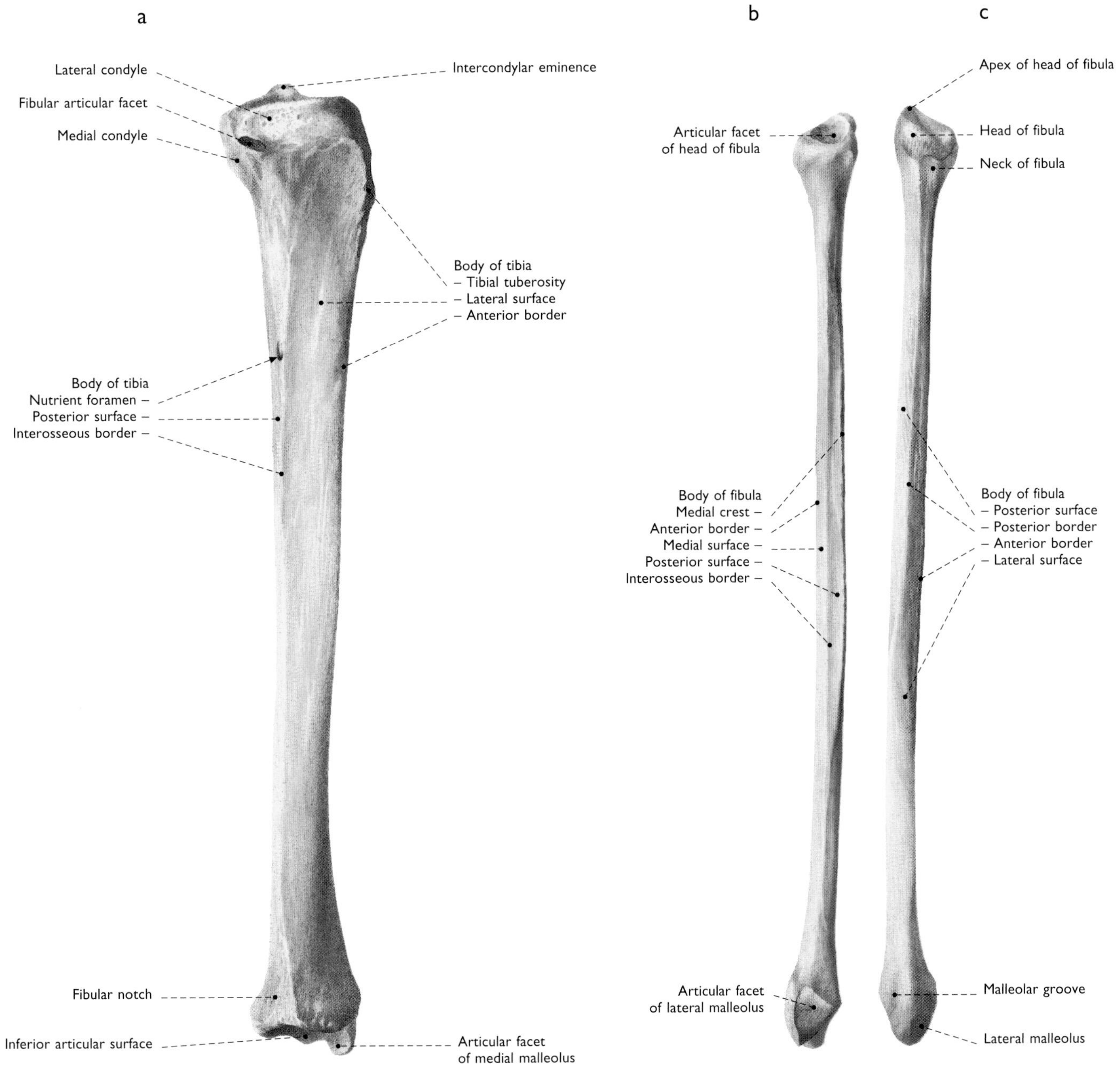
a
b
c
Lateral condyle
Fibular articular facet
Medial condyle
Intercondylar eminence
Body of tibia
– Tibial tuberosity
– Lateral surface
– Anterior border
Body of tibia
Nutrient foramen –
Posterior surface –
Interosseous border –
Fibular notch
Inferior articular surface
Articular facet
of medial malleolus
Articular facet
of head of fibula
Apex of head of fibula
Head of fibula
Neck of fibula
Body of fibula
Medial crest –
Anterior border –
Medial surface –
Posterior surface –
Interosseous border –
Body of fibula
– Posterior surface
– Posterior border
– Anterior border
– Lateral surface
Articular facet
of lateral malleolus
Malleolar groove
Lateral malleolus

197 Right tibia and fibula (40%)

a Tibia (= shin bone), lateral aspect
b Fibula (= calf bone), medial aspect
c Fibula (= calf bone), lateral aspect

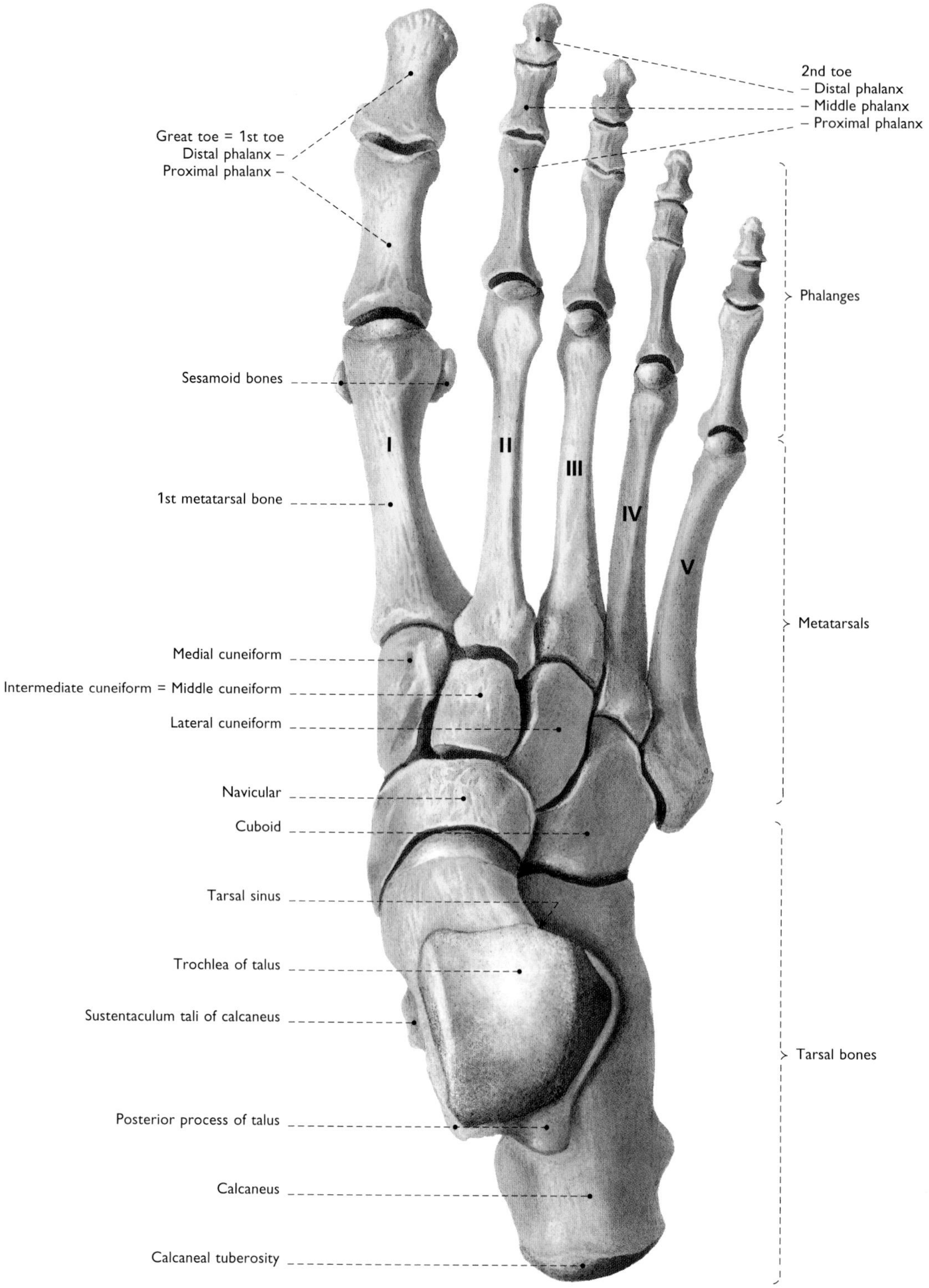
2nd toe
– Distal phalanx
– Middle phalanx
– Proximal phalanx
Great toe = 1st toe
Distal phalanx –
Proximal phalanx –
Phalanges
Sesamoid bones
I
II
III
IV
V
1st metatarsal bone
Metatarsals
Medial cuneiform
Intermediate cuneiform = Middle cuneiform
Lateral cuneiform
Navicular
Cuboid
Tarsal sinus
Trochlea of talus
Sustentaculum tali of calcaneus
Tarsal bones
Posterior process of talus
Calcaneus
Calcaneal tuberosity

198 Bones of the right foot (80%)
Dorsal aspect

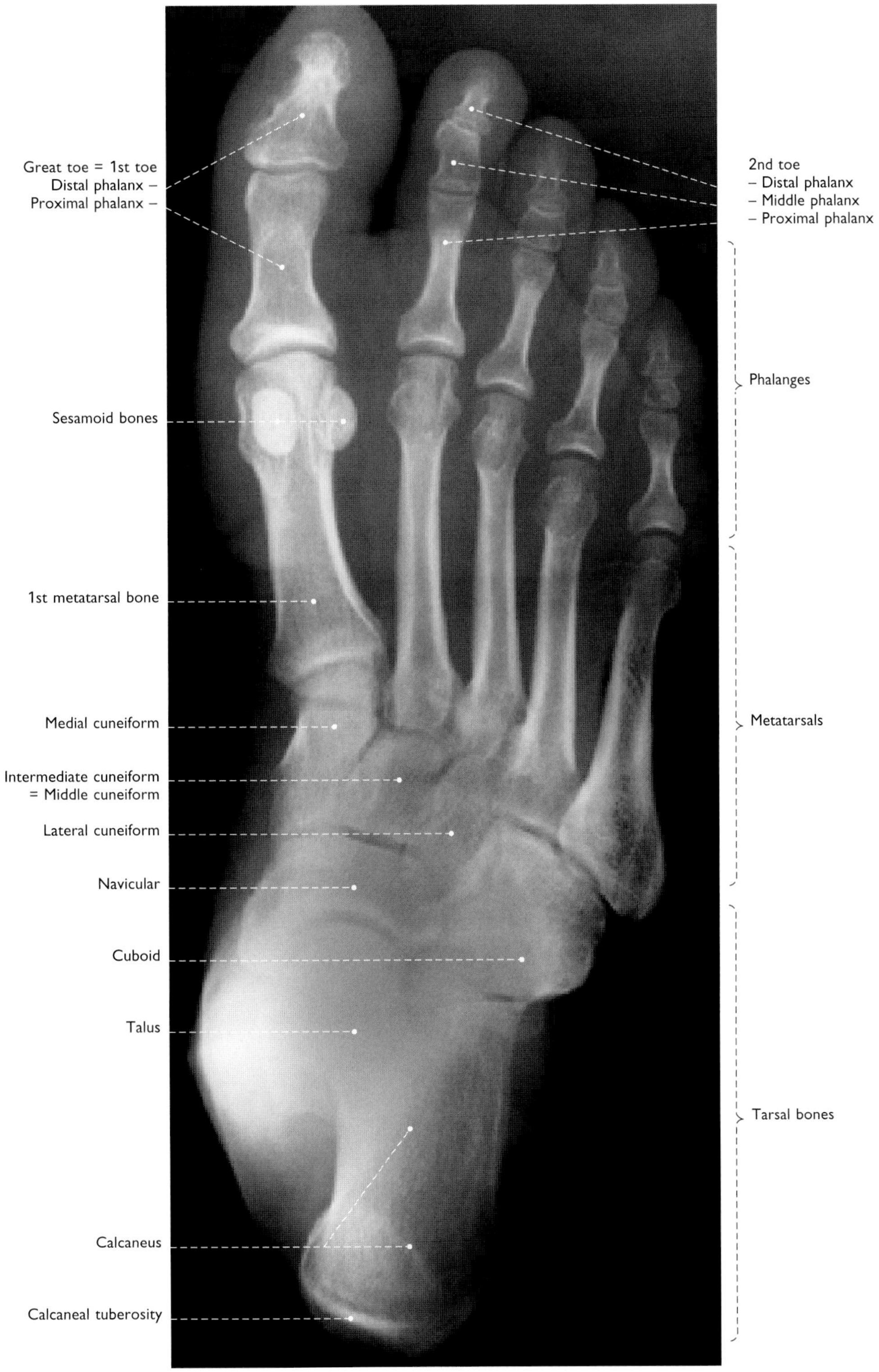
Great toe = 1st toe
Distal phalanx –
Proximal phalanx –
Sesamoid bones
1st metatarsal bone
Medial cuneiform
Intermediate cuneiform
= Middle cuneiform
Lateral cuneiform
Navicular
Cuboid
Talus
Calcaneus
Calcaneal tuberosity
2nd toe
– Distal phalanx
– Middle phalanx
– Proximal phalanx
Phalanges
Metatarsals
Tarsal bones

199 Bones of the right foot (80%)

Dorsoplantar radiograph

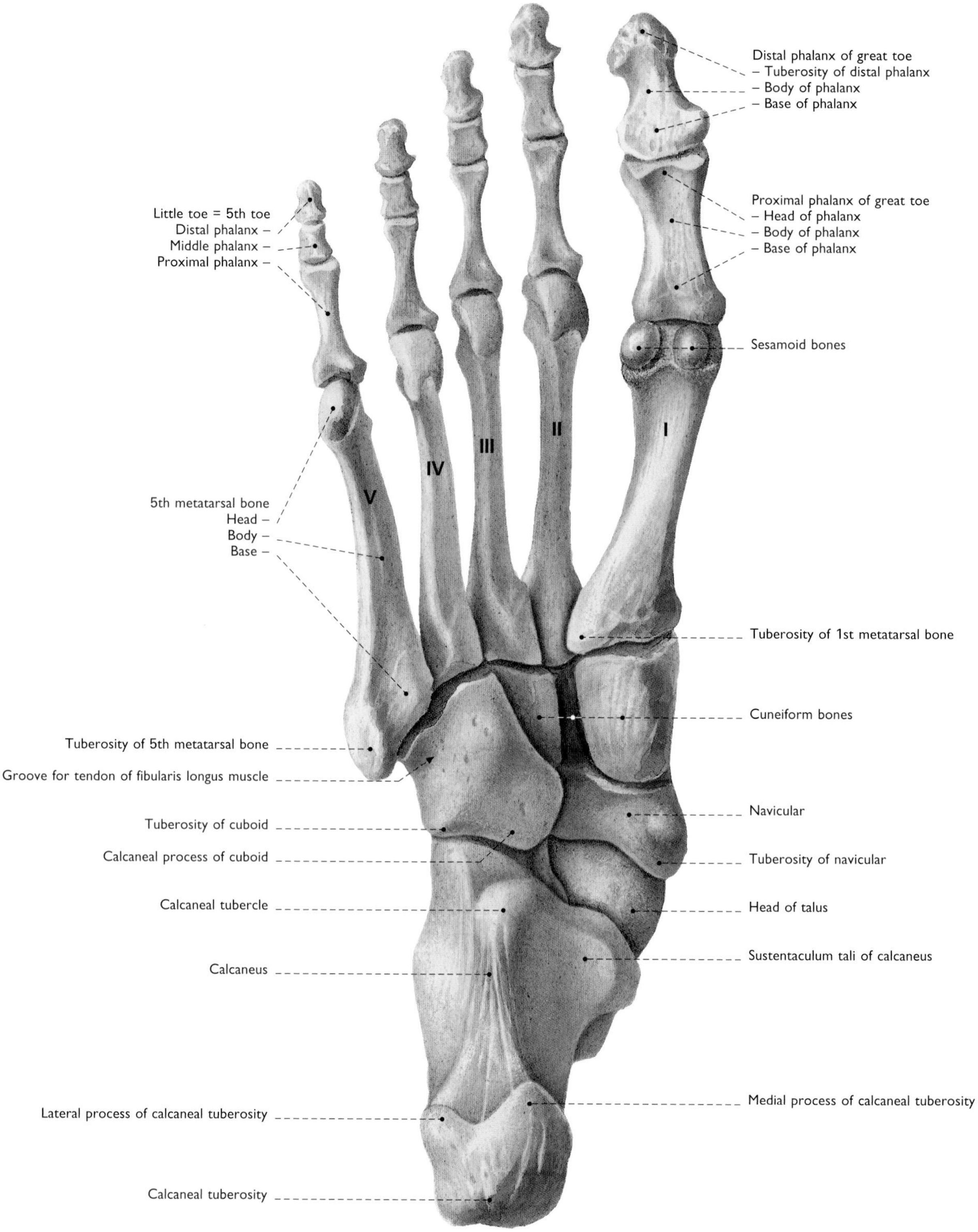
Distal phalanx of great toe
– Tuberosity of distal phalanx
– Body of phalanx
– Base of phalanx
Little toe = 5th toe
Distal phalanx –
Middle phalanx –
Proximal phalanx –
Proximal phalanx of great toe
– Head of phalanx
– Body of phalanx
– Base of phalanx
Sesamoid bones
I
II
III
IV
V
5th metatarsal bone
Head –
Body –
Base –
Tuberosity of 1st metatarsal bone
Cuneiform bones
Tuberosity of 5th metatarsal bone
Groove for tendon of fibularis longus muscle
Navicular
Tuberosity of cuboid
Calcaneal process of cuboid
Tuberosity of navicular
Calcaneal tubercle
Head of talus
Calcaneus
Sustentaculum tali of calcaneus
Medial process of calcaneal tuberosity
Lateral process of calcaneal tuberosity
Calcaneal tuberosity

200 Bones of the right foot (80%)

Plantar aspect

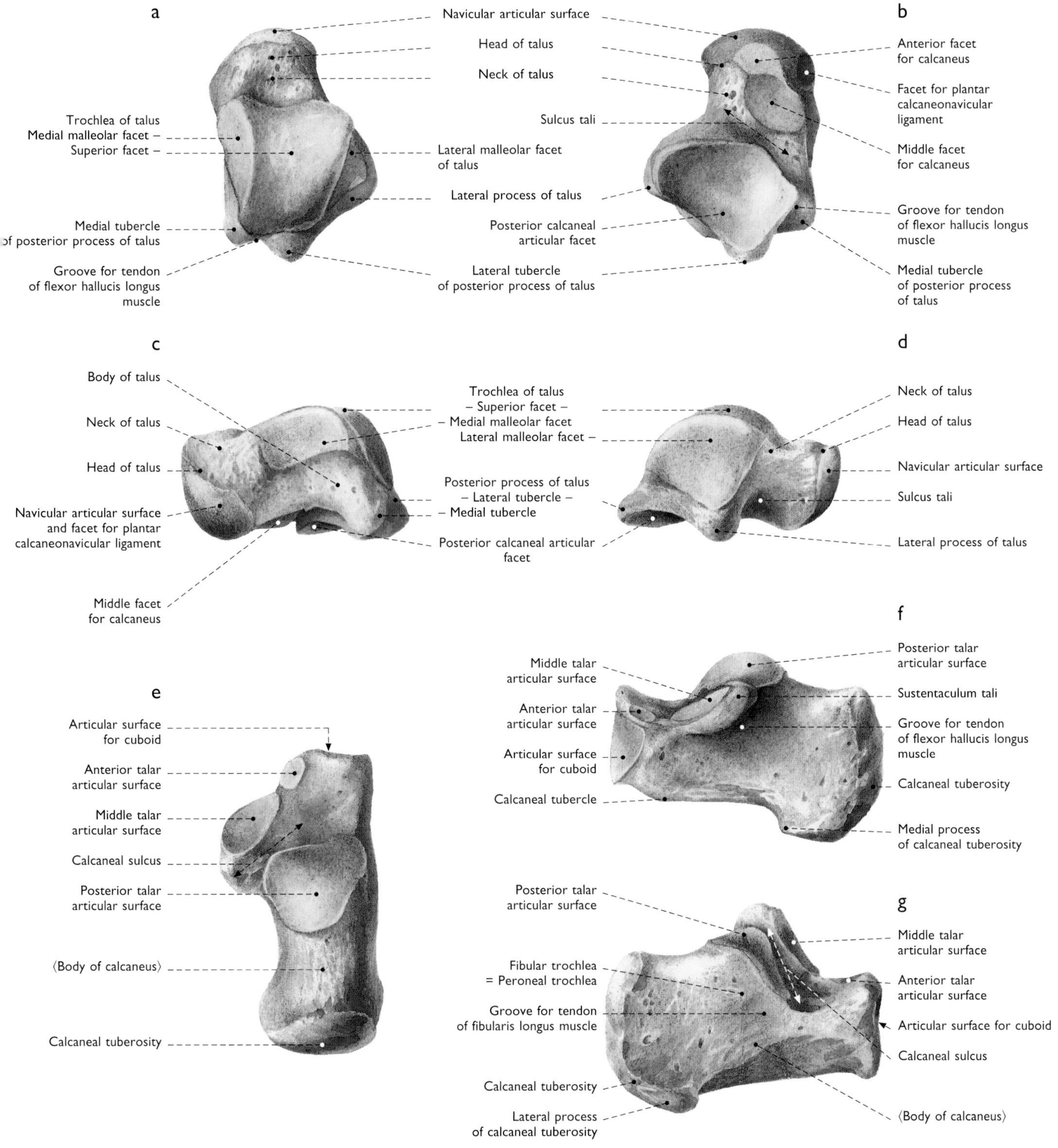
a
Navicular articular surface
Head of talus
Neck of talus
Trochlea of talus
Medial malleolar facet –
Superior facet –
Lateral malleolar facet of talus
Lateral process of talus
Medial tubercle of posterior process of talus
Groove for tendon of flexor hallucis longus muscle
Lateral tubercle of posterior process of talus
b
Anterior facet for calcaneus
Facet for plantar calcaneonavicular ligament
Sulcus tali
Middle facet for calcaneus
Posterior calcaneal articular facet
Groove for tendon of flexor hallucis longus muscle
Medial tubercle of posterior process of talus
c
Body of talus
Neck of talus
Head of talus
Navicular articular surface and facet for plantar calcaneonavicular ligament
Middle facet for calcaneus
Trochlea of talus
– Superior facet –
– Medial malleolar facet
Lateral malleolar facet –
Posterior process of talus
– Lateral tubercle –
– Medial tubercle
Posterior calcaneal articular facet
d
Neck of talus
Head of talus
Navicular articular surface
Sulcus tali
Lateral process of talus
e
Articular surface for cuboid
Anterior talar articular surface
Middle talar articular surface
Calcaneal sulcus
Posterior talar articular surface
(Body of calcaneus)
Calcaneal tuberosity
f
Middle talar articular surface
Anterior talar articular surface
Articular surface for cuboid
Calcaneal tubercle
Posterior talar articular surface
Sustentaculum tali
Groove for tendon of flexor hallucis longus muscle
Calcaneal tuberosity
Medial process of calcaneal tuberosity
g
Posterior talar articular surface
Fibular trochlea = Peroneal trochlea
Groove for tendon of fibularis longus muscle
Calcaneal tuberosity
Lateral process of calcaneal tuberosity
Middle talar articular surface
Anterior talar articular surface
Articular surface for cuboid
Calcaneal sulcus
(Body of calcaneus)

201 Right talus and calcaneus (75%)

a–d Talus (= ankle bone)
e–g Calcaneus (= heel bone)
a, e Proximal aspect
b Plantar aspect
c, f Medial aspect
d, g Lateral aspect

a

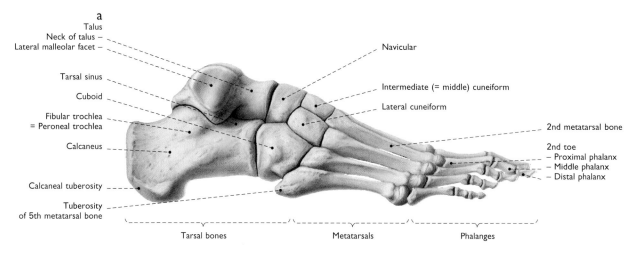

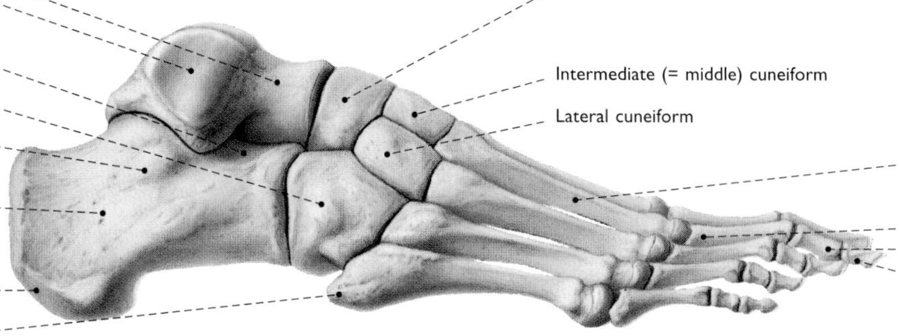
Talus
Neck of talus –
Lateral malleolar facet –
Tarsal sinus
Cuboid
Fibular trochlea
= Peroneal trochlea
Calcaneus
Calcaneal tuberosity
Tuberosity
of 5th metatarsal bone
Navicular
Intermediate (= middle) cuneiform
Lateral cuneiform
2nd metatarsal bone
2nd toe
– Proximal phalanx
– Middle phalanx
– Distal phalanx
Tarsal bones
Metatarsals
Phalanges

b

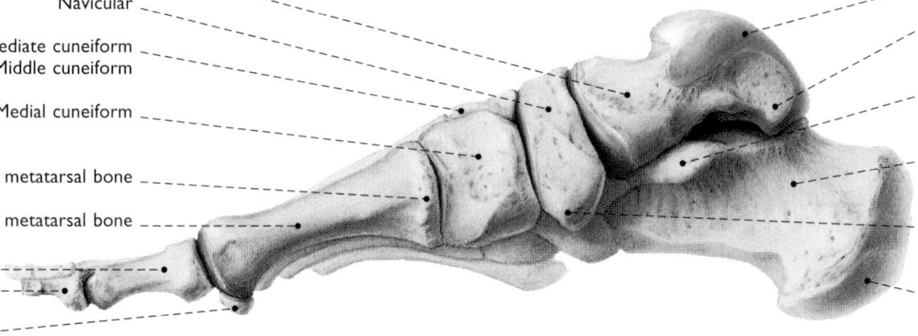
Neck of talus
Navicular
Intermediate cuneiform
= Middle cuneiform
Medial cuneiform
Tuberosity of 1st metatarsal bone
1st metatarsal bone
Great toe = 1st toe
Proximal phalanx –
Distal phalanx –
Sesamoid bone
Talus
– Superior facet
of talus
– Medial tubercle
of posterior process of talus
Sustentaculum tali
Calcaneus
Tuberosity of navicular
Calcaneal tuberosity
Phalanges
Metatarsals
Tarsal bones

c

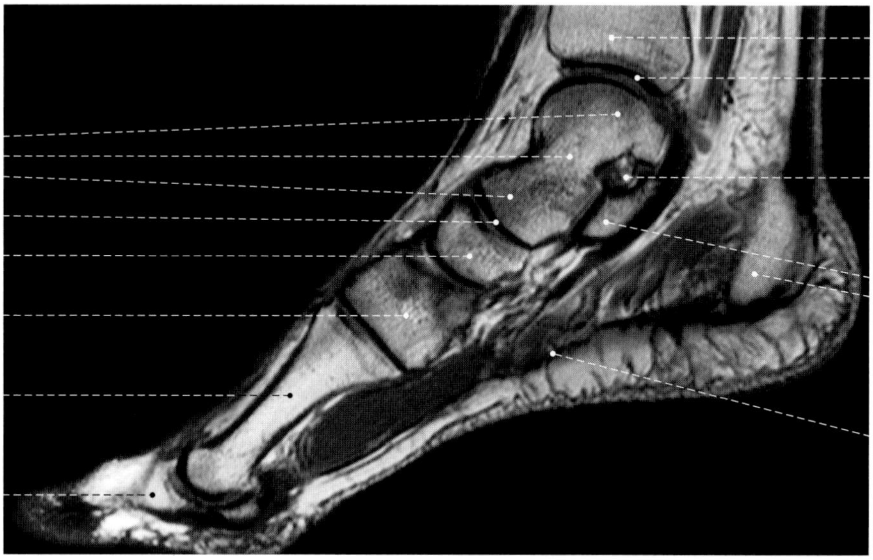
Talus
Trochlea of talus –
Neck of talus –
Head of talus –
Talocalcaneonavicular joint
Navicular
Medial cuneiform
1st metatarsal bone
Proximal phalanx
of great toe
Tibia
Ankle joint
⟨= Talocrural joint⟩
Tarsal sinus
with talocalcaneal
interosseous ligament
Calcaneus
– Sustentaculum tali
– Calcaneal tuberosity
Plantar aponeurosis

202 Bones of the right foot (45%)

a Lateral aspect
b Medial aspect
c Sagittal magnetic resonance image (MRI, T_1-weighted) through the medial part of the right foot, medial aspect

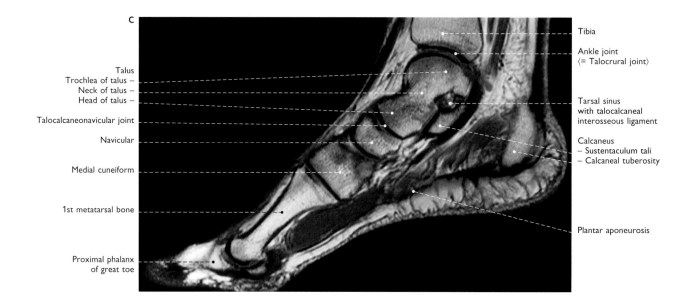

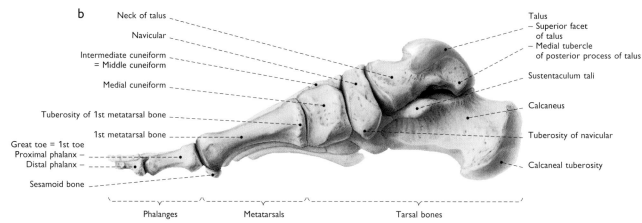

a

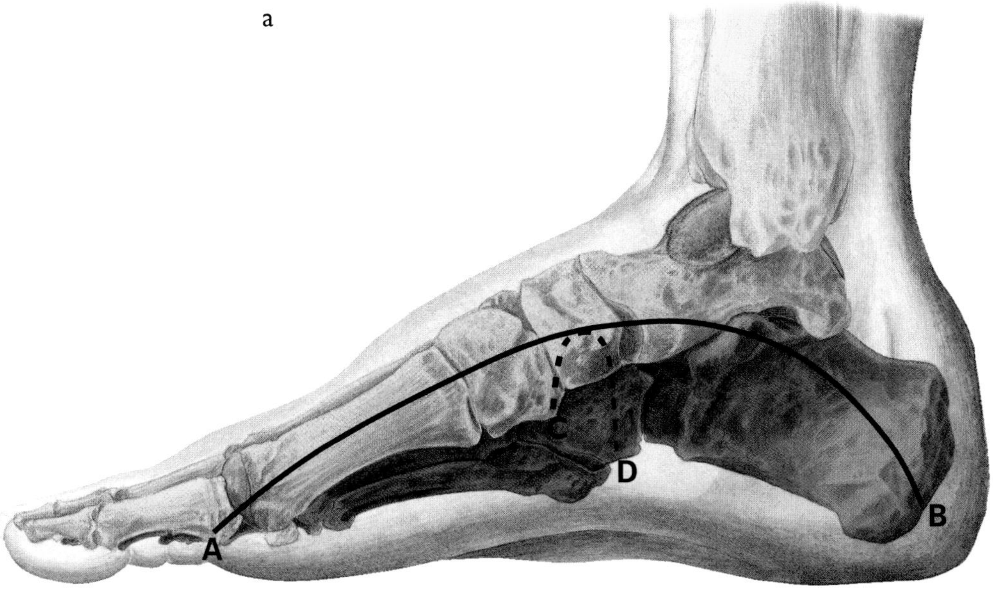
D
A
B

Bones of medial arch of foot

Bones of lateral arch of foot

b

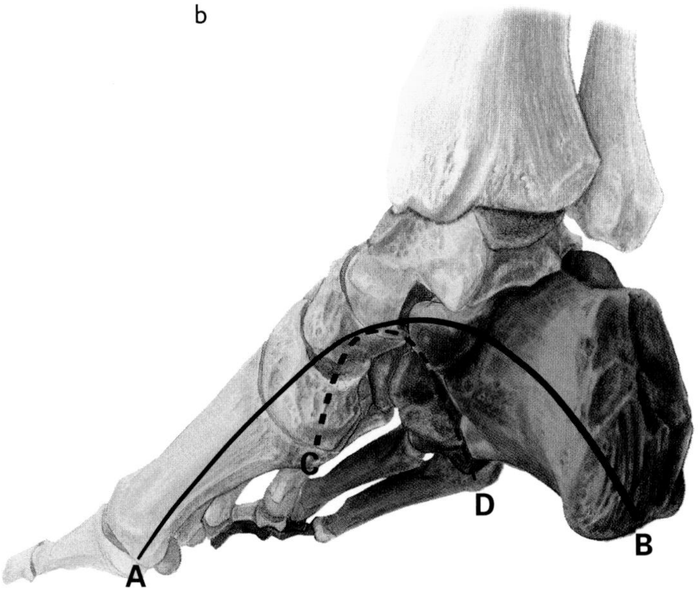
C
D
A
B

c

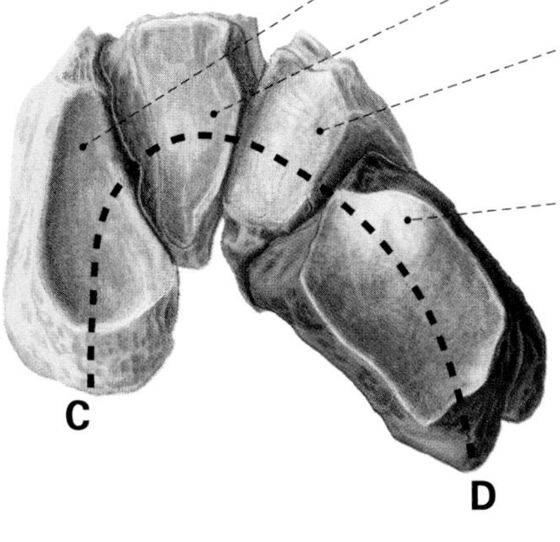
Medial cuneiform
Intermediate cuneiform = Middle cuneiform
Lateral cuneiform
Cuboid
C
D

203 Longitudinal and transverse arches of the skeleton of the right foot

The bones of the medial arch are illustrated in clear brown, those of the lateral arch in dark brown color. The longitudinal arch is shown by a continuous line (A–B), the transverse arch by a broken line (C–D).

a Medial aspect (55%)
b Mediodorsal aspect (55%)
c Proximal aspect of the cuneiform bones and the cuboid bone (85%)

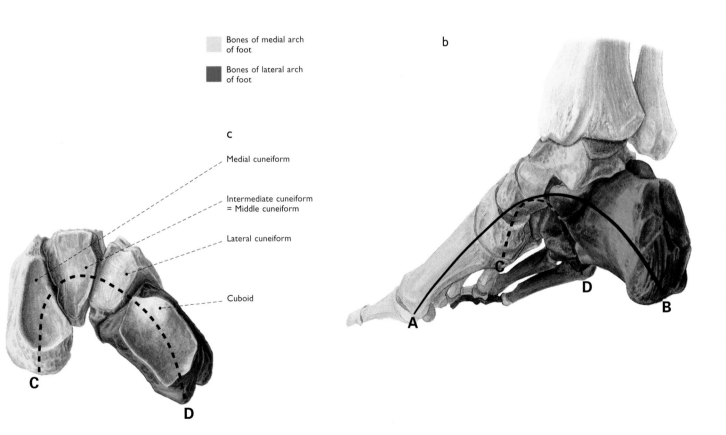

a

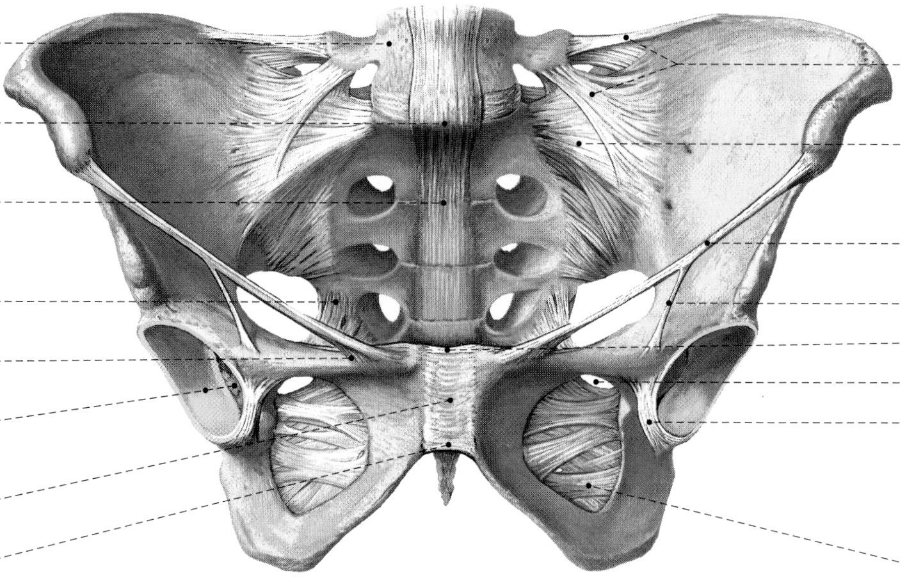
5th lumbar vertebra
Promontory of sacrum
Anterior longitudinal ligament
Sacrospinous ligament
Lacunar ligament (GIMBERNAT)
Lunate surface of acetabulum, Acetabular fossa
Pubic symphysis, Interpubic disc
Inferior pubic ligament
Iliolumbar ligament
Anterior sacro-iliac ligament
Inguinal ligament (POUPART)
Iliopectineal arch
Superior pubic ligament
Obturator canal
Transverse acetabular ligament
Obturator membrane

b

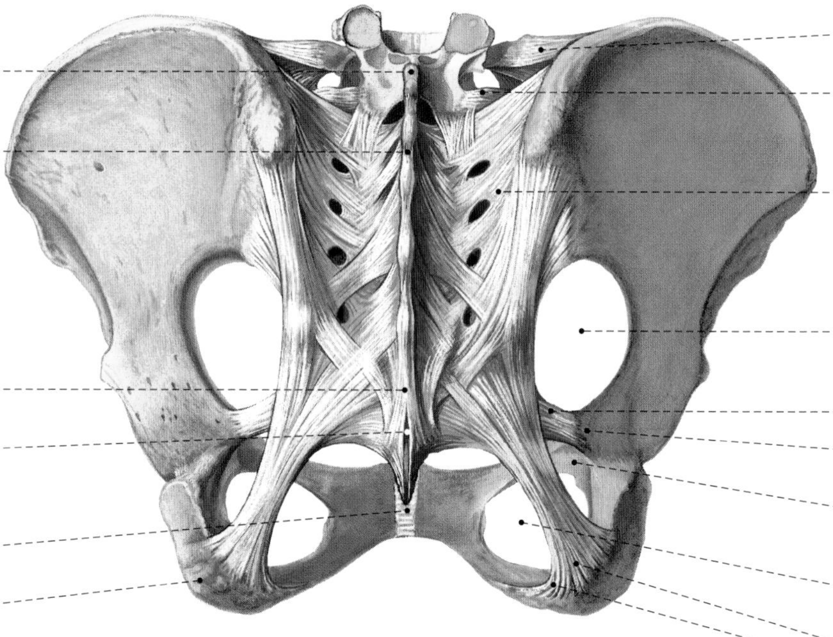
Spinous process of 5th lumbar vertebra
Supraspinous ligament
Superficial posterior sacrococcygeal ligament
Deep posterior sacrococcygeal ligament
Pubic symphysis
Ischial tuberosity
Iliolumbar ligament
Interosseous sacro-iliac ligament
Posterior sacro-iliac ligament
Greater sciatic foramen
Sacrospinous ligament
Ischial spine
Lesser sciatic foramen
Obturator foramen
Sacrotuberous ligament
– Falciform process

204 Joints and ligaments of the pelvic girdle of a female (40%)

a Ventral aspect
b The obturator membrane was removed. Dorsal aspect

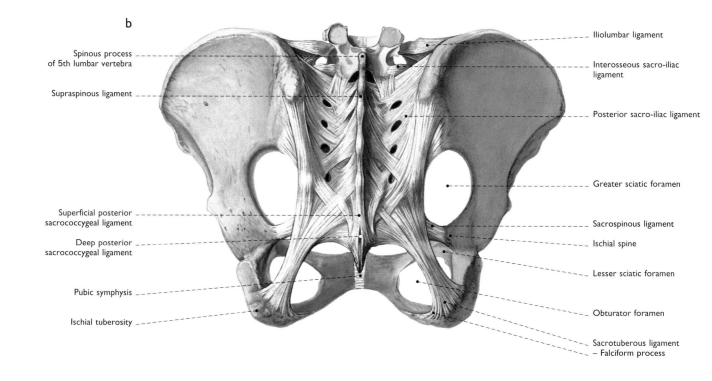

a

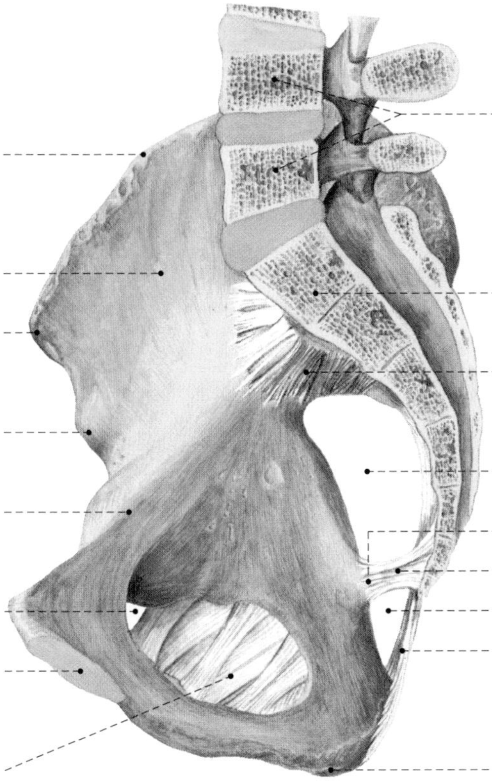
4th and 5th lumbar vertebrae
Iliac crest
Iliac fossa of ala of ilium
Sacrum,
1st sacral vertebra
Anterior superior iliac spine
Anterior sacro-iliac ligament
Anterior inferior iliac spine
Greater sciatic foramen
Arcuate line
Ischial spine
Sacrospinous ligament
Obturator canal
Lesser sciatic foramen
Sacrotuberous ligament
Symphysial surface
Obturator membrane
Ischial tuberosity

b

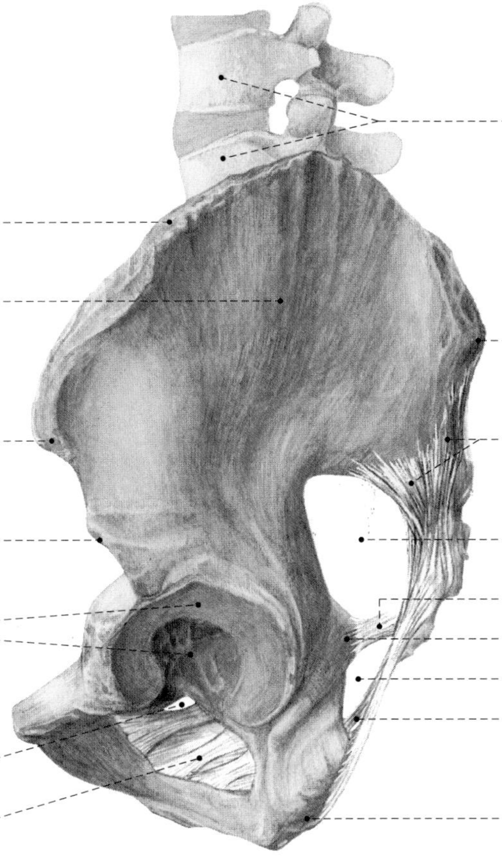
4th and 5th lumbar vertebrae
Iliac crest
Gluteal surface of ala of ilium
Posterior superior iliac spine
Anterior superior iliac spine
Posterior sacro-iliac ligament
Anterior inferior iliac spine
Greater sciatic foramen
Acetabulum
Lunate surface
Acetabular fossa
Sacrospinous ligament
Ischial spine
Lesser sciatic foramen
Sacrotuberous ligament
Obturator canal
Obturator membrane
Ischial tuberosity

205 Joints and ligaments of the pelvic girdle (45%)

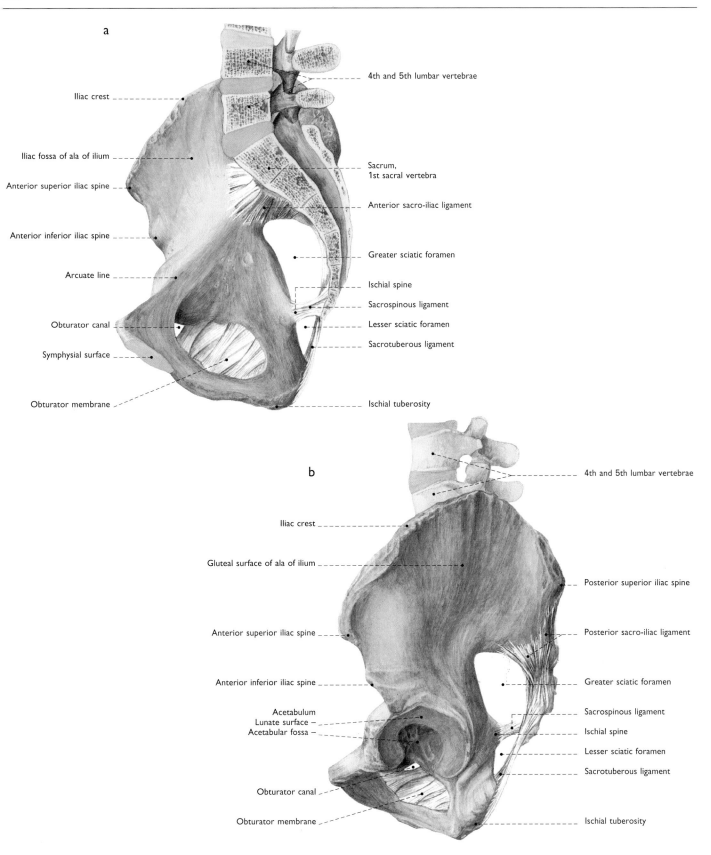

a Medial aspect of the right half of the pelvis
b Left lateral aspect of the pelvis

a

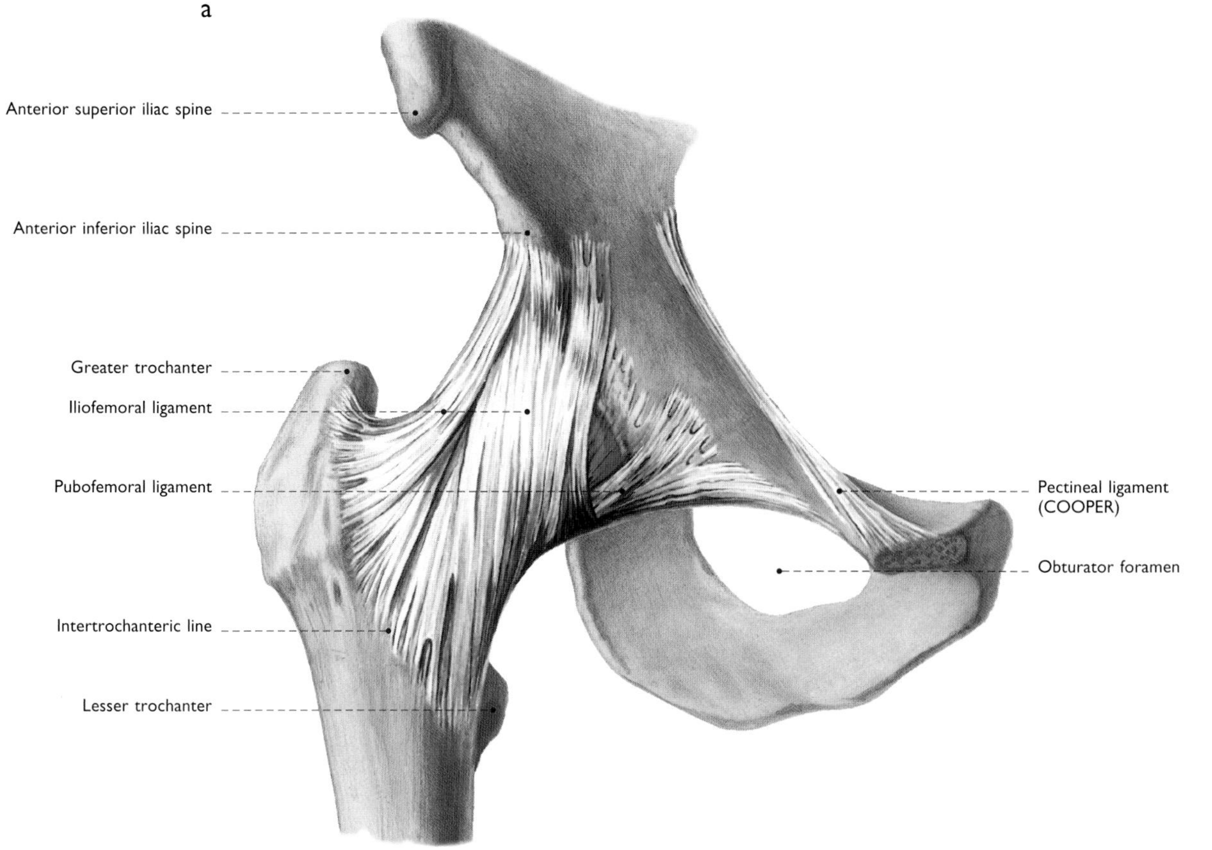
Anterior superior iliac spine
Anterior inferior iliac spine
Greater trochanter
Iliofemoral ligament
Pubofemoral ligament
Intertrochanteric line
Lesser trochanter
Pectineal ligament (COOPER)
Obturator foramen

b

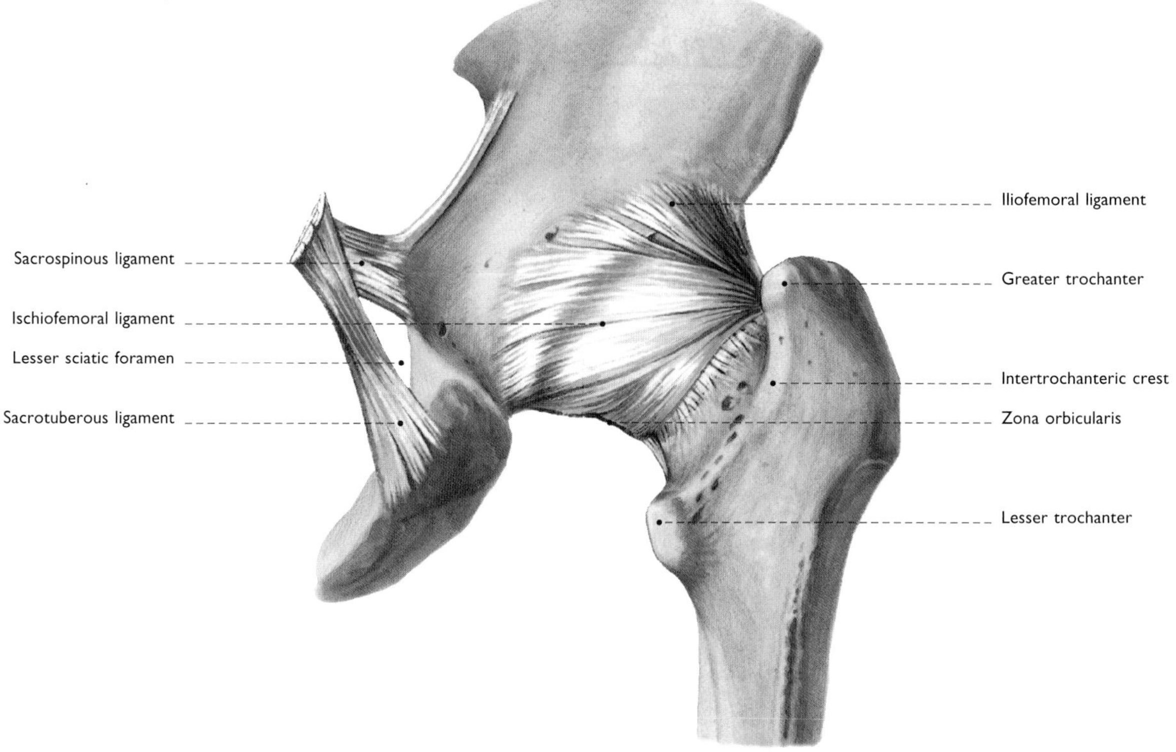
Iliofemoral ligament
Sacrospinous ligament
Greater trochanter
Ischiofemoral ligament
Lesser sciatic foramen
Intertrochanteric crest
Sacrotuberous ligament
Zona orbicularis
Lesser trochanter

206 Right hip joint (70%)

a Ventral aspect
b Dorsal aspect

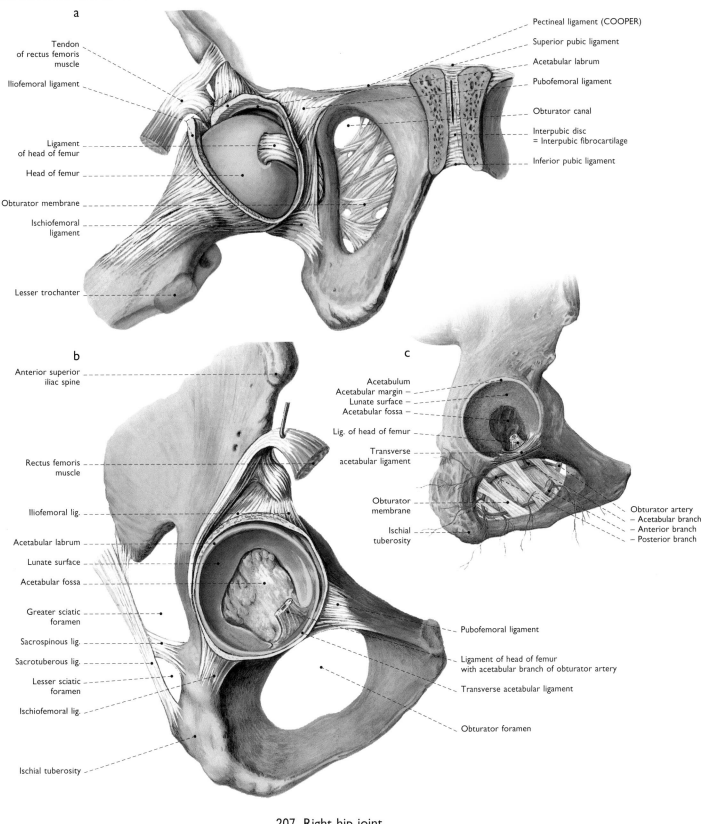

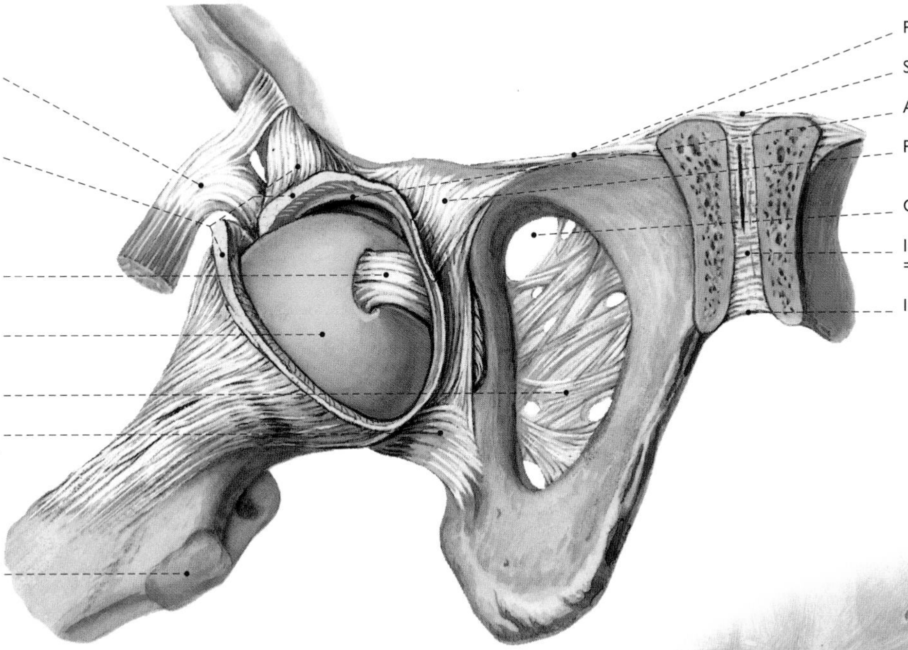
a
Tendon of rectus femoris muscle
Iliofemoral ligament
Ligament of head of femur
Head of femur
Obturator membrane
Ischiofemoral ligament
Lesser trochanter
Pectineal ligament (COOPER)
Superior pubic ligament
Acetabular labrum
Pubofemoral ligament
Obturator canal
Interpubic disc
= Interpubic fibrocartilage
Inferior pubic ligament

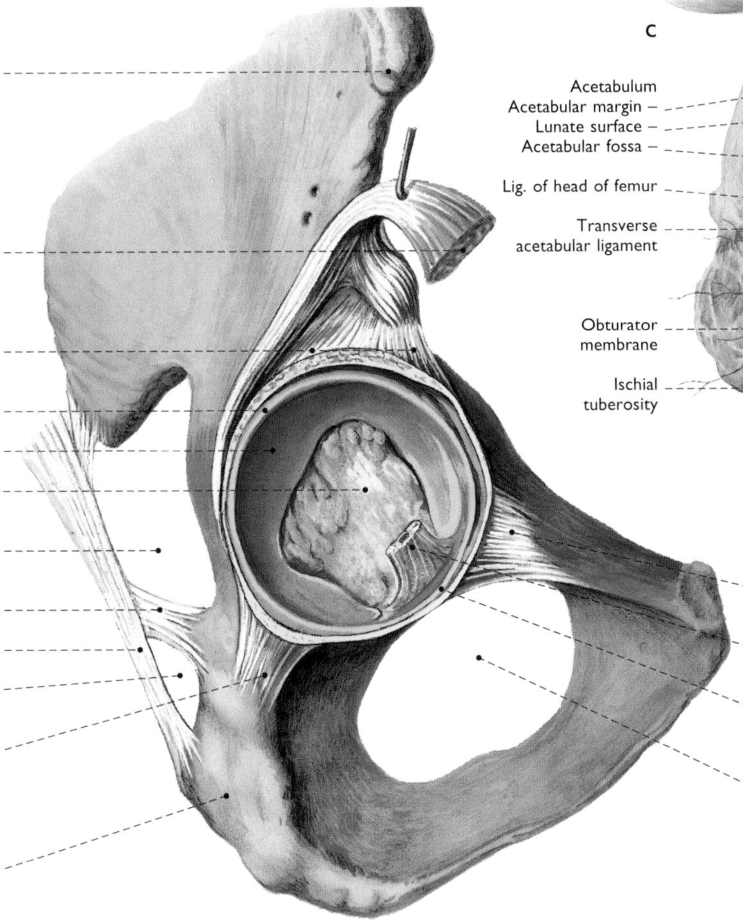
b
Anterior superior iliac spine
Rectus femoris muscle
Iliofemoral lig.
Acetabular labrum
Lunate surface
Acetabular fossa
Greater sciatic foramen
Sacrospinous lig.
Sacrotuberous lig.
Lesser sciatic foramen
Ischiofemoral lig.
Ischial tuberosity
Pubofemoral ligament
Ligament of head of femur with acetabular branch of obturator artery
Transverse acetabular ligament
Obturator foramen

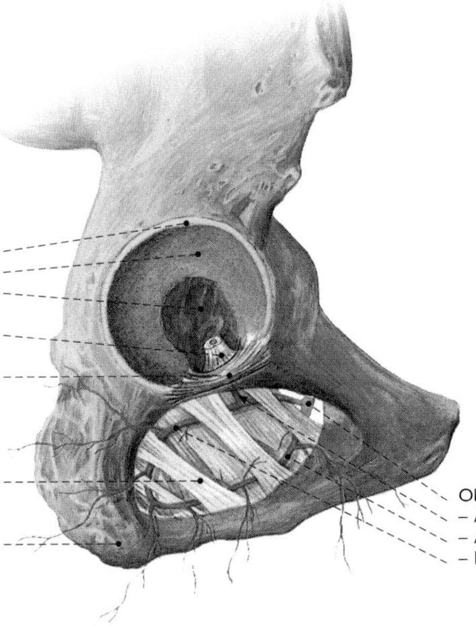
c
Acetabulum
Acetabular margin –
Lunate surface –
Acetabular fossa –
Lig. of head of femur
Transverse acetabular ligament
Obturator membrane
Ischial tuberosity
Obturator artery
– Acetabular branch
– Anterior branch
– Posterior branch

207 Right hip joint

a The femur was abducted and rotated outwards. The capsule of the hip joint was opened ventrally and the pubic symphysis cut frontally (60%). Ventral aspect

b View of the socket of hip joint (60%), ventrolateral aspect

c Ligament of the head of femur with acetabular artery (35%), ventrolateral aspect

a

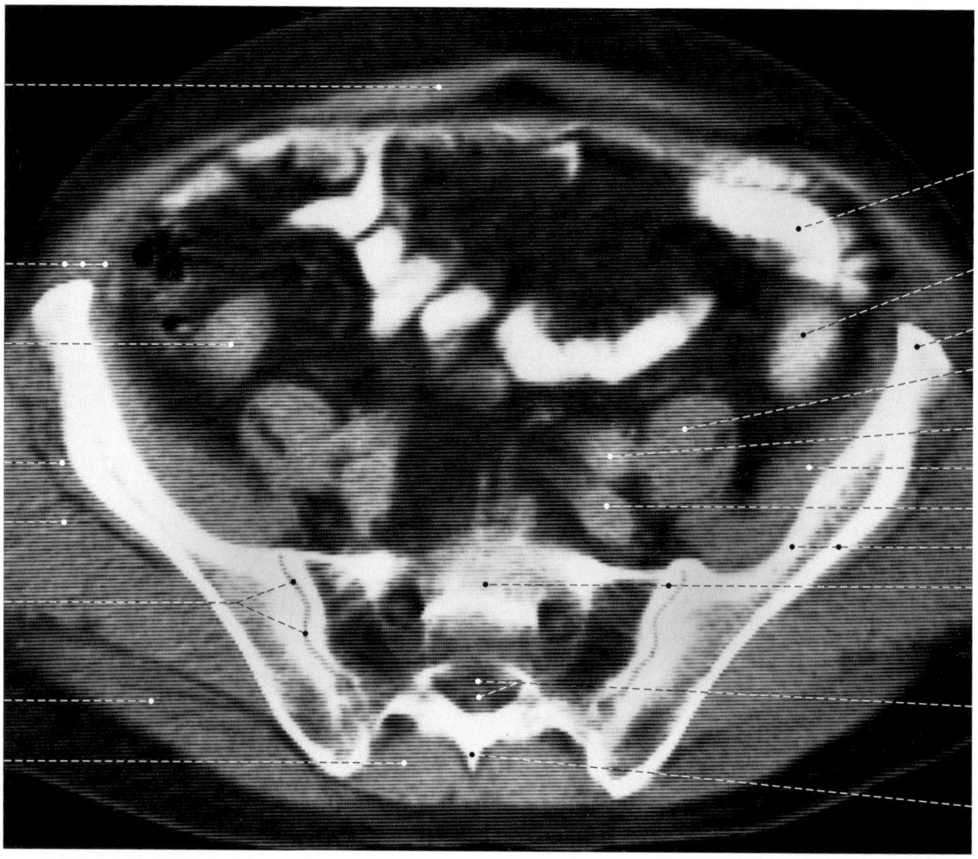
Rectus abdominis muscle
External and internal oblique muscles, Transversus abdominis m.
Cecum
Gluteus minimus muscle
Gluteus medius muscle
Sacro-iliac joint
Gluteus maximus muscle
Erector spinae muscle
Sigmoid colon
Descending colon
Iliac crest
Psoas major muscle
Common iliac artery
Iliacus muscle
Common iliac vein
Ilium
Sacrum (1st sacral vertebra)
Sacral canal, Cauda equina
Median sacral crest

b

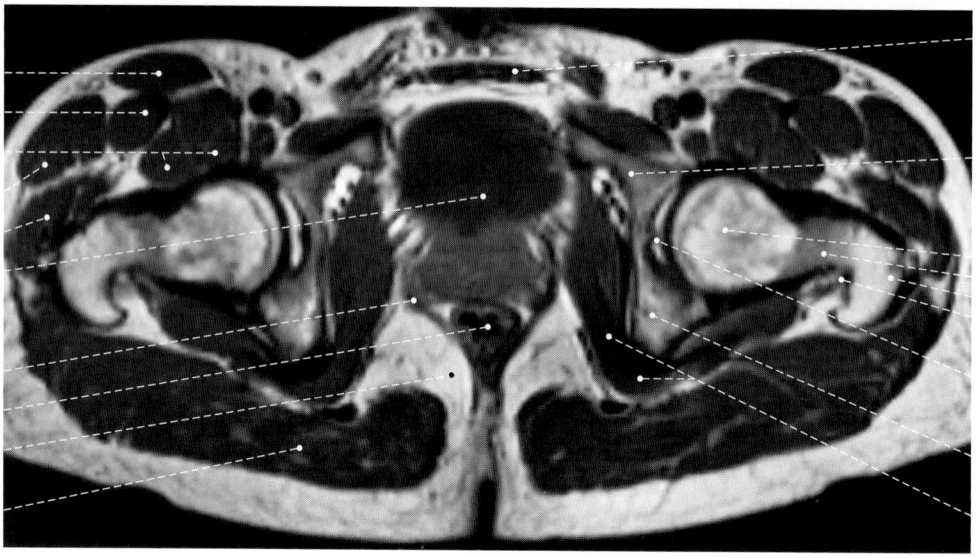
Sartorius muscle
Rectus femoris muscle
Iliopsoas muscle
Tensor fasciae latae muscle
Gluteus medius muscle
Urinary bladder
Levator ani muscle
Rectum
Ischio-anal fossa
Gluteus maximus muscle
Rectus abdominis muscle
Pubis
Femur
– Head of femur
– Neck of femur
– Greater trochanter
– Trochanteric fossa
Acetabular fossa
Ischium
Obturator internus muscle

208 Sacro-iliac and hip joints (40%)

Inferior aspect

a Axial (transverse) computed tomogram (CT) showing both sacro-iliac joints

b Axial (transverse) magnetic resonance image (MRI, T_1-weighted) showing both hip joints

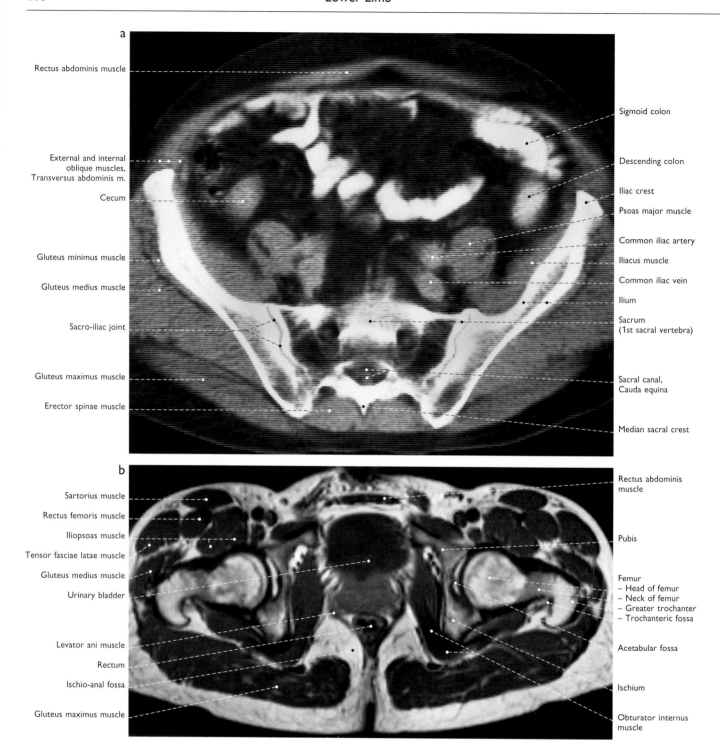

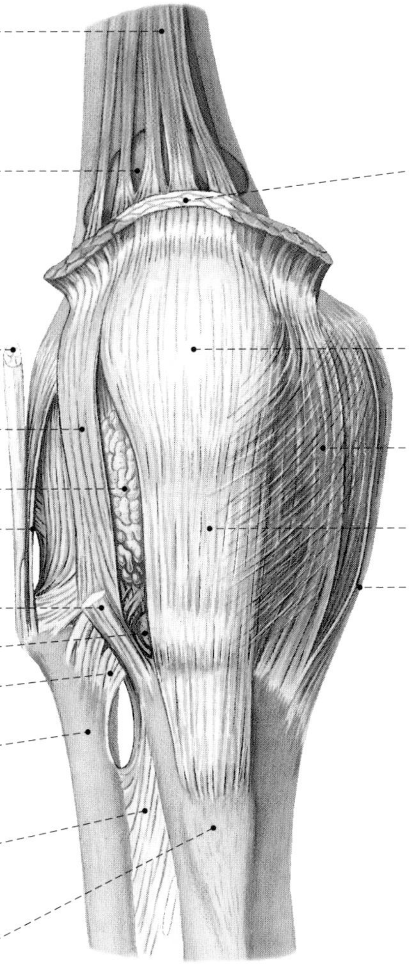
a
Articularis genus muscle
Suprapatellar bursa
Tendon
of quadriceps femoris muscle
Tendon
of biceps femoris muscle
Patella
Lateral patellar retinaculum
Medial patellar retinaculum
Infrapatellar fat pad
Fibular collateral ligament
Patellar ligament
Tibial collateral ligament
Iliotibial tract
Deep infrapatellar bursa
Anterior ligament
of fibular head
Fibula
Interosseous membrane
of leg
Tibial tuberosity

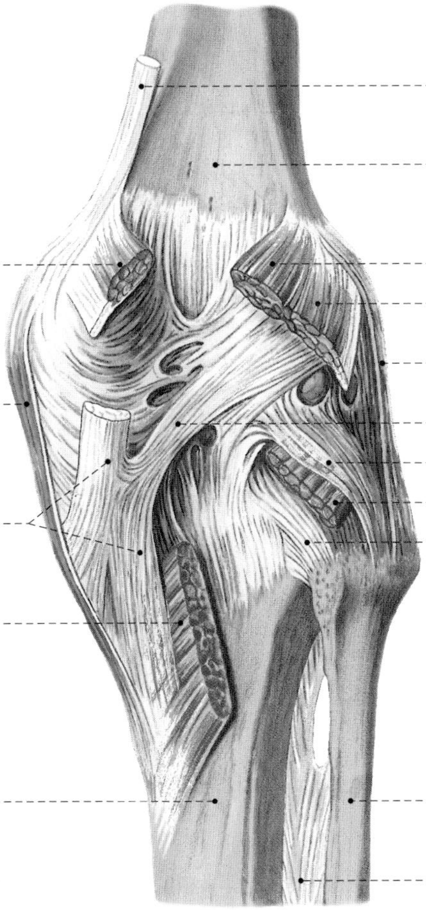
b
Tendon
of adductor magnus muscle
Popliteal surface
of femur
Medial head
of gastrocnemius muscle
Plantaris muscle
Lateral head
of gastrocnemius muscle
Fibular collateral ligament
Tibial collateral ligament
Oblique popliteal ligament
Arcuate popliteal ligament
Popliteus muscle
Tendons
of semimembranosus muscle
Posterior ligament
of fibular head
Popliteus muscle
Tibia
Fibula
Interosseous membrane
of leg

209 Right knee joint (70%)

a Ventral aspect
b Dorsal aspect

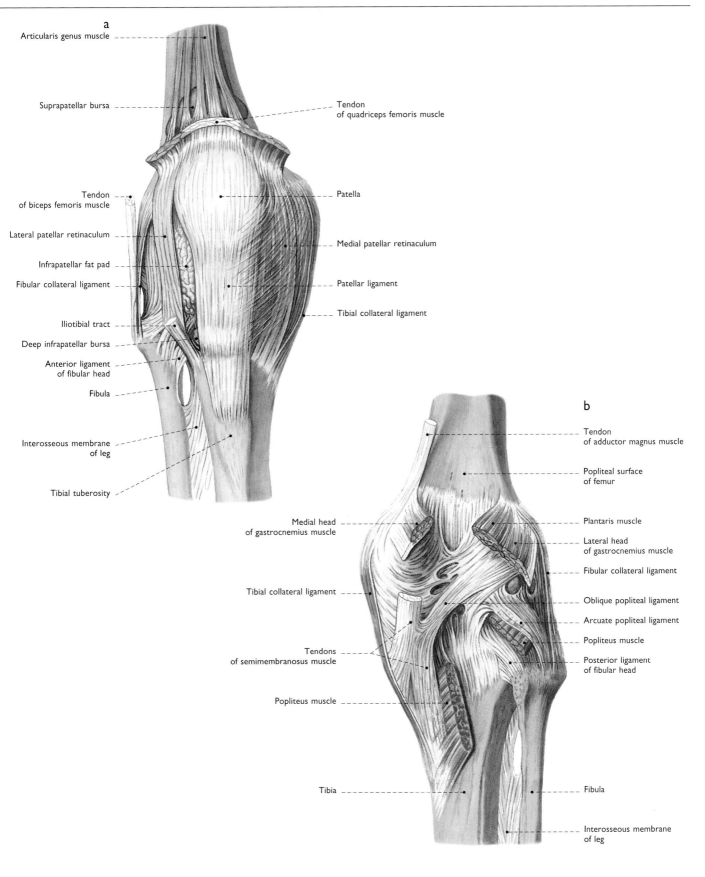

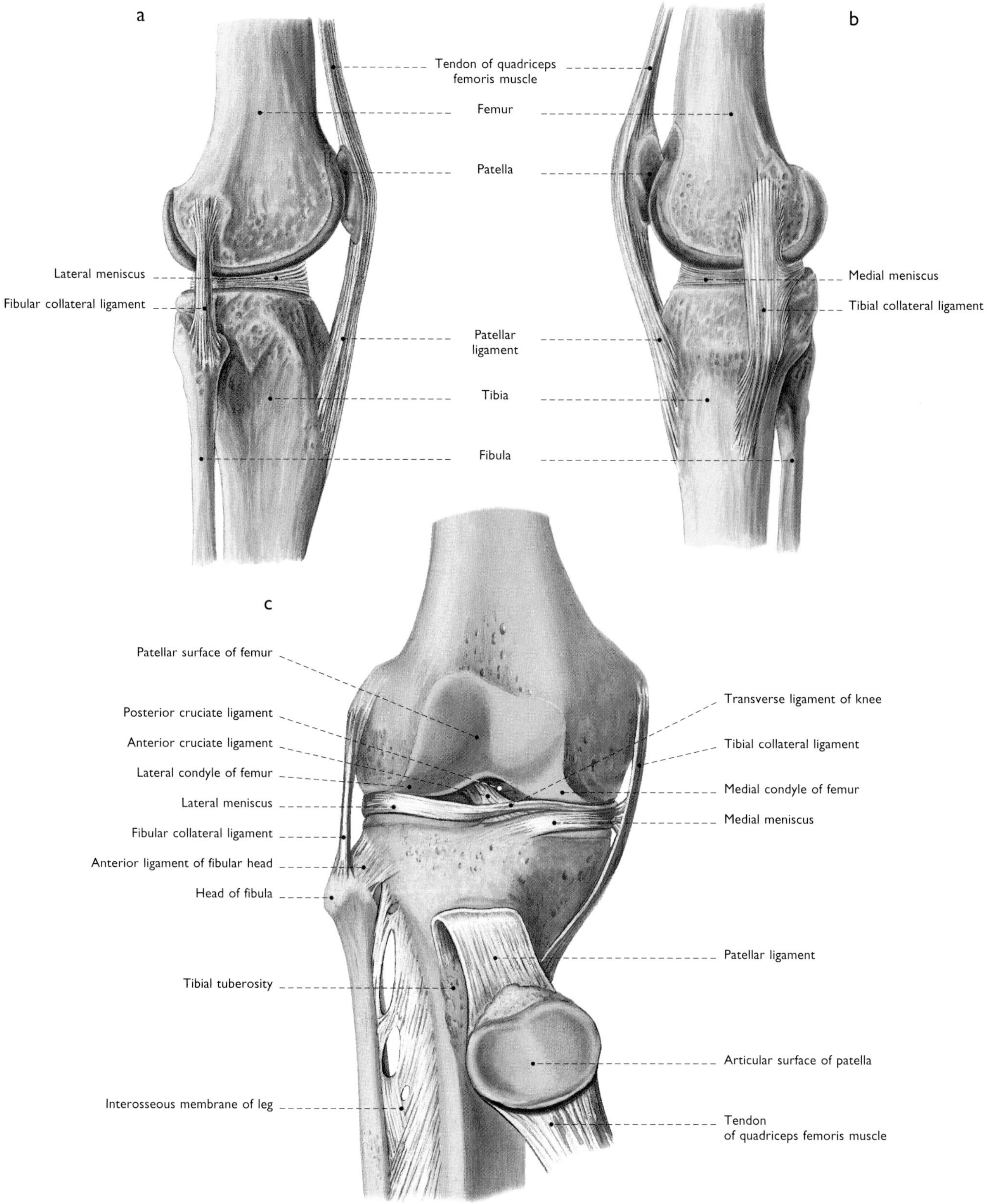
a
b
Tendon of quadriceps femoris muscle
Femur
Patella
Lateral meniscus
Fibular collateral ligament
Medial meniscus
Tibial collateral ligament
Patellar ligament
Tibia
Fibula
c
Patellar surface of femur
Posterior cruciate ligament
Anterior cruciate ligament
Lateral condyle of femur
Lateral meniscus
Fibular collateral ligament
Anterior ligament of fibular head
Head of fibula
Tibial tuberosity
Interosseous membrane of leg
Transverse ligament of knee
Tibial collateral ligament
Medial condyle of femur
Medial meniscus
Patellar ligament
Articular surface of patella
Tendon
of quadriceps femoris muscle

210 Right knee joint

The capsule was removed.
- a Lateral aspect (50%)
- b Medial aspect (50%)
- c The patella was turned downwards (70%). Ventral aspect

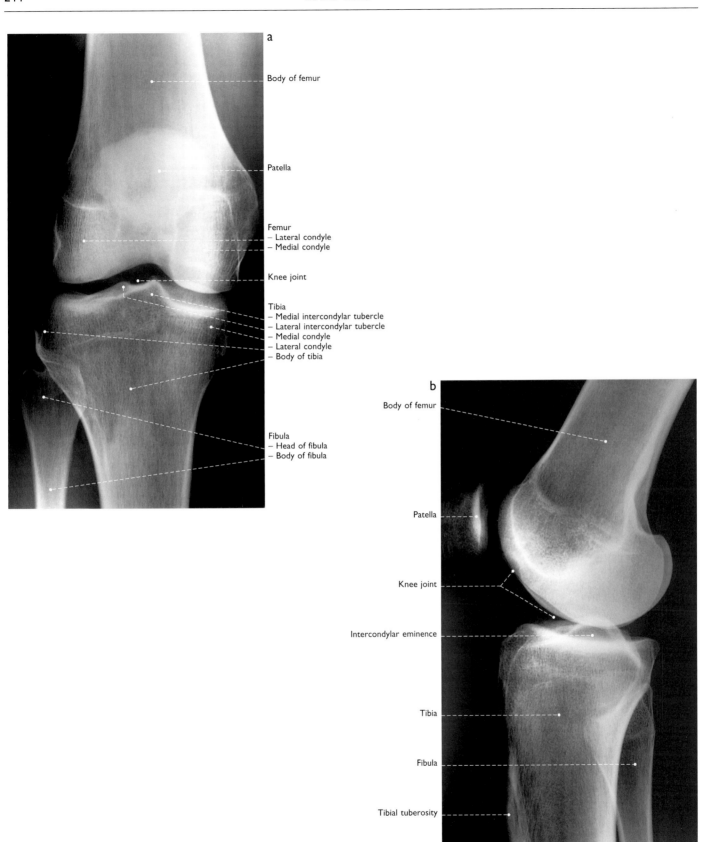

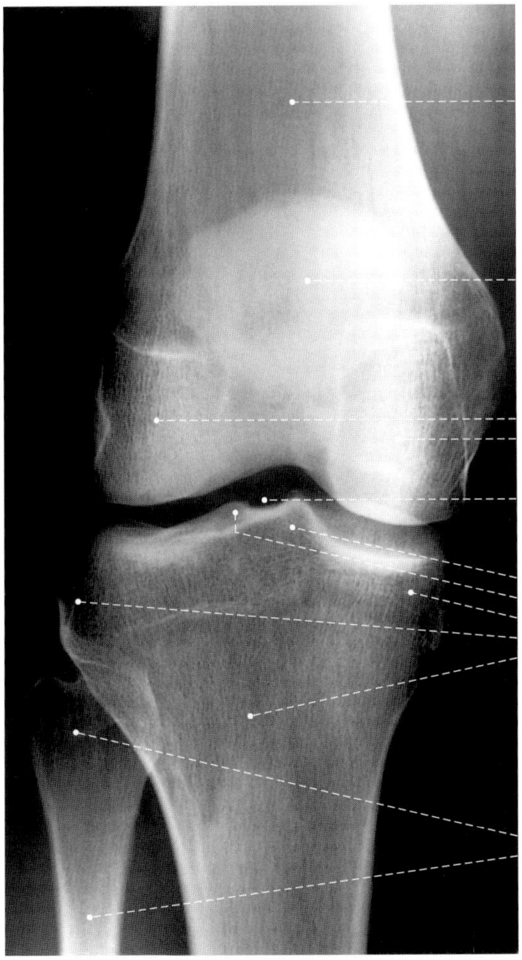
a
Body of femur
Patella
Femur
– Lateral condyle
– Medial condyle
Knee joint
Tibia
– Medial intercondylar tubercle
– Lateral intercondylar tubercle
– Medial condyle
– Lateral condyle
– Body of tibia
Fibula
– Head of fibula
– Body of fibula

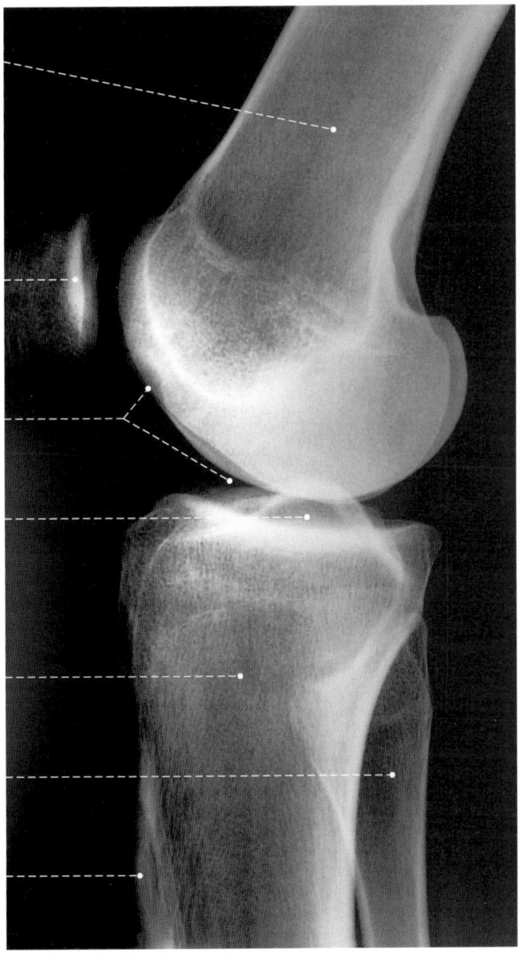
b
Body of femur
Patella
Knee joint
Intercondylar eminence
Tibia
Fibula
Tibial tuberosity

211 Right knee joint (80%)

a Anteroposterior radiograph
b Lateral radiograph

a

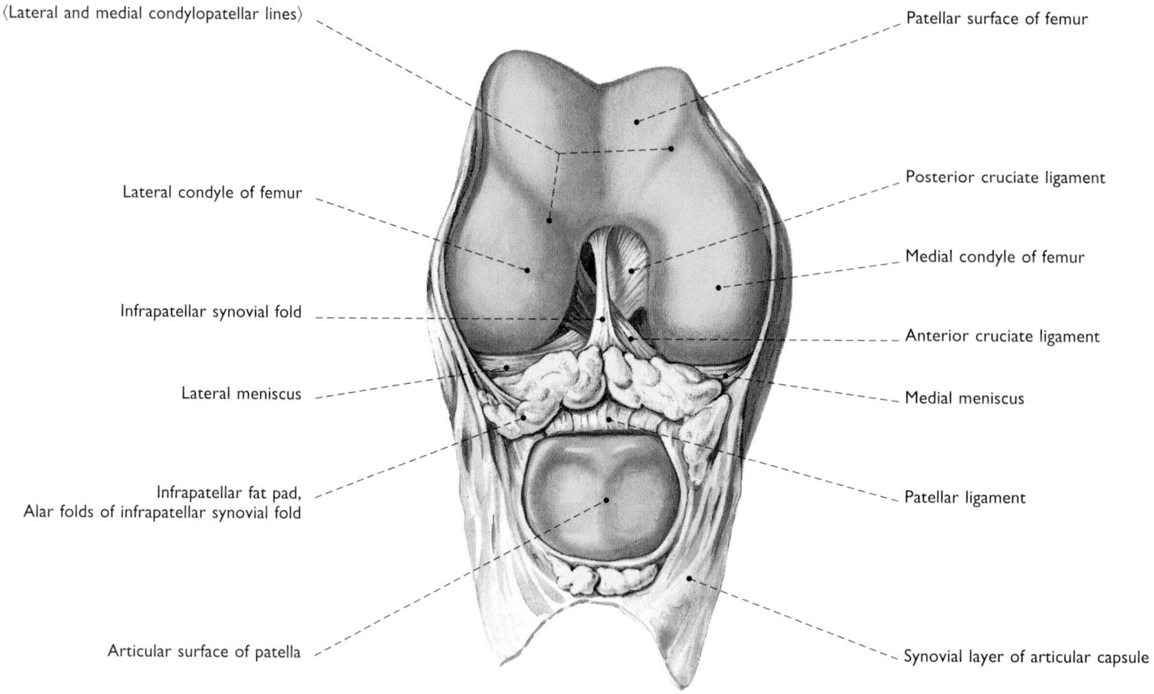
⟨Lateral and medial condylopatellar lines⟩
Patellar surface of femur
Lateral condyle of femur
Posterior cruciate ligament
Medial condyle of femur
Infrapatellar synovial fold
Anterior cruciate ligament
Lateral meniscus
Medial meniscus
Infrapatellar fat pad,
Alar folds of infrapatellar synovial fold
Patellar ligament
Articular surface of patella
Synovial layer of articular capsule

b

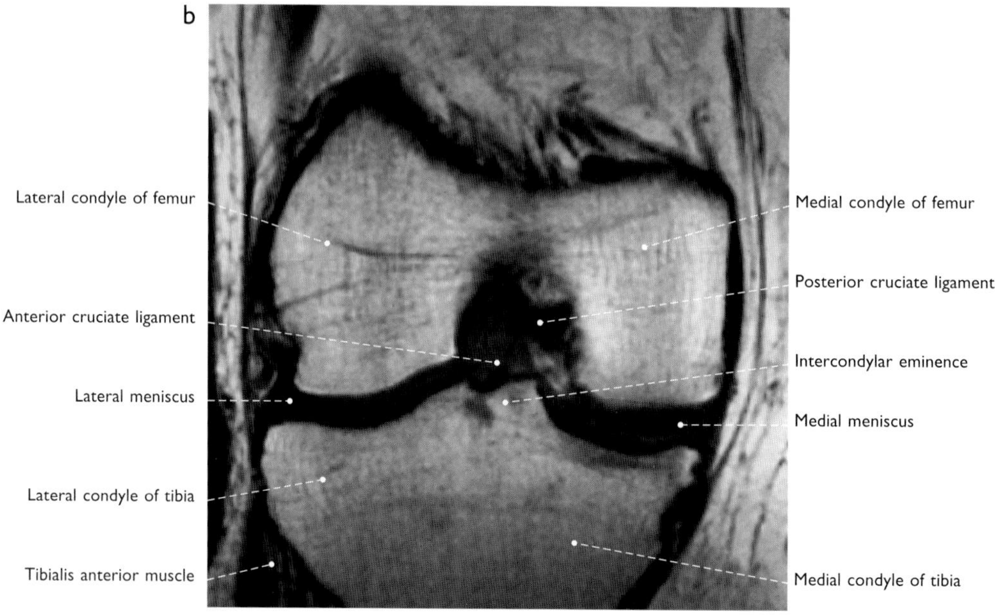
Lateral condyle of femur
Medial condyle of femur
Posterior cruciate ligament
Anterior cruciate ligament
Intercondylar eminence
Lateral meniscus
Medial meniscus
Lateral condyle of tibia
Tibialis anterior muscle
Medial condyle of tibia

212 Right knee joint

Ventral aspect

a The joint is flexed, the capsule was opened and the patella turned downwards (70%).

b Coronal magnetic resonance image (MRI, T_1-weighted) through ventral parts of the knee joint (90%)

a

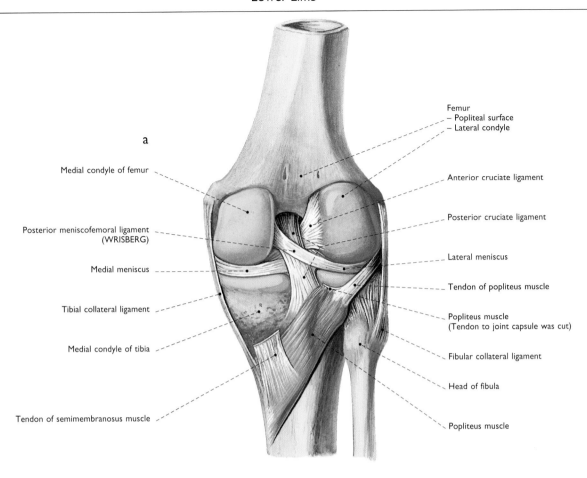

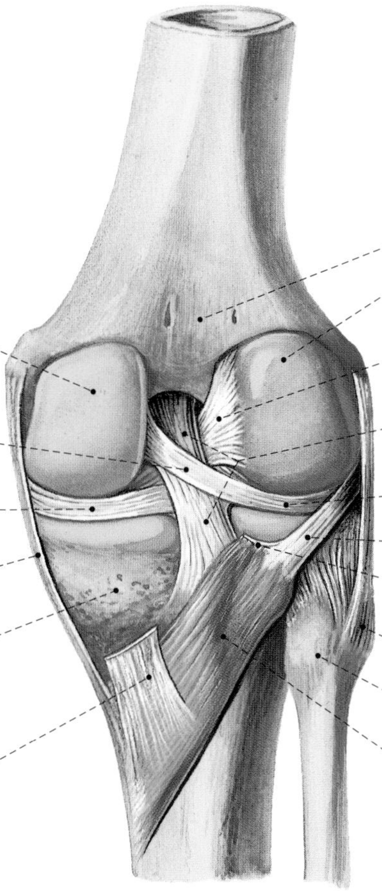
Femur
– Popliteal surface
– Lateral condyle
Medial condyle of femur
Anterior cruciate ligament
Posterior cruciate ligament
Posterior meniscofemoral ligament (WRISBERG)
Lateral meniscus
Medial meniscus
Tendon of popliteus muscle
Tibial collateral ligament
Popliteus muscle (Tendon to joint capsule was cut)
Medial condyle of tibia
Fibular collateral ligament
Head of fibula
Tendon of semimembranosus muscle
Popliteus muscle

b

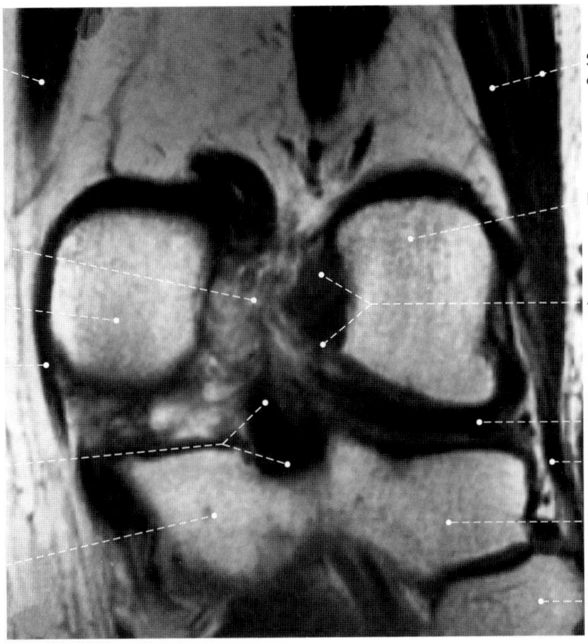
Sartorius muscle
Short and long heads of biceps femoris muscle
Lateral condyle of femur
Intercondylar fossa
Anterior cruciate ligament
Medial condyle of femur
Tibial collateral ligament
Lateral meniscus
Fibular collateral ligament
Posterior cruciate ligament
Lateral condyle of tibia
Medial condyle of tibia
Head of fibula

213 Right knee joint

Dorsal aspect

a The joint is extended, and the capsule was partially removed (70%).

b Coronal magnetic resonance image (MRI, T_1-weighted) through dorsal parts of the knee joint (90%)

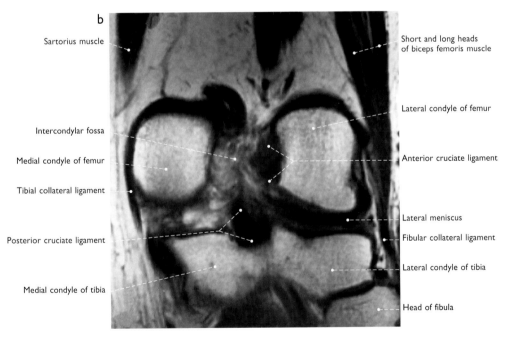

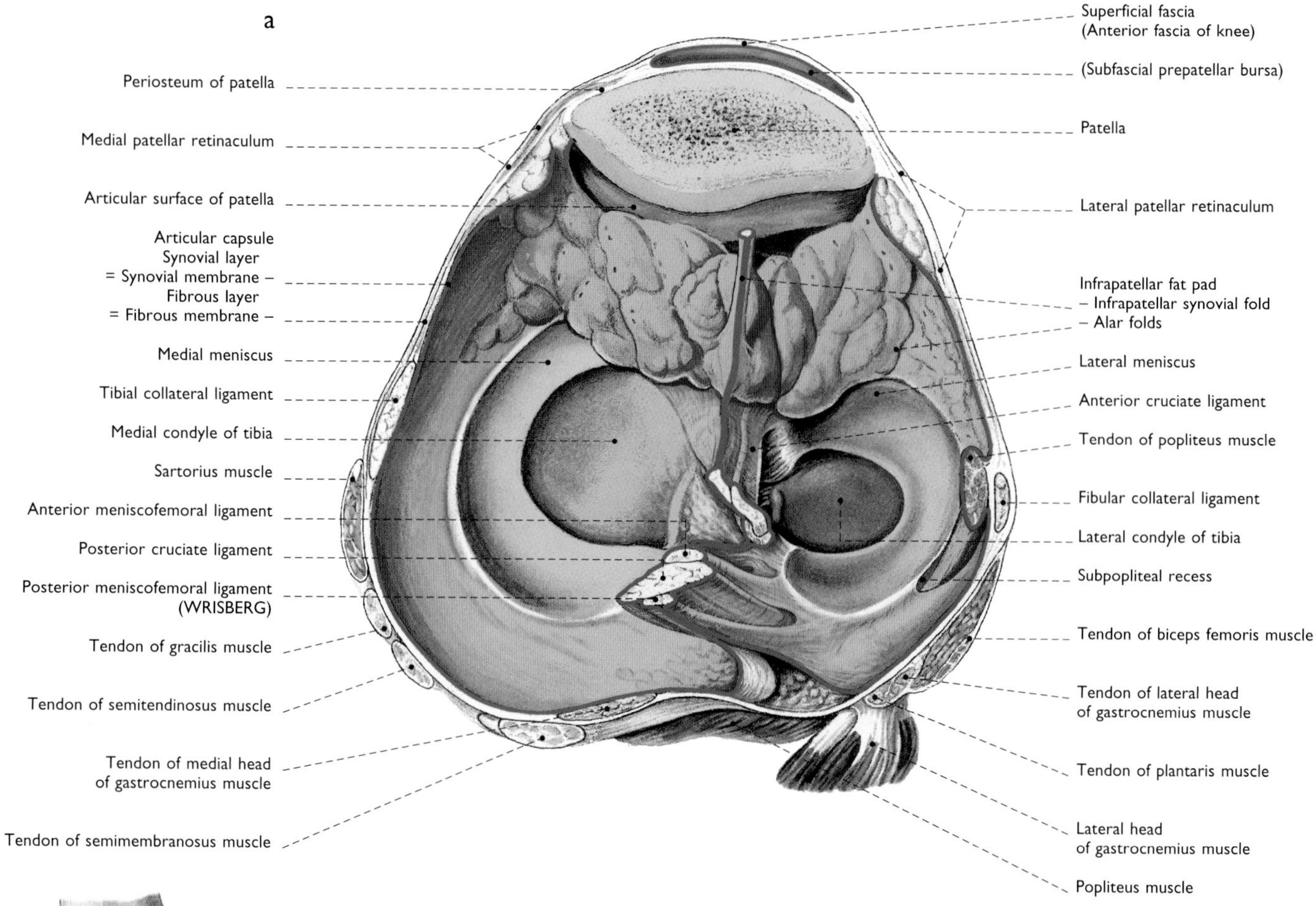
a
Superficial fascia
(Anterior fascia of knee)
(Subfascial prepatellar bursa)
Patella
Lateral patellar retinaculum
Infrapatellar fat pad
– Infrapatellar synovial fold
– Alar folds
Lateral meniscus
Anterior cruciate ligament
Tendon of popliteus muscle
Fibular collateral ligament
Lateral condyle of tibia
Subpopliteal recess
Tendon of biceps femoris muscle
Tendon of lateral head
of gastrocnemius muscle
Tendon of plantaris muscle
Lateral head
of gastrocnemius muscle
Popliteus muscle
Periosteum of patella
Medial patellar retinaculum
Articular surface of patella
Articular capsule
Synovial layer
= Synovial membrane –
Fibrous layer
= Fibrous membrane –
Medial meniscus
Tibial collateral ligament
Medial condyle of tibia
Sartorius muscle
Anterior meniscofemoral ligament
Posterior cruciate ligament
Posterior meniscofemoral ligament
(WRISBERG)
Tendon of gracilis muscle
Tendon of semitendinosus muscle
Tendon of medial head
of gastrocnemius muscle
Tendon of semimembranosus muscle

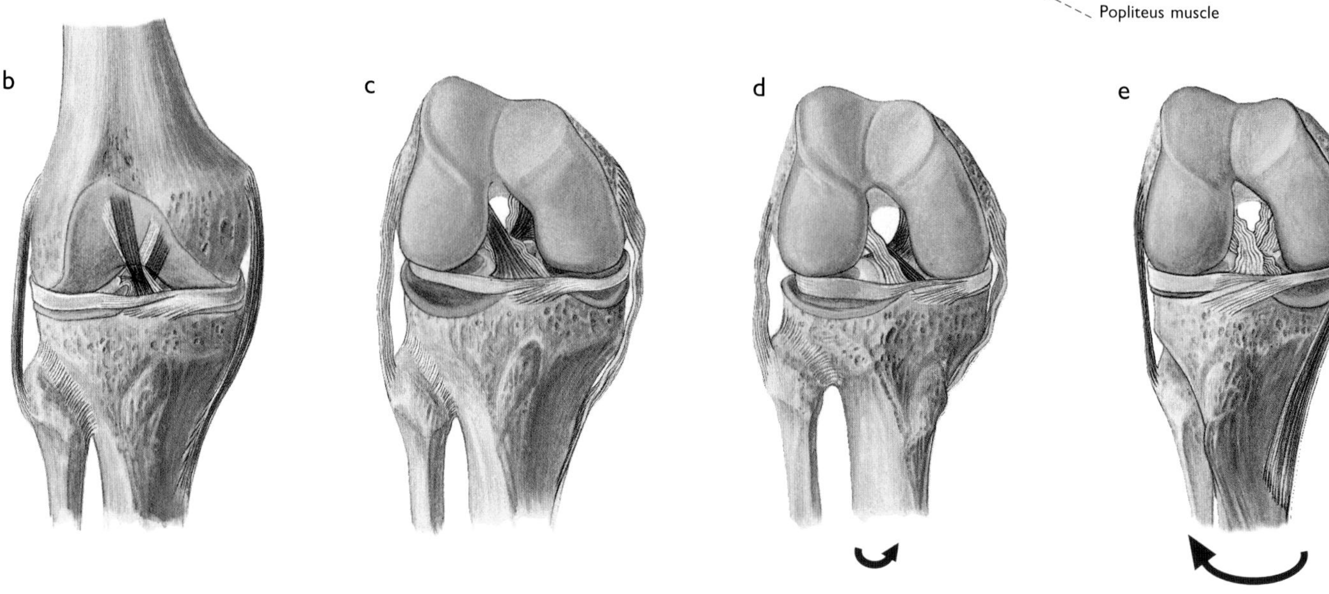
b
c
d
e

214 Right knee joint

a The joint was cut transversally through the middle of the patella.
The synovial membrane is colored greenish (100%).
Cranial aspect of the distal part

b–e State of tautening of the cruciate and collateral ligaments (50%)
(according to von LANZ and WACHSMUTH, 1972)

b knee in extension

c knee in flexion

d knee in flexion and medial rotation

e knee in flexion and lateral rotation.
The taut parts of ligaments are dark-colored. Ventral aspect

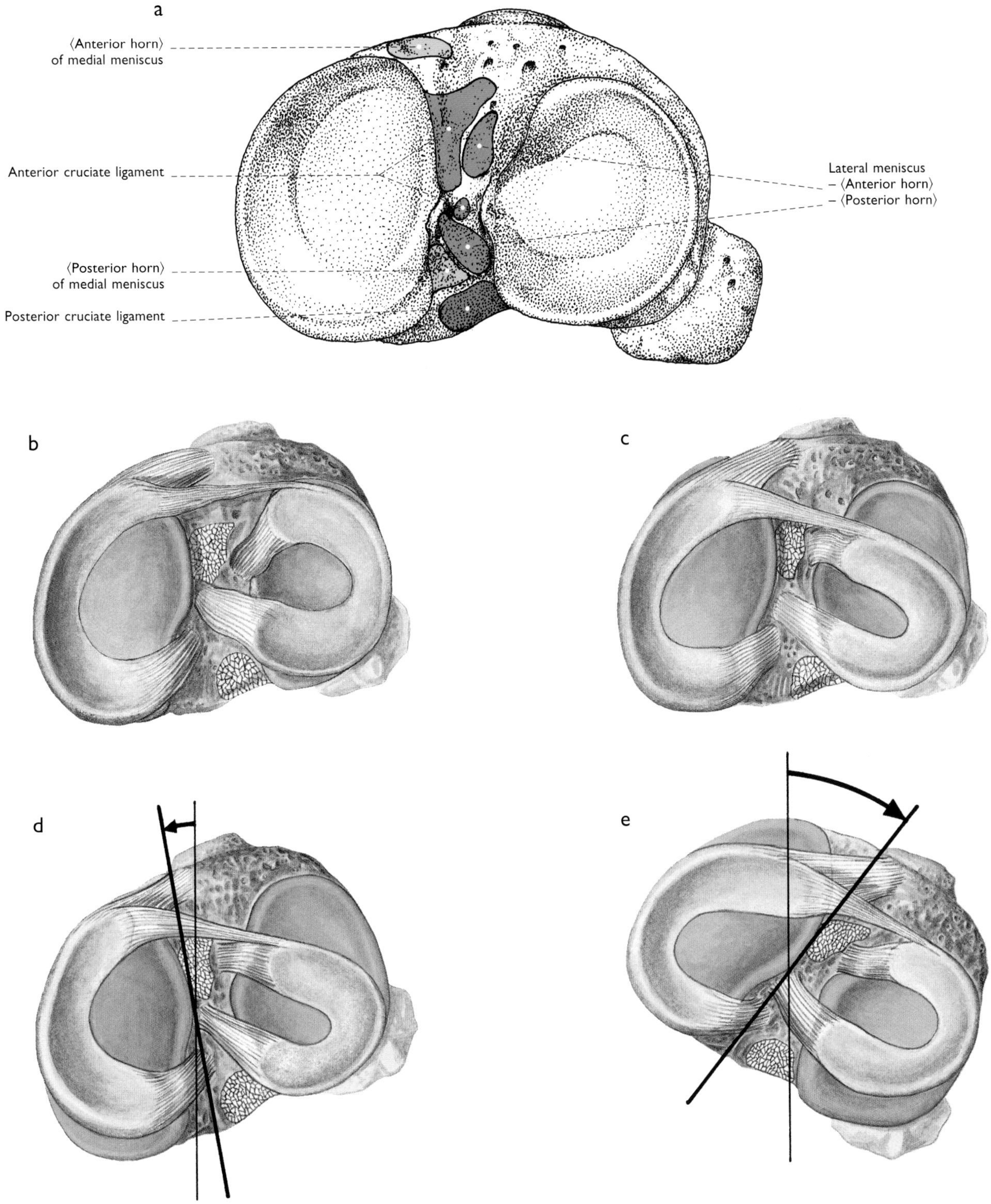
a
⟨Anterior horn⟩
of medial meniscus
Anterior cruciate ligament
⟨Posterior horn⟩
of medial meniscus
Posterior cruciate ligament
Lateral meniscus
– ⟨Anterior horn⟩
– ⟨Posterior horn⟩
b
c
d
e

215 Right knee joint

Cranial aspect

- a Insertions of the cruciate ligaments and menisci (100%), schematic representation
- b–e Position of the menisci (80%) (according to von LANZ and WACHSMUTH, 1972)
- b knee in extension
- c knee in flexion
- d knee in flexion and medial rotation
- e knee in flexion and lateral rotation

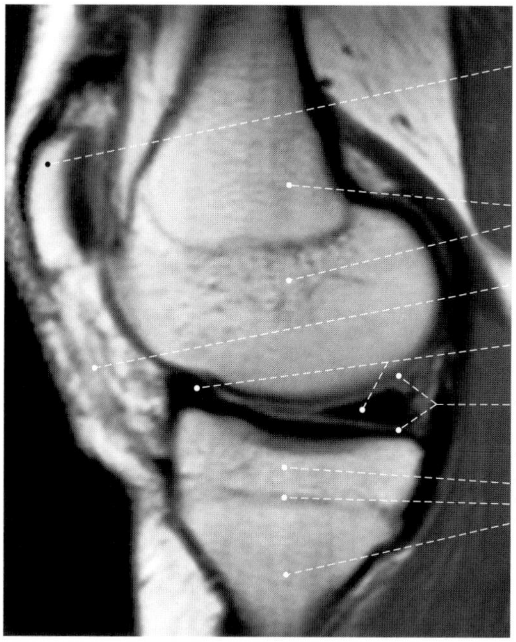
a
Patella
Femur
– Body of femur
– Medial condyle
Infrapatellar fat pad
Medial meniscus
Articular cartilage
Tibia
– Medial condyle
– Epiphysial line
– Body of tibia

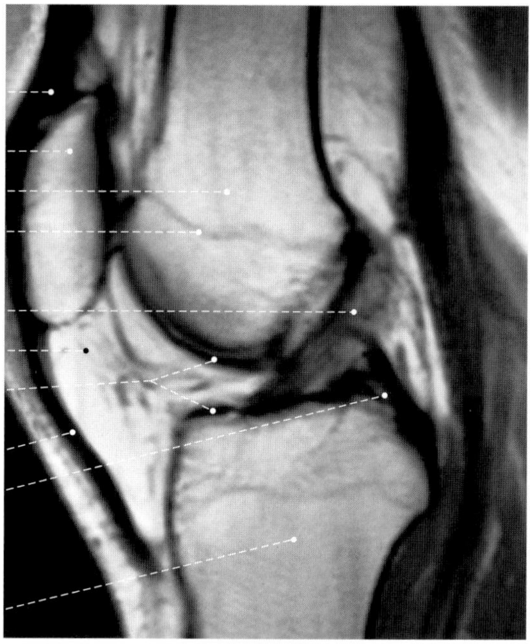
b
Quadriceps femoris muscle
Patella
Femur
Epiphysial line
Anterior cruciate ligament
Infrapatellar fat pad
Articular cartilage
Patellar ligament
Posterior cruciate ligament
Body of tibia

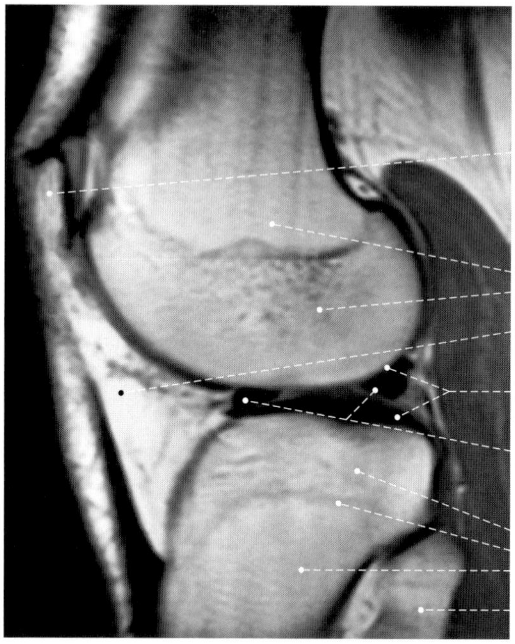
c
Patella
Femur
– Body of femur
– Lateral condyle
Infrapatellar fat pad
Articular cartilage
Lateral meniscus
Tibia
– Lateral condyle
– Epiphysial line
– Body of tibia
Head of fibula

216 Right knee joint (80%)

Sagittal magnetic resonance images (MRI, ^{1}H-weighted) through the

a medial part of the knee joint
b middle part of the knee joint
c lateral part of the knee joint.

Bones and fat can be well recognized.

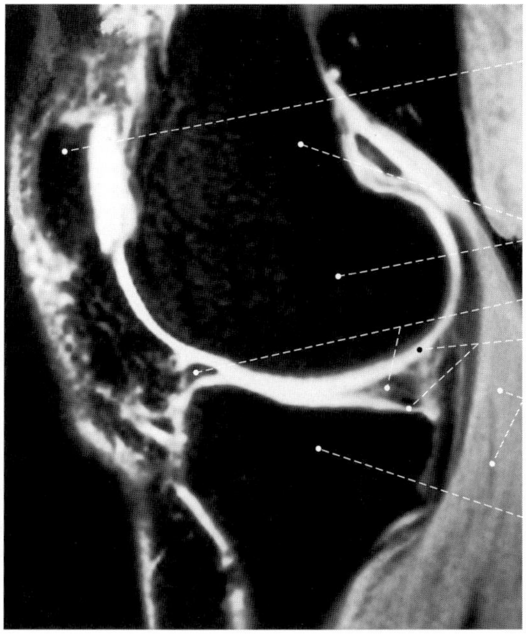
a
Patella
Femur
– Body of femur
– Medial condyle
Medial meniscus
Articular cartilage
Triceps surae muscle,
Medial head
of gastrocnemius muscle
Medial condyle of tibia

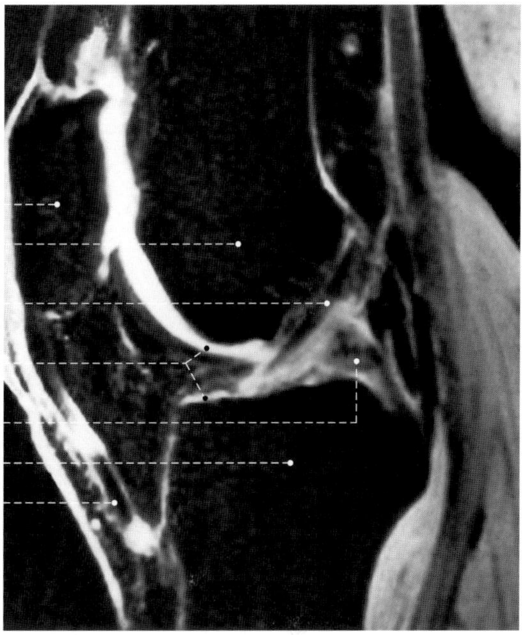
b
Patella
Femur
Anterior cruciate ligament
Articular cartilage
Posterior cruciate ligament
Tibia
Patellar ligament

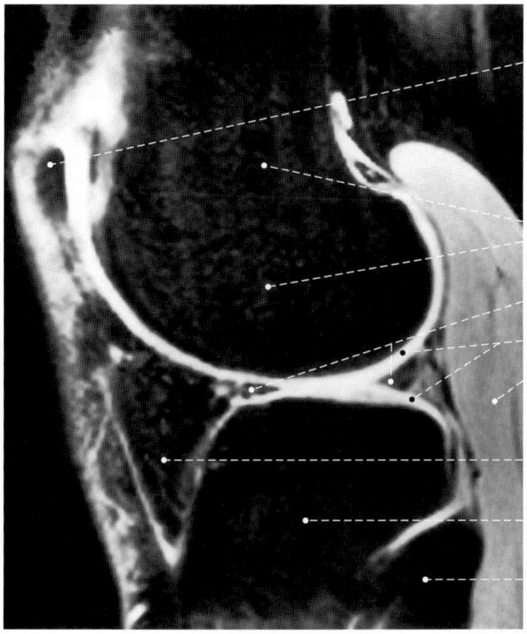
c
Patella
Femur
– Body of femur
– Lateral condyle
Lateral meniscus
Articular cartilage
Triceps surae muscle,
Lateral head
of gastrocnemius muscle
Infrapatellar fat pad
Lateral condyle of tibia
Head of fibula

217 Right knee joint (80%)

Sagittal magnetic resonance images (MRI, T_1-weighted, fat-suppressed) through the

a medial part of the knee joint
b middle part of the knee joint
c lateral part of the knee joint.

Cartilaginous and muscular structures can be well recognized.

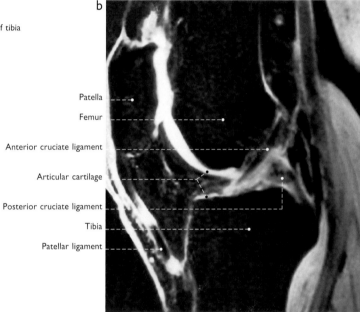

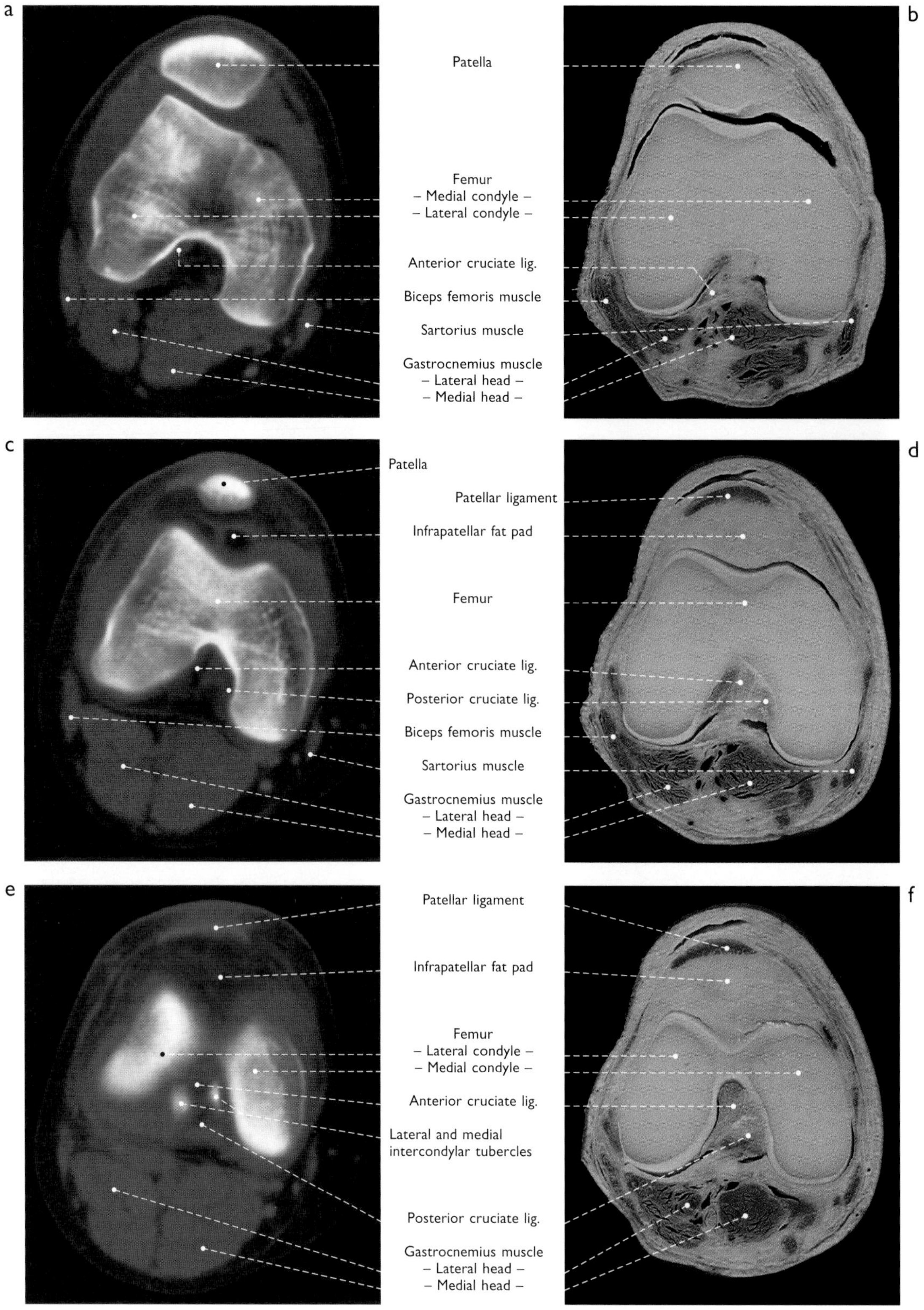
a
b
Patella
Femur
– Medial condyle –
– Lateral condyle –
Anterior cruciate lig.
Biceps femoris muscle
Sartorius muscle
Gastrocnemius muscle
– Lateral head –
– Medial head –
c
d
Patella
Patellar ligament
Infrapatellar fat pad
Femur
Anterior cruciate lig.
Posterior cruciate lig.
Biceps femoris muscle
Sartorius muscle
Gastrocnemius muscle
– Lateral head –
– Medial head –
e
f
Patellar ligament
Infrapatellar fat pad
Femur
– Lateral condyle –
– Medial condyle –
Anterior cruciate lig.
Lateral and medial
intercondylar tubercles
Posterior cruciate lig.
Gastrocnemius muscle
– Lateral head –
– Medial head –

218 Right knee joint (65%)

Inferior aspect

a, c, e Axial (transverse) magnetic resonance images (MRI, T_1-weighted)

b, d, f Transverse anatomical sections

through

a, b cranial parts

c, d middle parts

e, f caudal parts

of the knee joint

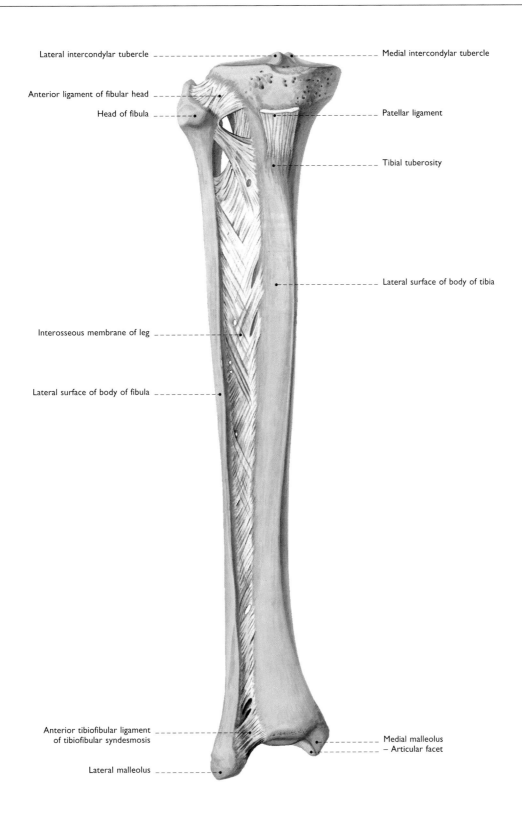

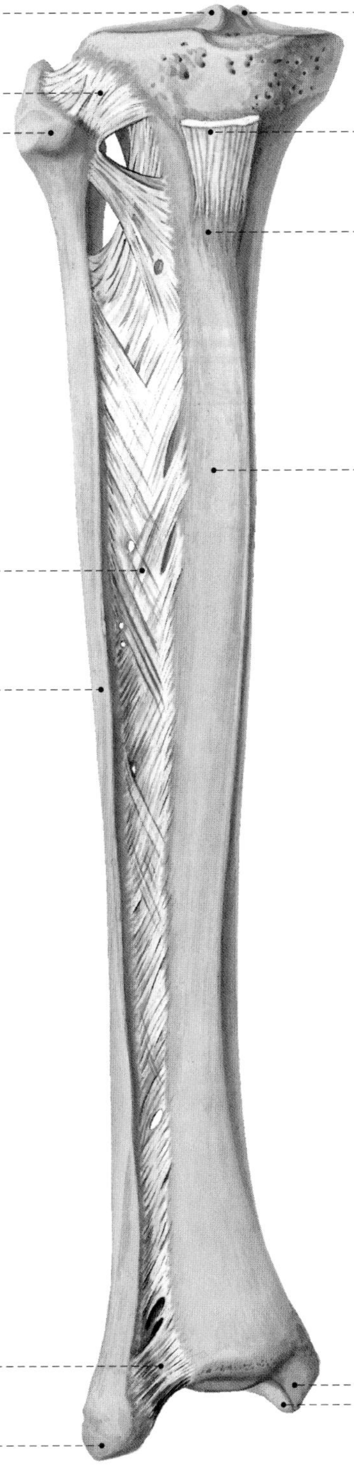
Lateral intercondylar tubercle
Medial intercondylar tubercle
Anterior ligament of fibular head
Head of fibula
Patellar ligament
Tibial tuberosity
Lateral surface of body of tibia
Interosseous membrane of leg
Lateral surface of body of fibula
Anterior tibiofibular ligament of tibiofibular syndesmosis
Medial malleolus
– Articular facet
Lateral malleolus

219 Tibiofibular joints and syndesmoses of the right leg (50%)

Ventral aspect

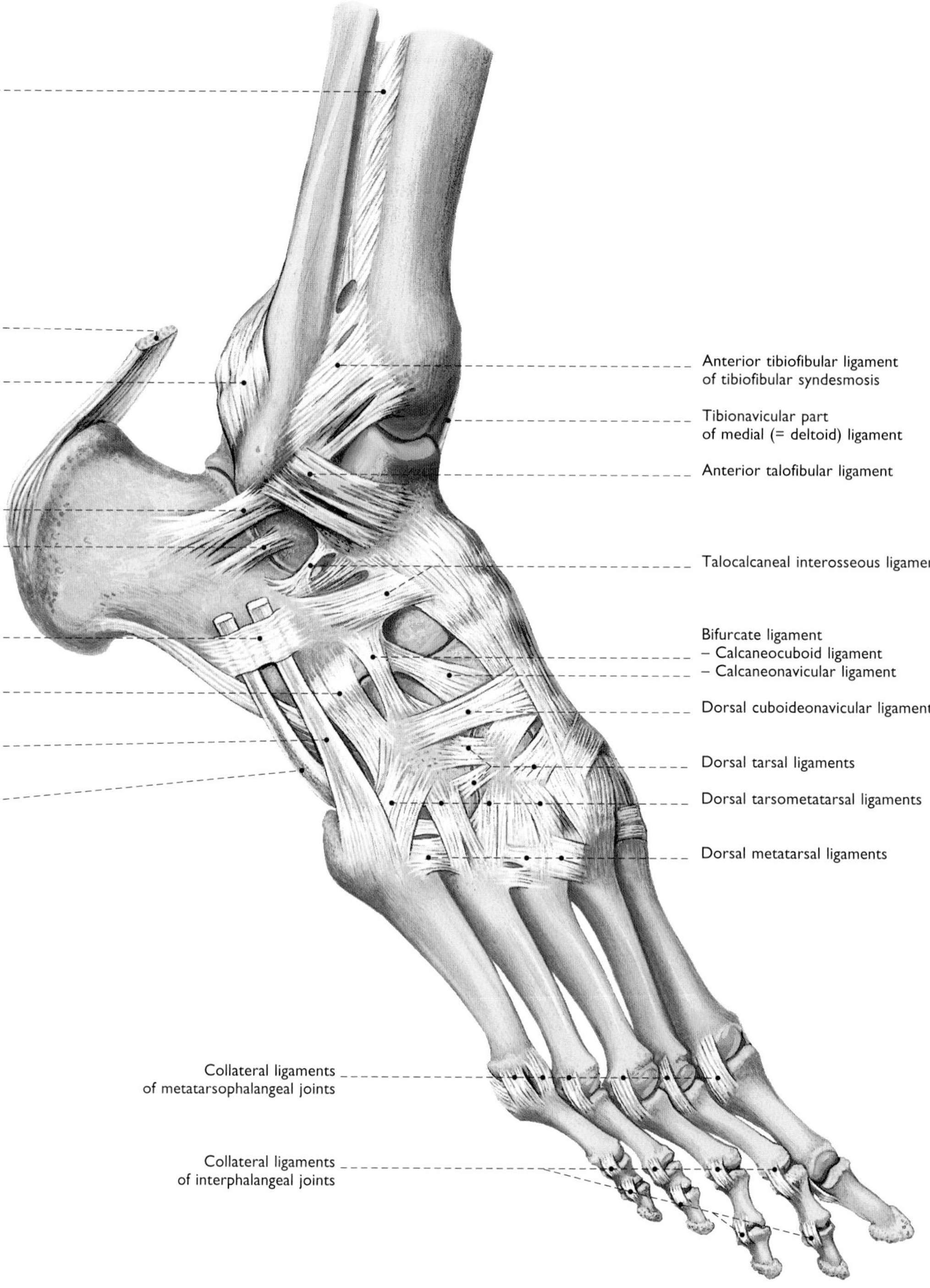
Interosseous membrane of leg
Calcaneal tendon (= Achilles tendon)
Posterior tibiofibular ligament
Calcaneofibular ligament
Lateral talocalcaneal ligament
Inferior fibular (= peroneal) retinaculum
Dorsal calcaneocuboid ligament
Tendon of fibularis brevis muscle
Tendon of fibularis longus muscle
Anterior tibiofibular ligament of tibiofibular syndesmosis
Tibionavicular part of medial (= deltoid) ligament
Anterior talofibular ligament
Talocalcaneal interosseous ligament
Bifurcate ligament
– Calcaneocuboid ligament
– Calcaneonavicular ligament
Dorsal cuboideonavicular ligament
Dorsal tarsal ligaments
Dorsal tarsometatarsal ligaments
Dorsal metatarsal ligaments
Collateral ligaments of metatarsophalangeal joints
Collateral ligaments of interphalangeal joints

220 Joints and ligaments of the right foot (70%)

Lateral aspect

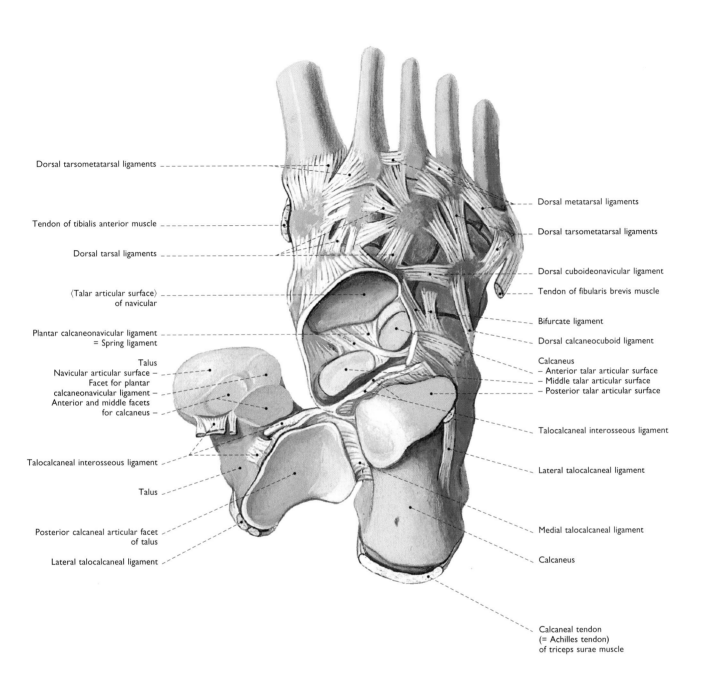

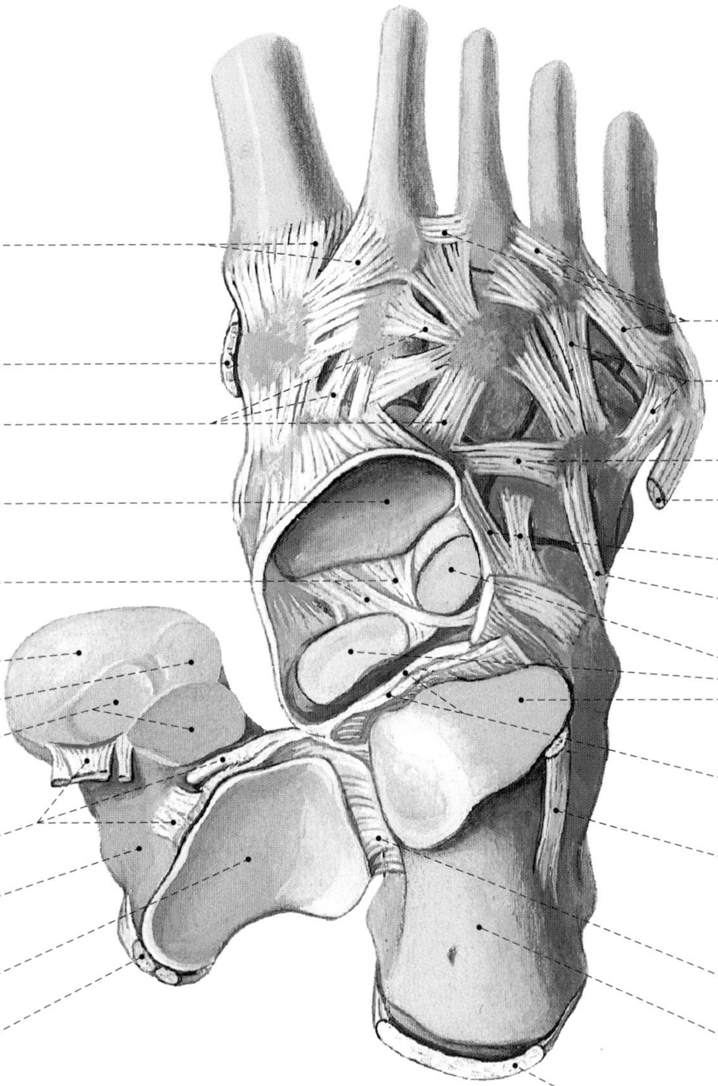
Dorsal tarsometatarsal ligaments
Tendon of tibialis anterior muscle
Dorsal tarsal ligaments
⟨Talar articular surface⟩ of navicular
Plantar calcaneonavicular ligament = Spring ligament
Talus
Navicular articular surface –
Facet for plantar calcaneonavicular ligament –
Anterior and middle facets for calcaneus –
Talocalcaneal interosseous ligament
Talus
Posterior calcaneal articular facet of talus
Lateral talocalcaneal ligament
Dorsal metatarsal ligaments
Dorsal tarsometatarsal ligaments
Dorsal cuboideonavicular ligament
Tendon of fibularis brevis muscle
Bifurcate ligament
Dorsal calcaneocuboid ligament
Calcaneus
– Anterior talar articular surface
– Middle talar articular surface
– Posterior talar articular surface
Talocalcaneal interosseous ligament
Lateral talocalcaneal ligament
Medial talocalcaneal ligament
Calcaneus
Calcaneal tendon (= Achilles tendon) of triceps surae muscle

221 Subtalar (= talocalcaneal), talocalcaneonavicular, and tarsometatarsal joints of the right foot (90%)

The talus was turned medially. Dorsal aspect

a

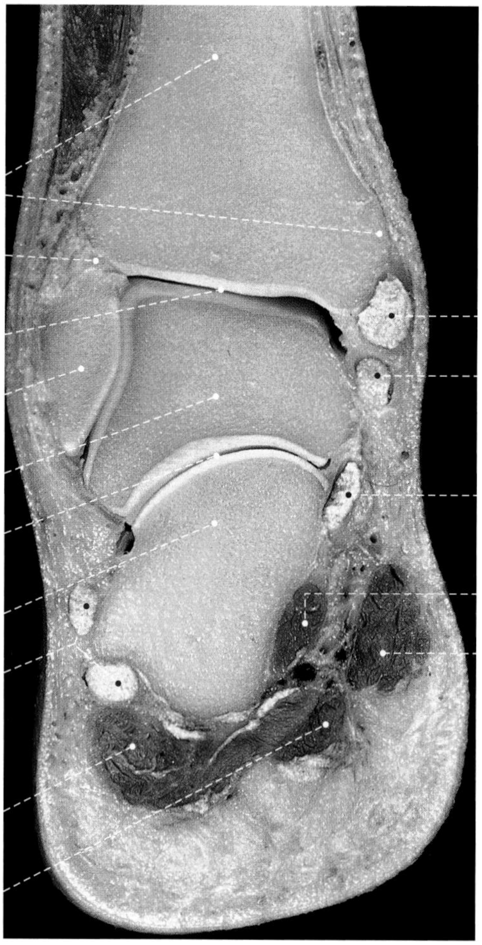
Tibia
Body of tibia –
Medial malleolus –
Tibiofibular syndesmosis
Ankle joint
⟨= Talocrural joint⟩
Lateral malleolus
of fibula
Talus
Subtalar joint
= Talocalcaneal joint
Calcaneus
Tendons
of fibularis brevis and
fibularis longus muscles
Abductor digiti minimi
muscle
Flexor digitorum brevis
muscle
Tendon
of tibialis posterior muscle
Tendon
of flexor digitorum longus muscle
Tendon
of flexor hallucis longus muscle
Quadratus plantae muscle
= Flexor accessorius muscle
Abductor hallucis muscle

b

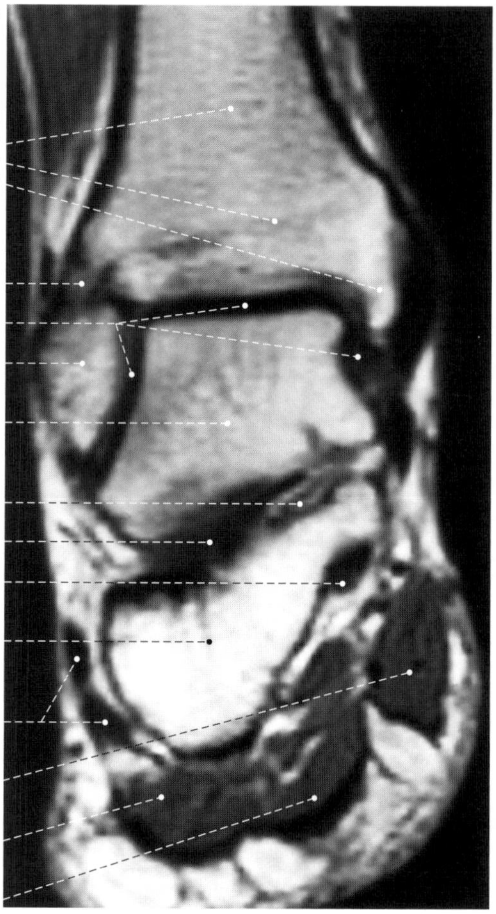
Tibia
Body of tibia –
Epiphysial line –
Medial malleolus –
Tibiofibular syndesmosis
Ankle joint ⟨= Talocrural joint⟩
Lateral malleolus of fibula
Talus
Talocalcaneal interosseous ligament
Subtalar joint = Talocalcaneal joint
Tendon
of flexor hallucis longus muscle
Calcaneus
Tendons of fibularis brevis and
fibularis longus muscles
Abductor hallucis muscle
Abductor digiti minimi muscle
Flexor digitorum brevis muscle

222 Bones, joints, and ligaments of the right foot (80%)

Coronal sections, distal aspect

a Anatomical section

b Magnetic resonance image (MRI, T_1-weighted)

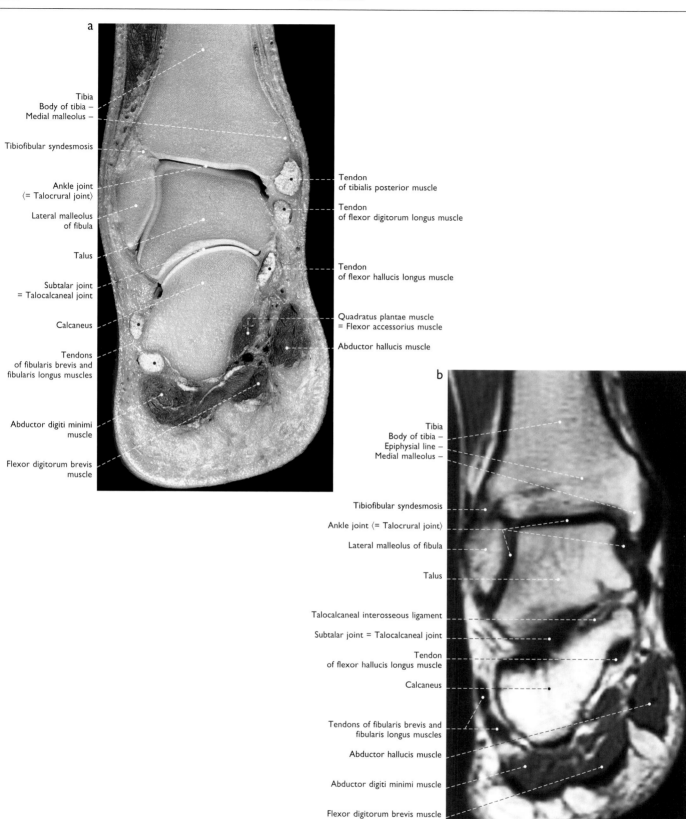

a

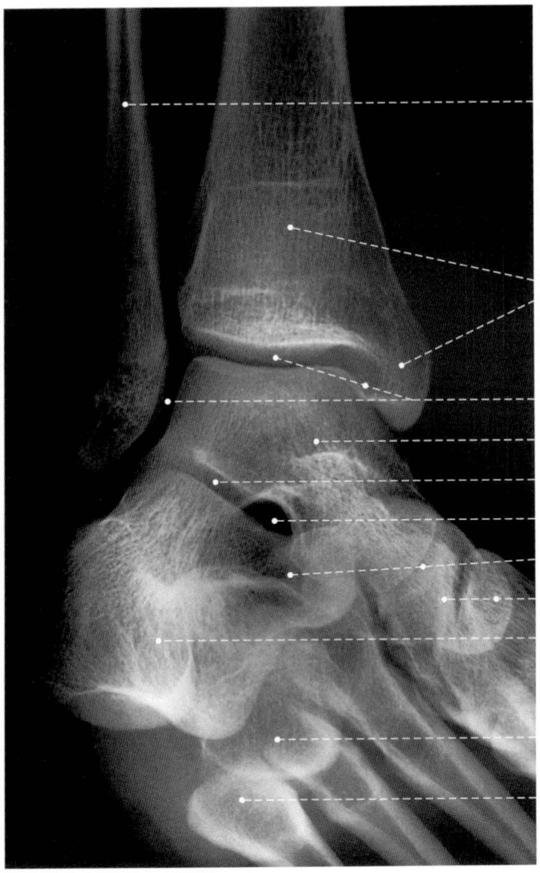
Body of fibula
Tibia
– Body of tibia
– Medial malleolus
Ankle joint ⟨= Talocrural joint⟩
Talus
Subtalar joint = Talocalcaneal joint
Tarsal sinus
Talocalcaneonavicular joint
Navicular
Calcaneus
Cuboid
Base
of 5th metatarsal bone

b

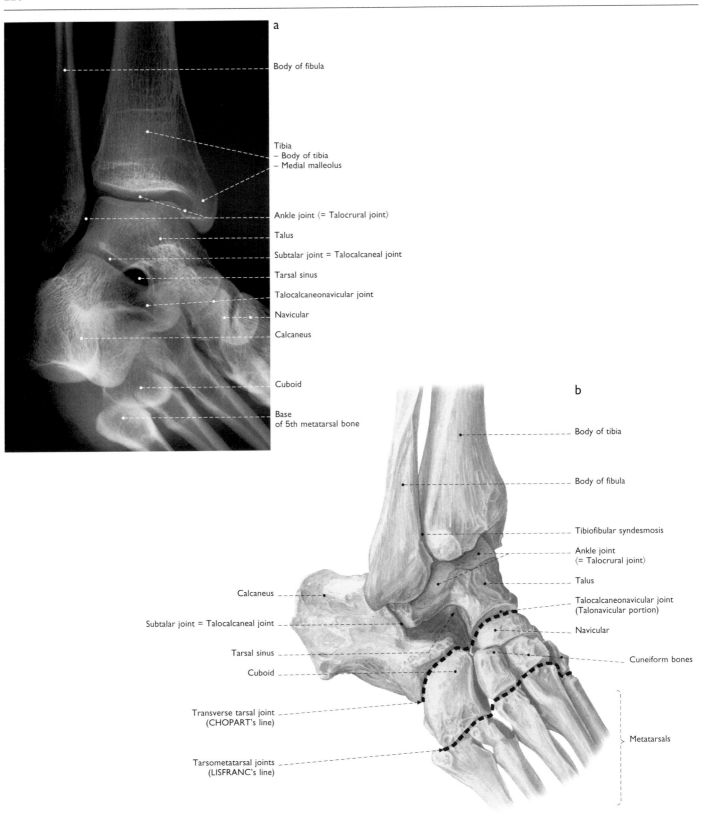

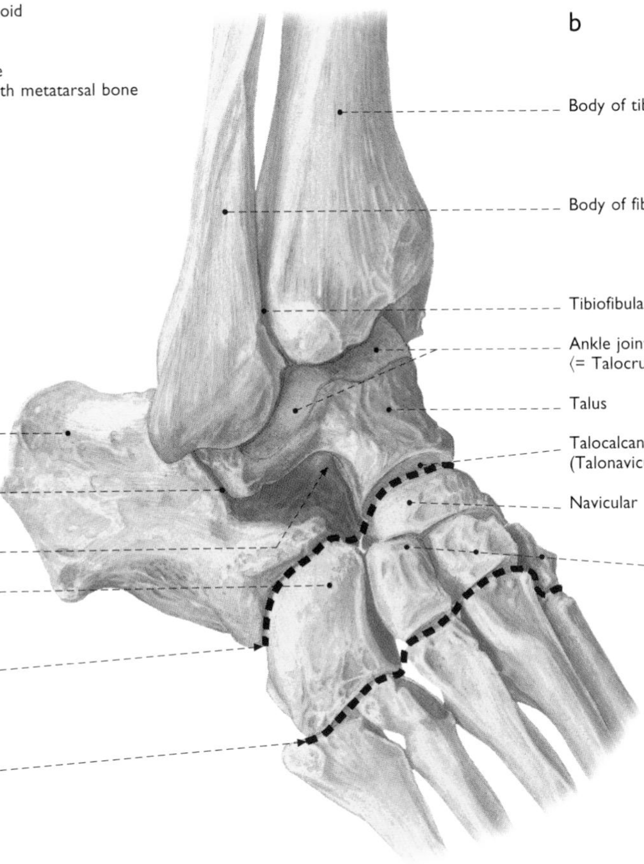
Body of tibia
Body of fibula
Tibiofibular syndesmosis
Ankle joint
⟨= Talocrural joint⟩
Talus
Talocalcaneonavicular joint
(Talonavicular portion)
Navicular
Cuneiform bones
Metatarsals
Calcaneus
Subtalar joint = Talocalcaneal joint
Tarsal sinus
Cuboid
Transverse tarsal joint
(CHOPART's line)
Tarsometatarsal joints
(LISFRANC's line)

223 Bones and joints of the right foot (75%)

Oblique laterodistal view

a Radiograph showing the ankle (= talocrural), subtalar (= talocalcaneal), and talocalcaneonavicular joints as well as the tarsal sinus

b Corresponding anatomical representation

a

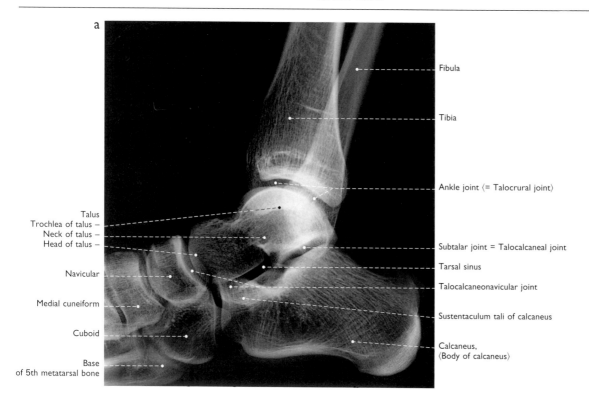

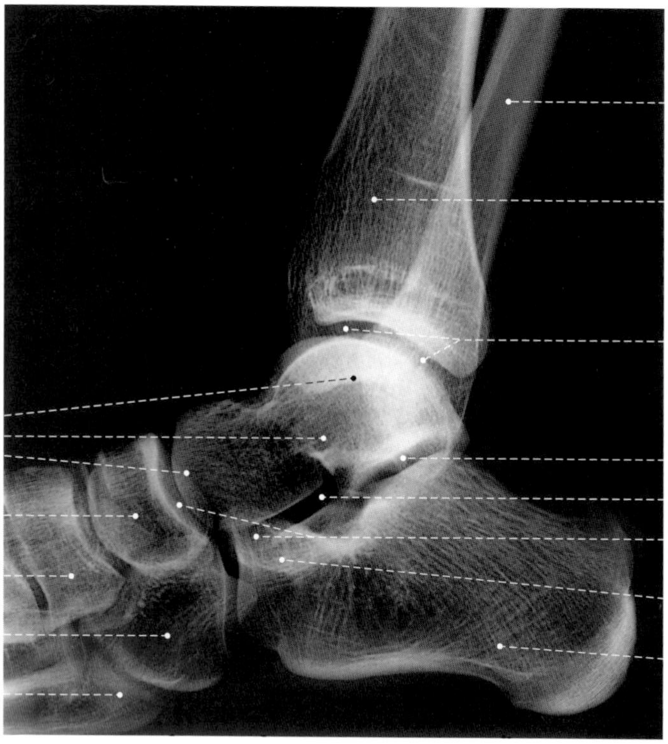
Fibula
Tibia
Ankle joint ⟨= Talocrural joint⟩
Talus
Trochlea of talus –
Neck of talus –
Head of talus –
Subtalar joint = Talocalcaneal joint
Tarsal sinus
Navicular
Talocalcaneonavicular joint
Medial cuneiform
Sustentaculum tali of calcaneus
Cuboid
Calcaneus,
⟨Body of calcaneus⟩
Base
of 5th metatarsal bone

b

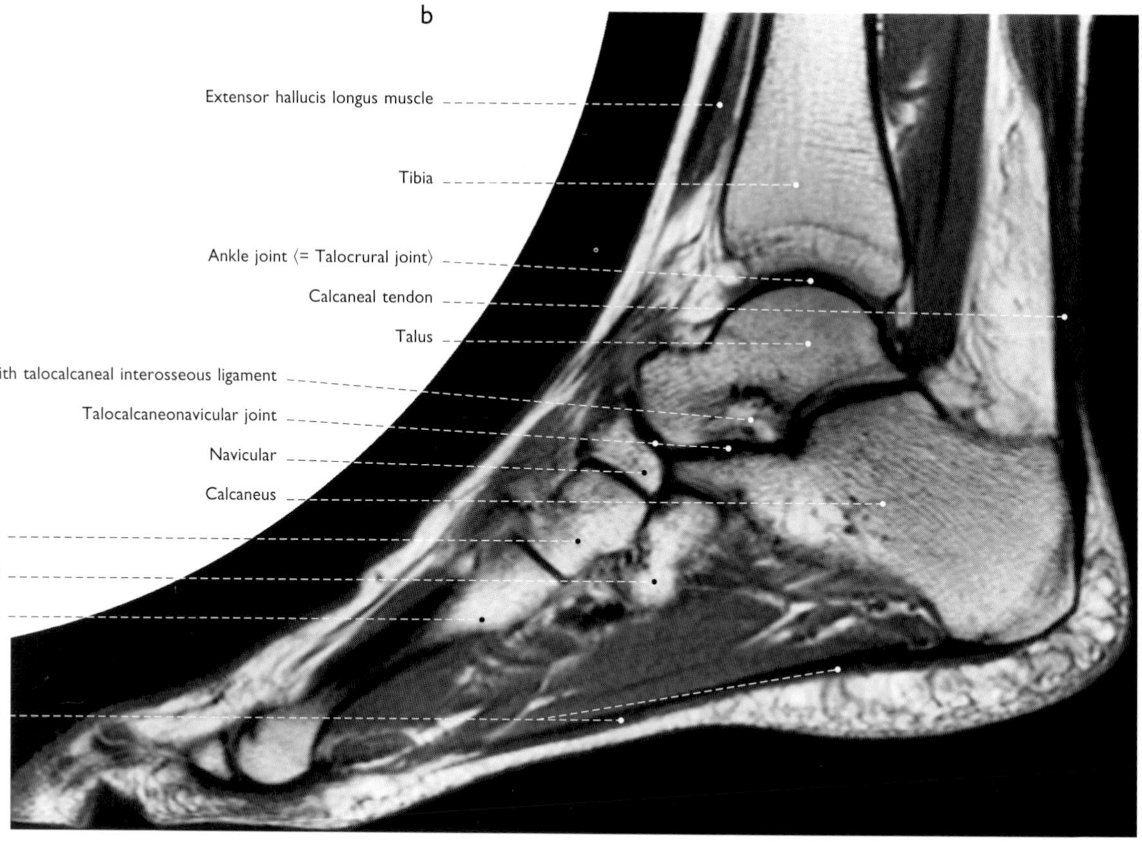
Extensor hallucis longus muscle
Tibia
Ankle joint ⟨= Talocrural joint⟩
Calcaneal tendon
Talus
Tarsal sinus with talocalcaneal interosseous ligament
Talocalcaneonavicular joint
Navicular
Calcaneus
Intermediate (= middle) cuneiform
Cuboid
2nd metatarsal bone
Plantar aponeurosis

224 Bones and joints of the right foot (70%)

a Mediolateral radiograph

b Sagittal magnetic resonance image (MRI, T_1-weighted) through the medial part of the bones of the right foot, medial aspect

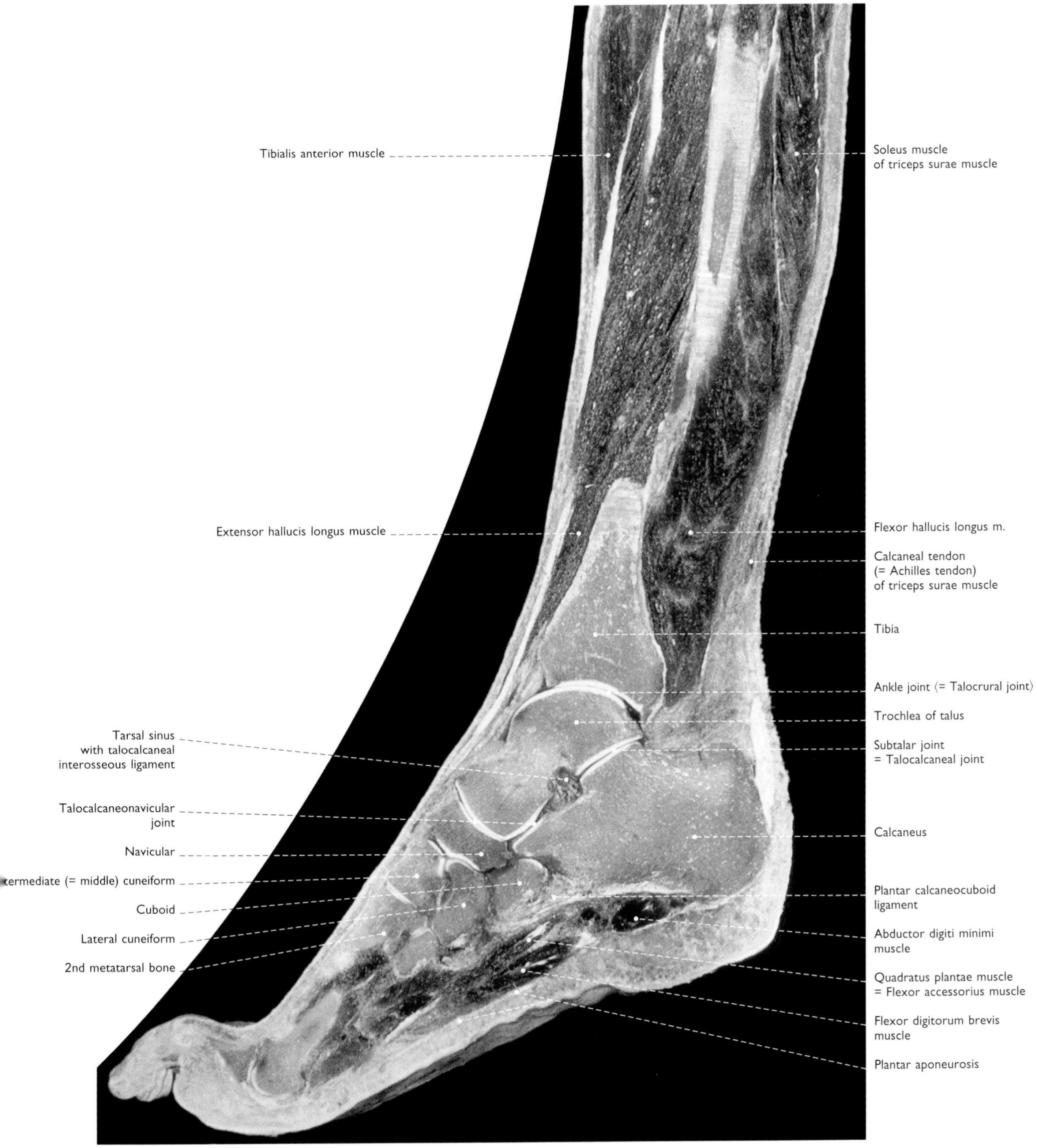
Tibialis anterior muscle
Soleus muscle of triceps surae muscle
Extensor hallucis longus muscle
Flexor hallucis longus m.
Calcaneal tendon (= Achilles tendon) of triceps surae muscle
Tibia
Ankle joint (= Talocrural joint)
Trochlea of talus
Tarsal sinus with talocalcaneal interosseous ligament
Subtalar joint = Talocalcaneal joint
Talocalcaneonavicular joint
Calcaneus
Navicular
termediate (= middle) cuneiform
Plantar calcaneocuboid ligament
Cuboid
Lateral cuneiform
Abductor digiti minimi muscle
2nd metatarsal bone
Quadratus plantae muscle = Flexor accessorius muscle
Flexor digitorum brevis muscle
Plantar aponeurosis

225 Bones and joints of the right foot (60%)

Sagittal anatomical section through the medial part of the bones of the right foot, medial aspect

a

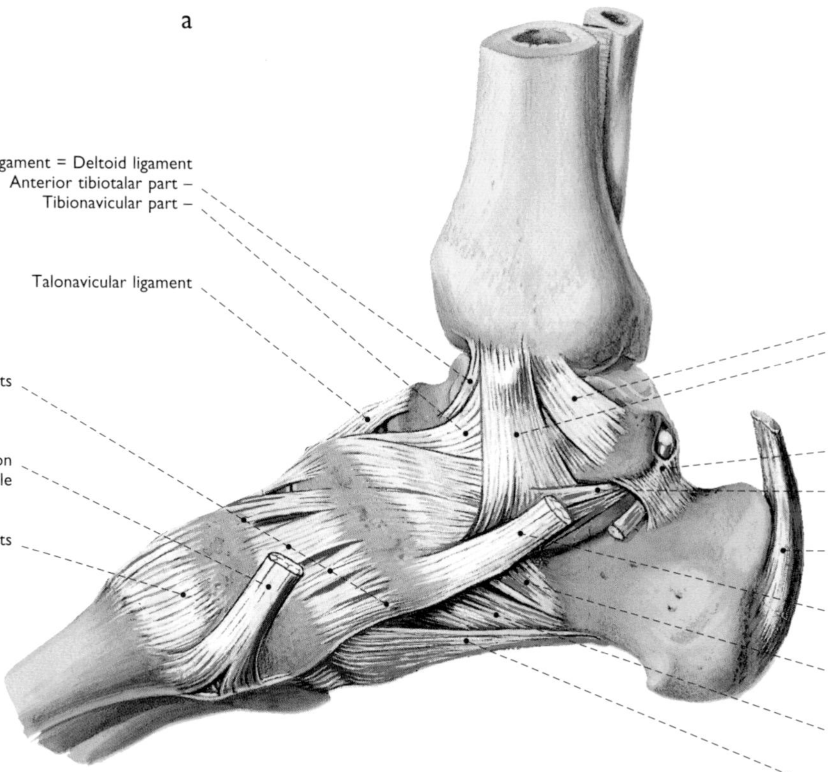
Medial ligament = Deltoid ligament
Anterior tibiotalar part –
Tibionavicular part –
Talonavicular ligament
Dorsal tarsal ligaments
Tendon
of tibialis anterior muscle
Dorsal tarsometatarsal ligaments
Medial ligament = Deltoid ligament
– Posterior tibiotalar part
– Tibiocalcaneal part
Posterior talocalcaneal ligament
Medial talocalcaneal ligament
Calcaneal tendon
(= Achilles tendon)
Tendon
of tibialis posterior muscle
Plantar calcaneonavicular ligament
= Spring ligament
Plantar calcaneocuboid ligament
= Short plantar ligament
Long plantar ligament

b

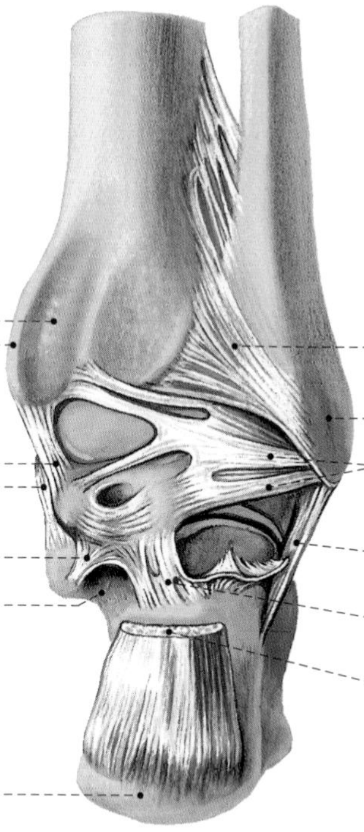
Tibia
Malleolar groove –
Medial malleolus –
Medial ligament = Deltoid ligament
Posterior tibiotalar part –
Tibiocalcaneal part –
Medial talocalcaneal ligament
Groove for tendon
of flexor hallucis longus muscle
Calcaneal tuberosity
Tibiofibular syndesmosis,
Posterior tibiofibular ligament
Lateral malleolus
Posterior talofibular ligament
Calcaneofibular ligament
Posterior talocalcaneal ligament
Calcaneal tendon
(= Achilles tendon)
of triceps surae muscle

226 Joints and ligaments of the right foot (60%)

a Medial aspect
b Dorsal aspect

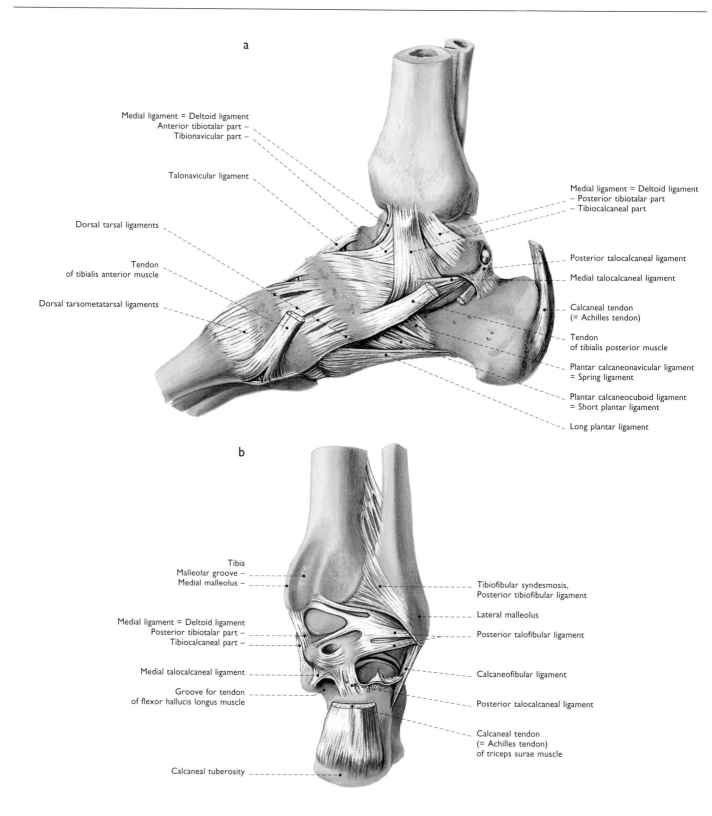

a

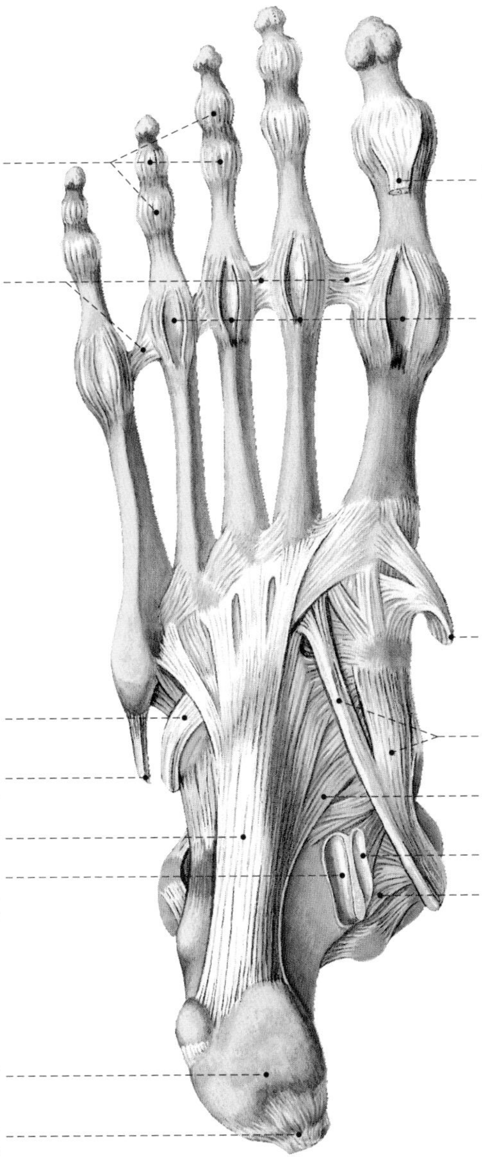
Plantar ligaments of interphalangeal joints of foot
Deep transverse metatarsal ligament
Tendon of fibularis longus muscle
Tendon of fibularis brevis muscle
Long plantar ligament
Groove for tendon of flexor hallucis longus muscle
Calcaneal tuberosity
Calcaneal tendon (= Achilles tendon) of triceps surae muscle
Tendon of flexor hallucis longus muscle
Plantar ligaments of metatarsophalangeal joints
Tendon of tibialis anterior muscle
Tendon of tibialis posterior muscle
Plantar calcaneonavicular ligament = Spring ligament
⟨Groove for tendon of flexor digitorum longus muscle⟩
Tibiocalcaneal part of deltoid (= medial) ligament

b

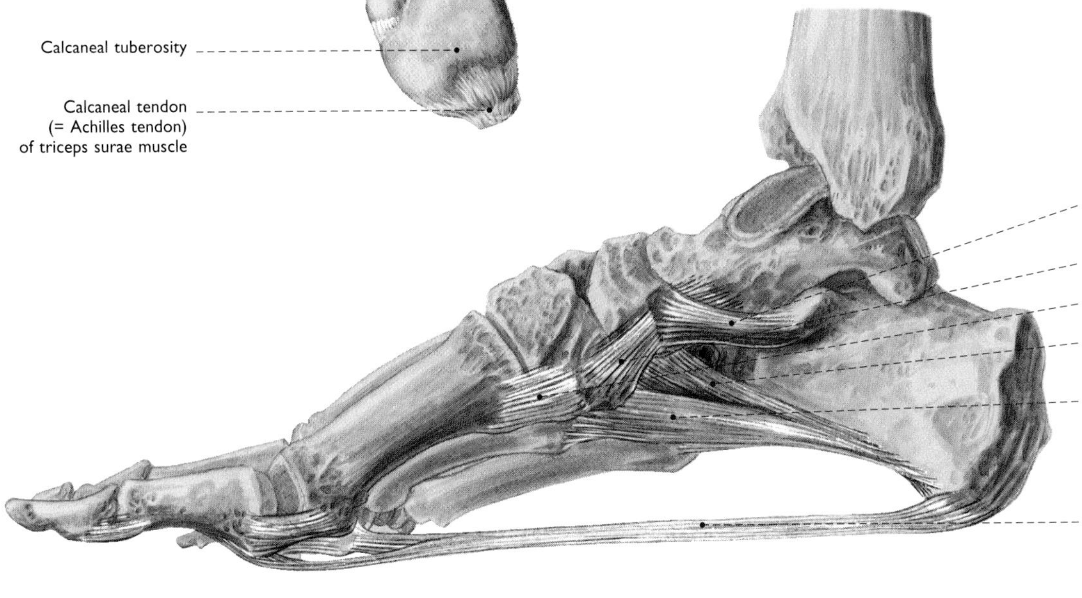
Plantar calcaneonavicular ligament = Spring ligament
Plantar cuneonavicular ligaments
Plantar tarsometatarsal ligaments
Plantar calcaneocuboid ligament = Short plantar ligament
Long plantar ligament
Plantar aponeurosis

227 Joints and ligaments of the right foot (60%)

a Plantar aspect
b Ligaments stabilizing the subtalar (= talocalcaneal) and talocalcaneonavicular joints, medial aspect

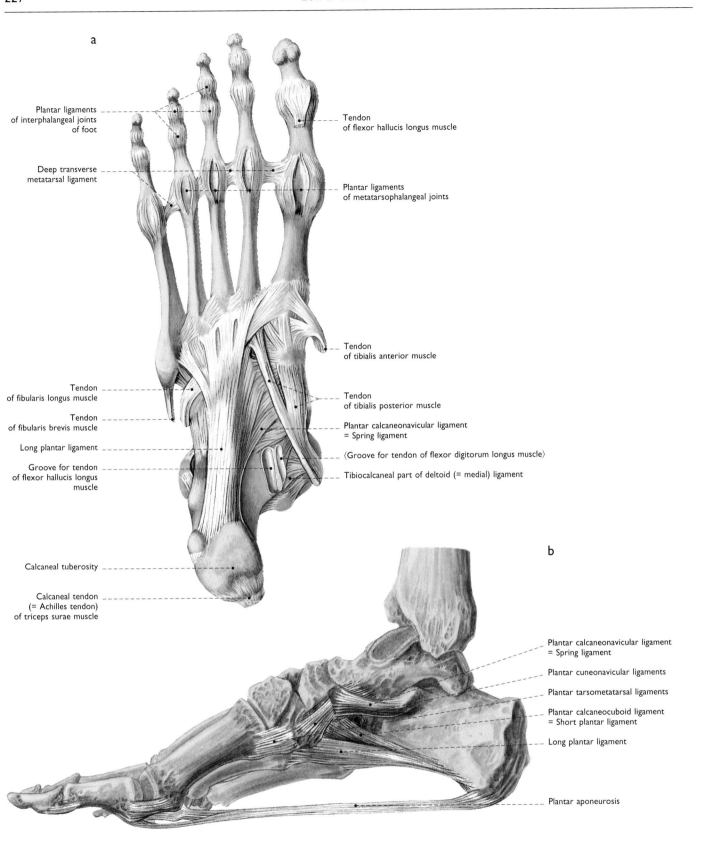

a

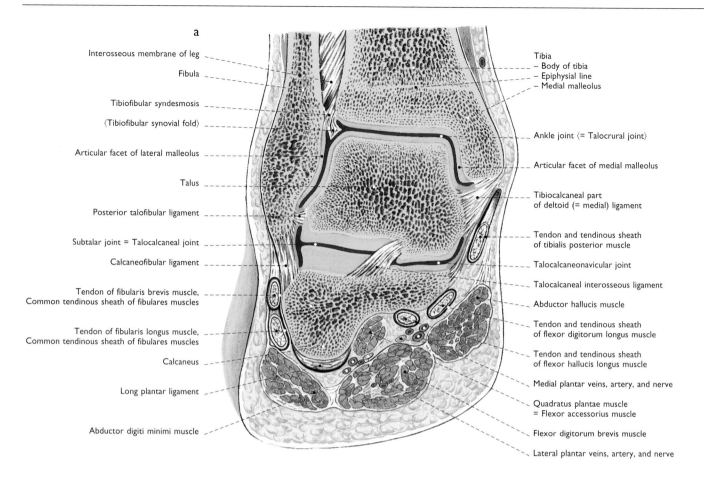

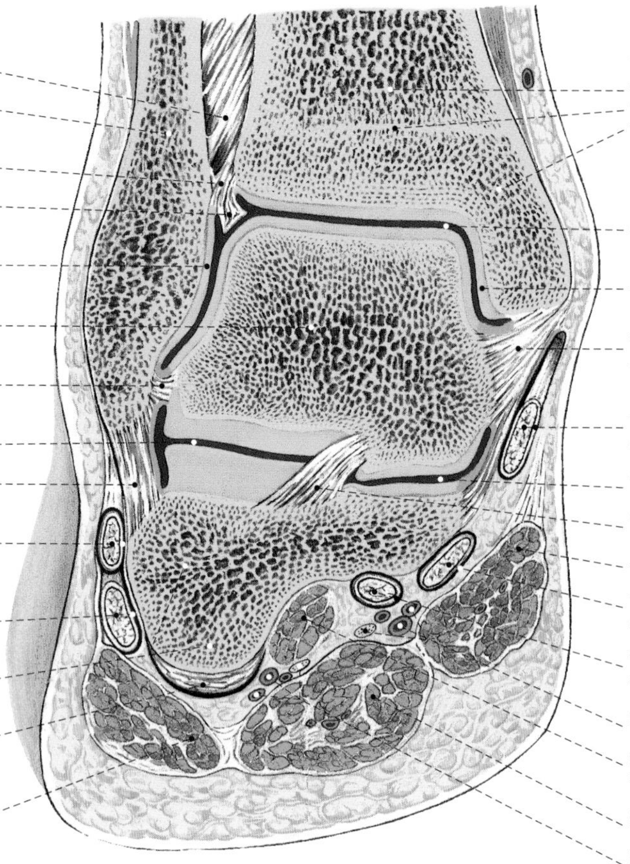
Interosseous membrane of leg
Fibula
Tibiofibular syndesmosis
⟨Tibiofibular synovial fold⟩
Articular facet of lateral malleolus
Talus
Posterior talofibular ligament
Subtalar joint = Talocalcaneal joint
Calcaneofibular ligament
Tendon of fibularis brevis muscle, Common tendinous sheath of fibulares muscles
Tendon of fibularis longus muscle, Common tendinous sheath of fibulares muscles
Calcaneus
Long plantar ligament
Abductor digiti minimi muscle
Tibia
– Body of tibia
– Epiphysial line
– Medial malleolus
Ankle joint ⟨= Talocrural joint⟩
Articular facet of medial malleolus
Tibiocalcaneal part of deltoid (= medial) ligament
Tendon and tendinous sheath of tibialis posterior muscle
Talocalcaneonavicular joint
Talocalcaneal interosseous ligament
Abductor hallucis muscle
Tendon and tendinous sheath of flexor digitorum longus muscle
Tendon and tendinous sheath of flexor hallucis longus muscle
Medial plantar veins, artery, and nerve
Quadratus plantae muscle = Flexor accessorius muscle
Flexor digitorum brevis muscle
Lateral plantar veins, artery, and nerve

b

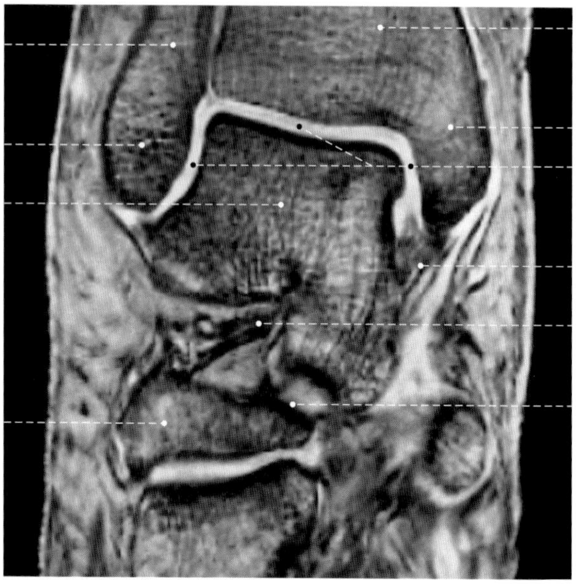
Body of fibula
Lateral malleolus
Talus
Calcaneus
Body of tibia
Medial malleolus
Ankle joint ⟨= Talocrural joint⟩
Tibiocalcaneal part of deltoid (= medial) ligament
Talocalcaneal interosseous ligament
Talocalcaneonavicular joint

228 Ankle (= talocrural), subtalar, and talocalcaneonavicular joints of the right foot (100%)

Coronal sections, distal aspect

a Anatomical section

b Magnetic resonance image (MRI, T_2-weighted)

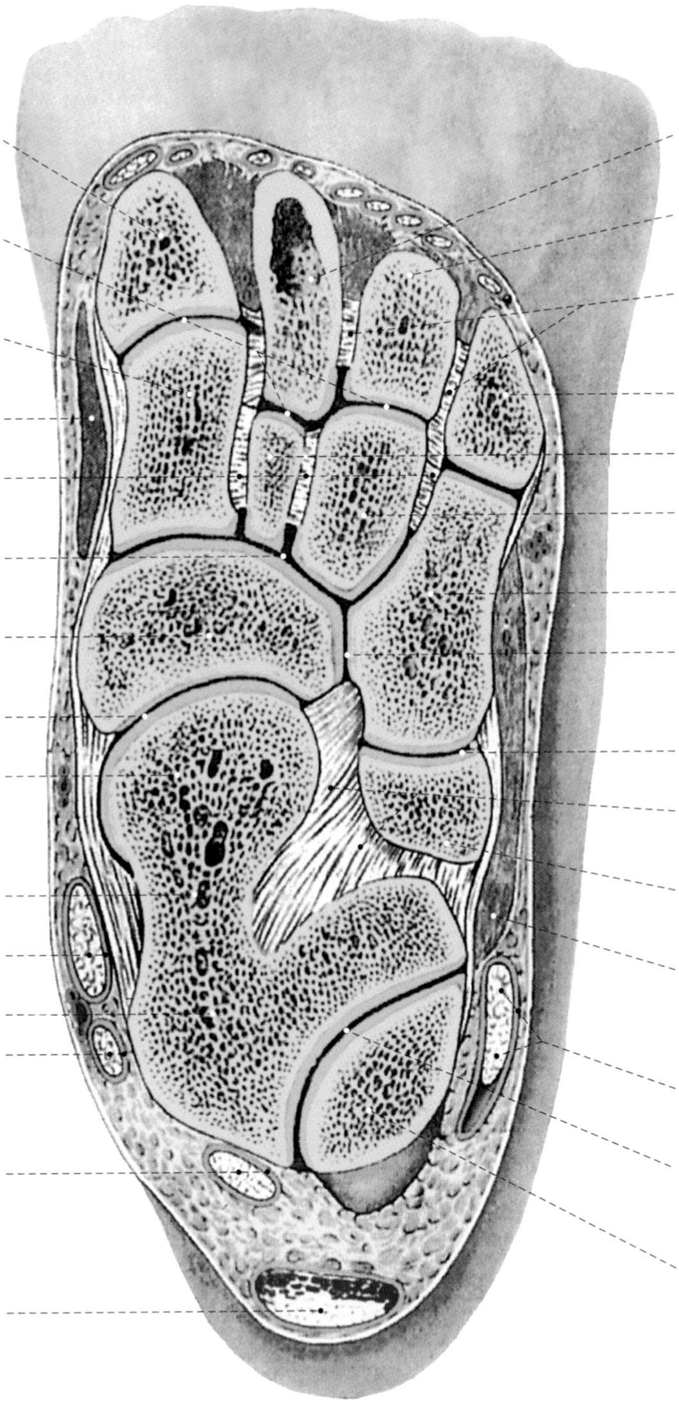
1st metatarsal bone
Tarsometatarsal joints I–III
Medial cuneiform
Abductor hallucis muscle
Tarsal interosseous ligaments
Cuneonavicular joint
Navicular
Talocalcaneonavicular joint
(Talonavicular portion)
Head of talus
Neck of talus
Tendon and tendinous sheath
of tibialis posterior muscle
Body of talus
Tendon and tendinous sheath
of flexor digitorum longus muscle
Tendon and tendinous sheath
of flexor hallucis longus muscle
Calcaneal tendon
(= Achilles tendon)
of triceps surae muscle
2nd metatarsal bone
3rd metatarsal bone
Metatarsal interosseous ligaments
4th metatarsal bone
Intermediate cuneiform
= Middle cuneiform
Lateral cuneiform
Cuboid
⟨Cuboideonavicular joint⟩
Calcaneocuboid joint
Talocalcaneal interosseous ligament
in tarsal sinus
Calcaneus
Extensor digitorum brevis muscle
Tendons and common tendinous sheath
of fibulares muscles
Subtalar joint
= Talocalcaneal joint
Calcaneus

229 Joints of the right foot (100%)

Axial (horizontal) section through the right foot, proximal aspect of the plantar part

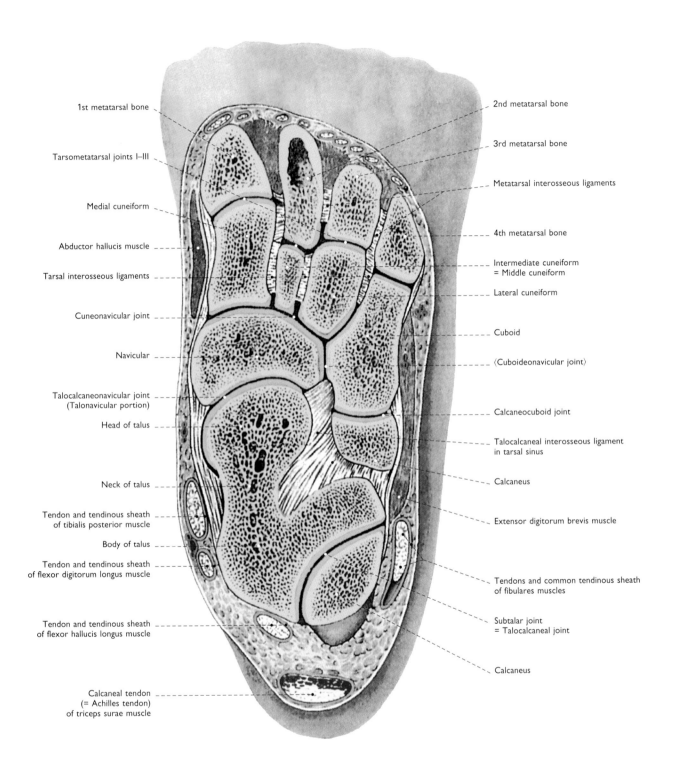

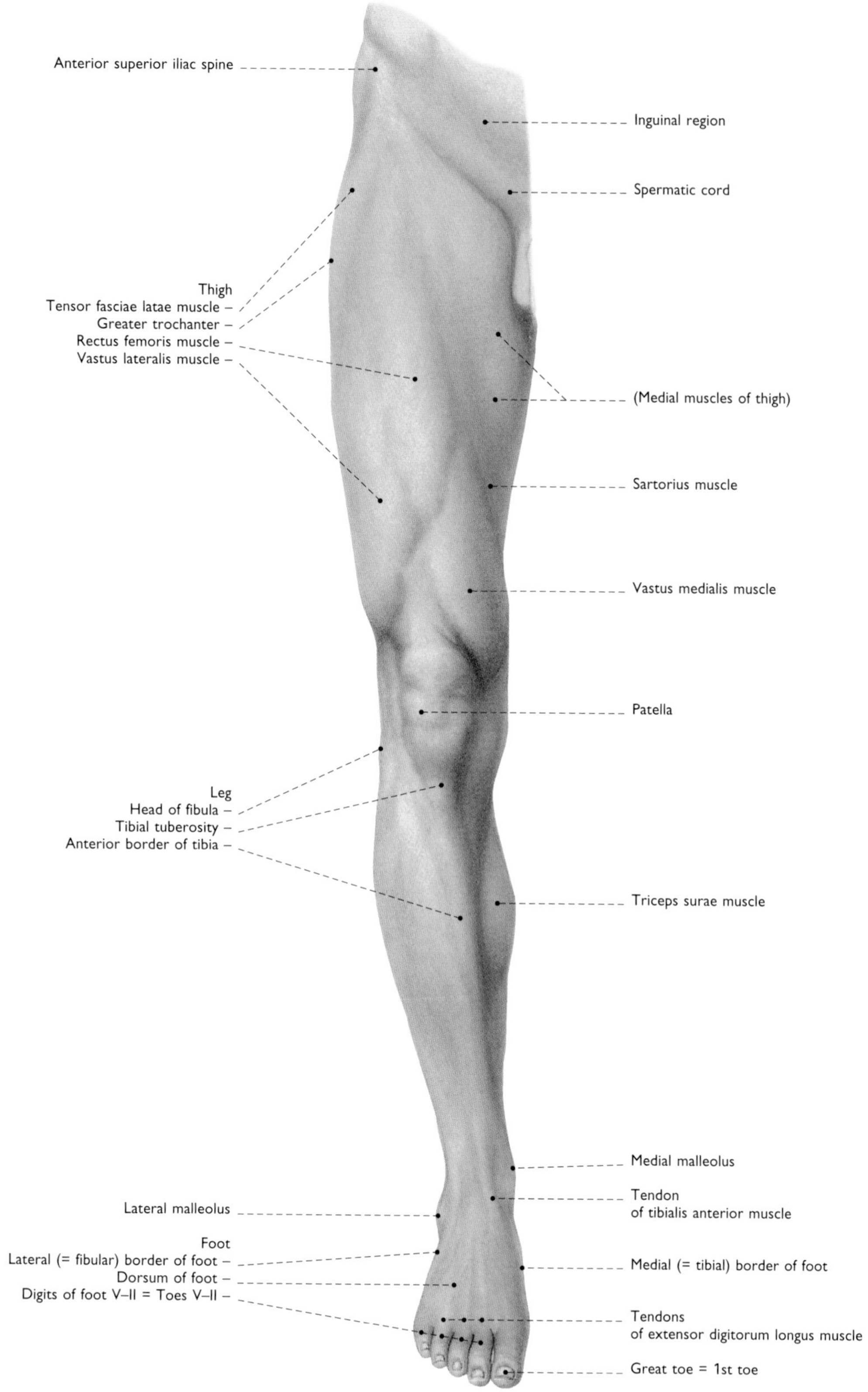

Anterior superior iliac spine
Inguinal region
Spermatic cord
Thigh
Tensor fasciae latae muscle
Greater trochanter
Rectus femoris muscle
Vastus lateralis muscle
(Medial muscles of thigh)
Sartorius muscle
Vastus medialis muscle
Patella
Leg
Head of fibula
Tibial tuberosity
Anterior border of tibia
Triceps surae muscle
Medial malleolus
Tendon
of tibialis anterior muscle
Lateral malleolus
Foot
Lateral (= fibular) border of foot
Dorsum of foot
Digits of foot V–II = Toes V–II
Medial (= tibial) border of foot
Tendons
of extensor digitorum longus muscle
Great toe = 1st toe

230 Surface anatomy of the right lower limb (20%)

Ventral aspect

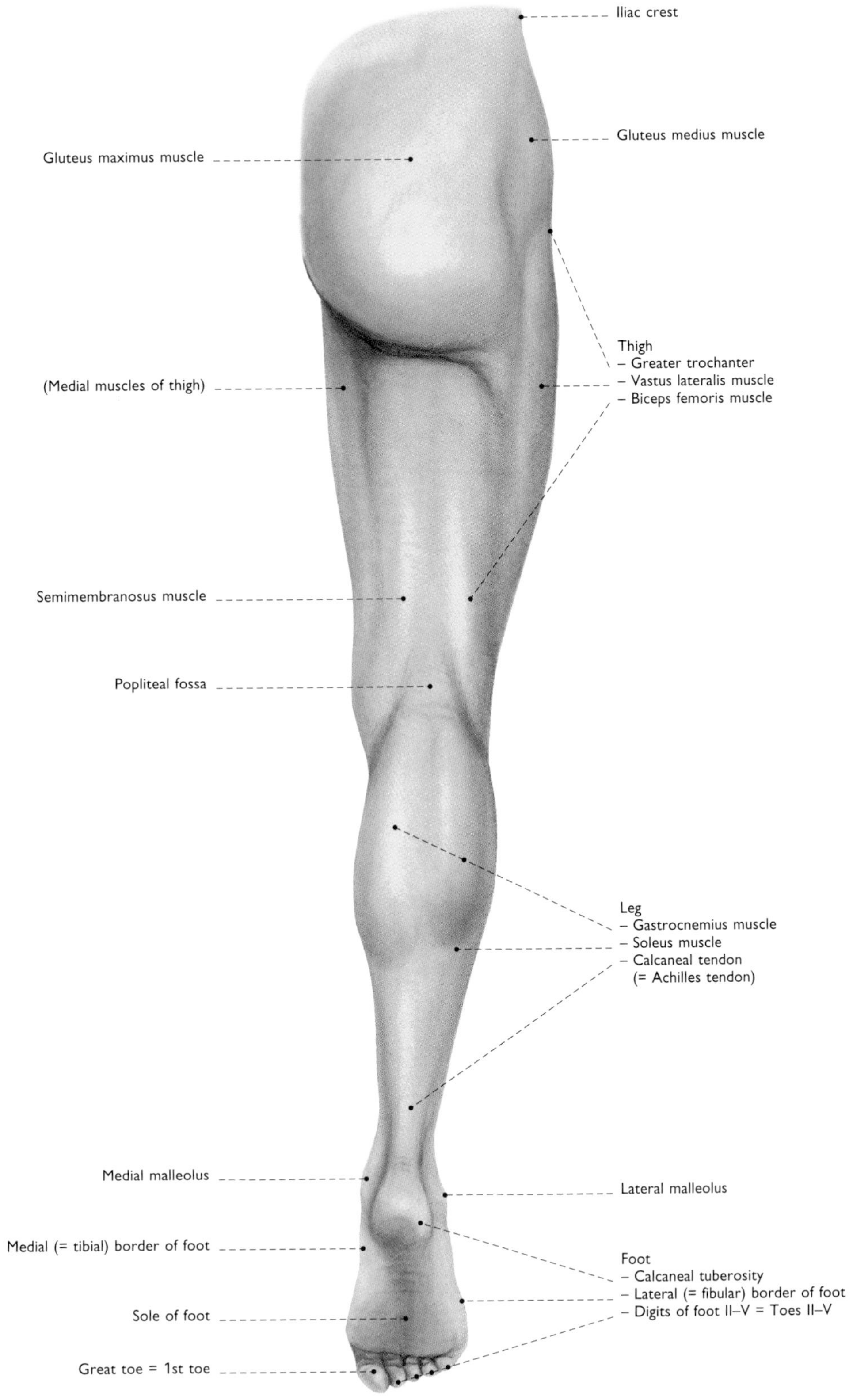
Iliac crest
Gluteus medius muscle
Gluteus maximus muscle
Thigh
– Greater trochanter
– Vastus lateralis muscle
– Biceps femoris muscle
(Medial muscles of thigh)
Semimembranosus muscle
Popliteal fossa
Leg
– Gastrocnemius muscle
– Soleus muscle
– Calcaneal tendon
(= Achilles tendon)
Medial malleolus
Lateral malleolus
Medial (= tibial) border of foot
Foot
– Calcaneal tuberosity
– Lateral (= fibular) border of foot
– Digits of foot II–V = Toes II–V
Sole of foot
Great toe = 1st toe

231 Surface anatomy of the right lower limb (20%)

Dorsal aspect

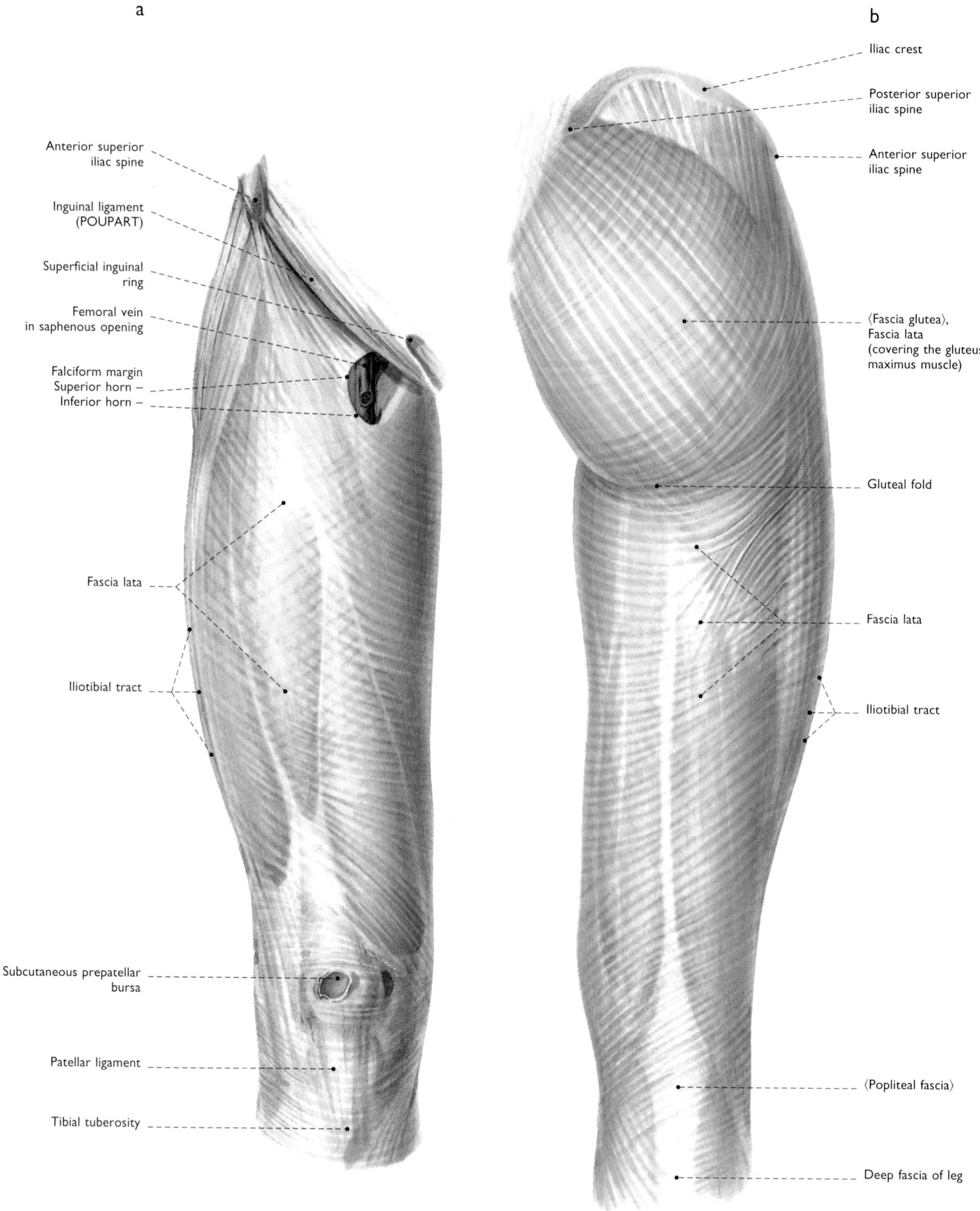
a
Anterior superior iliac spine
Inguinal ligament (POUPART)
Superficial inguinal ring
Femoral vein in saphenous opening
Falciform margin
Superior horn –
Inferior horn –
Fascia lata
Iliotibial tract
Subcutaneous prepatellar bursa
Patellar ligament
Tibial tuberosity
b
Iliac crest
Posterior superior iliac spine
Anterior superior iliac spine
⟨Fascia glutea⟩, Fascia lata (covering the gluteus maximus muscle)
Gluteal fold
Fascia lata
Iliotibial tract
⟨Popliteal fascia⟩
Deep fascia of leg

232 Fascia lata of the right thigh (30%)

a The cribriform fascia in the saphenous opening was removed (cf. fig. 249b). Ventral aspect

b Dorsal aspect

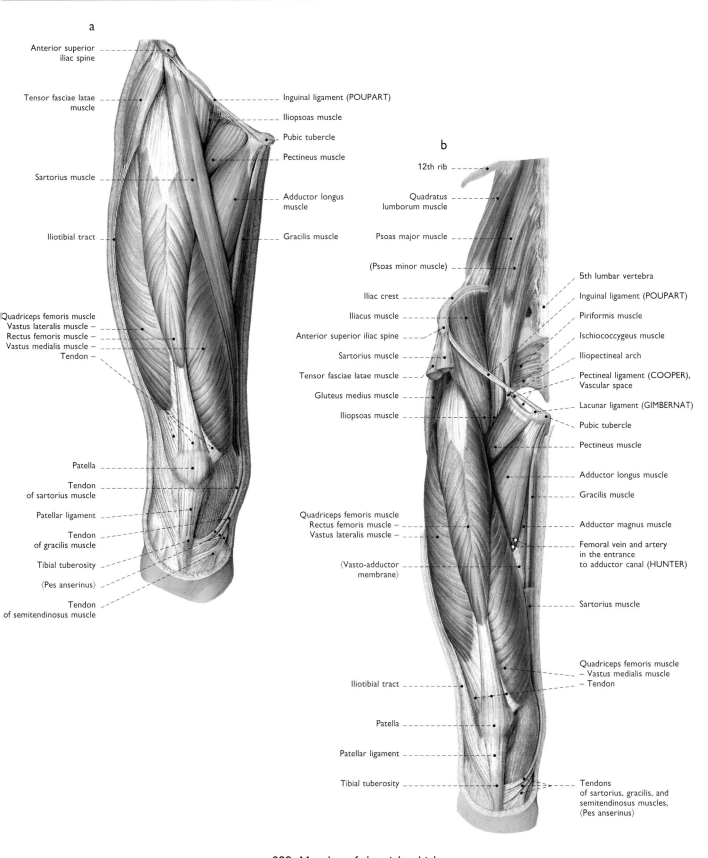

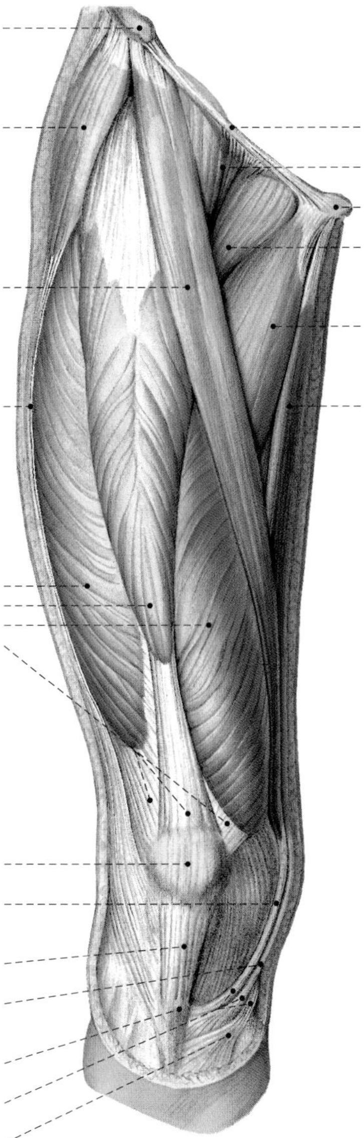
a
Anterior superior iliac spine
Tensor fasciae latae muscle
Sartorius muscle
Iliotibial tract
Quadriceps femoris muscle
Vastus lateralis muscle –
Rectus femoris muscle –
Vastus medialis muscle –
Tendon –
Patella
Tendon of sartorius muscle
Patellar ligament
Tendon of gracilis muscle
Tibial tuberosity
⟨Pes anserinus⟩
Tendon of semitendinosus muscle
Inguinal ligament (POUPART)
Iliopsoas muscle
Pubic tubercle
Pectineus muscle
Adductor longus muscle
Gracilis muscle

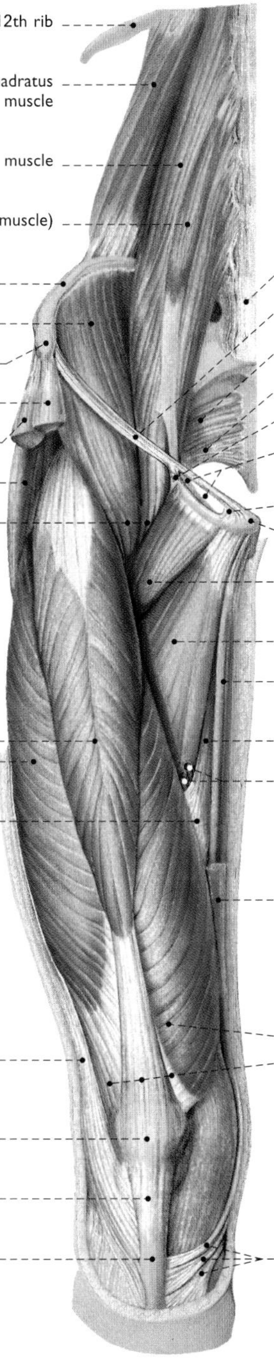
b
12th rib
Quadratus lumborum muscle
Psoas major muscle
(Psoas minor muscle)
Iliac crest
Iliacus muscle
Anterior superior iliac spine
Sartorius muscle
Tensor fasciae latae muscle
Gluteus medius muscle
Iliopsoas muscle
Quadriceps femoris muscle
Rectus femoris muscle –
Vastus lateralis muscle –
⟨Vasto-adductor membrane⟩
Iliotibial tract
Patella
Patellar ligament
Tibial tuberosity
5th lumbar vertebra
Inguinal ligament (POUPART)
Piriformis muscle
Ischiococcygeus muscle
Iliopectineal arch
Pectineal ligament (COOPER), Vascular space
Lacunar ligament (GIMBERNAT)
Pubic tubercle
Pectineus muscle
Adductor longus muscle
Gracilis muscle
Adductor magnus muscle
Femoral vein and artery in the entrance to adductor canal (HUNTER)
Sartorius muscle
Quadriceps femoris muscle
– Vastus medialis muscle
– Tendon
Tendons of sartorius, gracilis, and semitendinosus muscles, ⟨Pes anserinus⟩

233 Muscles of the right thigh (25%)

Ventral aspect

a Anterior muscles of thigh

b The sartorius and tensor fasciae latae muscles were partially removed. Some muscles of the pelvis are additionally shown.

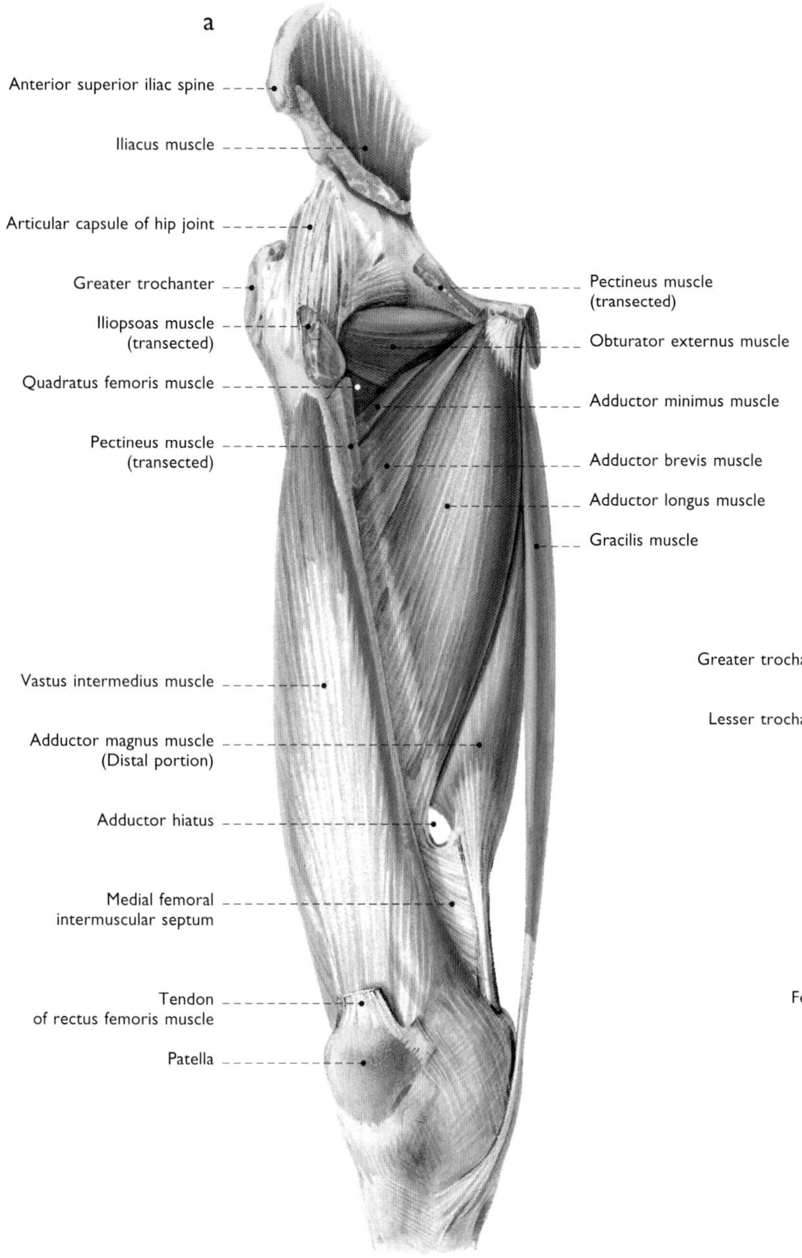
a
Anterior superior iliac spine
Iliacus muscle
Articular capsule of hip joint
Greater trochanter
Iliopsoas muscle (transected)
Quadratus femoris muscle
Pectineus muscle (transected)
Vastus intermedius muscle
Adductor magnus muscle (Distal portion)
Adductor hiatus
Medial femoral intermuscular septum
Tendon of rectus femoris muscle
Patella
Pectineus muscle (transected)
Obturator externus muscle
Adductor minimus muscle
Adductor brevis muscle
Adductor longus muscle
Gracilis muscle

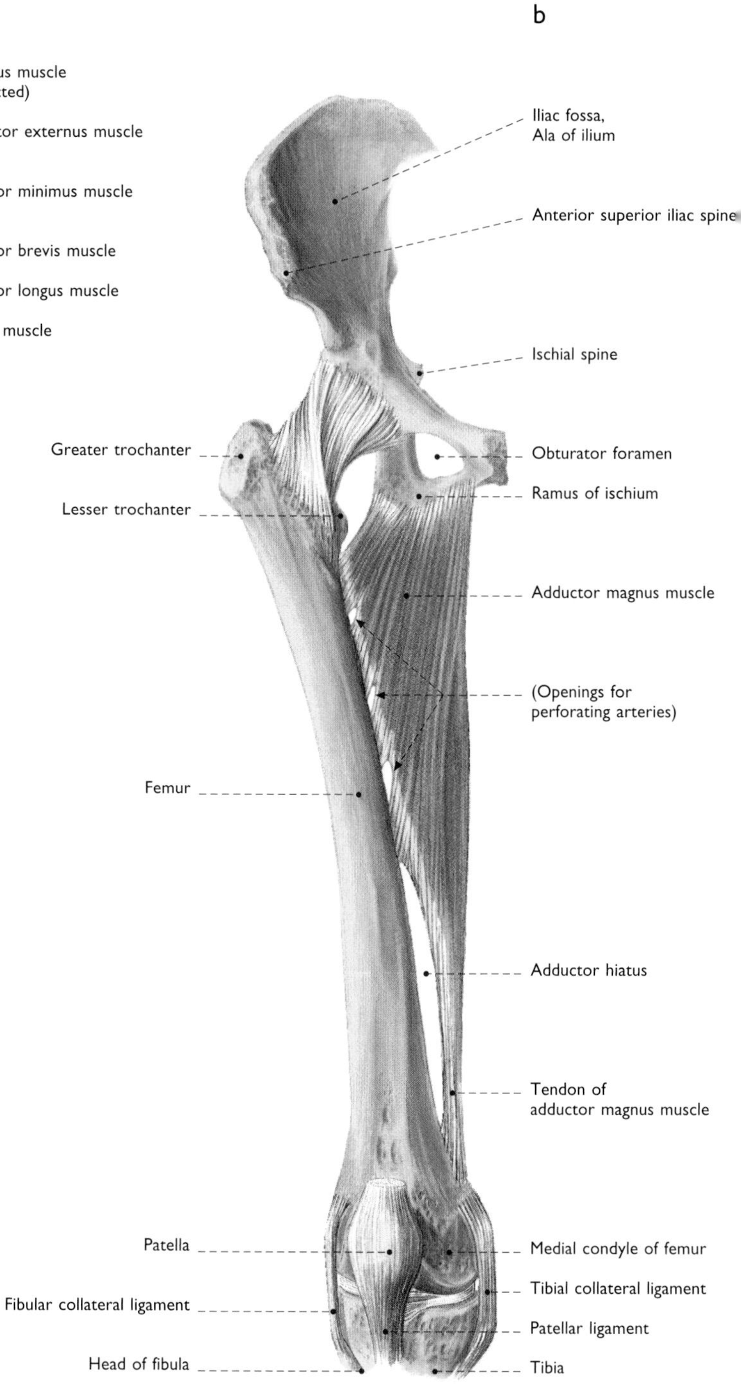
b
Iliac fossa, Ala of ilium
Anterior superior iliac spine
Ischial spine
Obturator foramen
Ramus of ischium
Adductor magnus muscle
(Openings for perforating arteries)
Adductor hiatus
Tendon of adductor magnus muscle
Medial condyle of femur
Tibial collateral ligament
Patellar ligament
Tibia
Greater trochanter
Lesser trochanter
Femur
Patella
Fibular collateral ligament
Head of fibula

234 Muscles of the right thigh (25%)

Ventral aspect

a Medial muscles (adductors) of thigh and deep part of the quadriceps femoris muscle

b Adductor magnus muscle

a

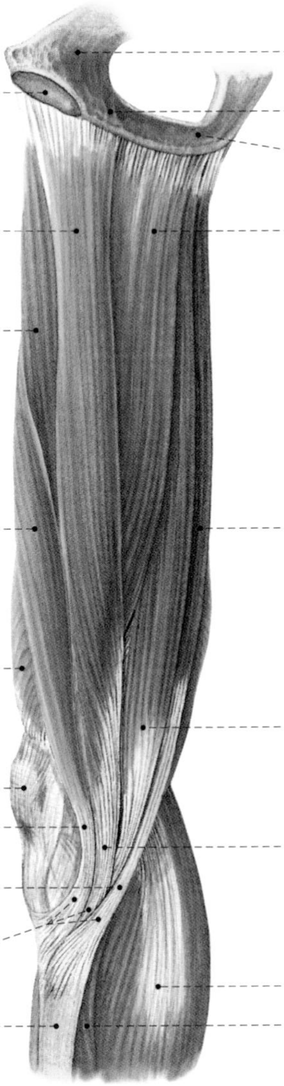
Superior pubic ramus
Symphysial surface
of pubis
Inferior pubic ramus
Ramus of ischium
Gracilis muscle
Adductor magnus muscle
Adductor longus muscle
Sartorius muscle
Semitendinosus muscle
Vastus medialis muscle
Semimembranosus muscle
Patella
Tendon
of sartorius muscle
Tendon
of gracilis muscle
Tendon
of semitendinosus muscle
(Pes anserinus)
Triceps surae muscle
– Medial head
of gastrocnemius muscle
Tibia
– Soleus muscle

b

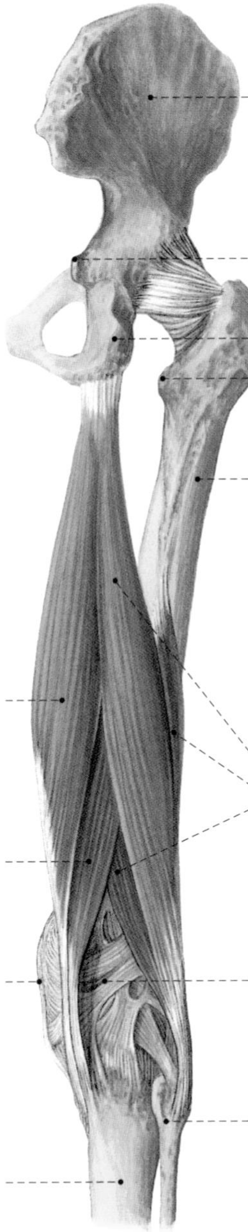
Gluteal surface of ilium
Ischial spine
Greater trochanter
Ischial tuberosity
Lesser trochanter
Femur
Semitendinosus
muscle
Biceps femoris muscle
– Long head
– Short head
Semimembranosus muscle
Tibial collateral ligament
Oblique popliteal
ligament
Head of fibula
Tibia

235 Muscles of the right thigh (25%)

a Medial muscles (adductors) of thigh,
medial aspect

b Posterior muscles of thigh ('hamstrings'), dorsal aspect

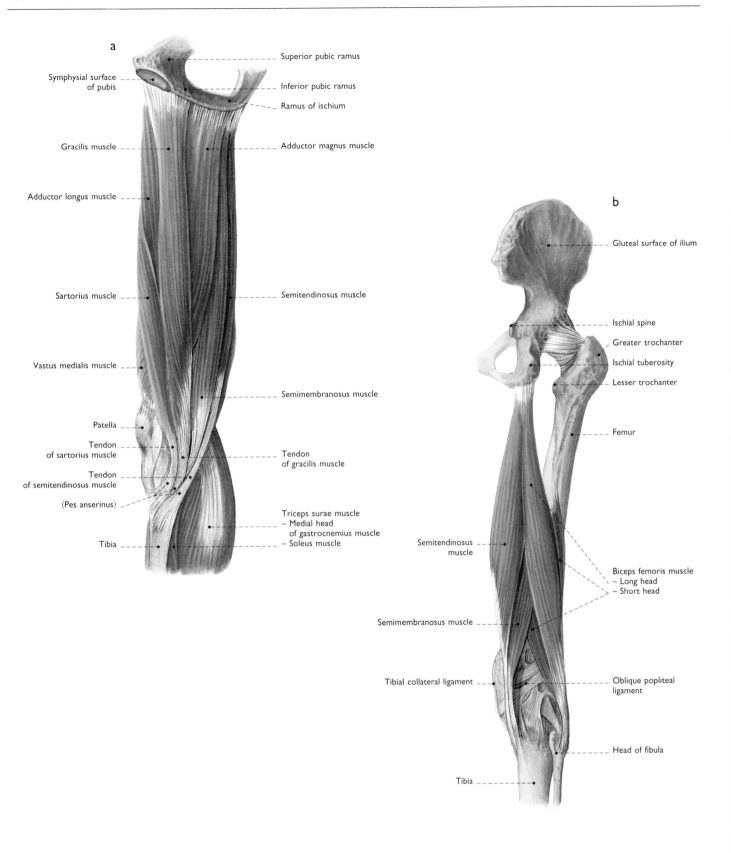

a

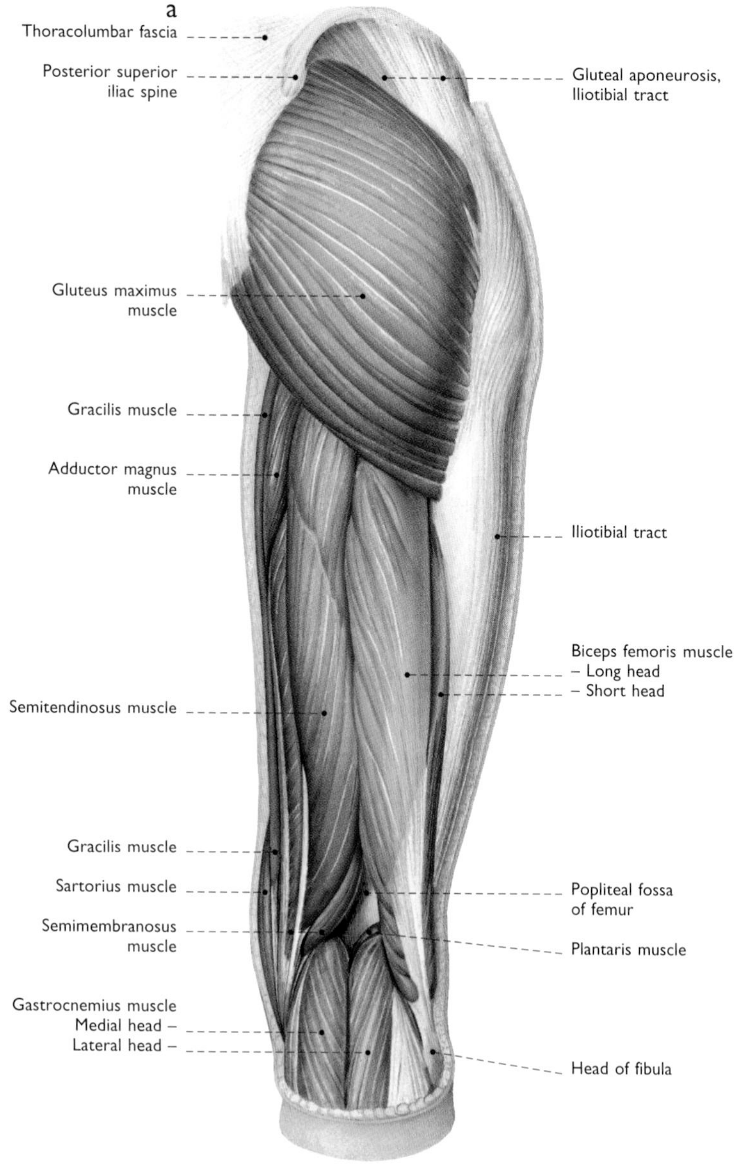
Thoracolumbar fascia
Posterior superior iliac spine
Gluteus maximus muscle
Gracilis muscle
Adductor magnus muscle
Semitendinosus muscle
Gracilis muscle
Sartorius muscle
Semimembranosus muscle
Gastrocnemius muscle
Medial head –
Lateral head –
Gluteal aponeurosis, Iliotibial tract
Iliotibial tract
Biceps femoris muscle
– Long head
– Short head
Popliteal fossa of femur
Plantaris muscle
Head of fibula

b

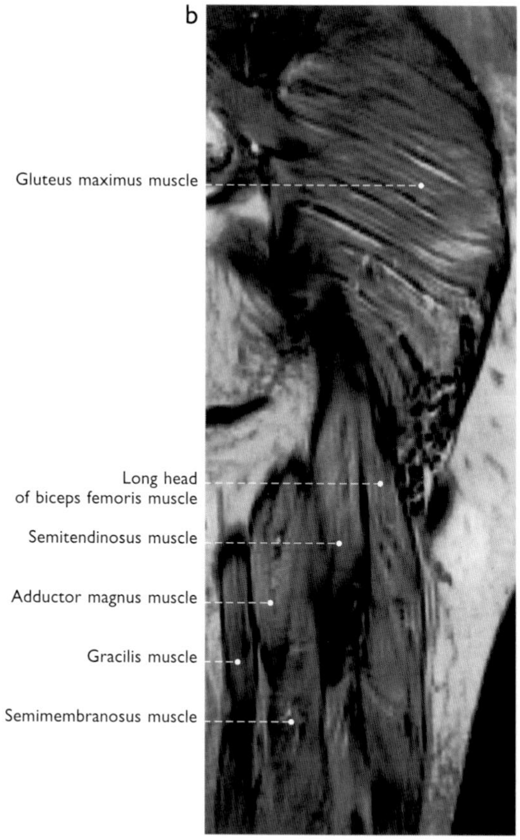
Gluteus maximus muscle
Long head of biceps femoris muscle
Semitendinosus muscle
Adductor magnus muscle
Gracilis muscle
Semimembranosus muscle

236 Muscles of the right thigh and superficial layer of the muscles of the hip

a Dorsal aspect (20%)
b Coronal magnetic resonance image (MRI, T_1-weighted)

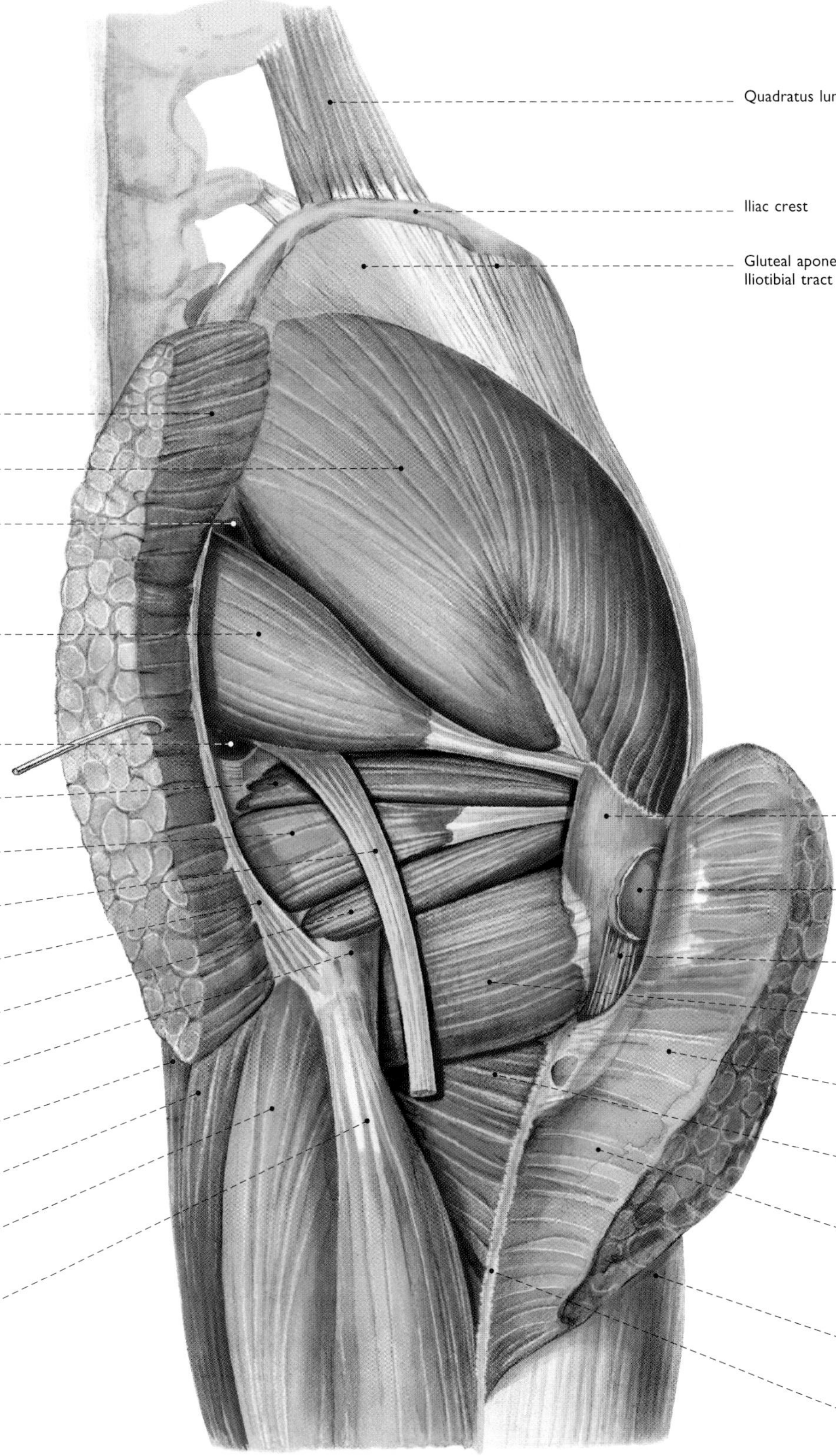
Quadratus lumborum muscle
Iliac crest
Gluteal aponeurosis,
Iliotibial tract
Gluteus maximus muscle
Gluteus medius muscle
⟨Suprapiriform foramen⟩
Piriformis muscle
⟨Infrapiriform foramen⟩
Gemellus superior muscle
Obturator internus muscle
Sciatic nerve
Sacrotuberous ligament
Gemellus inferior muscle
Ischial tuberosity
Gracilis muscle
Adductor magnus muscle
Semitendinosus muscle
Long head
of biceps femoris muscle
Greater trochanter
of femur
Trochanteric bursa
of gluteus maximus muscle
Tendon
of vastus lateralis muscle
Quadratus femoris muscle
Gluteus maximus muscle
Adductor minimus muscle
Gluteus maximus muscle
Vastus lateralis muscle
Medial lip of linea aspera

237 Muscles of the right hip (50%)

Deep layer. The gluteus maximus muscle was divided and turned up.
Dorsal aspect

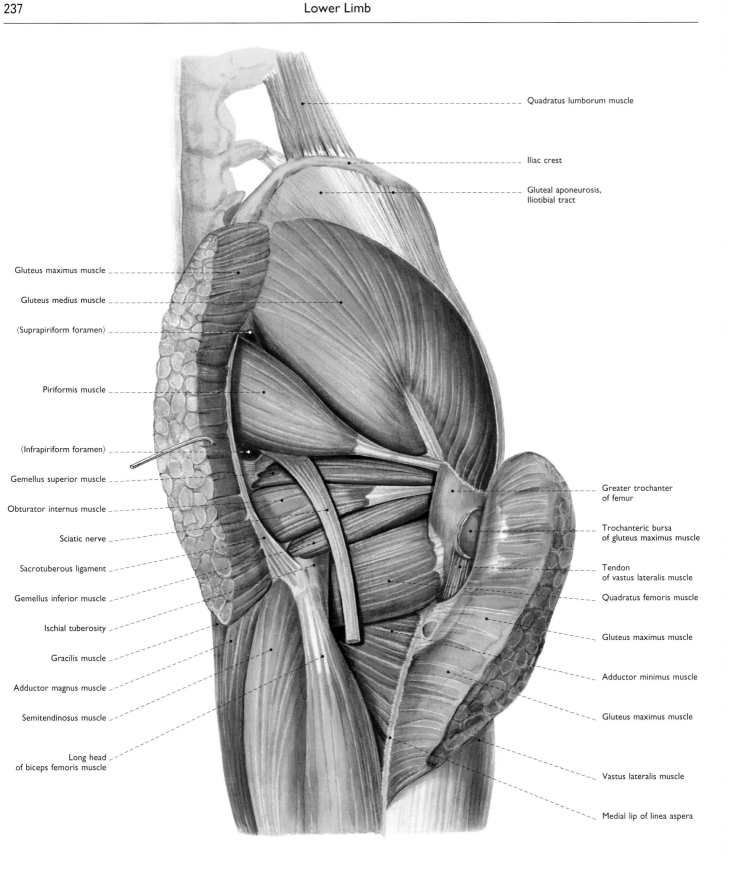

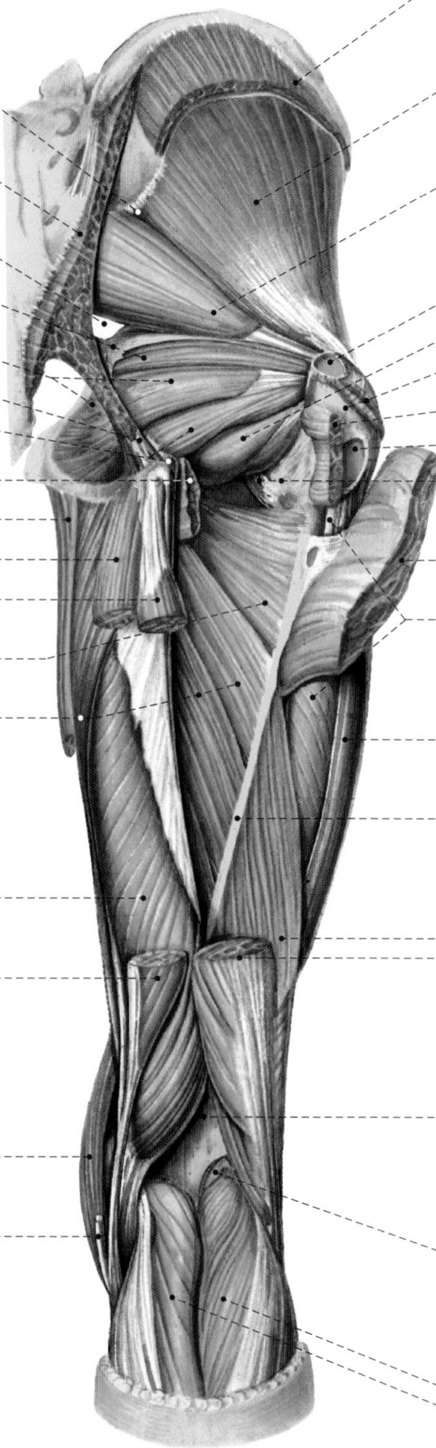
Gluteus medius muscle
Gluteus minimus muscle
Piriformis muscle
Trochanteric bursa of gluteus medius muscle
Obturator externus muscle
Greater trochanter of femur,
Gluteus medius muscle
Quadratus femoris muscle
Trochanteric bursa of gluteus maximus muscle
Tendon of iliopsoas muscle,
Lesser trochanter of femur
Gluteus maximus muscle
Vastus lateralis muscle
Iliotibial tract
Linea aspera
Biceps femoris muscle
– Short head
– Long head
Popliteal surface of femur
Plantaris muscle
Gastrocnemius muscle
– Lateral head
– Medial head
⟨Suprapiriform foramen⟩
Gluteus maximus muscle
⟨Infrapiriform foramen⟩
Ischial spine,
Gemellus superior muscle
Obturator internus muscle
Sacrotuberous ligament
Gemellus inferior muscle,
Ischial tuberosity
Quadratus femoris muscle
Gracilis muscle
Semitendinosus muscle
Long head
of biceps femoris muscle
Adductor minimus muscle
Adductor magnus muscle
Semimembranosus muscle
Semitendinosus muscle
Sartorius muscle
Tendon
of gracilis muscle

238 Muscles of the right thigh and hip (30%)

Deep muscular layer. The superficial muscles were partially removed. Dorsal aspect

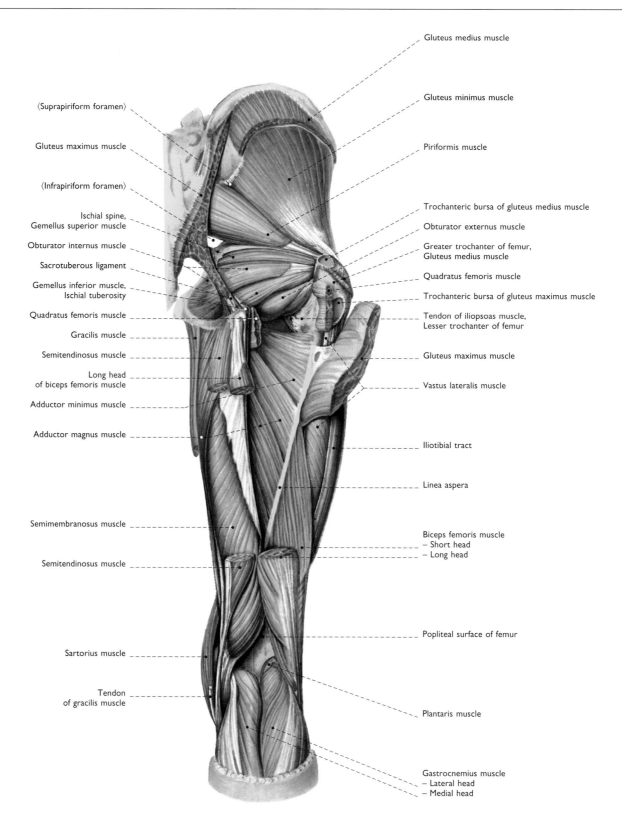

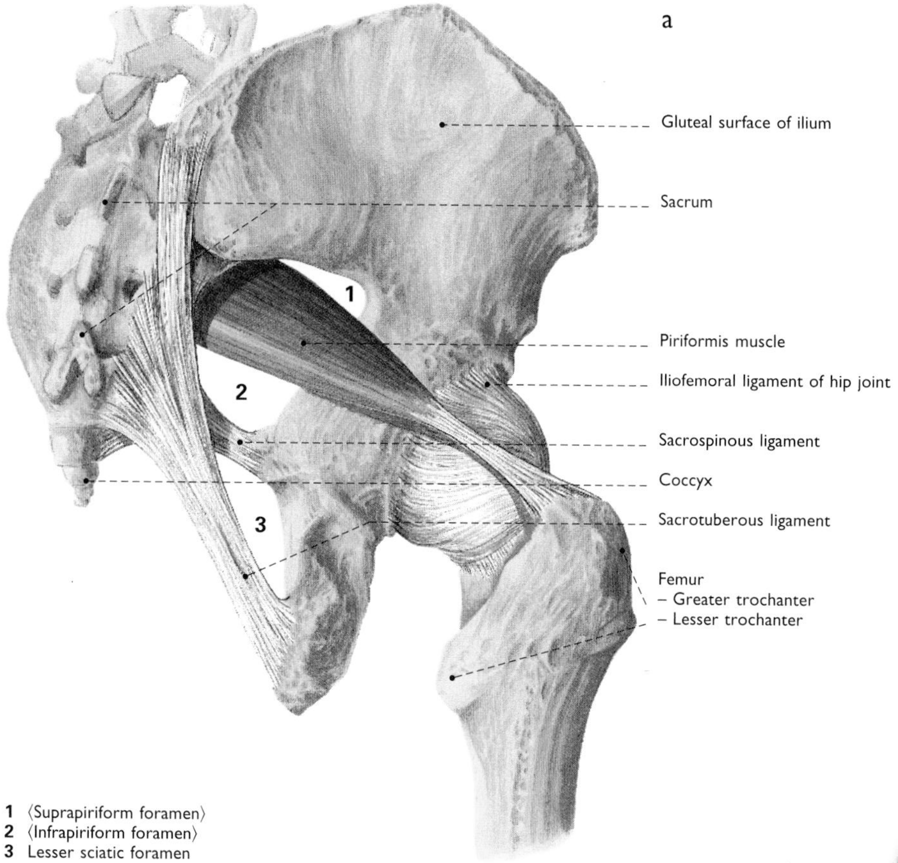
a
Gluteal surface of ilium
Sacrum
Piriformis muscle
Iliofemoral ligament of hip joint
Sacrospinous ligament
Coccyx
Sacrotuberous ligament
Femur
– Greater trochanter
– Lesser trochanter
1
2
3

1 ⟨Suprapiriform foramen⟩
2 ⟨Infrapiriform foramen⟩
3 Lesser sciatic foramen

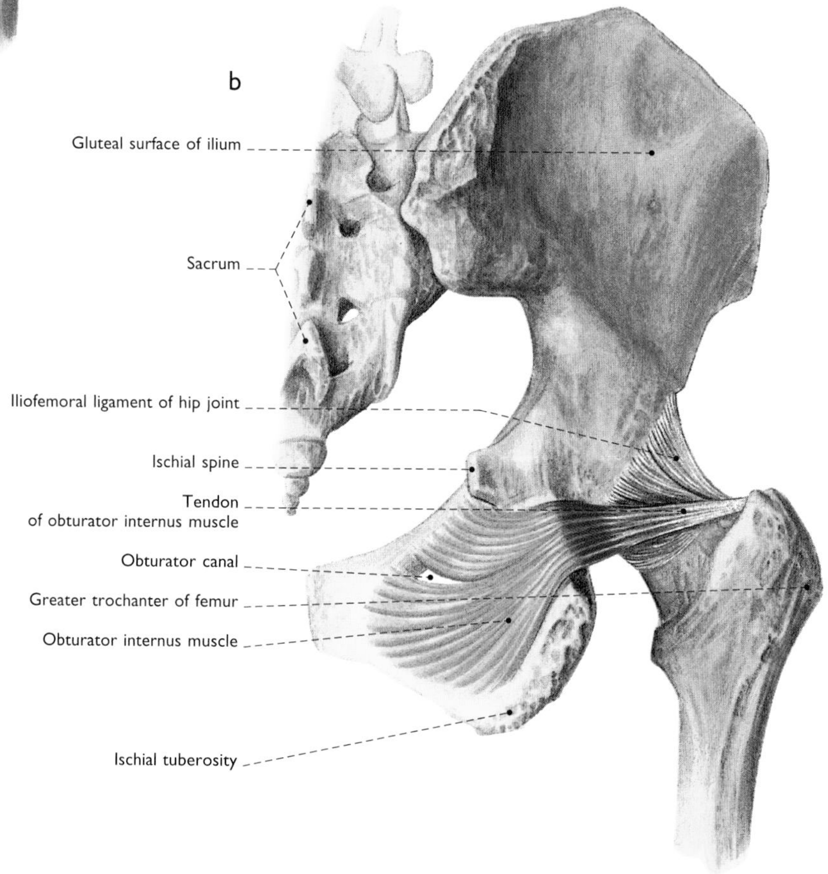
b
Gluteal surface of ilium
Sacrum
Iliofemoral ligament of hip joint
Ischial spine
Tendon
of obturator internus muscle
Obturator canal
Greater trochanter of femur
Obturator internus muscle
Ischial tuberosity

239 Muscles of the right hip (40%)

a Piriformis muscle, dorsolateral aspect
b Obturator internus muscle, dorsal aspect

a

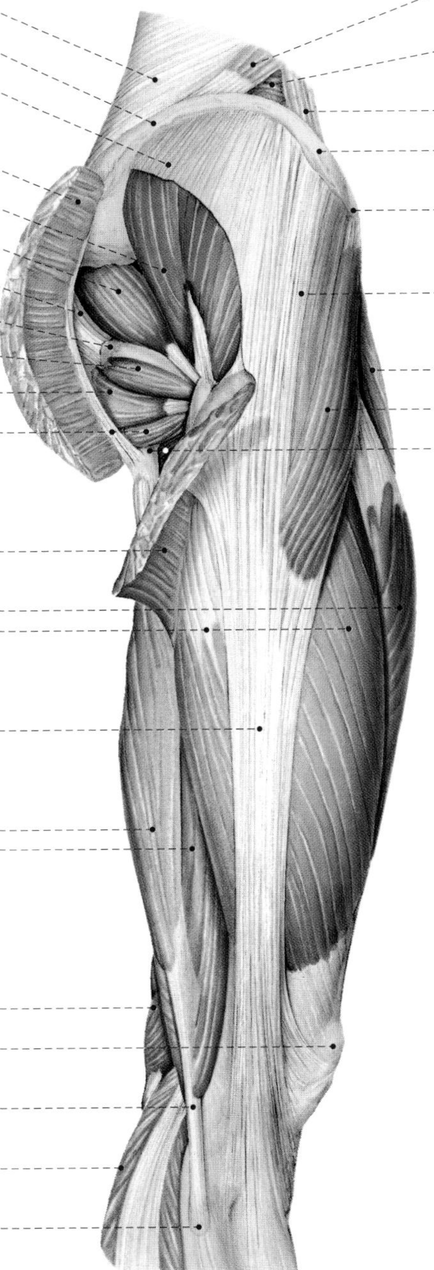
Thoracolumbar fascia
Iliac crest
Gluteal aponeurosis
Gluteus maximus muscle
Gluteus medius muscle
Piriformis muscle
Sacrospinous ligament
Ischial spine
Gemellus superior muscle
Obturator internus muscle
Sacrotuberous ligament,
Gemellus inferior muscle
Gluteus maximus muscle
Quadriceps femoris muscle
Rectus femoris muscle –
Vastus lateralis muscle –
Iliotibial tract
Biceps femoris muscle
Long head –
Short head –
Semimembranosus muscle
Patella
Tendon
of biceps femoris muscle
Lateral head
of gastrocnemius muscle
Head of fibula
Latissimus dorsi muscle
Internal oblique muscle,
(Inferior lumbar triangle, PETIT)
External oblique muscle
Iliac crest
Anterior superior iliac spine
Iliotibial tract
Sartorius muscle
Tensor fasciae latae muscle
Ischial tuberosity,
Quadratus femoris muscle

b

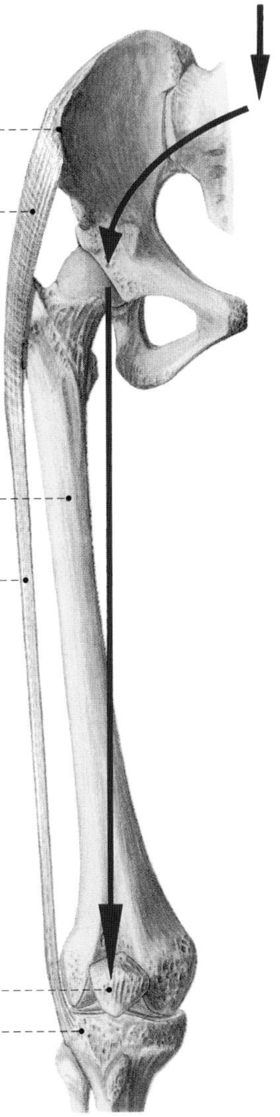
Anterior superior iliac spine
Tensor fasciae latae muscle
Femur
Iliotibial tract
Patella
Lateral condyle of tibia

240 Muscles of the right thigh and hip (20%)

a The gluteus maximus muscle was divided and turned up. Lateral aspect

b Tensor fasciae latae muscle and iliotibial tract, ventral aspect. The arrow indicates the weight line in erect posture.

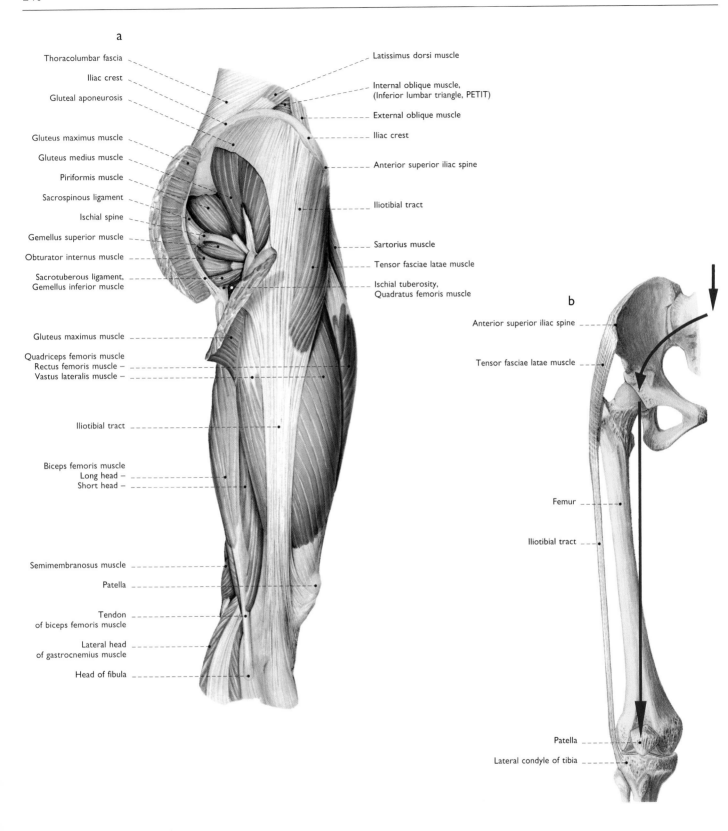

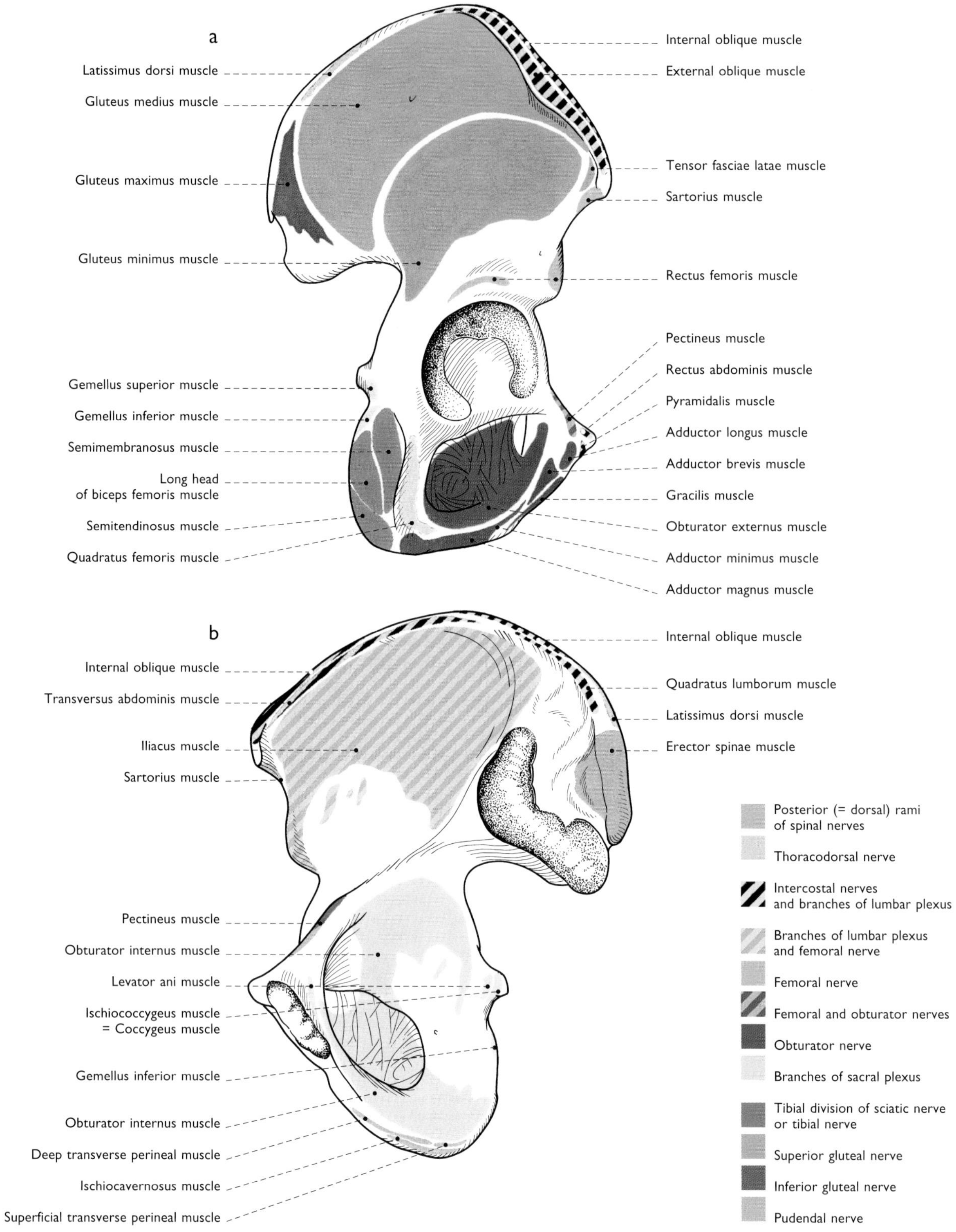
a
Latissimus dorsi muscle
Gluteus medius muscle
Gluteus maximus muscle
Gluteus minimus muscle
Gemellus superior muscle
Gemellus inferior muscle
Semimembranosus muscle
Long head of biceps femoris muscle
Semitendinosus muscle
Quadratus femoris muscle
Internal oblique muscle
External oblique muscle
Tensor fasciae latae muscle
Sartorius muscle
Rectus femoris muscle
Pectineus muscle
Rectus abdominis muscle
Pyramidalis muscle
Adductor longus muscle
Adductor brevis muscle
Gracilis muscle
Obturator externus muscle
Adductor minimus muscle
Adductor magnus muscle
b
Internal oblique muscle
Transversus abdominis muscle
Iliacus muscle
Sartorius muscle
Pectineus muscle
Obturator internus muscle
Levator ani muscle
Ischiococcygeus muscle = Coccygeus muscle
Gemellus inferior muscle
Obturator internus muscle
Deep transverse perineal muscle
Ischiocavernosus muscle
Superficial transverse perineal muscle
Internal oblique muscle
Quadratus lumborum muscle
Latissimus dorsi muscle
Erector spinae muscle
Posterior (= dorsal) rami of spinal nerves
Thoracodorsal nerve
Intercostal nerves and branches of lumbar plexus
Branches of lumbar plexus and femoral nerve
Femoral nerve
Femoral and obturator nerves
Obturator nerve
Branches of sacral plexus
Tibial division of sciatic nerve or tibial nerve
Superior gluteal nerve
Inferior gluteal nerve
Pudendal nerve

241 Muscle attachments to the right hip bone

The colors indicate the innervation of the muscles attaching to the

a outer surface

b inner surface.

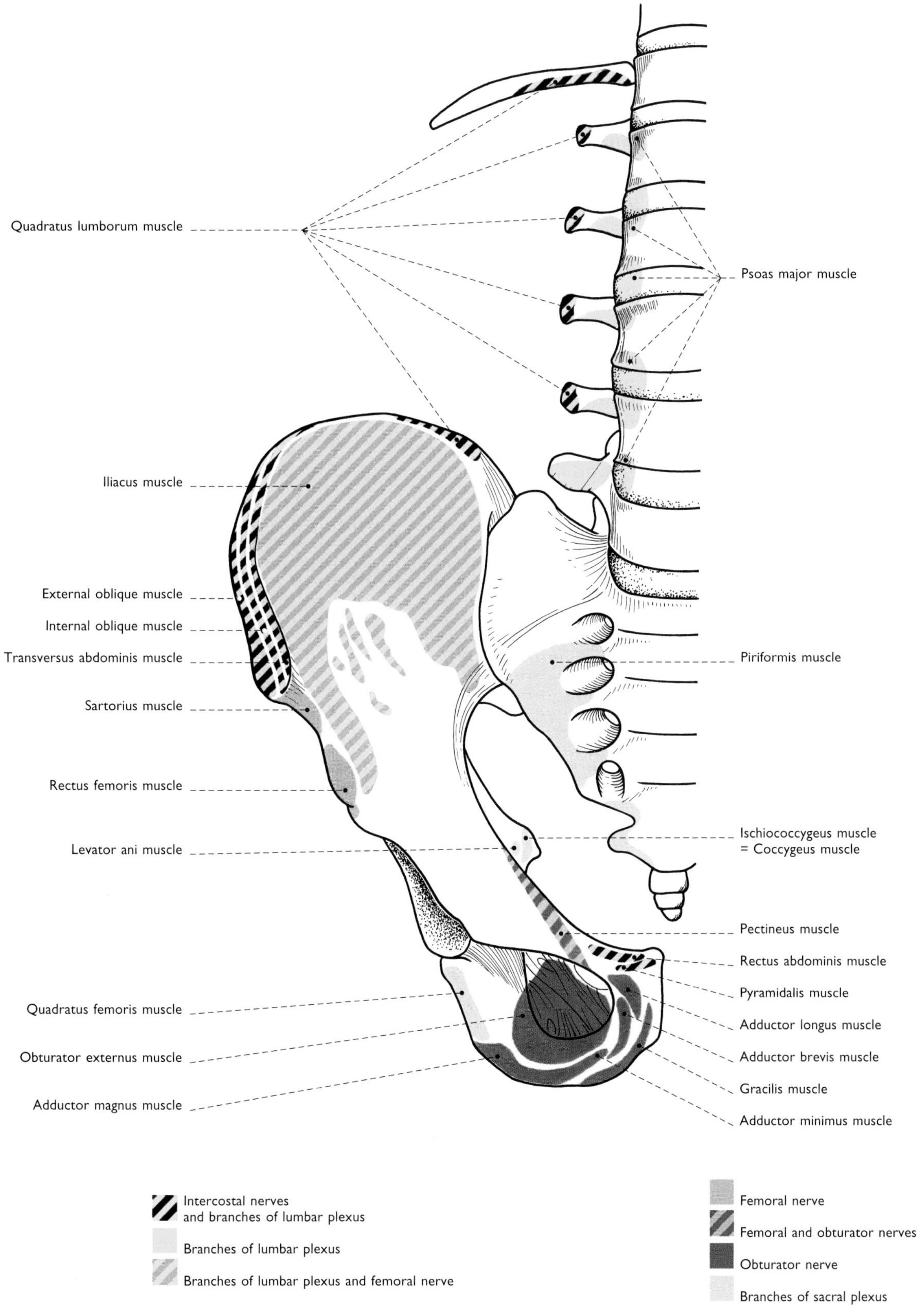
Quadratus lumborum muscle
Psoas major muscle
Iliacus muscle
External oblique muscle
Internal oblique muscle
Transversus abdominis muscle
Piriformis muscle
Sartorius muscle
Rectus femoris muscle
Ischiococcygeus muscle = Coccygeus muscle
Levator ani muscle
Pectineus muscle
Rectus abdominis muscle
Pyramidalis muscle
Quadratus femoris muscle
Adductor longus muscle
Obturator externus muscle
Adductor brevis muscle
Gracilis muscle
Adductor magnus muscle
Adductor minimus muscle
Intercostal nerves and branches of lumbar plexus
Branches of lumbar plexus
Branches of lumbar plexus and femoral nerve
Femoral nerve
Femoral and obturator nerves
Obturator nerve
Branches of sacral plexus

242 Muscle attachments to the lumbar spine and the pelvic girdle on the right side

The colors indicate the innervation.
Ventral aspect

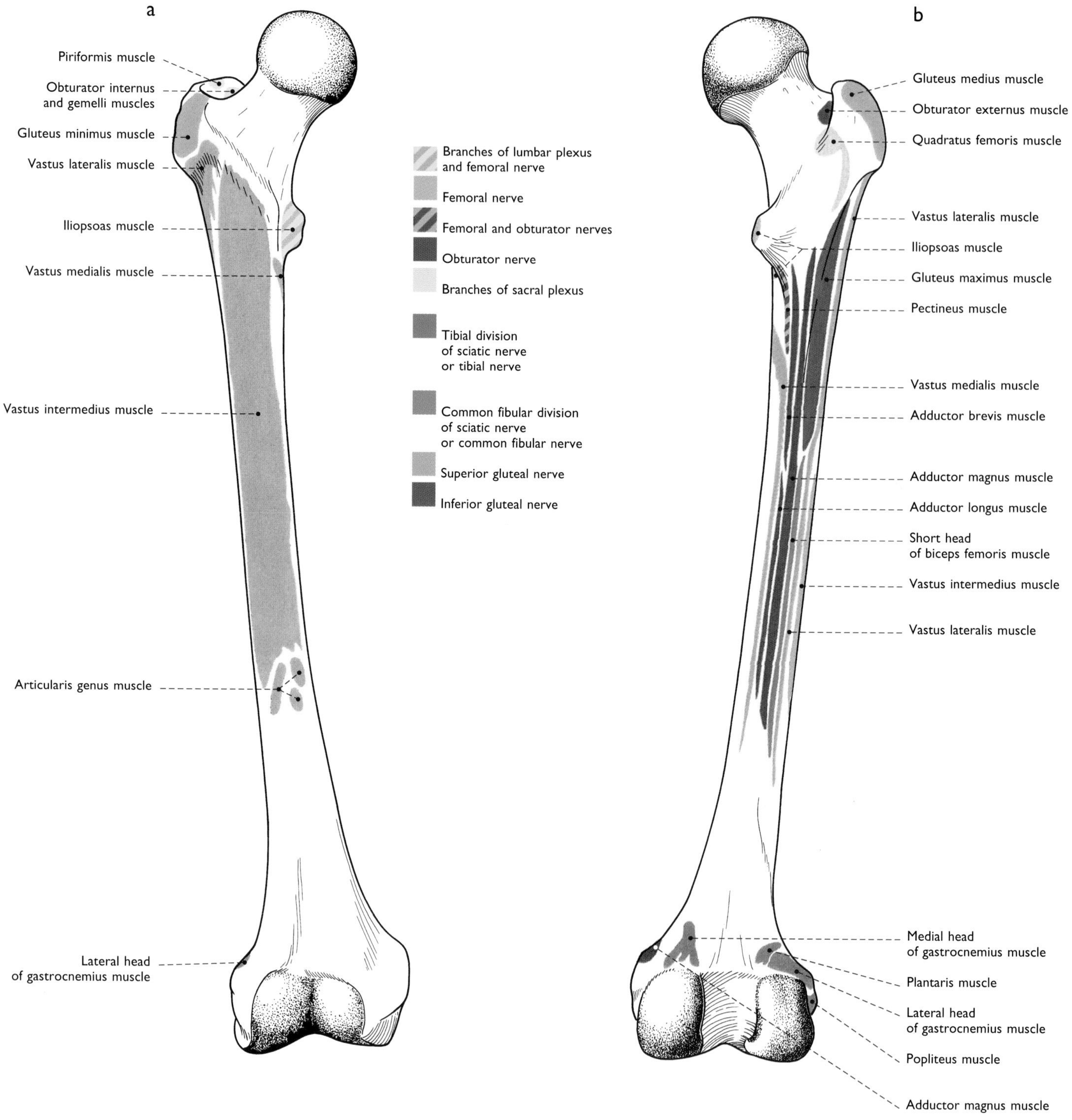
a
Piriformis muscle
Obturator internus and gemelli muscles
Gluteus minimus muscle
Vastus lateralis muscle
Iliopsoas muscle
Vastus medialis muscle
Vastus intermedius muscle
Articularis genus muscle
Lateral head of gastrocnemius muscle
Branches of lumbar plexus and femoral nerve
Femoral nerve
Femoral and obturator nerves
Obturator nerve
Branches of sacral plexus
Tibial division of sciatic nerve or tibial nerve
Common fibular division of sciatic nerve or common fibular nerve
Superior gluteal nerve
Inferior gluteal nerve
b
Gluteus medius muscle
Obturator externus muscle
Quadratus femoris muscle
Vastus lateralis muscle
Iliopsoas muscle
Gluteus maximus muscle
Pectineus muscle
Vastus medialis muscle
Adductor brevis muscle
Adductor magnus muscle
Adductor longus muscle
Short head of biceps femoris muscle
Vastus intermedius muscle
Vastus lateralis muscle
Medial head of gastrocnemius muscle
Plantaris muscle
Lateral head of gastrocnemius muscle
Popliteus muscle
Adductor magnus muscle

243 Muscle attachments to the right thigh bone (= femur)

The colors indicate the innervation of the muscles attaching to the

a ventral surface
b dorsal surface.

a

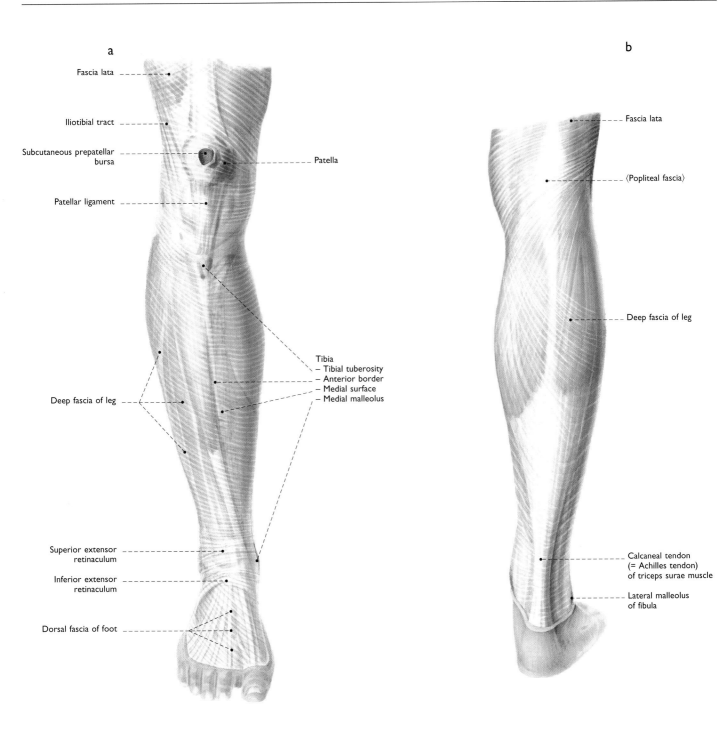

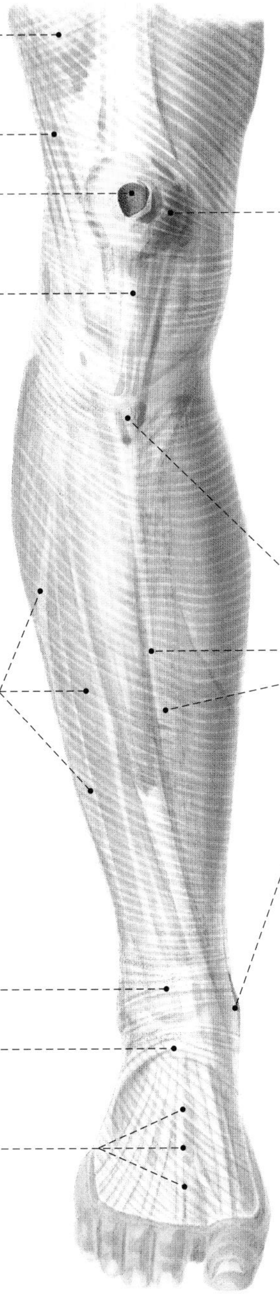
Fascia lata
Iliotibial tract
Subcutaneous prepatellar bursa
Patella
Patellar ligament
Tibia
– Tibial tuberosity
– Anterior border
– Medial surface
– Medial malleolus
Deep fascia of leg
Superior extensor retinaculum
Inferior extensor retinaculum
Dorsal fascia of foot

b

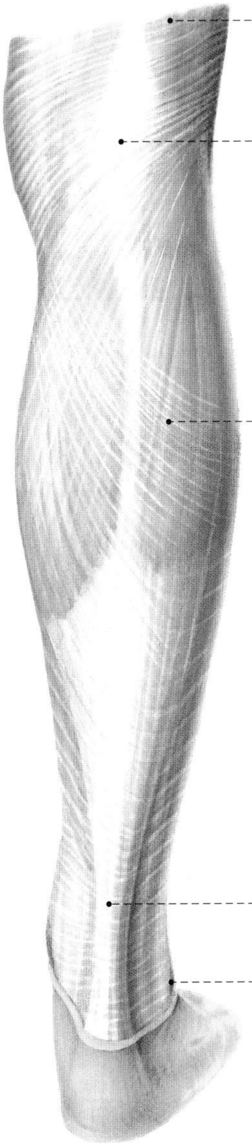
Fascia lata
⟨Popliteal fascia⟩
Deep fascia of leg
Calcaneal tendon
(= Achilles tendon)
of triceps surae muscle
Lateral malleolus
of fibula

244 Fasciae of the right leg and the dorsum of foot (25%)

a Ventral aspect
b Dorsal aspect

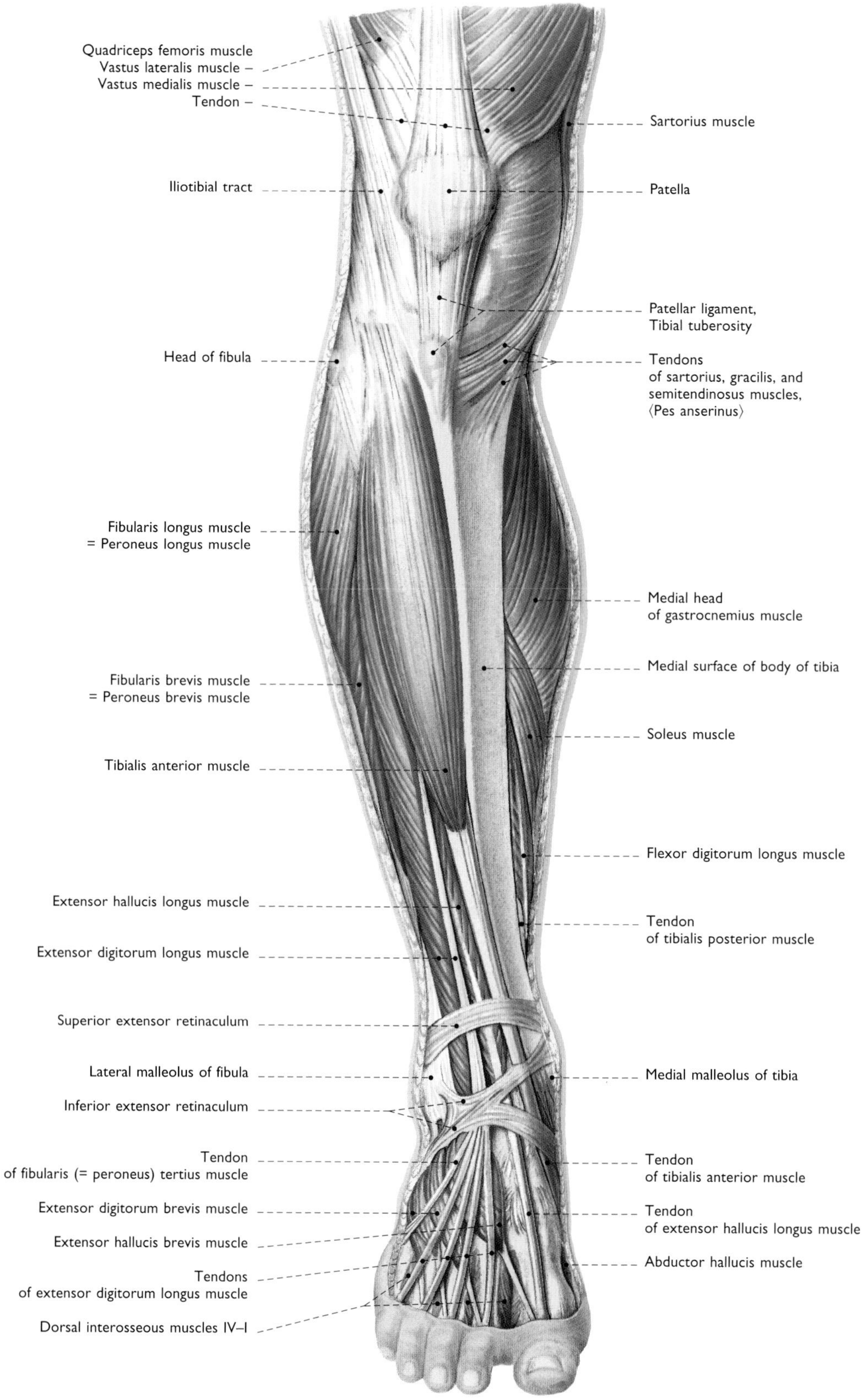
Quadriceps femoris muscle
Vastus lateralis muscle –
Vastus medialis muscle –
Tendon –
Sartorius muscle
Iliotibial tract
Patella
Patellar ligament,
Tibial tuberosity
Head of fibula
Tendons
of sartorius, gracilis, and
semitendinosus muscles,
⟨Pes anserinus⟩
Fibularis longus muscle
= Peroneus longus muscle
Medial head
of gastrocnemius muscle
Medial surface of body of tibia
Fibularis brevis muscle
= Peroneus brevis muscle
Soleus muscle
Tibialis anterior muscle
Flexor digitorum longus muscle
Extensor hallucis longus muscle
Tendon
of tibialis posterior muscle
Extensor digitorum longus muscle
Superior extensor retinaculum
Lateral malleolus of fibula
Medial malleolus of tibia
Inferior extensor retinaculum
Tendon
of fibularis (= peroneus) tertius muscle
Tendon
of tibialis anterior muscle
Extensor digitorum brevis muscle
Tendon
of extensor hallucis longus muscle
Extensor hallucis brevis muscle
Abductor hallucis muscle
Tendons
of extensor digitorum longus muscle
Dorsal interosseous muscles IV–I

245 Muscles of the right leg and the dorsum of foot (30%)

Ventral aspect

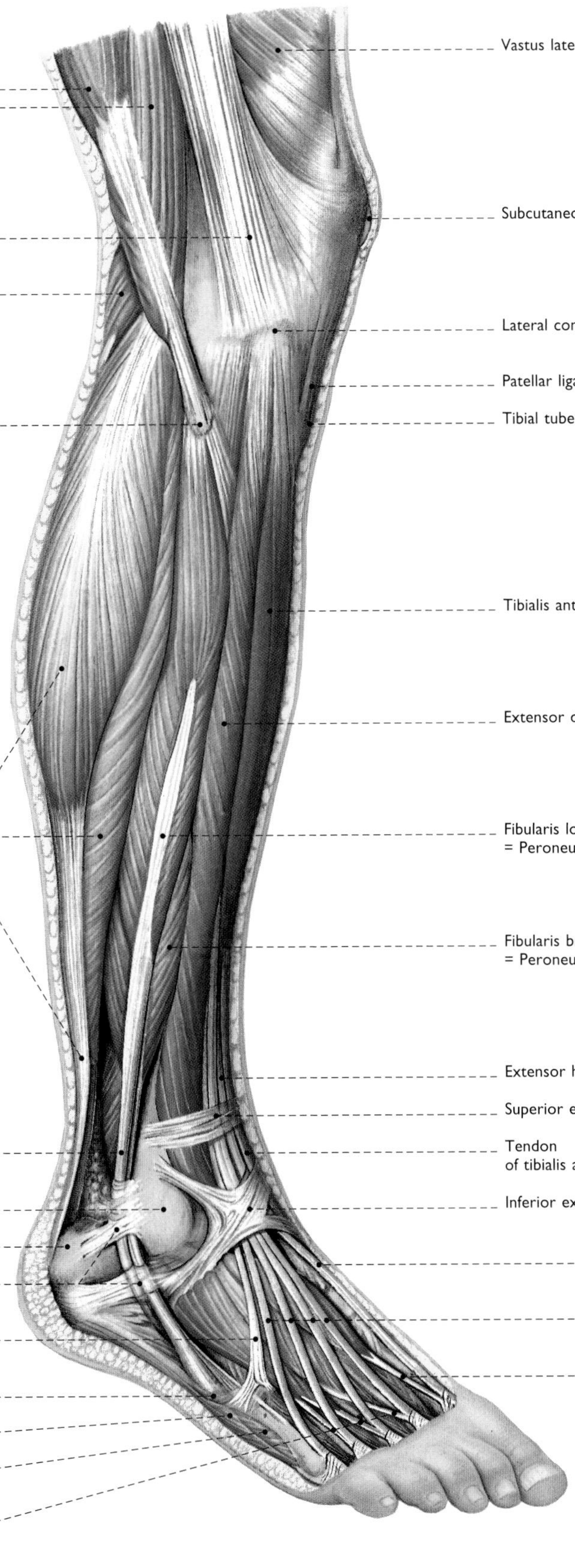
Biceps femoris muscle
Long head –
Short head –
Iliotibial tract
Semimembranosus muscle
Head of fibula
Triceps surae muscle
Lateral head
of gastrocnemius muscle –
Soleus muscle –
Calcaneal tendon
(= Achilles tendon) –
Tendon
of fibularis (= peroneus) longus muscle
Lateral malleolus of fibula
Calcaneal tuberosity
Superior and inferior
fibular (= peroneal) retinacula
Tendon
of fibularis (= peroneus) tertius muscle
Tuberosity of 5th metatarsal bone
Abductor digiti minimi muscle
(Opponens digiti minimi muscle)
Tendons
of extensor digitorum brevis muscle
Vastus lateralis muscle
Subcutaneous prepatellar bursa
Lateral condyle of tibia
Patellar ligament
Tibial tuberosity
Tibialis anterior muscle
Extensor digitorum longus muscle
Fibularis longus muscle
= Peroneus longus muscle
Fibularis brevis muscle
= Peroneus brevis muscle
Extensor hallucis longus muscle
Superior extensor retinaculum
Tendon
of tibialis anterior muscle
Inferior extensor retinaculum
Tendon
of extensor hallucis longus muscle
Tendons
of extensor digitorum longus muscle
Tendon
of extensor hallucis brevis muscle

246 Muscles of the right leg and the dorsum of foot (30%)

Lateral aspect

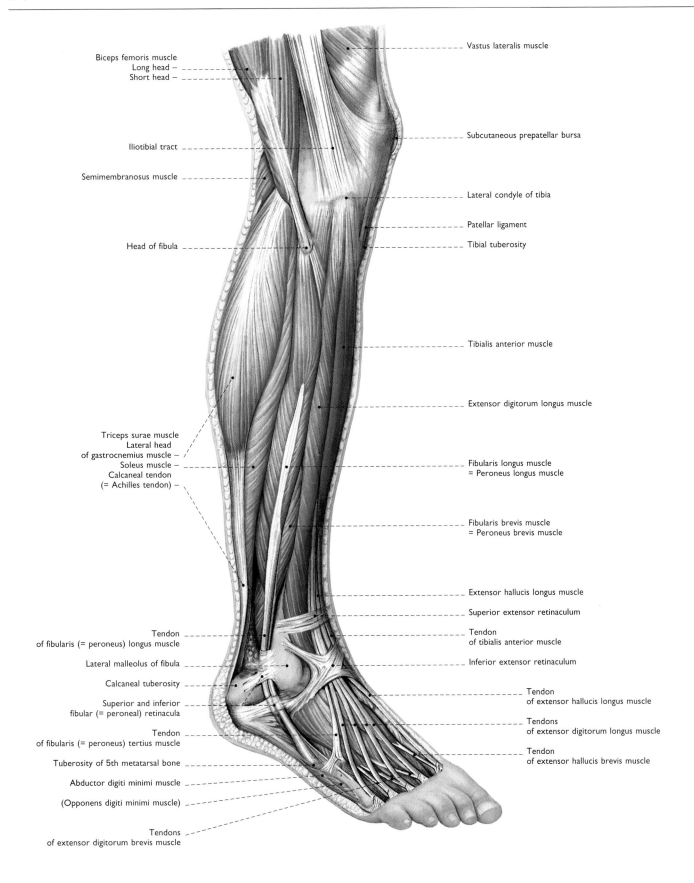

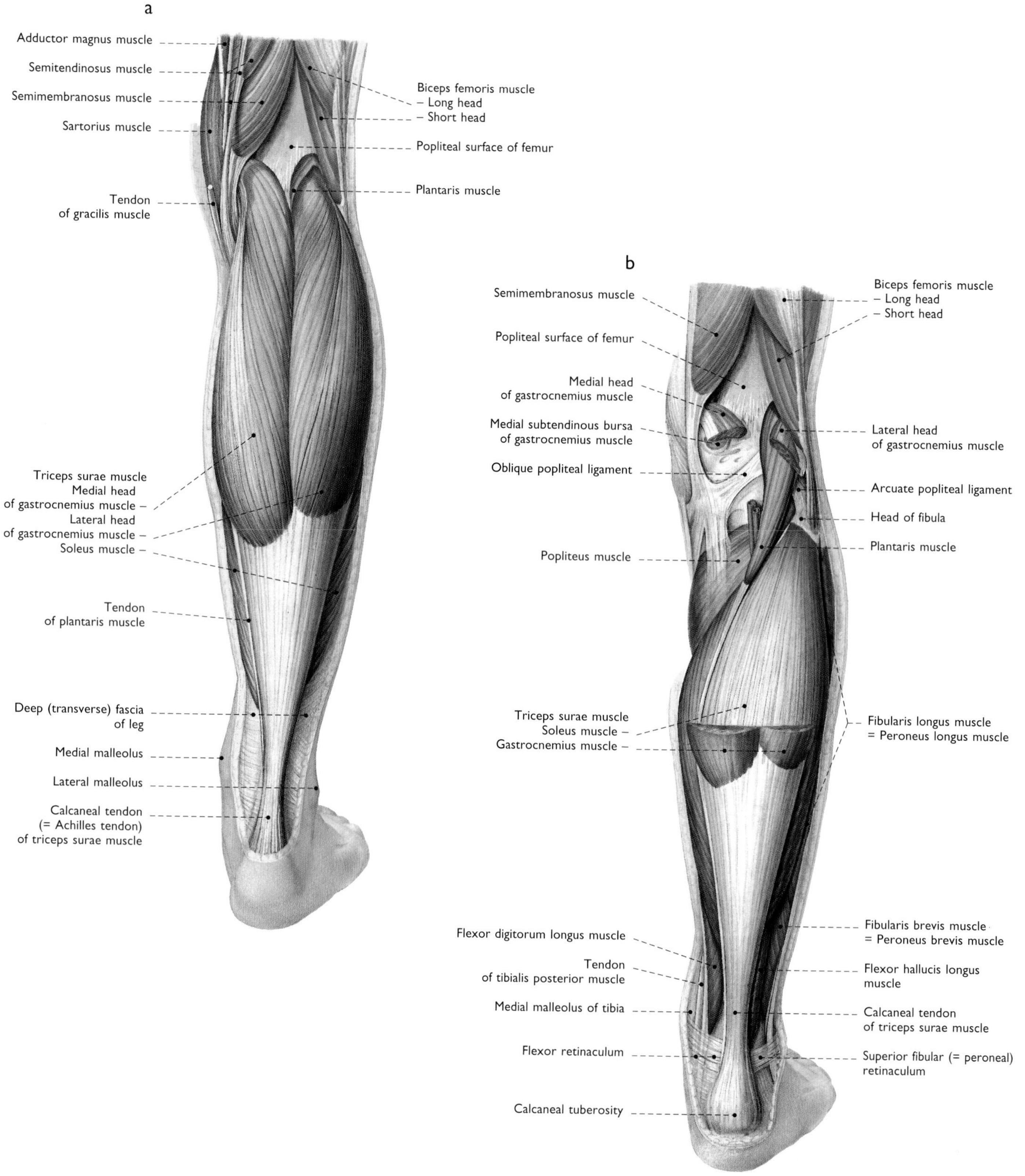
a
Adductor magnus muscle
Semitendinosus muscle
Semimembranosus muscle
Sartorius muscle
Tendon of gracilis muscle
Biceps femoris muscle
– Long head
– Short head
Popliteal surface of femur
Plantaris muscle
Triceps surae muscle
Medial head of gastrocnemius muscle –
Lateral head of gastrocnemius muscle –
Soleus muscle –
Tendon of plantaris muscle
Deep (transverse) fascia of leg
Medial malleolus
Lateral malleolus
Calcaneal tendon (= Achilles tendon) of triceps surae muscle
b
Semimembranosus muscle
Popliteal surface of femur
Medial head of gastrocnemius muscle
Medial subtendinous bursa of gastrocnemius muscle
Oblique popliteal ligament
Popliteus muscle
Biceps femoris muscle
– Long head
– Short head
Lateral head of gastrocnemius muscle
Arcuate popliteal ligament
Head of fibula
Plantaris muscle
Triceps surae muscle
Soleus muscle –
Gastrocnemius muscle –
Fibularis longus muscle = Peroneus longus muscle
Flexor digitorum longus muscle
Tendon of tibialis posterior muscle
Medial malleolus of tibia
Flexor retinaculum
Calcaneal tuberosity
Fibularis brevis muscle = Peroneus brevis muscle
Flexor hallucis longus muscle
Calcaneal tendon of triceps surae muscle
Superior fibular (= peroneal) retinaculum

247 Muscles of the right leg (25%)

Dorsal aspect

a Most superficial layer

b Superficial layer after partial removal of the gastrocnemius muscle

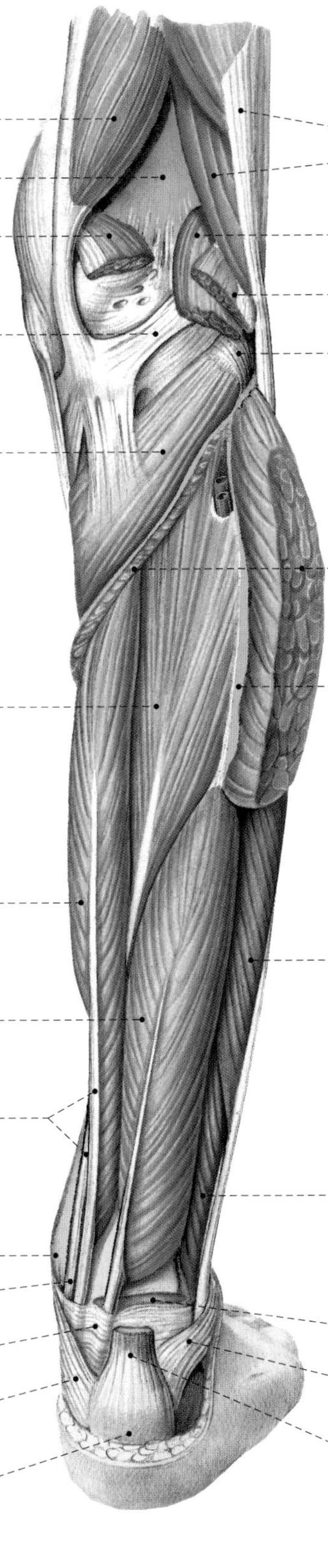
Semimembranosus muscle
Popliteal surface of femur
Medial head
of gastrocnemius muscle
Oblique popliteal ligament
Popliteus muscle
Tibialis posterior muscle
Flexor digitorum longus muscle
Flexor hallucis longus muscle
⟨Crural chiasm⟩
Medial malleolus of tibia
Tendon
of tibialis posterior muscle
Flexor retinaculum
Deep (transverse) fascia of leg
Calcaneal tuberosity
Biceps femoris muscle
– Long head
– Short head
Plantaris muscle
Lateral head
of gastrocnemius muscle
Arcuate popliteal ligament
Soleus muscle
(cut surfaces)
Posterior surface of body of tibia
Fibularis longus muscle
= Peroneus longus muscle
Fibularis brevis muscle
= Peroneus brevis muscle
Ankle joint
⟨= Talocrural joint⟩
Superior fibular (= peroneal) retinaculum
Calcaneal tendon
(= Achilles tendon)
of triceps surae muscle

248 Muscles of the right leg (30%)

Deep layer, dorsal aspect

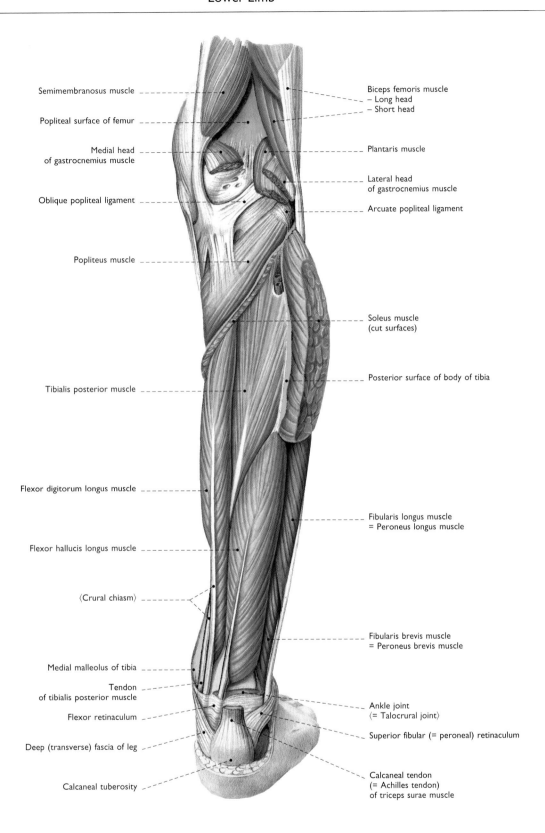

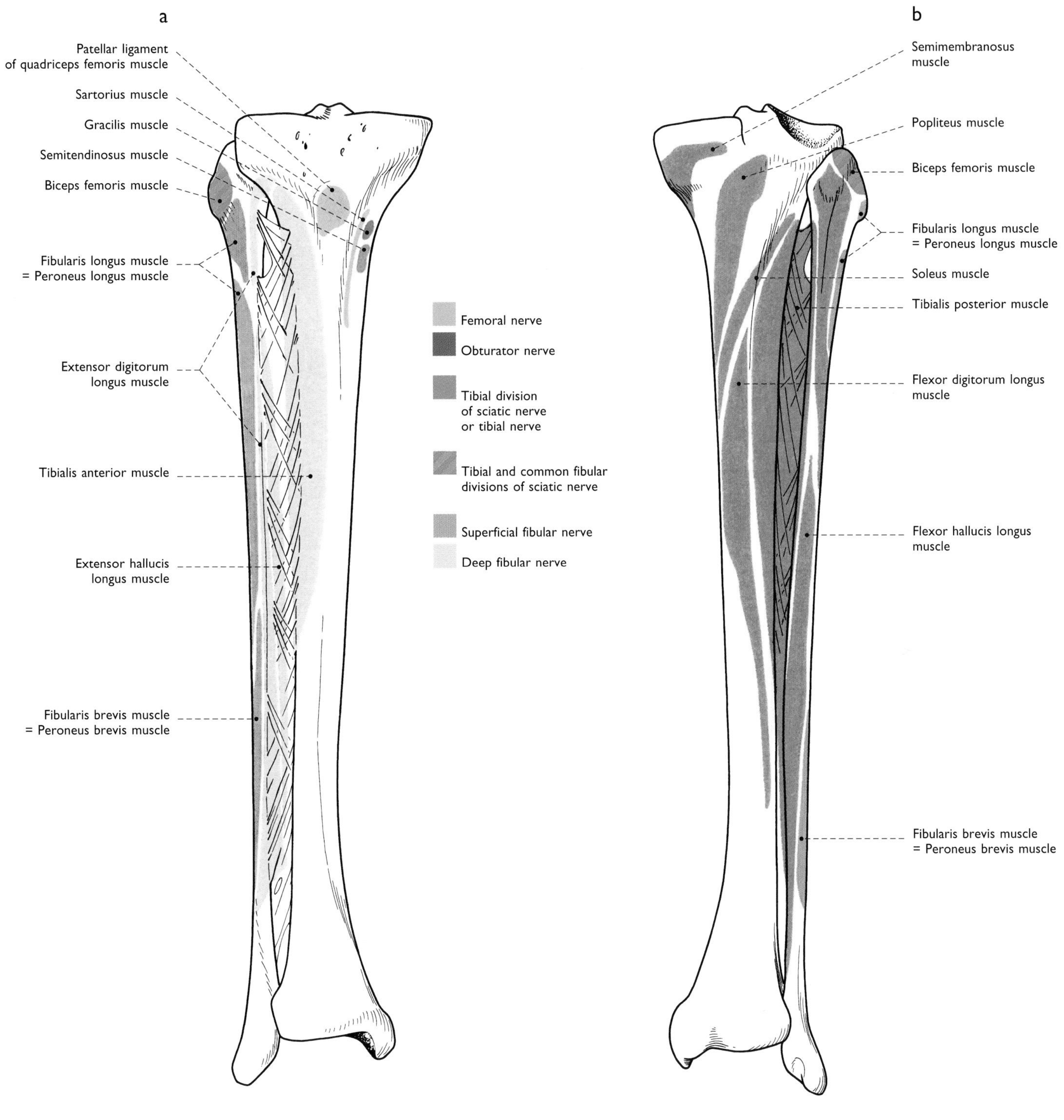
a
Patellar ligament of quadriceps femoris muscle
Sartorius muscle
Gracilis muscle
Semitendinosus muscle
Biceps femoris muscle
Fibularis longus muscle = Peroneus longus muscle
Extensor digitorum longus muscle
Tibialis anterior muscle
Extensor hallucis longus muscle
Fibularis brevis muscle = Peroneus brevis muscle
Femoral nerve
Obturator nerve
Tibial division of sciatic nerve or tibial nerve
Tibial and common fibular divisions of sciatic nerve
Superficial fibular nerve
Deep fibular nerve
b
Semimembranosus muscle
Popliteus muscle
Biceps femoris muscle
Fibularis longus muscle = Peroneus longus muscle
Soleus muscle
Tibialis posterior muscle
Flexor digitorum longus muscle
Flexor hallucis longus muscle
Fibularis brevis muscle = Peroneus brevis muscle

249 Muscle attachments to the right tibia, fibula, and the interosseous membrane of leg

The colors indicate the innervation of the muscles attaching to the

a ventral surface

b dorsal surface.

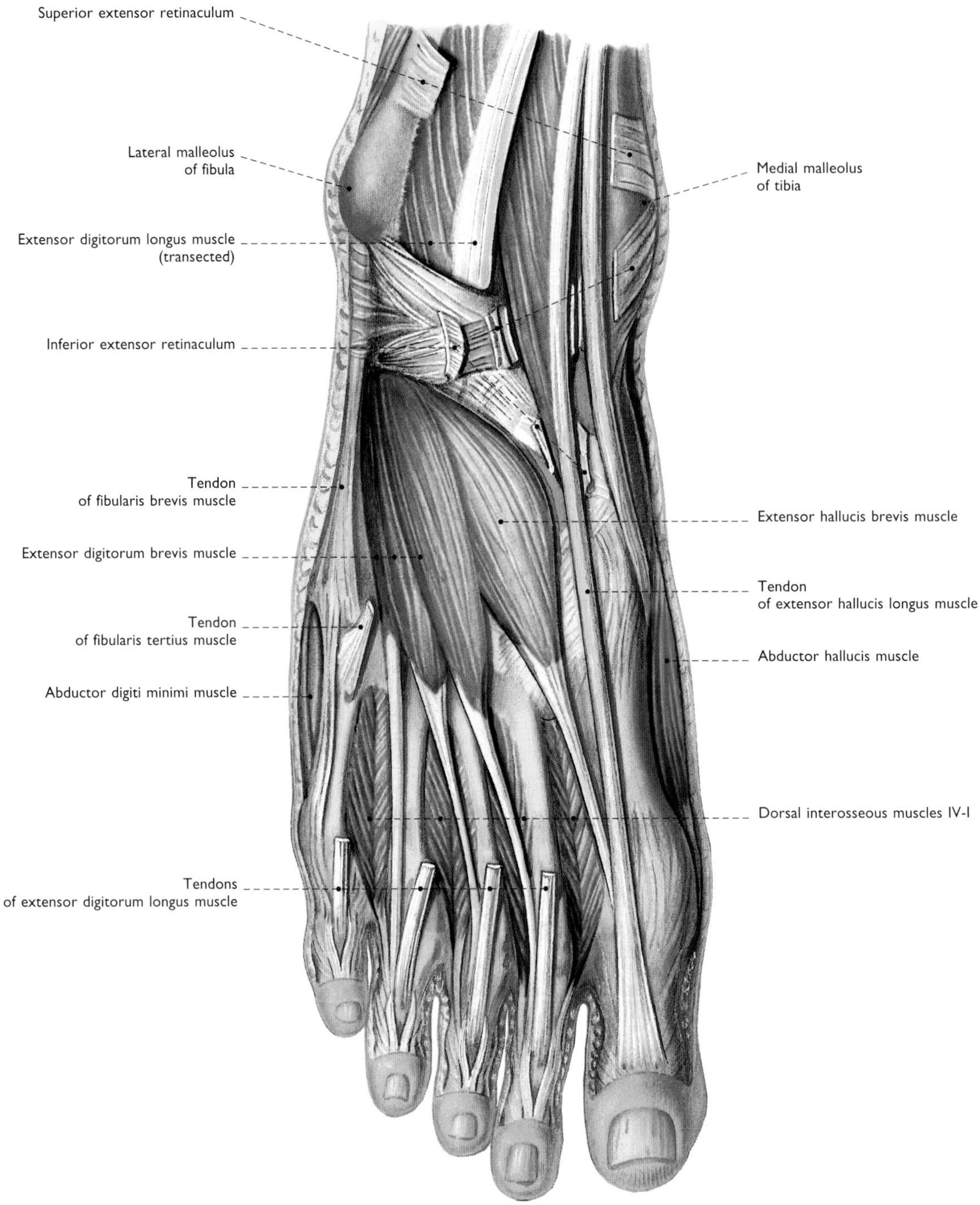
Superior extensor retinaculum
Lateral malleolus of fibula
Extensor digitorum longus muscle (transected)
Inferior extensor retinaculum
Tendon of fibularis brevis muscle
Extensor digitorum brevis muscle
Tendon of fibularis tertius muscle
Abductor digiti minimi muscle
Tendons of extensor digitorum longus muscle
Medial malleolus of tibia
Extensor hallucis brevis muscle
Tendon of extensor hallucis longus muscle
Abductor hallucis muscle
Dorsal interosseous muscles IV-I

250 Muscles of the dorsum of the right foot (75%)

The extensor digitorum longus muscle and the extensor retinacula were partially removed. Ventral aspect

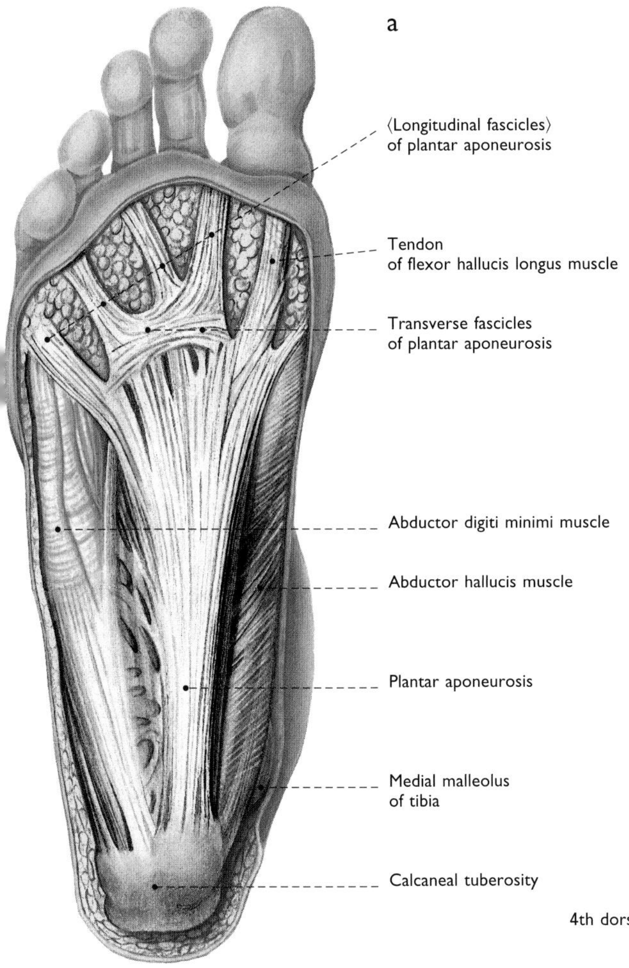
a
⟨Longitudinal fascicles⟩ of plantar aponeurosis
Tendon of flexor hallucis longus muscle
Transverse fascicles of plantar aponeurosis
Abductor digiti minimi muscle
Abductor hallucis muscle
Plantar aponeurosis
Medial malleolus of tibia
Calcaneal tuberosity

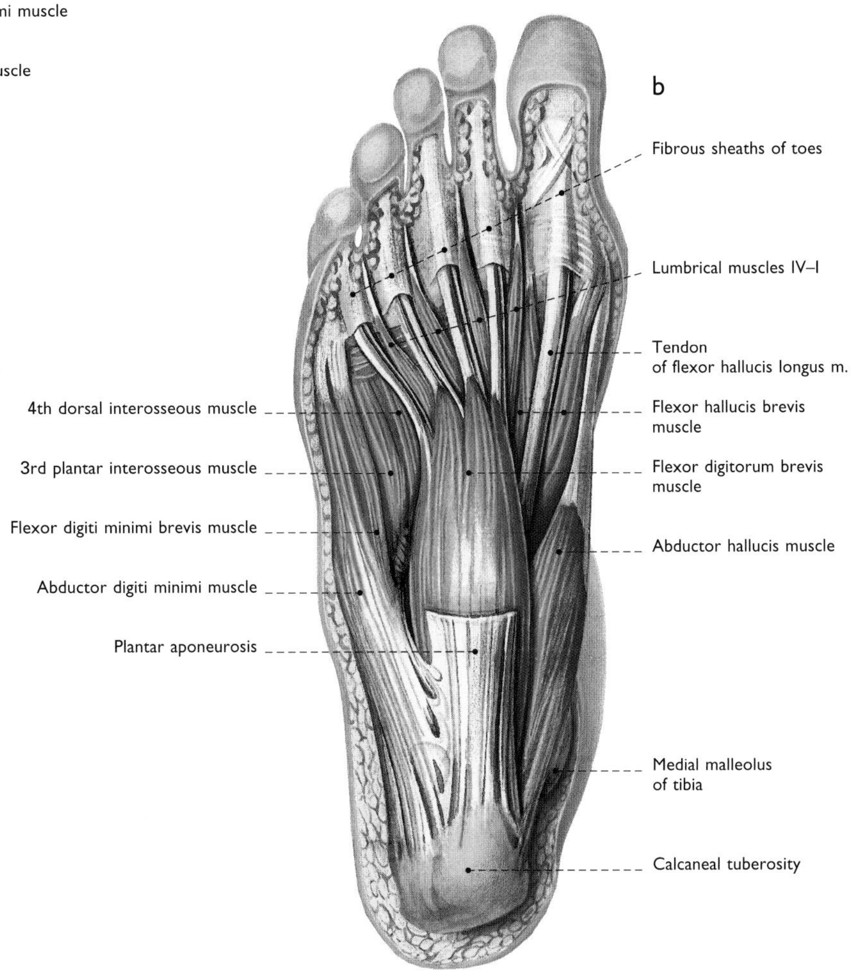
b
Fibrous sheaths of toes
Lumbrical muscles IV–I
Tendon of flexor hallucis longus m.
4th dorsal interosseous muscle
Flexor hallucis brevis muscle
3rd plantar interosseous muscle
Flexor digitorum brevis muscle
Flexor digiti minimi brevis muscle
Abductor hallucis muscle
Abductor digiti minimi muscle
Plantar aponeurosis
Medial malleolus of tibia
Calcaneal tuberosity

251 Muscles of the sole of the right foot (50%)

Plantar aspect

a Plantar aponeurosis and superficial muscles

b Superficial layer after partial removal of the plantar aponeurosis

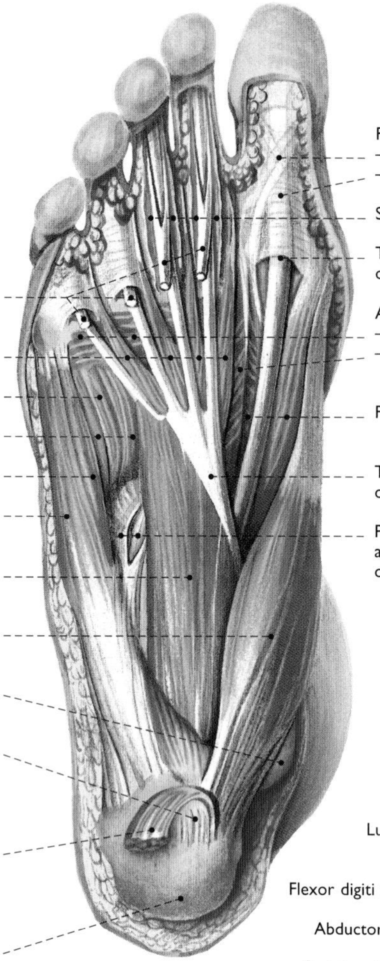
a
Fibrous sheath of great toe
– Cruciform part
– Anular part
Synovial sheaths of toes
Tendon
of flexor hallucis longus muscle
Adductor hallucis muscle
– Transverse head
– Oblique head
Flexor hallucis brevis muscle
Tendon
of flexor digitorum longus muscle
Plantar tendinous sheath
and tendon
of fibularis longus muscle
Tendons
of flexor digitorum brevis muscle
Lumbrical muscles IV–I
4th dorsal interosseous muscle
3rd + 2nd plantar interosseous mm.
Flexor digiti minimi brevis muscle
Abductor digiti minimi muscle
Quadratus plantae muscle
= Flexor accessorius muscle
Abductor hallucis muscle
Medial malleolus
of tibia
Plantar aponeurosis
(cut and retracted)
Flexor digitorum brevis
muscle
(cut and retracted)
Calcaneal tuberosity

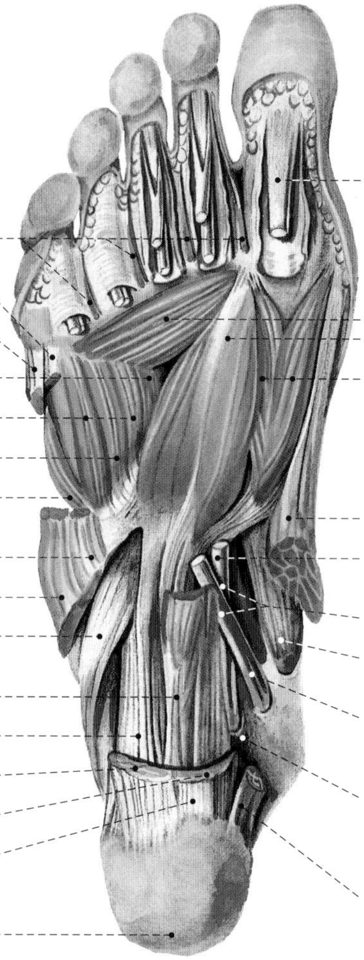
b
Tendon
of flexor hallucis longus musc
Adductor hallucis muscle
– Transverse head
– Oblique head
Flexor hallucis brevis muscle
Abductor hallucis muscle
Tendon
of flexor hallucis longus muscle
⟨Plantar chiasm⟩
Tendon
of tibialis posterior muscle
Tendon
of flexor digitorum longus m.
Flexor retinaculum
Abductor hallucis muscle
Lumbrical muscles IV–I
Flexor digiti minimi brevis muscle
Abductor digiti minimi muscle
3rd dorsal interosseous muscle
3rd and 2nd plantar interosseous muscles
4th dorsal interosseous muscle
(Opponens digiti minimi muscle)
Flexor digiti minimi brevis muscle
Abductor digiti minimi muscle
Tendon
of fibularis longus muscle
Quadratus plantae muscle
Long plantar ligament
Abductor digiti minimi muscle
Flexor digitorum brevis muscle
Plantar aponeurosis
Calcaneal tuberosity

252 Muscles of the sole of the right foot (50%)

Plantar aspect

a Deep layer after partial removal of the plantar aponeurosis and the flexor digitorum brevis muscle

b Deepest layer after extensive removal of the muscles of the superficial and deep layers

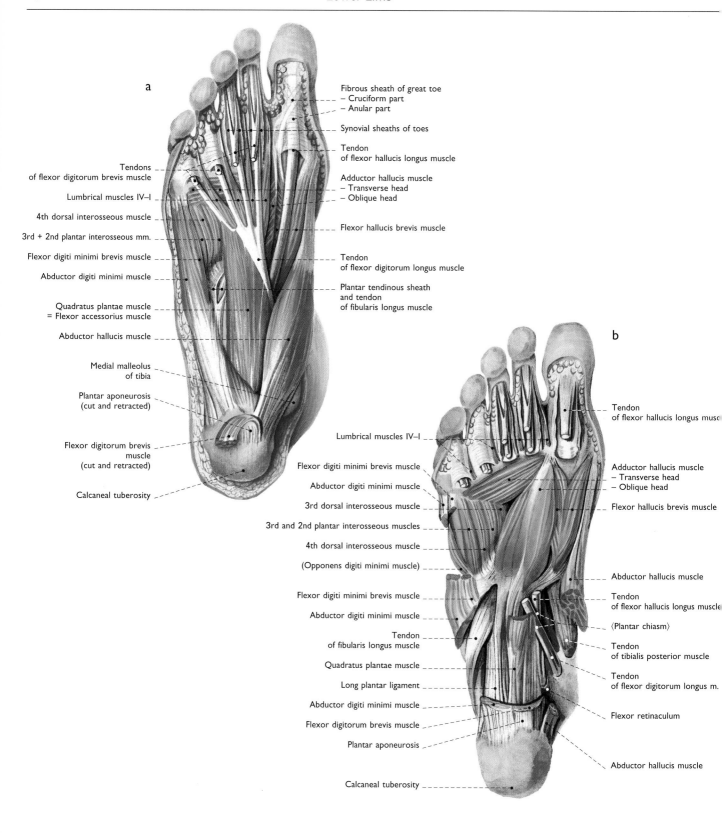

a

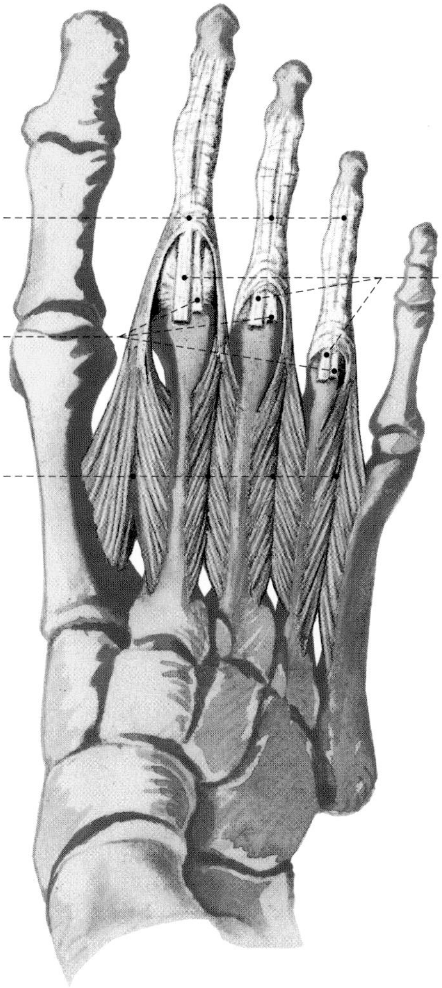
⟨Dorsal digital expansions⟩
Tendons
of extensor digitorum longus muscle
Tendons
of extensor digitorum brevis
muscle
Dorsal interosseous muscles I–IV

b

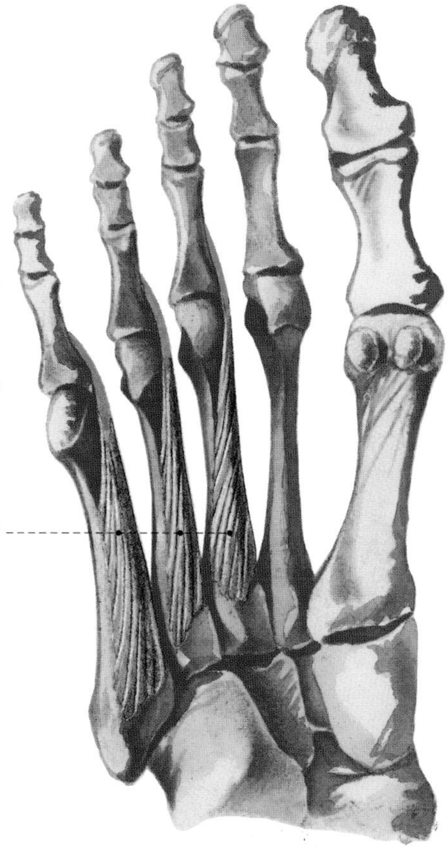
Plantar interosseous muscles III–I

253 Interosseous muscles of the right foot (75%)

a Dorsal interosseous muscles, dorsal aspect
b Plantar interosseous muscles, plantar aspect

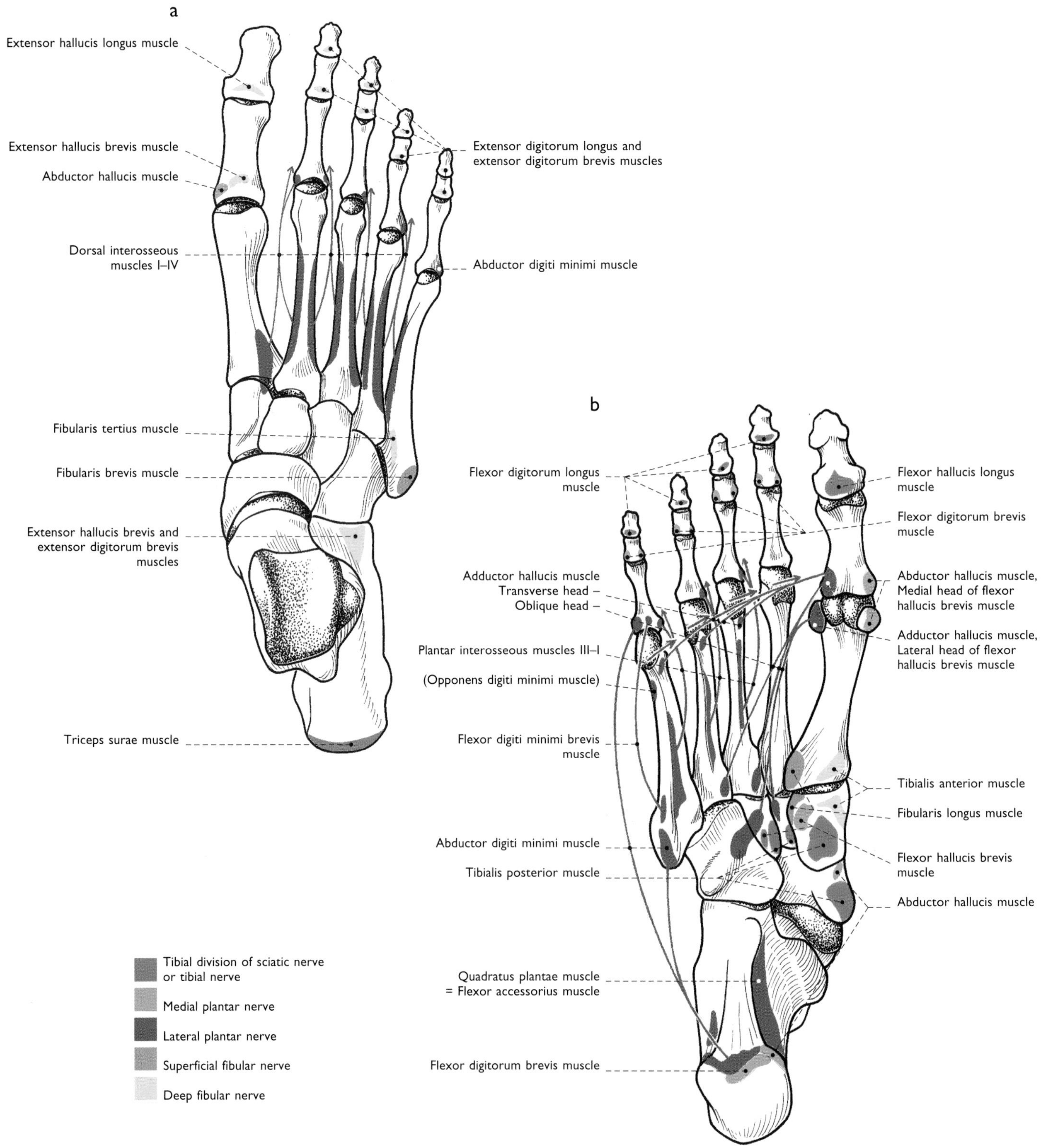
a
Extensor hallucis longus muscle
Extensor hallucis brevis muscle
Abductor hallucis muscle
Dorsal interosseous muscles I–IV
Fibularis tertius muscle
Fibularis brevis muscle
Extensor hallucis brevis and extensor digitorum brevis muscles
Triceps surae muscle
Extensor digitorum longus and extensor digitorum brevis muscles
Abductor digiti minimi muscle
b
Flexor digitorum longus muscle
Adductor hallucis muscle
Transverse head –
Oblique head –
Plantar interosseous muscles III–I
(Opponens digiti minimi muscle)
Flexor digiti minimi brevis muscle
Abductor digiti minimi muscle
Tibialis posterior muscle
Quadratus plantae muscle = Flexor accessorius muscle
Flexor digitorum brevis muscle
Flexor hallucis longus muscle
Flexor digitorum brevis muscle
Abductor hallucis muscle, Medial head of flexor hallucis brevis muscle
Adductor hallucis muscle, Lateral head of flexor hallucis brevis muscle
Tibialis anterior muscle
Fibularis longus muscle
Flexor hallucis brevis muscle
Abductor hallucis muscle
Tibial division of sciatic nerve or tibial nerve
Medial plantar nerve
Lateral plantar nerve
Superficial fibular nerve
Deep fibular nerve

254 Muscle attachments to the bones of the right foot

The colors indicate the innervation of the muscles attaching to the

a dorsal surface

b plantar surface.

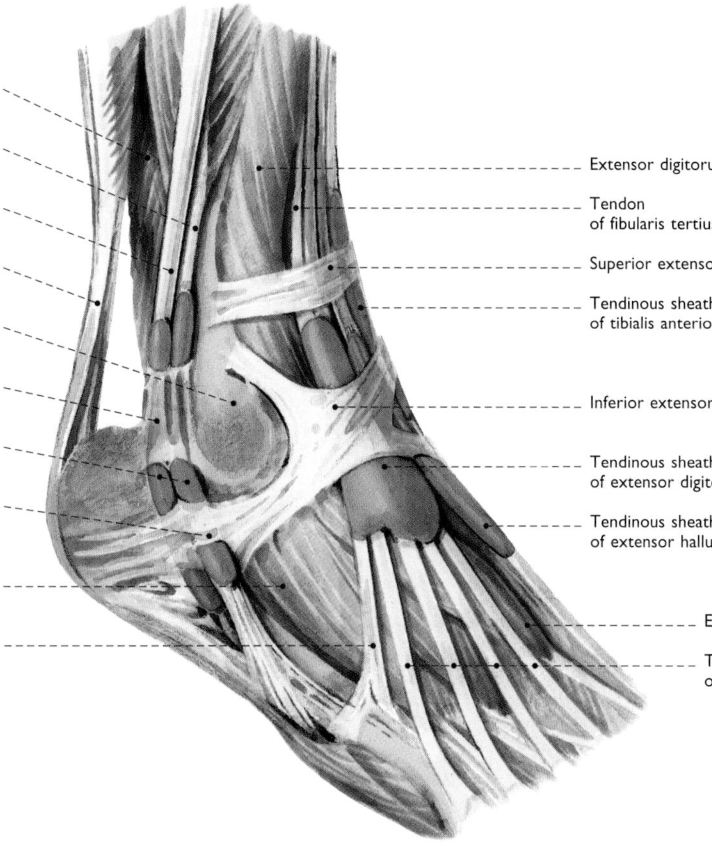
a
Flexor hallucis longus muscle
Tendon of fibularis brevis muscle
Tendon of fibularis longus muscle
Calcaneal tendon (= Achilles tendon) of triceps surae muscle
Lateral malleolus of fibula
Superior fibular (= peroneal) retinaculum
Common tendinous sheath of fibulares muscles
Inferior fibular (= peroneal) retinaculum
Extensor digitorum brevis muscle
Tendon of fibularis tertius muscle
Extensor digitorum longus muscle
Tendon of fibularis tertius muscle
Superior extensor retinaculum
Tendinous sheath of tibialis anterior muscle
Inferior extensor retinaculum
Tendinous sheath of extensor digitorum longus muscle
Tendinous sheath of extensor hallucis longus muscle
Extensor hallucis brevis muscle
Tendons of extensor digitorum longus muscle

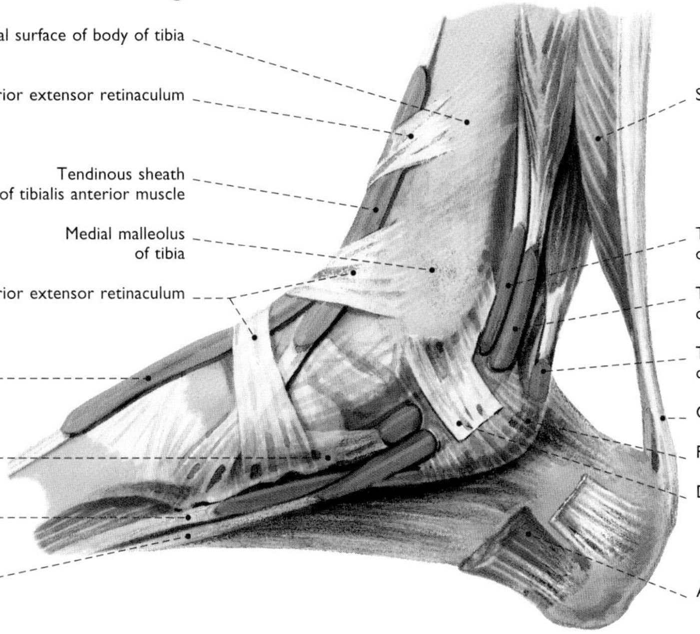
b
Medial surface of body of tibia
Superior extensor retinaculum
Tendinous sheath of tibialis anterior muscle
Medial malleolus of tibia
Inferior extensor retinaculum
Tedinous sheath of extensor hallucis longus muscle
Tendon of tibialis posterior muscle
Tendon of flexor hallucis longus muscle
Tendon of flexor digitorum longus muscle
Soleus muscle
Tendinous sheath of tibialis posterior muscle
Tendinous sheath of flexor digitorum longus muscle
Tendinous sheath of flexor hallucis longus muscle
Calcaneal tendon (= Achilles tendon)
Flexor retinaculum
Deep fascia of leg
Abductor hallucis muscle

255 Tarsal tendinous sheaths of the right foot (50%)

a Lateral aspect
b Medial aspect

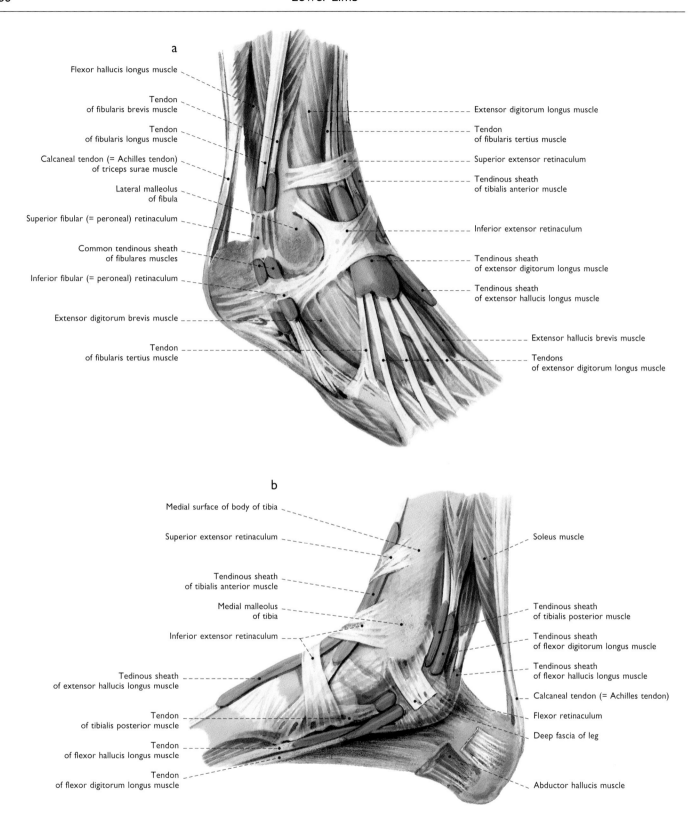

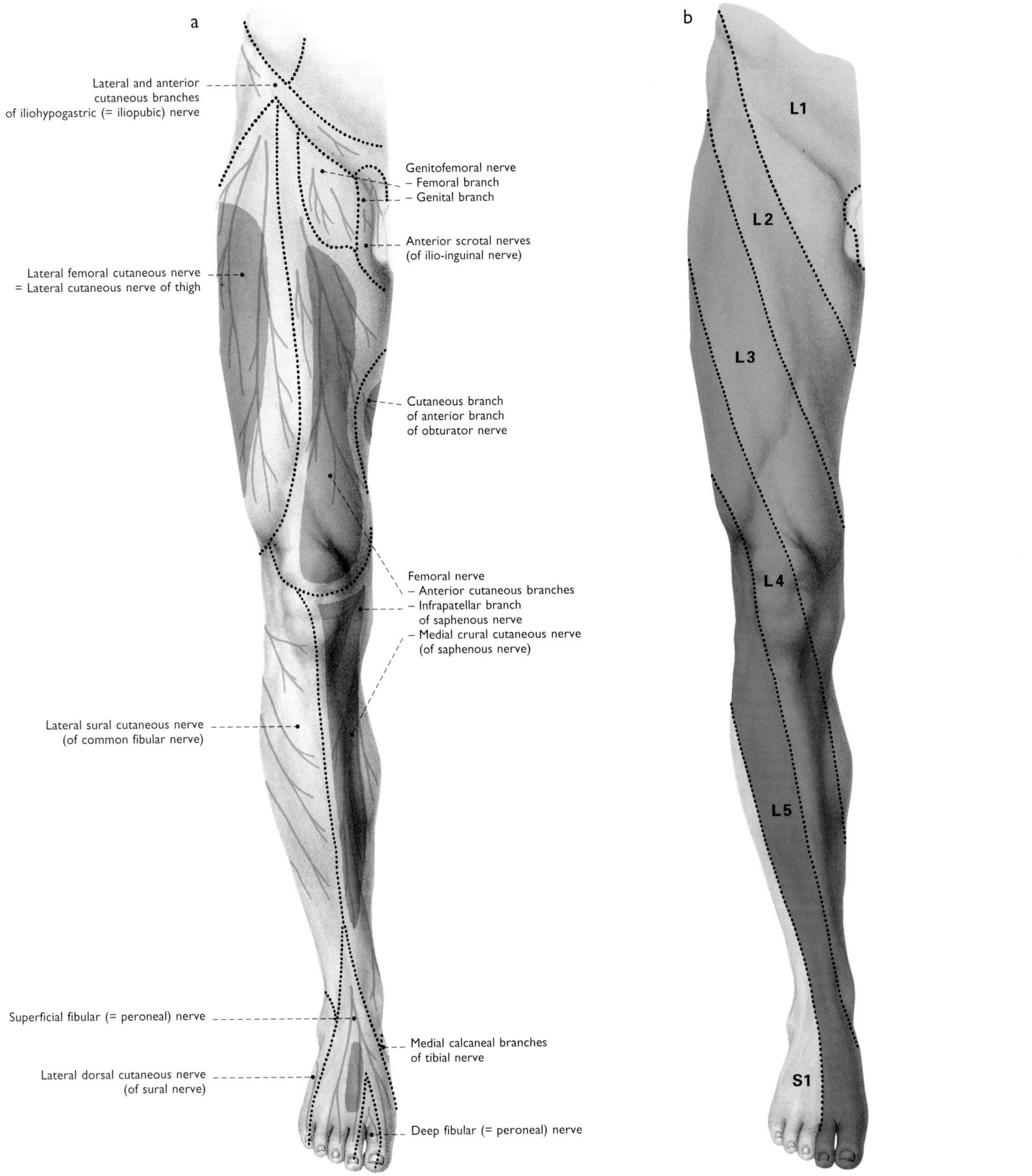
a
Lateral and anterior cutaneous branches of iliohypogastric (= iliopubic) nerve
Genitofemoral nerve
– Femoral branch
– Genital branch
Anterior scrotal nerves (of ilio-inguinal nerve)
Lateral femoral cutaneous nerve = Lateral cutaneous nerve of thigh
Cutaneous branch of anterior branch of obturator nerve
Femoral nerve
– Anterior cutaneous branches
– Infrapatellar branch of saphenous nerve
– Medial crural cutaneous nerve (of saphenous nerve)
Lateral sural cutaneous nerve (of common fibular nerve)
Superficial fibular (= peroneal) nerve
Medial calcaneal branches of tibial nerve
Lateral dorsal cutaneous nerve (of sural nerve)
Deep fibular (= peroneal) nerve
b
L1
L2
L3
L4
L5
S1

256 Cutaneous and segmental innervation of the right lower limb (20%)

Schematic representations, ventral aspect

a Cutaneous nerves and areas of distribution, the autonomic areas of the different nerves are given in a darker gray.

b Segmental innervation (dermatomes)

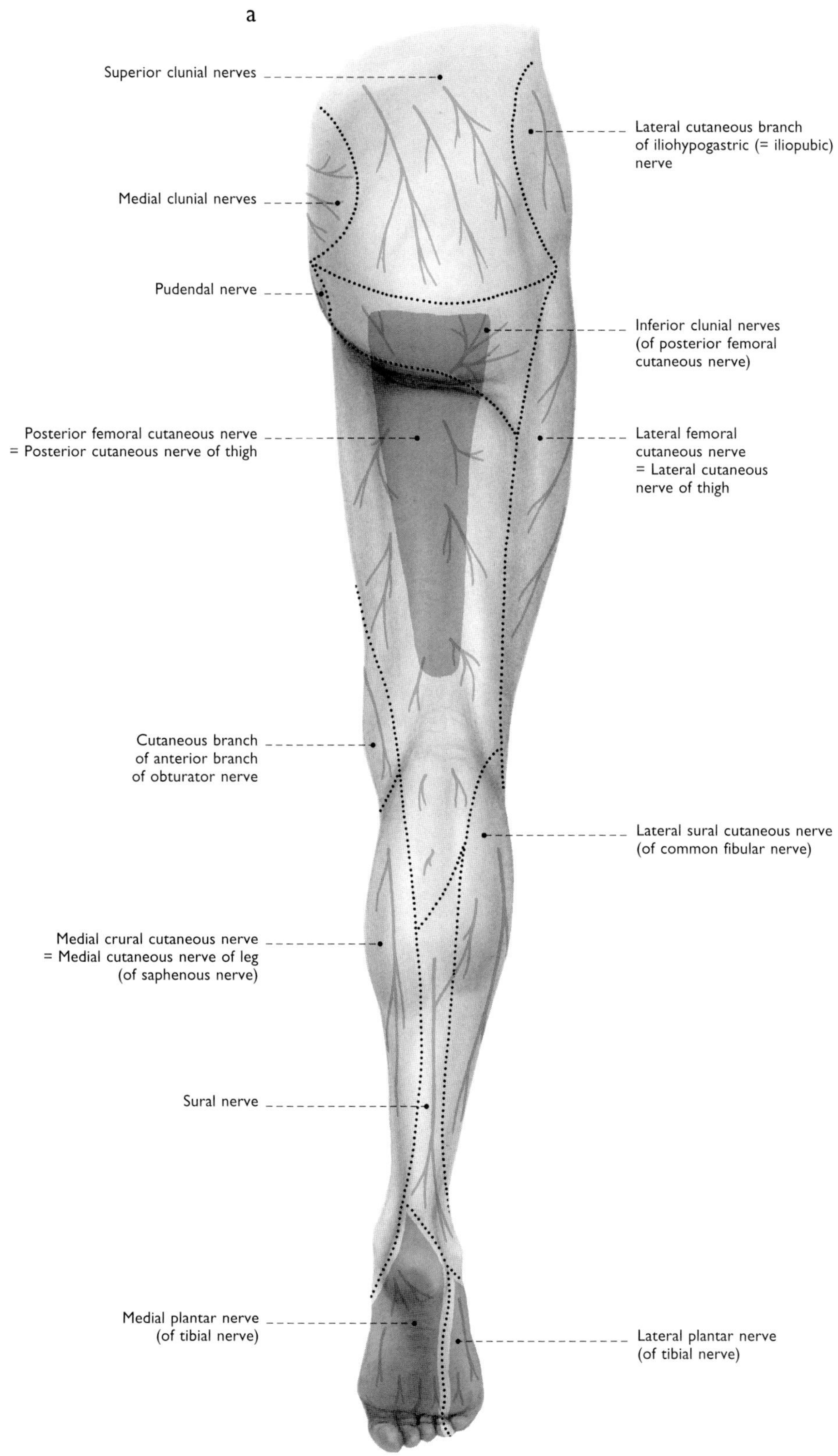
a
Superior clunial nerves
Medial clunial nerves
Pudendal nerve
Posterior femoral cutaneous nerve
= Posterior cutaneous nerve of thigh
Cutaneous branch
of anterior branch
of obturator nerve
Medial crural cutaneous nerve
= Medial cutaneous nerve of leg
(of saphenous nerve)
Sural nerve
Medial plantar nerve
(of tibial nerve)
Lateral cutaneous branch
of iliohypogastric (= iliopubic)
nerve
Inferior clunial nerves
(of posterior femoral
cutaneous nerve)
Lateral femoral
cutaneous nerve
= Lateral cutaneous
nerve of thigh
Lateral sural cutaneous nerve
(of common fibular nerve)
Lateral plantar nerve
(of tibial nerve)

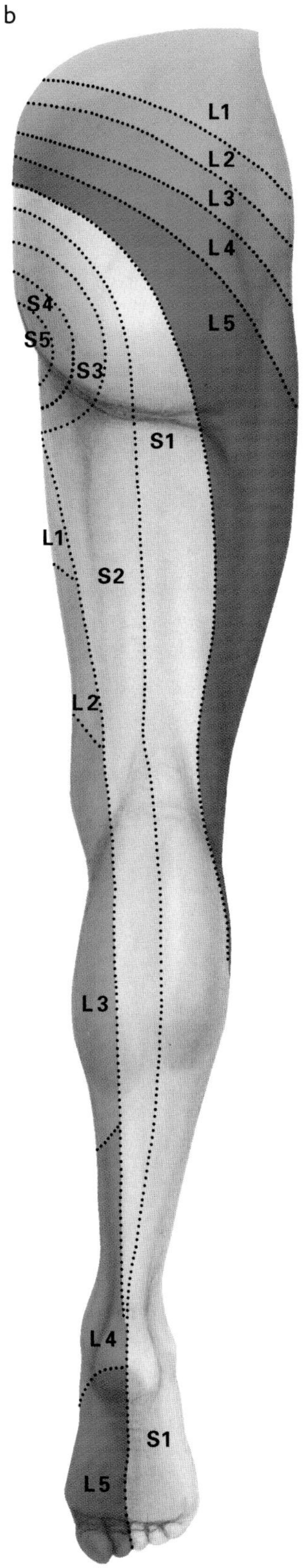
b
L1
L2
L3
L4
L5
S4
S5
S3
S1
L1
S2
L2
L3
L4
S1
L5

257 Cutaneous and segmental innervation of the right lower limb (20%)

Schematic representations, dorsal aspect

a Cutaneous nerves and areas of distribution, the autonomic areas of the different nerves are given in a darker gray.

b Segmental innervation (dermatomes)

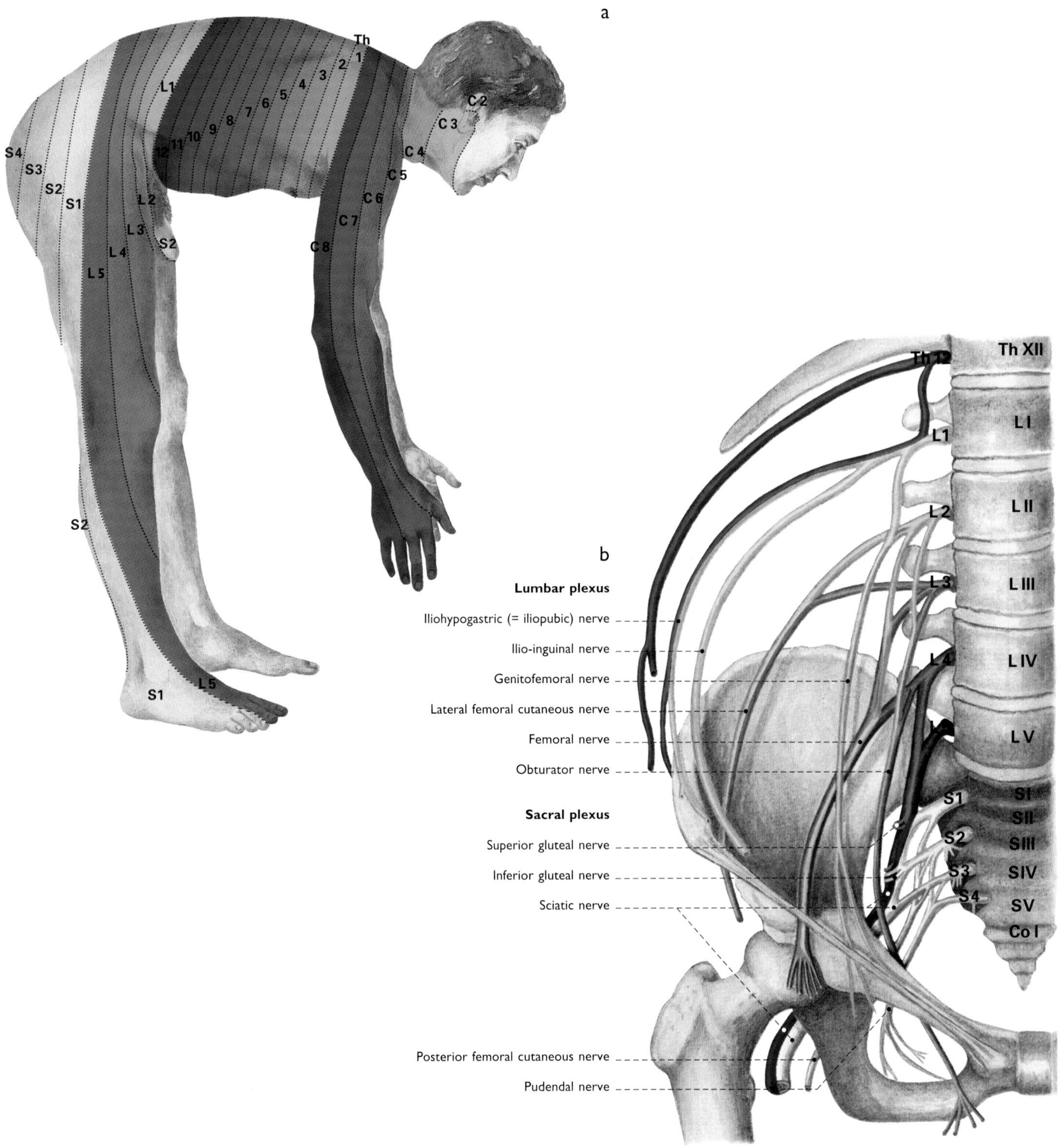
a
Th
1
2
3
4
5
6
7
8
9
10
11
12
C2
C3
C4
C5
C6
C7
C8
L1
L2
L3
L4
L5
S1
S2
S3
S4
b
Lumbar plexus
Iliohypogastric (= iliopubic) nerve
Ilio-inguinal nerve
Genitofemoral nerve
Lateral femoral cutaneous nerve
Femoral nerve
Obturator nerve
Sacral plexus
Superior gluteal nerve
Inferior gluteal nerve
Sciatic nerve
Posterior femoral cutaneous nerve
Pudendal nerve
Th 12
Th XII
L I
L II
L III
L IV
L V
SI
SII
SIII
SIV
SV
Co I

258 Segmental innervation and lumbosacral plexus

a Segmental innervation (dermatomes) of the upper limb, trunk, and lower limb (according to von LANZ and WACHSMUTH, 1972)

b Plan of the lumbosacral plexus

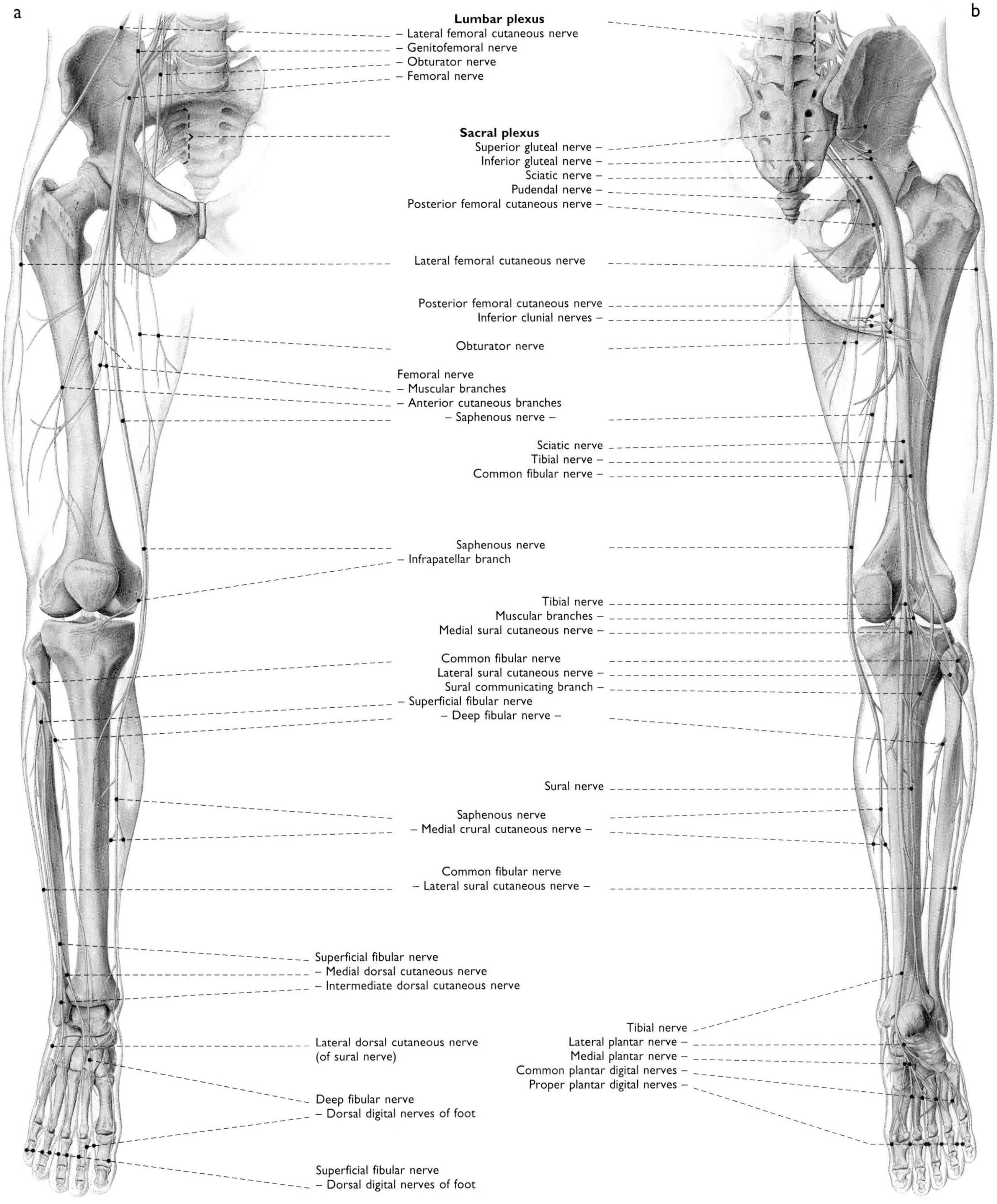
a
b
Lumbar plexus
– Lateral femoral cutaneous nerve
– Genitofemoral nerve
– Obturator nerve
– Femoral nerve
Sacral plexus
Superior gluteal nerve –
Inferior gluteal nerve –
Sciatic nerve –
Pudendal nerve –
Posterior femoral cutaneous nerve –
Lateral femoral cutaneous nerve
Posterior femoral cutaneous nerve
Inferior clunial nerves –
Obturator nerve
Femoral nerve
– Muscular branches
– Anterior cutaneous branches
– Saphenous nerve –
Sciatic nerve
Tibial nerve –
Common fibular nerve –
Saphenous nerve
– Infrapatellar branch
Tibial nerve
Muscular branches –
Medial sural cutaneous nerve –
Common fibular nerve
Lateral sural cutaneous nerve –
Sural communicating branch –
– Superficial fibular nerve
– Deep fibular nerve –
Sural nerve
Saphenous nerve
– Medial crural cutaneous nerve –
Common fibular nerve
– Lateral sural cutaneous nerve –
Superficial fibular nerve
– Medial dorsal cutaneous nerve
– Intermediate dorsal cutaneous nerve
Tibial nerve
Lateral plantar nerve –
Medial plantar nerve –
Common plantar digital nerves –
Proper plantar digital nerves –
Lateral dorsal cutaneous nerve
(of sural nerve)
Deep fibular nerve
– Dorsal digital nerves of foot
Superficial fibular nerve
– Dorsal digital nerves of foot

259 Nerves of the right lower limb (20%)

Schematic representations

a Ventral aspect

b Dorsal aspect

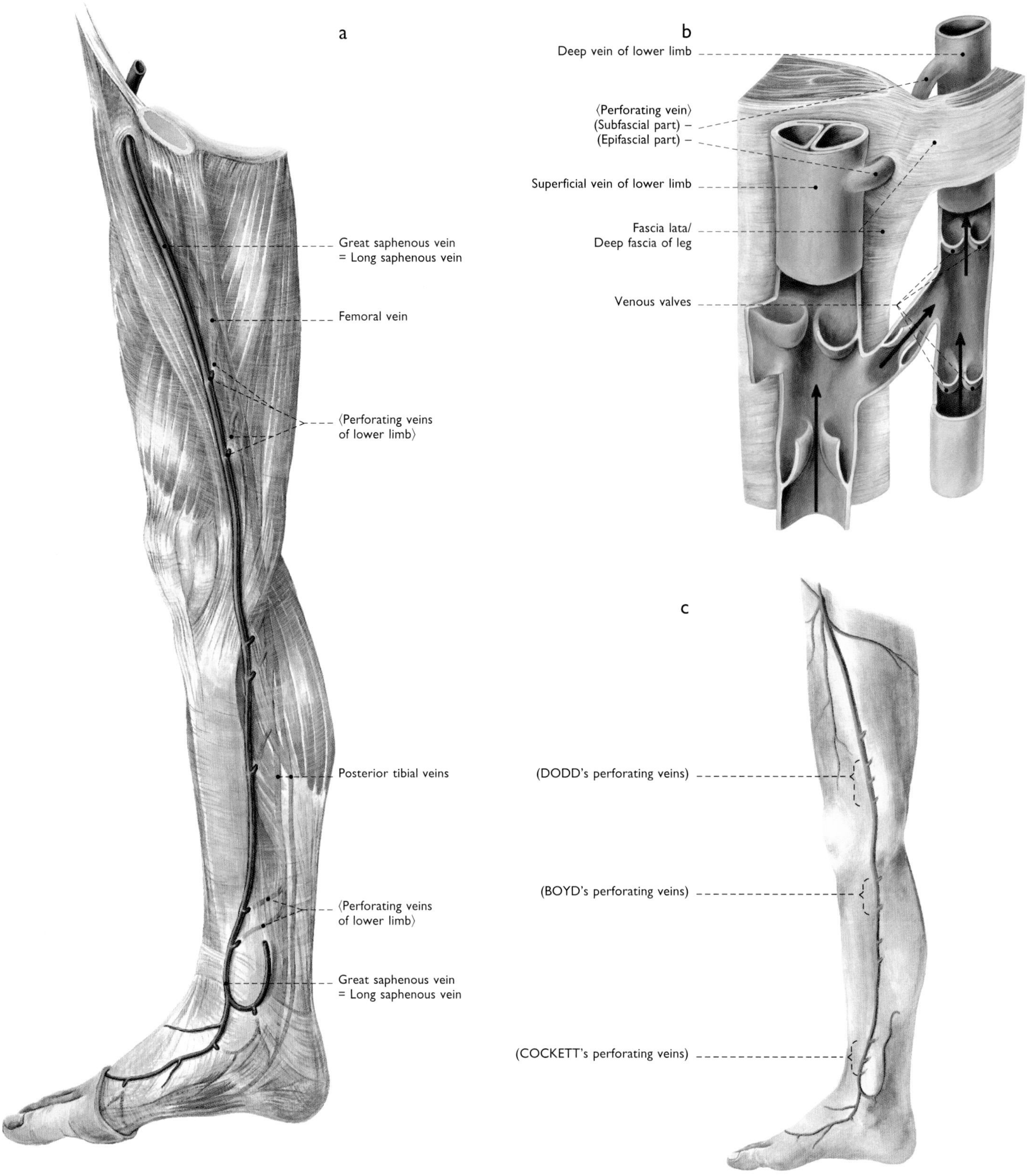
a
Great saphenous vein
= Long saphenous vein
Femoral vein
⟨Perforating veins
of lower limb⟩
Posterior tibial veins
⟨Perforating veins
of lower limb⟩
Great saphenous vein
= Long saphenous vein
b
Deep vein of lower limb
⟨Perforating vein⟩
(Subfascial part) –
(Epifascial part) –
Superficial vein of lower limb
Fascia lata/
Deep fascia of leg
Venous valves
c
(DODD's perforating veins)
(BOYD's perforating veins)
(COCKETT's perforating veins)

260 Veins of the right lower limb

a Superficial and deep veins of the lower limb (20%), medial aspect
b Connection between superficial and deep veins of the lower limb by perforating veins (200%), schematic representation
c Main localization of perforating veins over the lower limb (10%), medial aspect

a

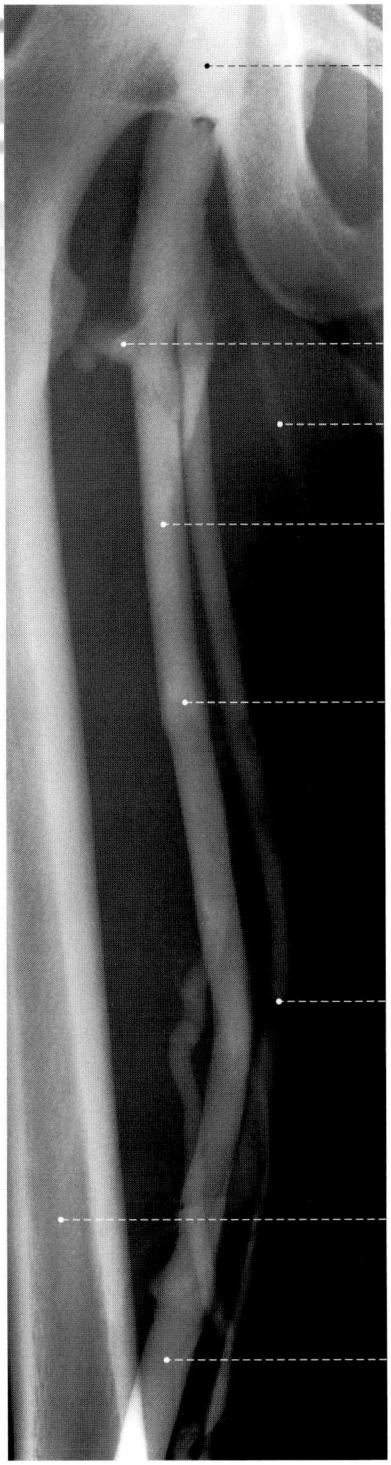
External iliac vein
Lateral circumflex femoral vein
Great saphenous vein
= Long saphenous vein
Femoral vein
Venous valve
Venous valve
Body of femur
Femoral vein

b

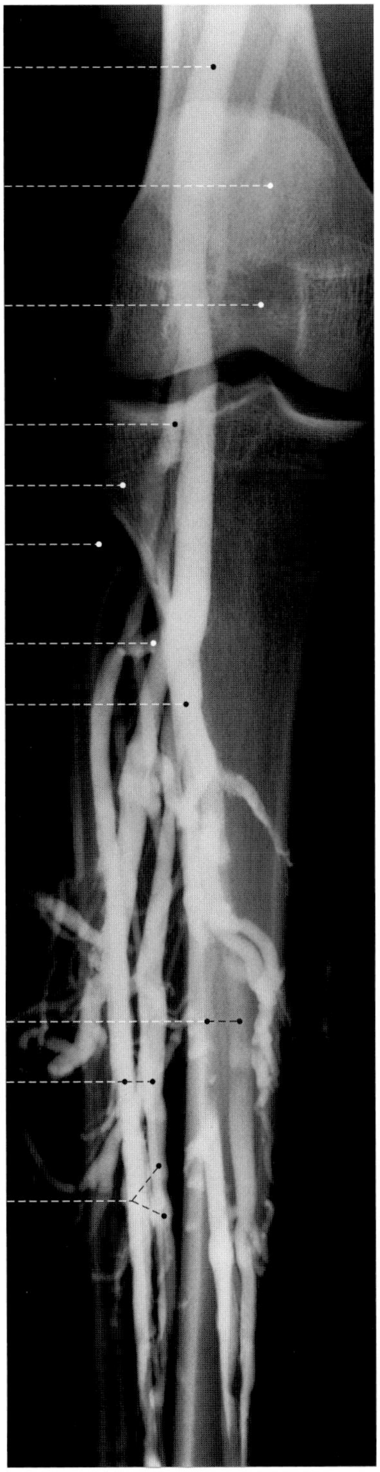
Popliteal vein
Patella
Femur
Small saphenous vein
= Short saphenous vein
Tibia
Head of fibula
Anterior tibial vein
Posterior tibial vein
Posterior tibial veins
Fibular veins
= Peroneal veins
Venous valves

261 Veins of the right lower limb (45%)

a Anteroposterior venogram of the thigh
b Anteroposterior venogram of the leg

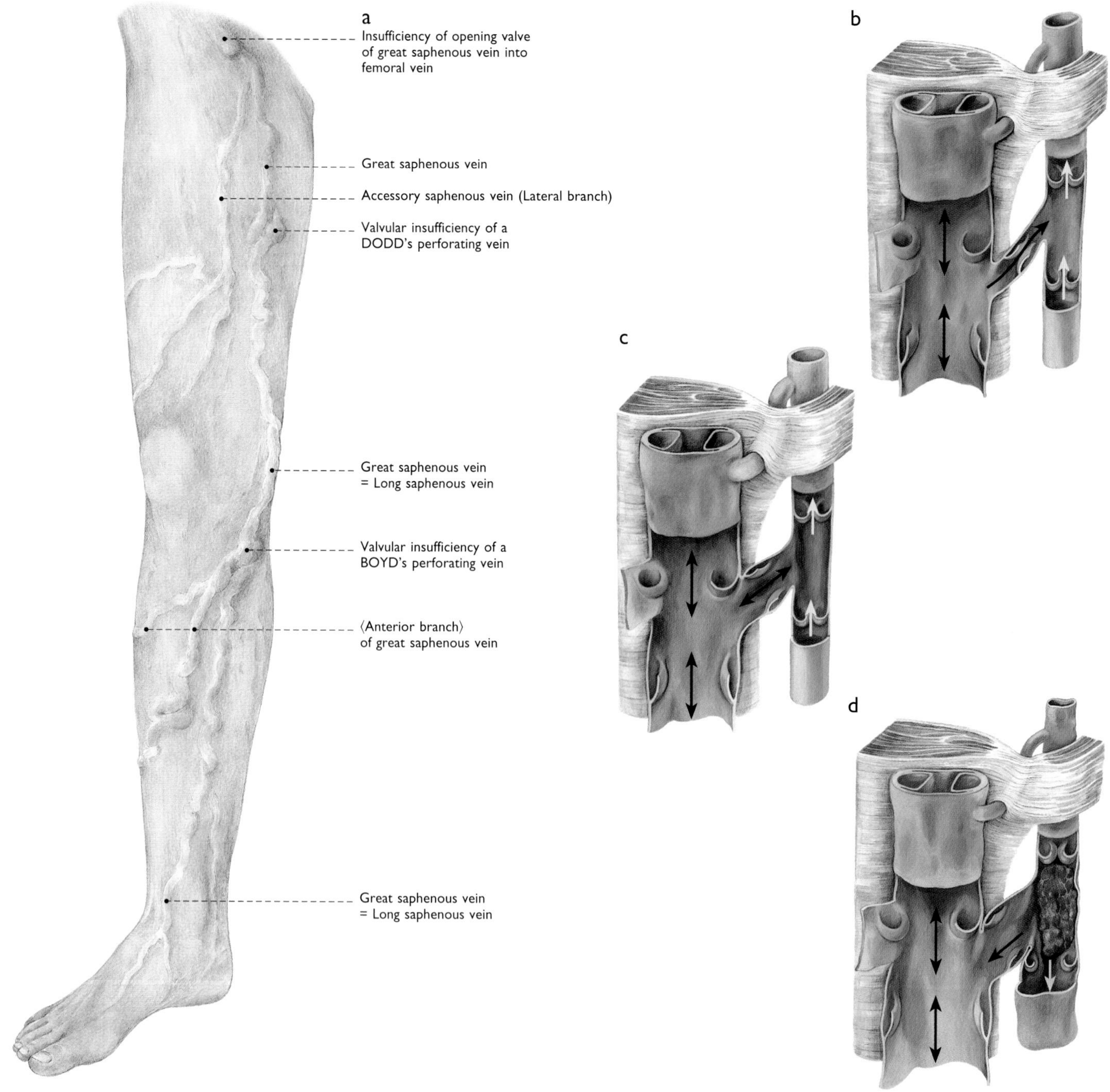
a
Insufficiency of opening valve of great saphenous vein into femoral vein
Great saphenous vein
Accessory saphenous vein (Lateral branch)
Valvular insufficiency of a DODD's perforating vein
Great saphenous vein = Long saphenous vein
Valvular insufficiency of a BOYD's perforating vein
⟨Anterior branch⟩ of great saphenous vein
Great saphenous vein = Long saphenous vein
b
c
d

262 Veins of the right lower limb

a Varicosis involving trunk and branches of the great saphenous vein at thigh and leg of the right lower limb

b–d Representation of three main causes for varicosis (cf. fig. 260b)

b Weakness of connective tissue based on genetic disposition results in dilatation and valvular insufficiency of **superficial veins**. The perforating and deep veins are not affected.

c Valvular insufficiency of **perforating veins** leads to an additional volume load and, thereby, to the dilatation of superficial veins.

d **Deep vein thrombosis** forces a collateral circulation and, thus, results in the dilatation and valvular insufficiency of perforating and superficial veins.

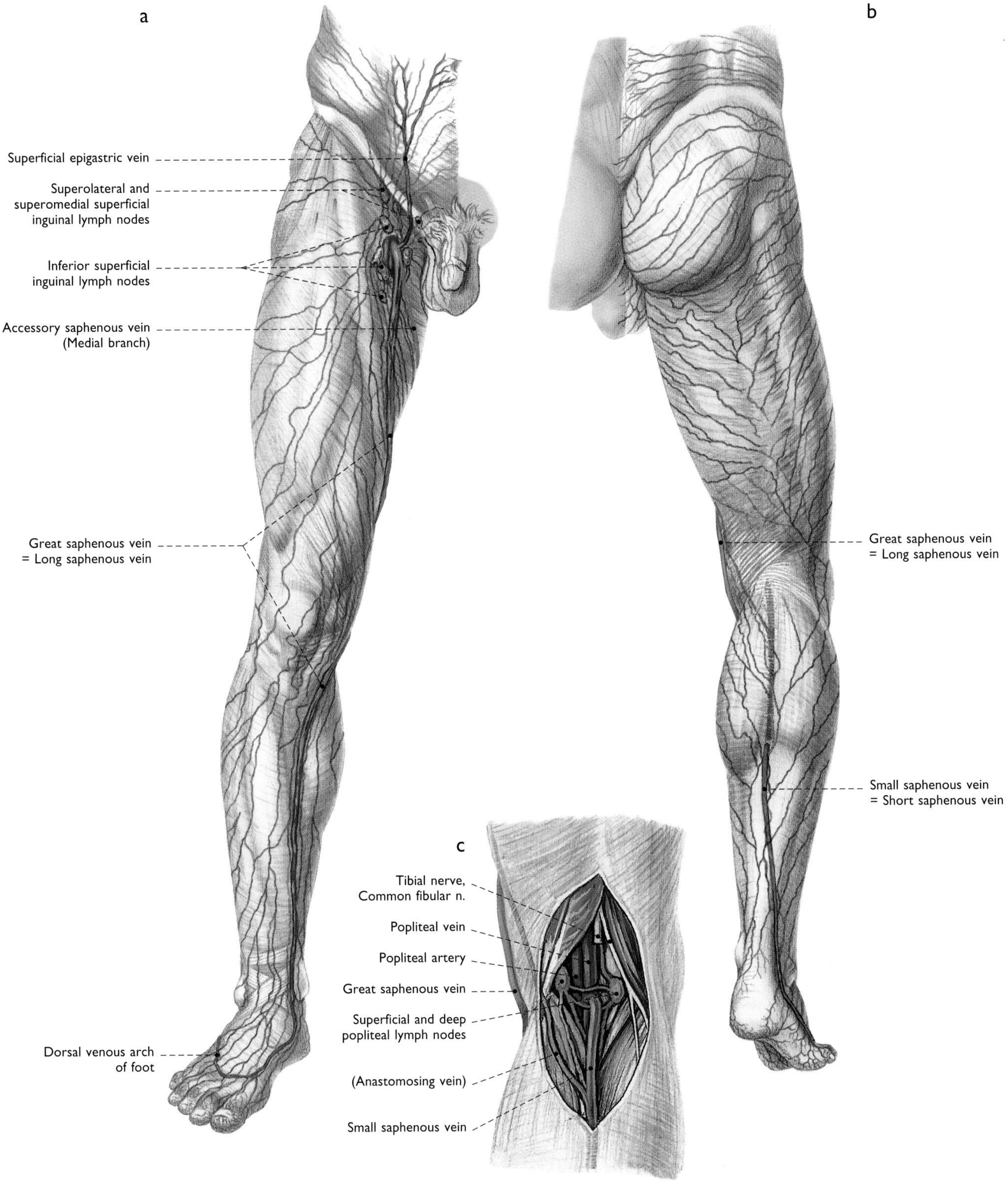
a
b
Superficial epigastric vein
Superolateral and superomedial superficial inguinal lymph nodes
Inferior superficial inguinal lymph nodes
Accessory saphenous vein (Medial branch)
Great saphenous vein = Long saphenous vein
Dorsal venous arch of foot
Great saphenous vein = Long saphenous vein
Small saphenous vein = Short saphenous vein
c
Tibial nerve, Common fibular n.
Popliteal vein
Popliteal artery
Great saphenous vein
Superficial and deep popliteal lymph nodes
(Anastomosing vein)
Small saphenous vein

263 Lymphatic vessels and lymph nodes of the right lower limb

a Ventral aspect (20%)
b Dorsal aspect (20%)
c Lymphatic vessels of the popliteal fossa (30%), dorsal aspect

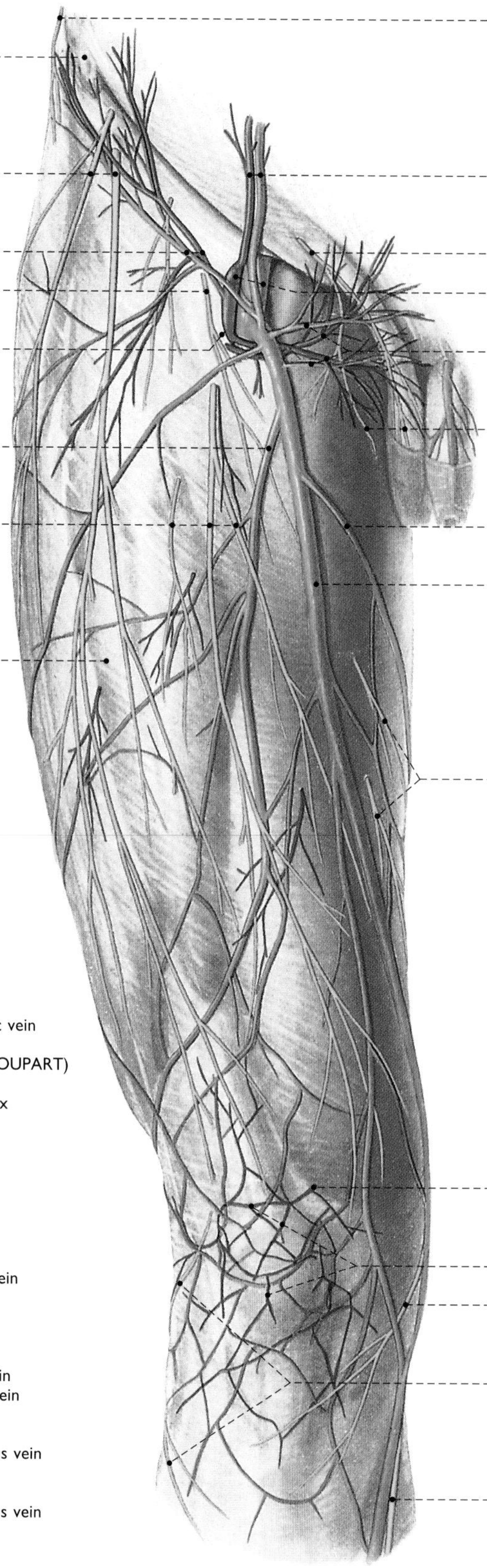
a
Anterior superior iliac spine
Lateral femoral cutaneous nerve
= Lateral cutaneous nerve of thigh
Superficial circumflex iliac vein and artery
Femoral branch
of genitofemoral nerve
Falciform margin
of saphenous opening
Accessory saphenous vein
(Lateral branch)
Anterior cutaneous branches
of femoral nerve
Fascia lata
Lateral cutaneous branch
of iliohypogastric (= iliopubic)
nerve
Superficial epigastric
artery and vein
Ilio-inguinal nerve
Femoral artery and vein
External pudendal veins,
Superficial external
pudendal artery
Anterior scrotal nerves
(of ilio-inguinal nerve)
Accessory saphenous vein
(Medial branch)
Great saphenous vein
= Long saphenous vein
Cutaneous branches
of anterior branch
of obturator nerve
Articular branch
of descending genicular artery
Patellar anastomosis
Infrapatellar branch
of saphenous nerve
Lateral sural cutaneous nerve
(of common fibular nerve)
Saphenous nerve

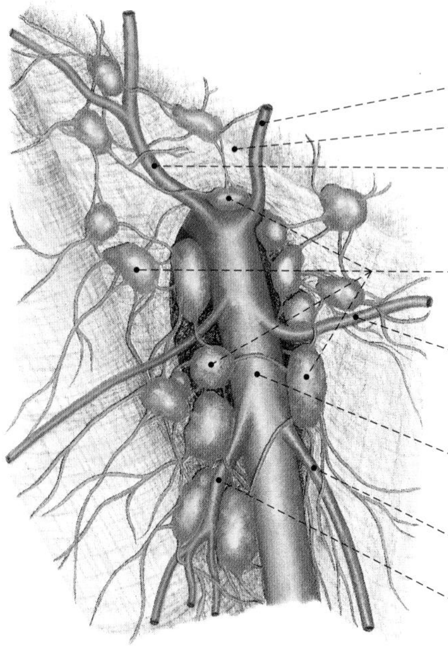
b
Superficial epigastric vein
Inguinal ligament (POUPART)
Superficial circumflex
iliac vein
Superficial inguinal
lymph nodes
External pudendal vein
Great saphenous vein
= Long saphenous vein
Accessory saphenous vein
(Medial branch)
Accessory saphenous vein
(Lateral branch)

264 Subcutaneous blood vessels, nerves, and lymph nodes of the right thigh

a Ventral aspect (30%)

b Superficial veins and lymph nodes in and around the saphenous opening (70%)

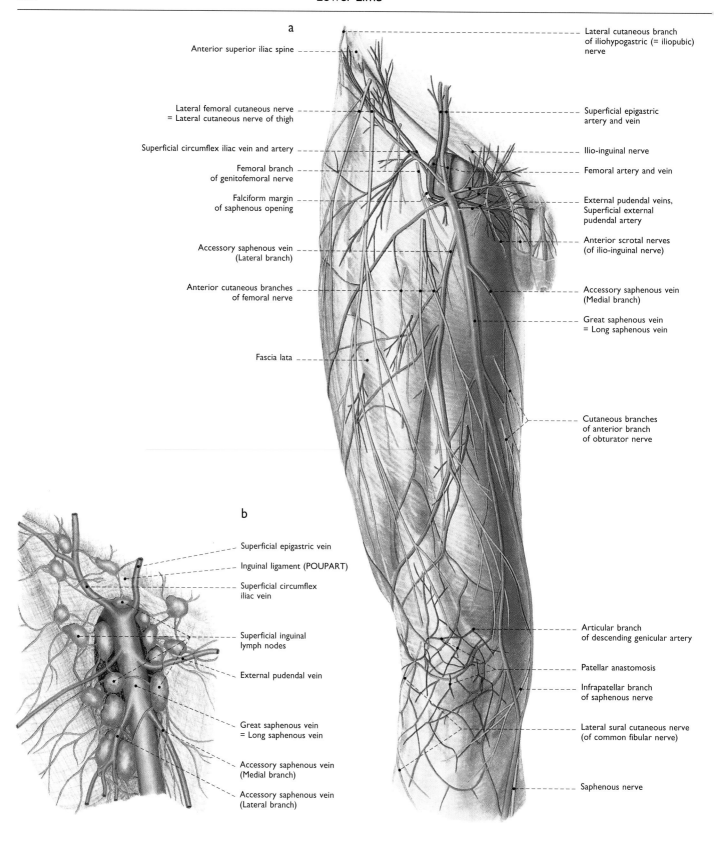

a

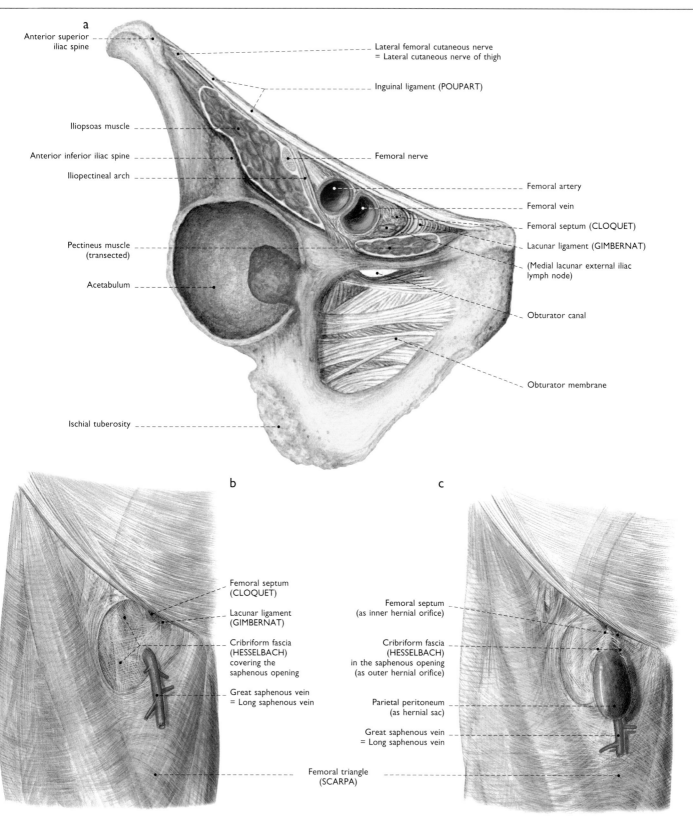

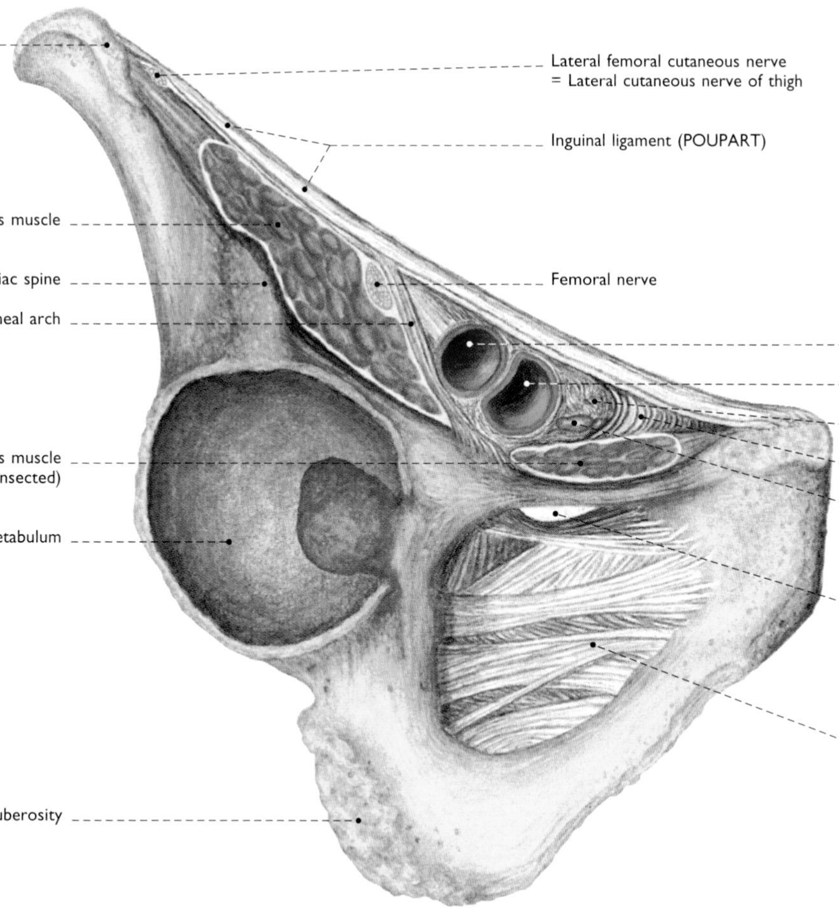
Anterior superior iliac spine
Lateral femoral cutaneous nerve = Lateral cutaneous nerve of thigh
Inguinal ligament (POUPART)
Iliopsoas muscle
Anterior inferior iliac spine
Femoral nerve
Iliopectineal arch
Femoral artery
Femoral vein
Femoral septum (CLOQUET)
Pectineus muscle (transected)
Lacunar ligament (GIMBERNAT)
(Medial lacunar external iliac lymph node)
Acetabulum
Obturator canal
Obturator membrane
Ischial tuberosity

b

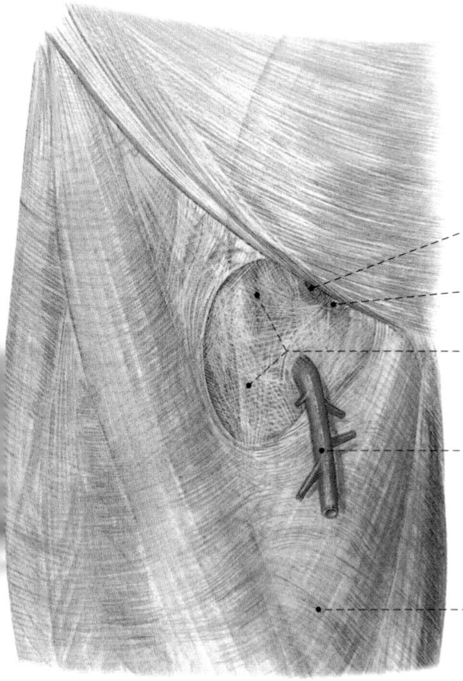
Femoral septum (CLOQUET)
Lacunar ligament (GIMBERNAT)
Cribriform fascia (HESSELBACH) covering the saphenous opening
Great saphenous vein = Long saphenous vein
Femoral triangle (SCARPA)

c

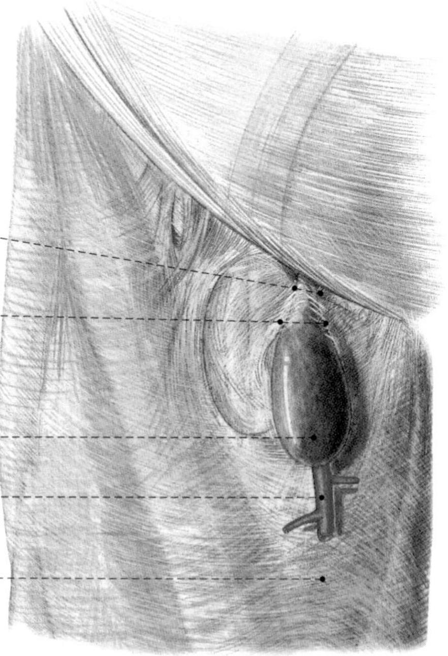
Femoral septum (as inner hernial orifice)
Cribriform fascia (HESSELBACH) in the saphenous opening (as outer hernial orifice)
Parietal peritoneum (as hernial sac)
Great saphenous vein = Long saphenous vein

265 Inguinal region and femoral triangle

a Structures passing posterior to the inguinal ligament (60%) (according to von LANZ and WACHSMUTH, 1972), inferior (distal) aspect

b, c Femoral triangle, saphenous opening, and femoral hernia (30%), ventral aspect

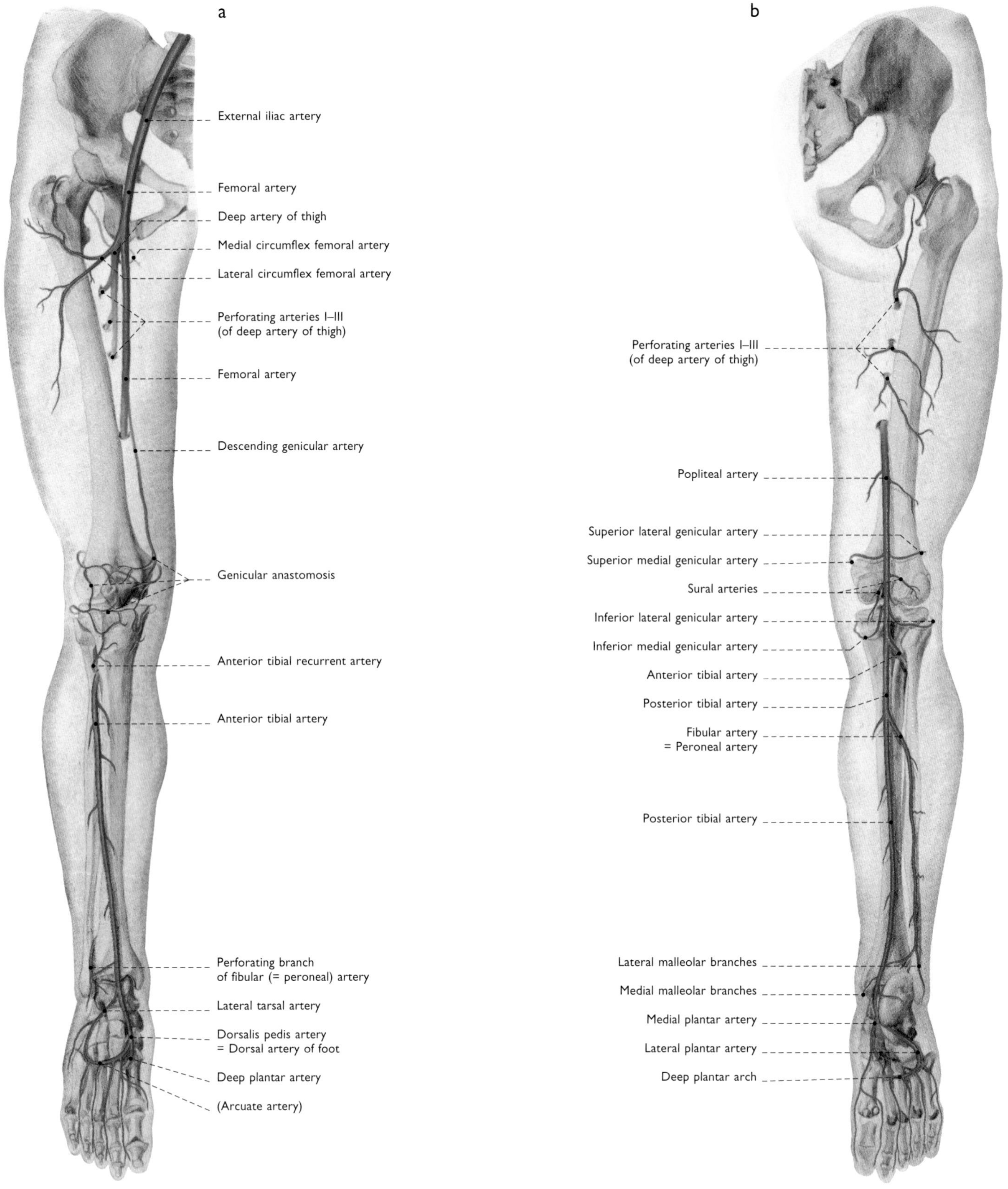
a
External iliac artery
Femoral artery
Deep artery of thigh
Medial circumflex femoral artery
Lateral circumflex femoral artery
Perforating arteries I–III (of deep artery of thigh)
Femoral artery
Descending genicular artery
Genicular anastomosis
Anterior tibial recurrent artery
Anterior tibial artery
Perforating branch of fibular (= peroneal) artery
Lateral tarsal artery
Dorsalis pedis artery = Dorsal artery of foot
Deep plantar artery
(Arcuate artery)
b
Perforating arteries I–III (of deep artery of thigh)
Popliteal artery
Superior lateral genicular artery
Superior medial genicular artery
Sural arteries
Inferior lateral genicular artery
Inferior medial genicular artery
Anterior tibial artery
Posterior tibial artery
Fibular artery = Peroneal artery
Posterior tibial artery
Lateral malleolar branches
Medial malleolar branches
Medial plantar artery
Lateral plantar artery
Deep plantar arch

266 Arteries of the right lower limb (20%)

Schematic representations
a Ventral aspect
b Dorsal aspect

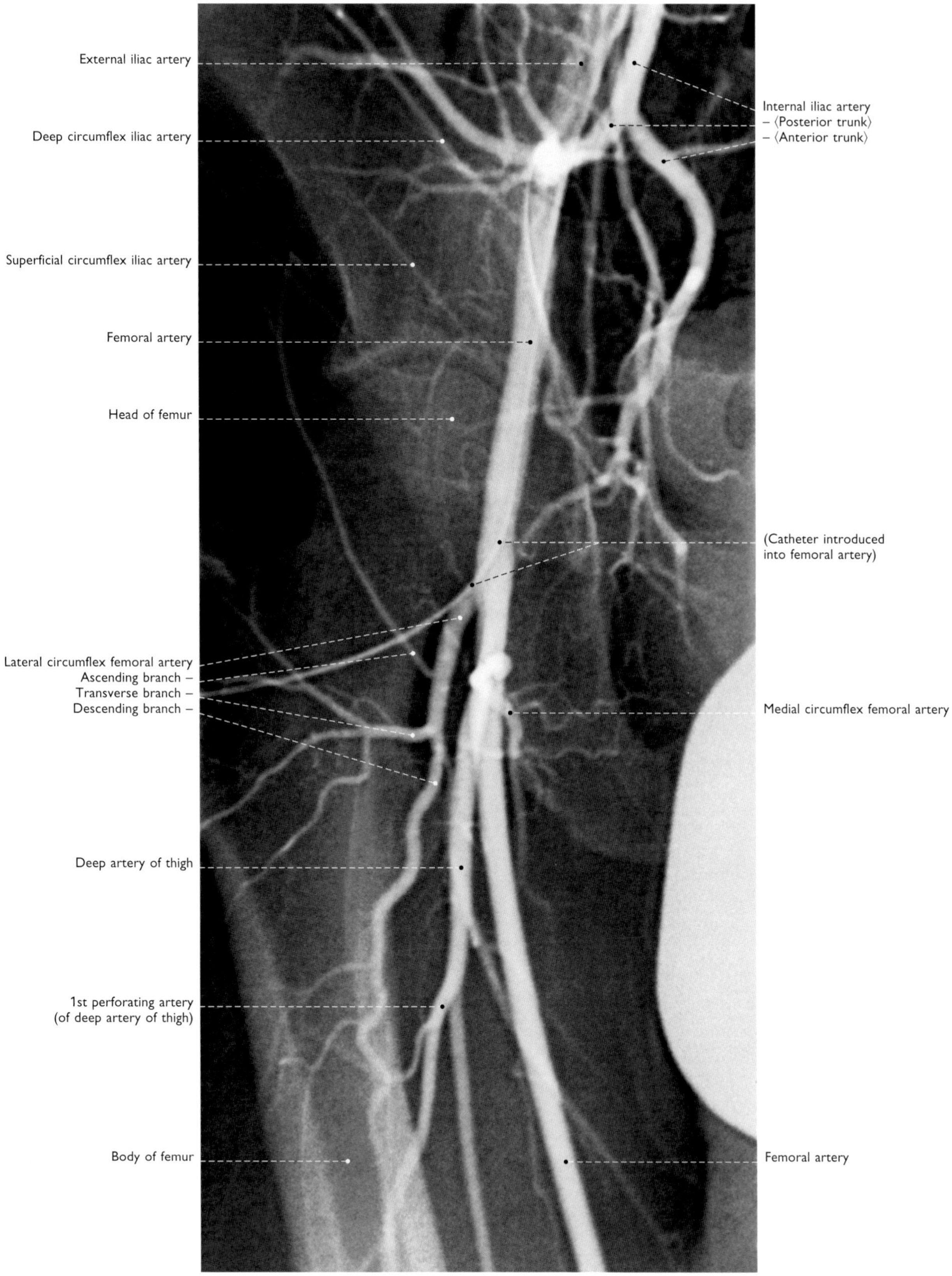
External iliac artery
Deep circumflex iliac artery
Superficial circumflex iliac artery
Femoral artery
Head of femur
Lateral circumflex femoral artery
Ascending branch –
Transverse branch –
Descending branch –
Deep artery of thigh
1st perforating artery
(of deep artery of thigh)
Body of femur
Internal iliac artery
– (Posterior trunk)
– (Anterior trunk)
(Catheter introduced
into femoral artery)
Medial circumflex femoral artery
Femoral artery

267 Arteries of the right lower limb (80%)

Anteroposterior arteriogram of pelvic and femoral arteries

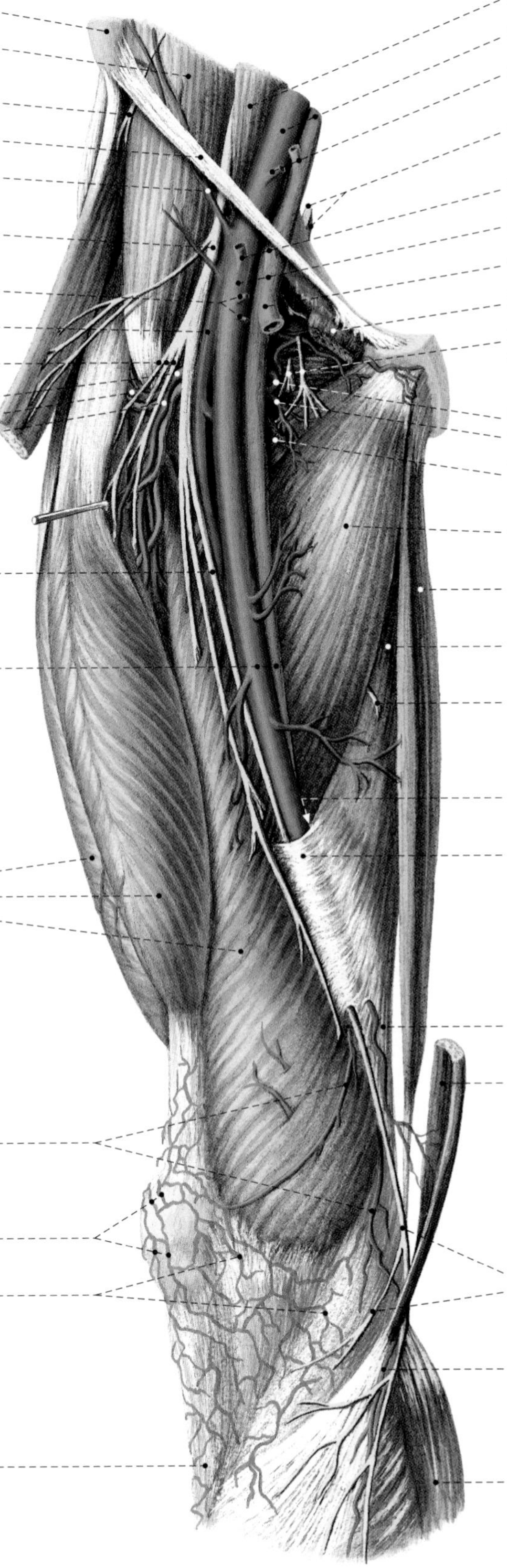

Anterior superior iliac spine
Iliacus muscle
Lateral femoral cutaneous nerve
Inguinal ligament (POUPART)
Deep circumflex iliac artery
Femoral nerve
Superficial and deep external pudendal arteries
Deep artery of thigh
Muscular branches of femoral nerve
Lateral circumflex femoral artery
Ascending branch –
Descending branch –
Saphenous nerve
Femoral artery and vein
Quadriceps femoris muscle
Vastus lateralis muscle –
Rectus femoris muscle –
Vastus medialis muscle –
Descending genicular artery
Patellar anastomosis
Genicular anastomosis
Tibial tuberosity
Psoas major muscle
External iliac artery and vein
Inferior epigastric artery and vein
Obturator nerve and artery
Superficial epigastric artery and vein
Femoral artery and vein
Great (= long) saphenous vein
Pectineus muscle
Posterior and anterior branches of obturator nerve
Medial circumflex femoral artery
– Superficial branch
Pectineus muscle
Adductor longus muscle
Gracilis muscle
Adductor magnus muscle
Cutaneous branch of anterior branch of obturator nerve
Adductor canal (HUNTER)
⟨Vasto-adductor membrane⟩
Tendon of adductor magnus muscle
Sartorius muscle
Saphenous nerve
– Infrapatellar branch
Saphenous branch of descending genicular artery
Medial head of gastrocnemius muscle

268 Blood vessels and nerves of the right thigh and knee (30%)

The sartorius and pectineus muscles were partially removed.
Ventral aspect

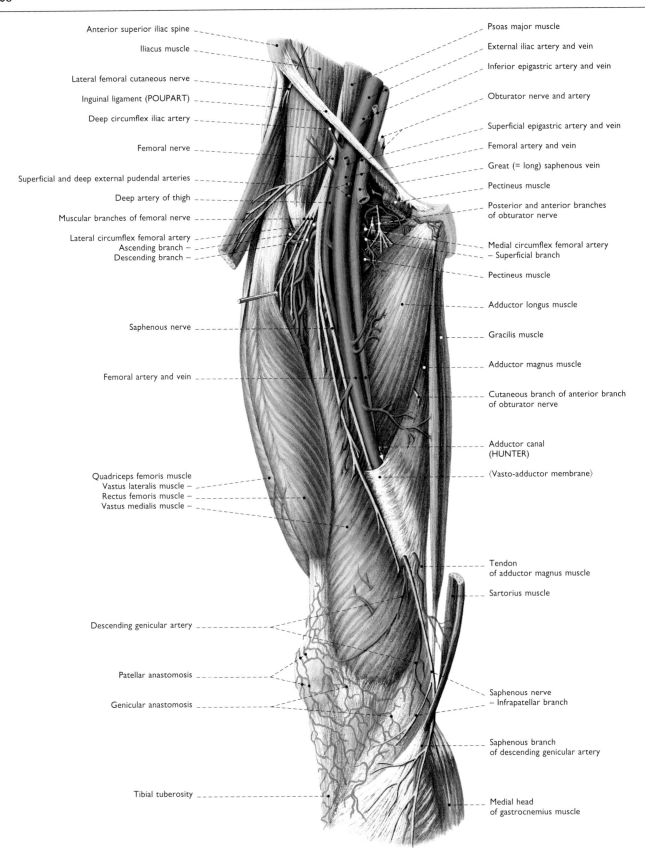

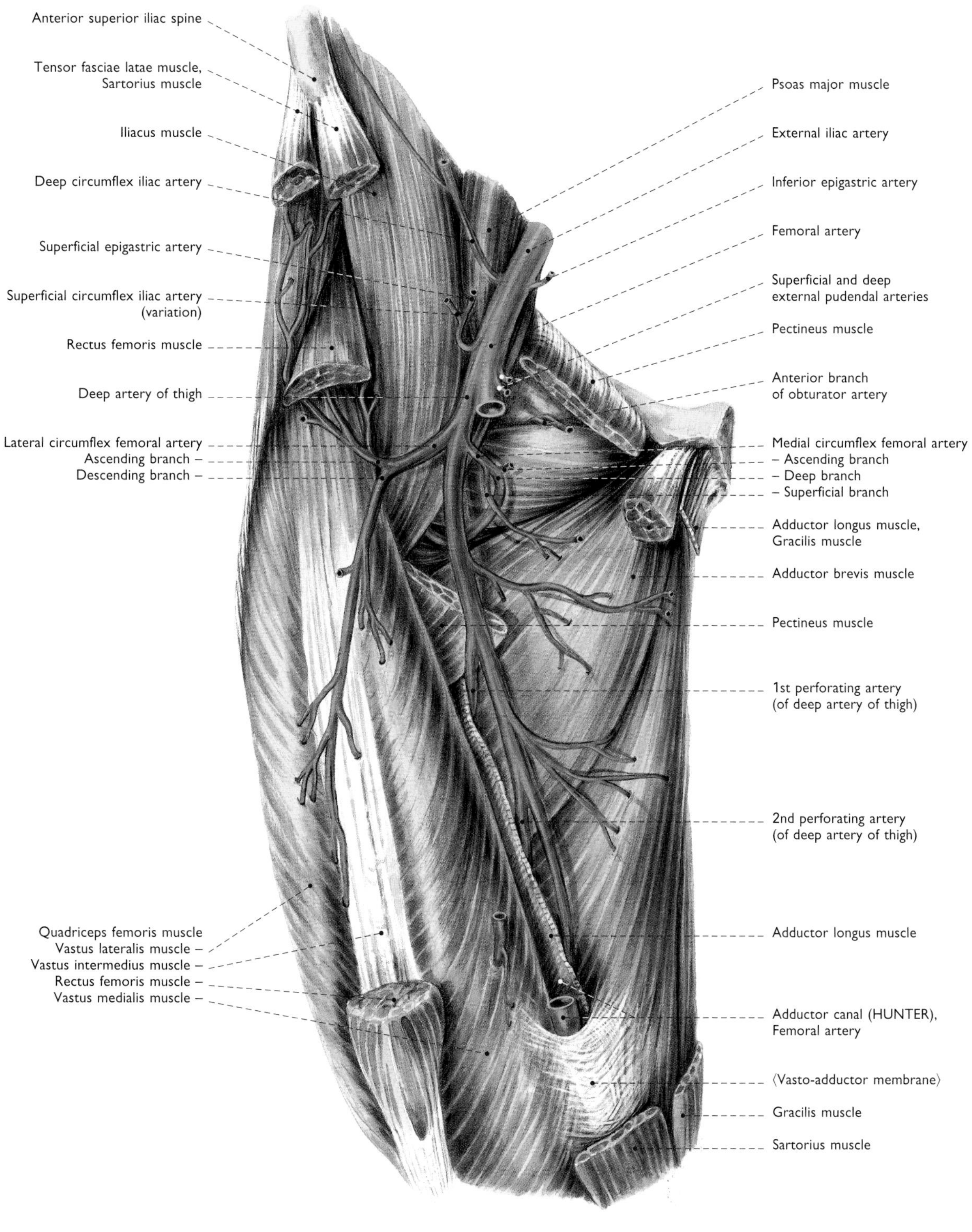
Anterior superior iliac spine
Tensor fasciae latae muscle, Sartorius muscle
Iliacus muscle
Deep circumflex iliac artery
Superficial epigastric artery
Superficial circumflex iliac artery (variation)
Rectus femoris muscle
Deep artery of thigh
Lateral circumflex femoral artery
Ascending branch –
Descending branch –
Quadriceps femoris muscle
Vastus lateralis muscle –
Vastus intermedius muscle –
Rectus femoris muscle –
Vastus medialis muscle –
Psoas major muscle
External iliac artery
Inferior epigastric artery
Femoral artery
Superficial and deep external pudendal arteries
Pectineus muscle
Anterior branch of obturator artery
Medial circumflex femoral artery
– Ascending branch
– Deep branch
– Superficial branch
Adductor longus muscle, Gracilis muscle
Adductor brevis muscle
Pectineus muscle
1st perforating artery (of deep artery of thigh)
2nd perforating artery (of deep artery of thigh)
Adductor longus muscle
Adductor canal (HUNTER), Femoral artery
⟨Vasto-adductor membrane⟩
Gracilis muscle
Sartorius muscle

269 Deep artery of thigh and its branches in the right thigh (40%)

The superficial muscles were partially removed.
Ventral aspect

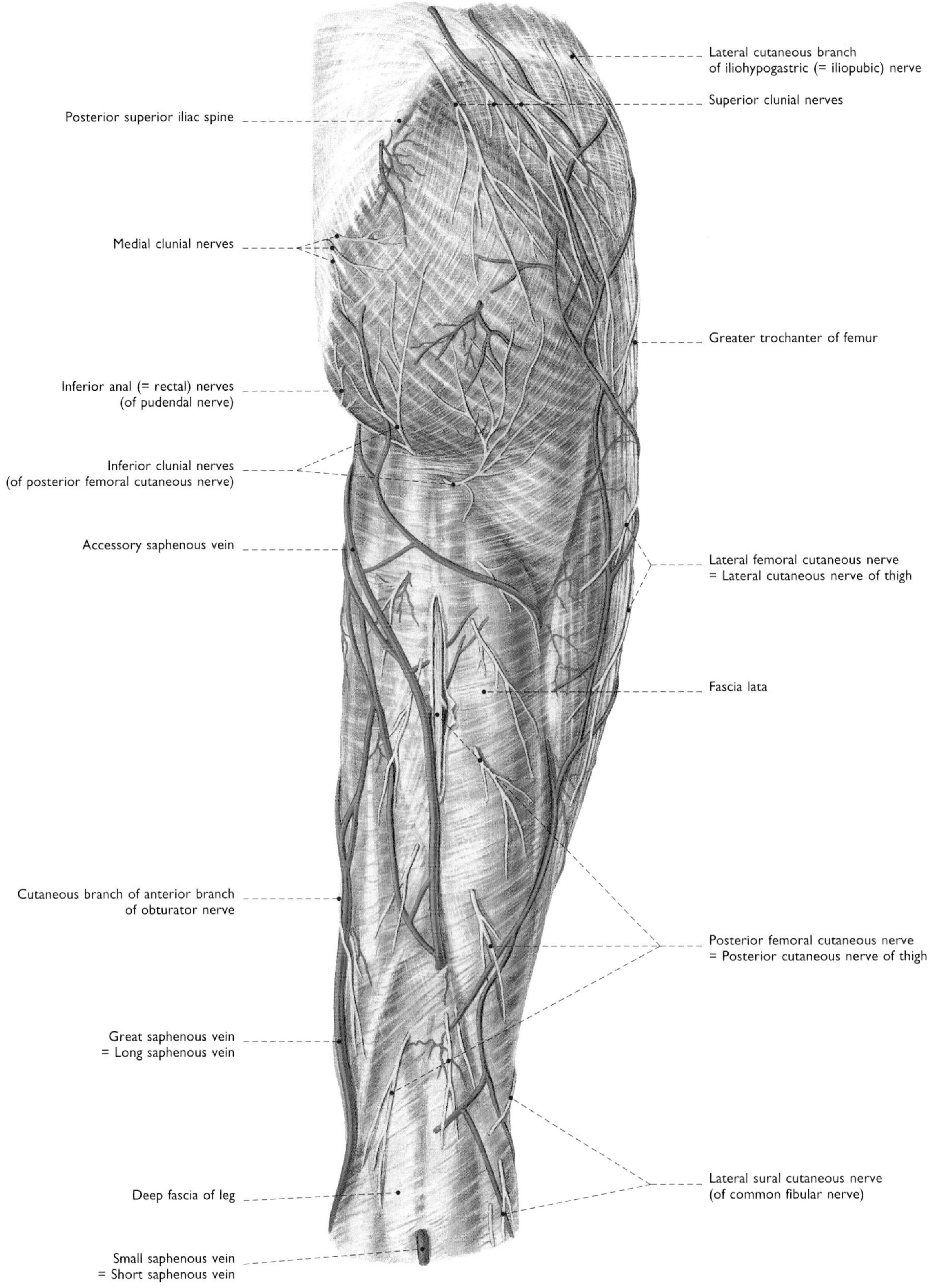
Lateral cutaneous branch
of iliohypogastric (= iliopubic) nerve
Superior clunial nerves
Posterior superior iliac spine
Medial clunial nerves
Greater trochanter of femur
Inferior anal (= rectal) nerves
(of pudendal nerve)
Inferior clunial nerves
(of posterior femoral cutaneous nerve)
Accessory saphenous vein
Lateral femoral cutaneous nerve
= Lateral cutaneous nerve of thigh
Fascia lata
Cutaneous branch of anterior branch
of obturator nerve
Posterior femoral cutaneous nerve
= Posterior cutaneous nerve of thigh
Great saphenous vein
= Long saphenous vein
Deep fascia of leg
Lateral sural cutaneous nerve
(of common fibular nerve)
Small saphenous vein
= Short saphenous vein

270 Subcutaneous blood vessels and nerves of the gluteal region, thigh, and popliteal fossa of the right side (30%)

Dorsal aspect

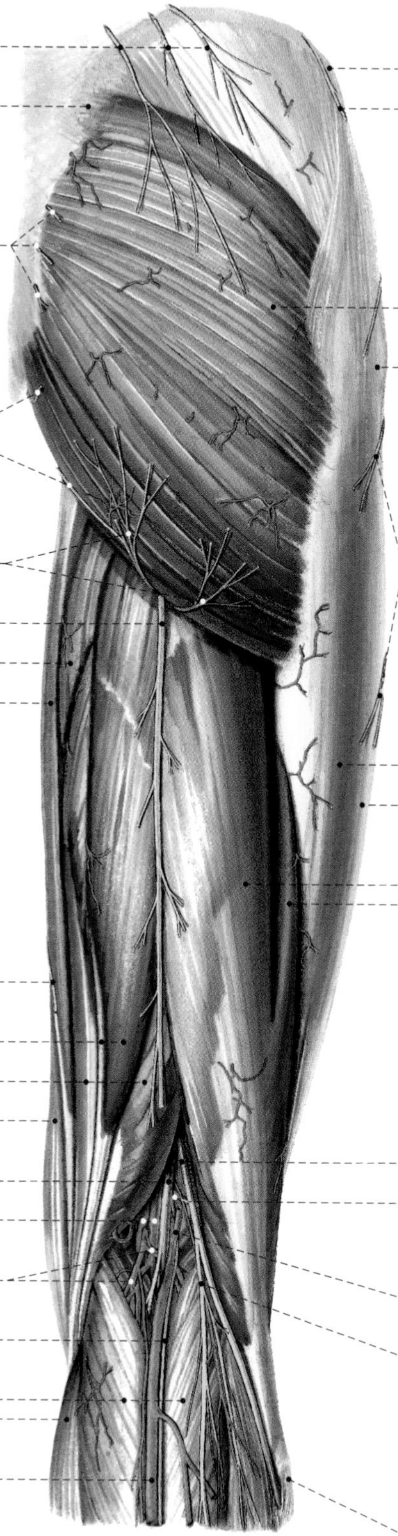
Superior clunial nerves
Posterior superior iliac spine
Medial clunial nerves
Pudendal nerve
Inferior anal (= rectal) nerves –
Perineal nerves –
Inferior clunial nerves
(of posterior femoral cutaneous nerve)
Posterior femoral cutaneous nerve
Adductor magnus muscle
Gracilis muscle
Cutaneous branch of anterior branch
of obturator nerve
Semitendinosus muscle
Semimembranosus muscle
Sartorius muscle
Tibial nerve
Popliteal artery and vein
Sural arteries
Medial sural cutaneous nerve (of tibial nerve)
Triceps surae muscle
Gastrocnemius muscle –
Soleus muscle –
Small saphenous vein
= Short saphenous vein
Iliac crest
Lateral cutaneous branch
of iliohypogastric (= iliopubic) nerve
Gluteus maximus muscle
Greater trochanter of femur
Branches
of lateral femoral cutaneous nerve
Vastus lateralis muscle
Iliotibial tract
Biceps femoris muscle
– Long head
– Short head
Common fibular (= peroneal) nerve
Superior lateral genicular artery
Accessory saphenous vein
Lateral sural cutaneous nerve
(of common fibular nerve)
Head of fibula

271 **Blood vessels and nerves of the gluteal region, thigh, and popliteal fossa of the right side** (30%)

The fasciae of the lower limb were removed.

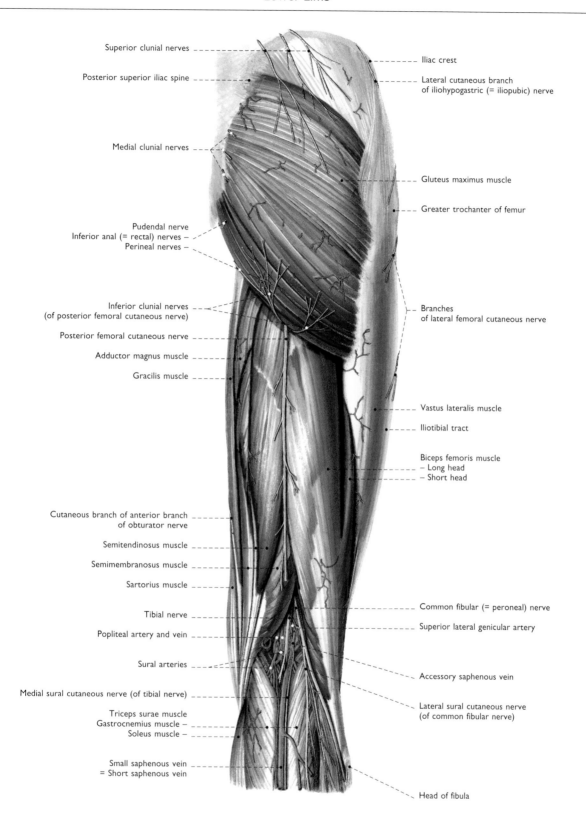

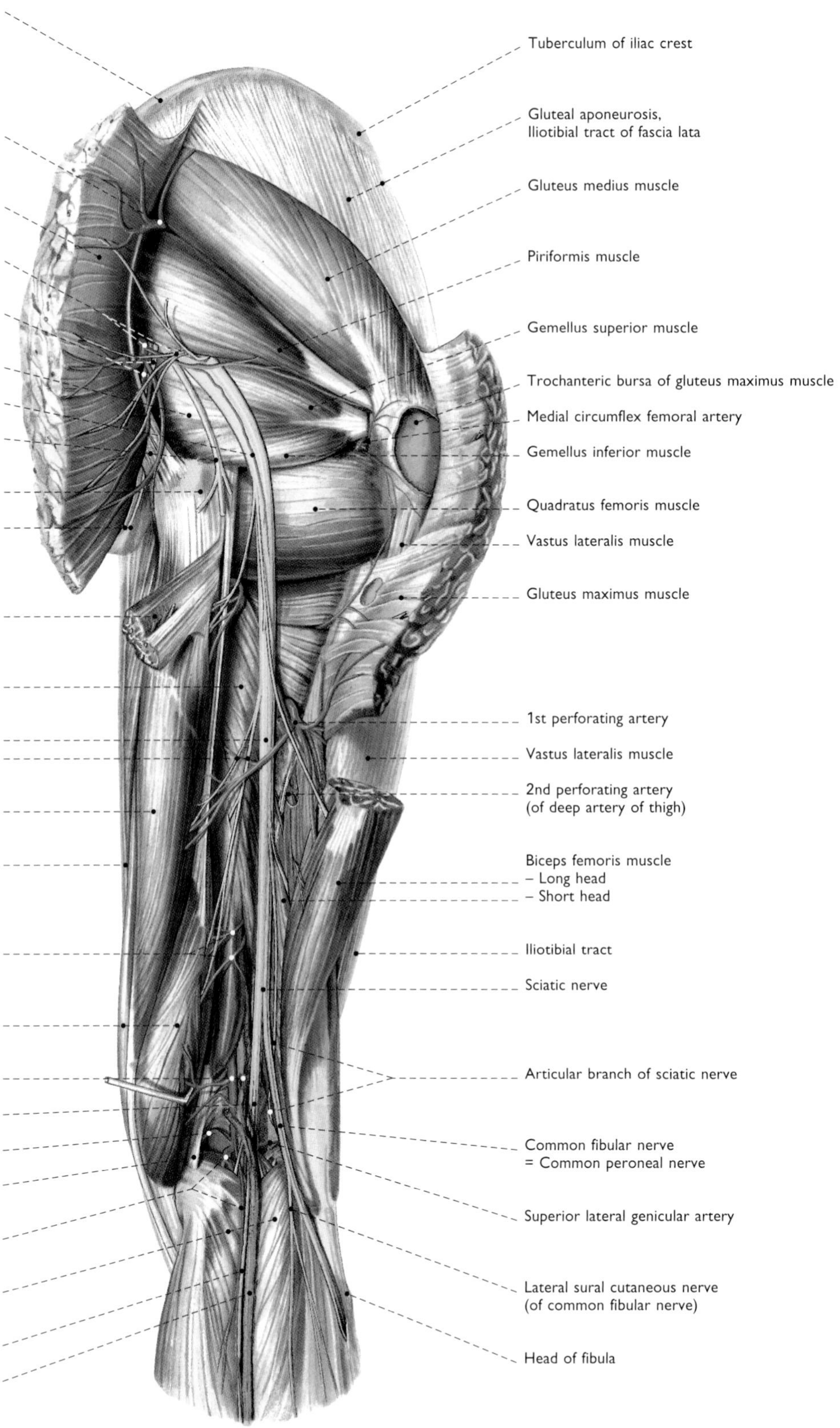
Iliac crest
Superior gluteal artery
Gluteus maximus muscle
Inferior gluteal nerve and artery
Pudendal nerve, Internal pudendal artery
Obturator internus muscle
Artery to sciatic nerve
Sacrotuberous ligament, Posterior femoral cutaneous nerve
Ischial tuberosity
Internal pudendal artery, Pudendal nerve
Long head of biceps femoris muscle
Adductor magnus muscle
Sciatic nerve
Muscular branches –
Semitendinosus muscle
Gracilis muscle
3rd perforating artery (of deep artery of thigh)
Semimembranosus muscle
Popliteal artery and vein
Tibial nerve
Superior medial genicular artery
Tendon of adductor magnus muscle
Sural arteries
Medial and lateral heads of gastrocnemius muscle
Medial sural cutaneous nerve
Small saphenous vein = Short saphenous vein
Tuberculum of iliac crest
Gluteal aponeurosis, Iliotibial tract of fascia lata
Gluteus medius muscle
Piriformis muscle
Gemellus superior muscle
Trochanteric bursa of gluteus maximus muscle
Medial circumflex femoral artery
Gemellus inferior muscle
Quadratus femoris muscle
Vastus lateralis muscle
Gluteus maximus muscle
1st perforating artery
Vastus lateralis muscle
2nd perforating artery (of deep artery of thigh)
Biceps femoris muscle
– Long head
– Short head
Iliotibial tract
Sciatic nerve
Articular branch of sciatic nerve
Common fibular nerve = Common peroneal nerve
Superior lateral genicular artery
Lateral sural cutaneous nerve (of common fibular nerve)
Head of fibula

272 **Blood vessels and nerves of the gluteal region, thigh, and popliteal fossa of the right side** (30%)

The gluteus maximus muscle and the long head of the biceps femoris muscle were divided. Dorsal aspect

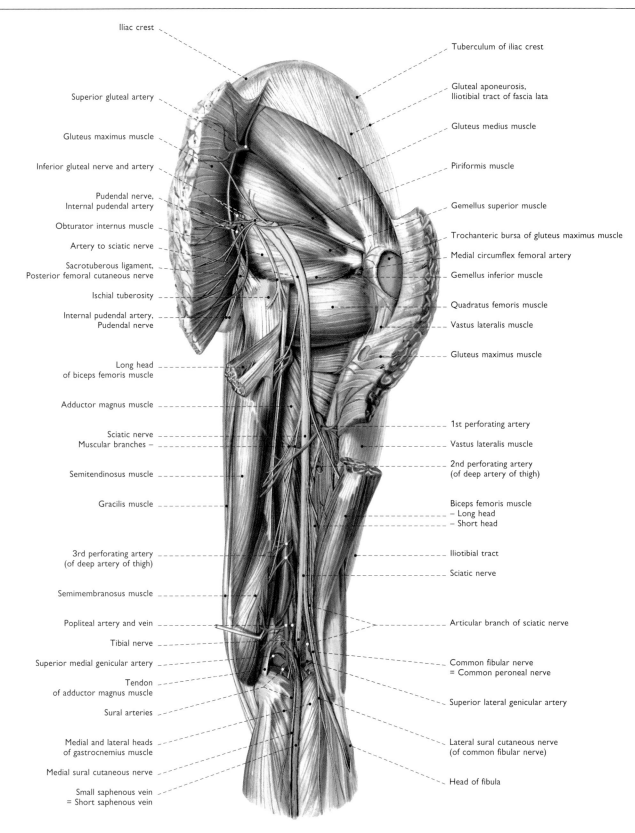

a

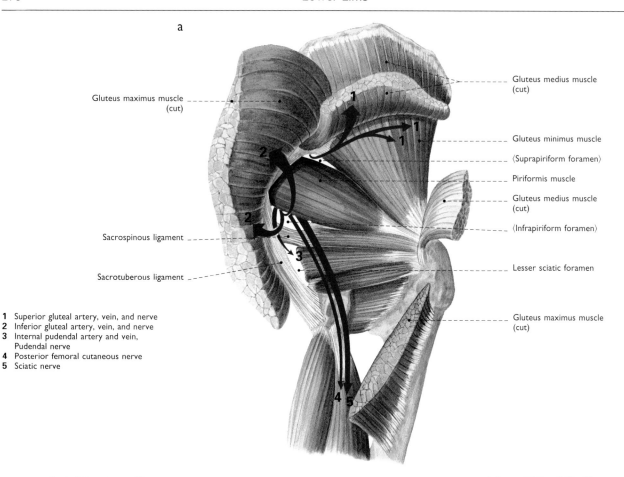

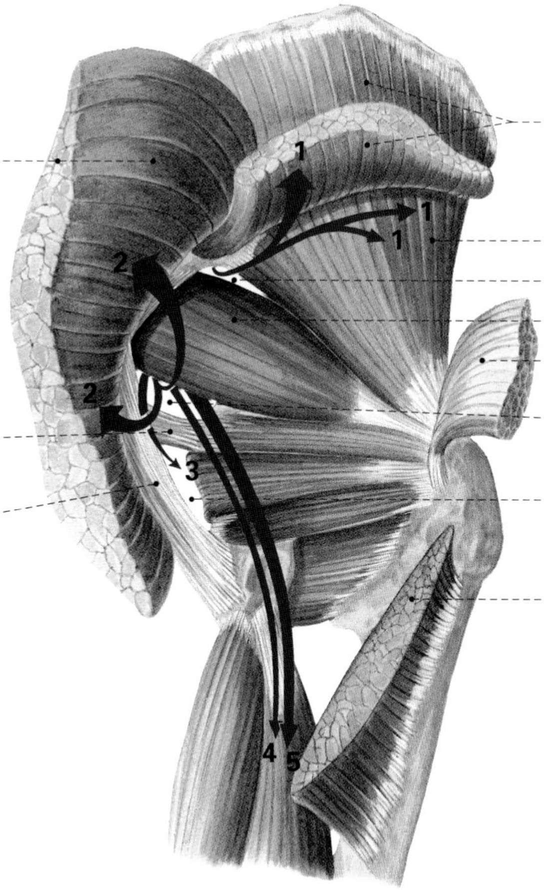
Gluteus maximus muscle (cut)
Sacrospinous ligament
Sacrotuberous ligament
Gluteus medius muscle (cut)
Gluteus minimus muscle
⟨Suprapiriform foramen⟩
Piriformis muscle
Gluteus medius muscle (cut)
⟨Infrapiriform foramen⟩
Lesser sciatic foramen
Gluteus maximus muscle (cut)
1
1
1
2
2
3
4
5

1 Superior gluteal artery, vein, and nerve
2 Inferior gluteal artery, vein, and nerve
3 Internal pudendal artery and vein, Pudendal nerve
4 Posterior femoral cutaneous nerve
5 Sciatic nerve

b

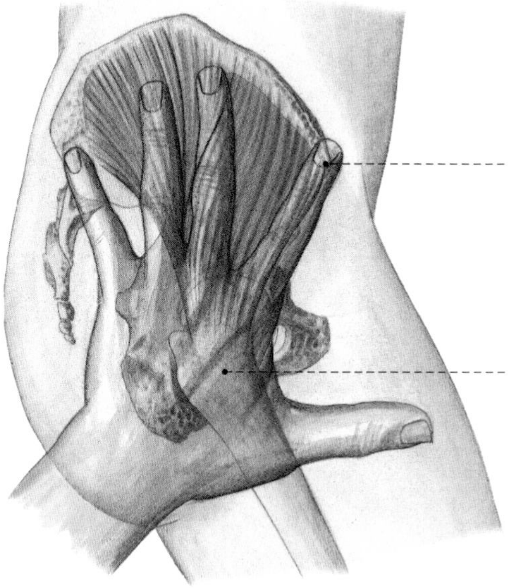
Anterior superior iliac spine
Greater trochanter of femur

c

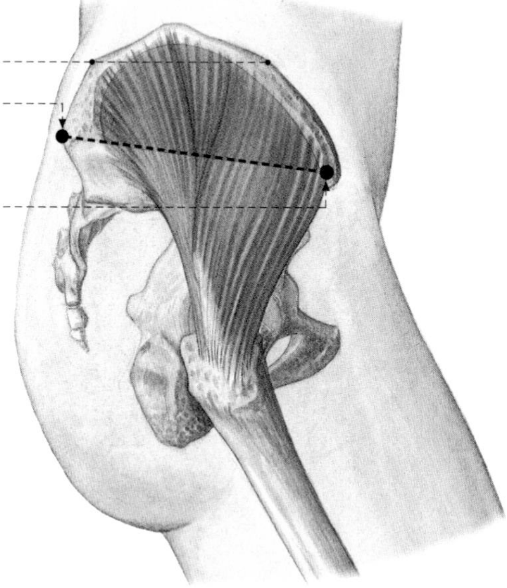
Iliac crest
Posterior superior iliac spine
Anterior superior iliac spine

273 Gluteal region and intragluteal injection

a The gluteus maximus and medius muscles were divided and retracted. The arteries and nerves passing through the greater sciatic foramen above and below the piriformis muscle are given by arrows (35%) (according to von LANZ and WACHSMUTH, 1972). Dorsal aspect

b, c Intragluteal injection according to von HOCHSTETTER (b) and to von LANZ and WACHSMUTH (c). The injection areas are indicated by red color (20%). Lateral aspect

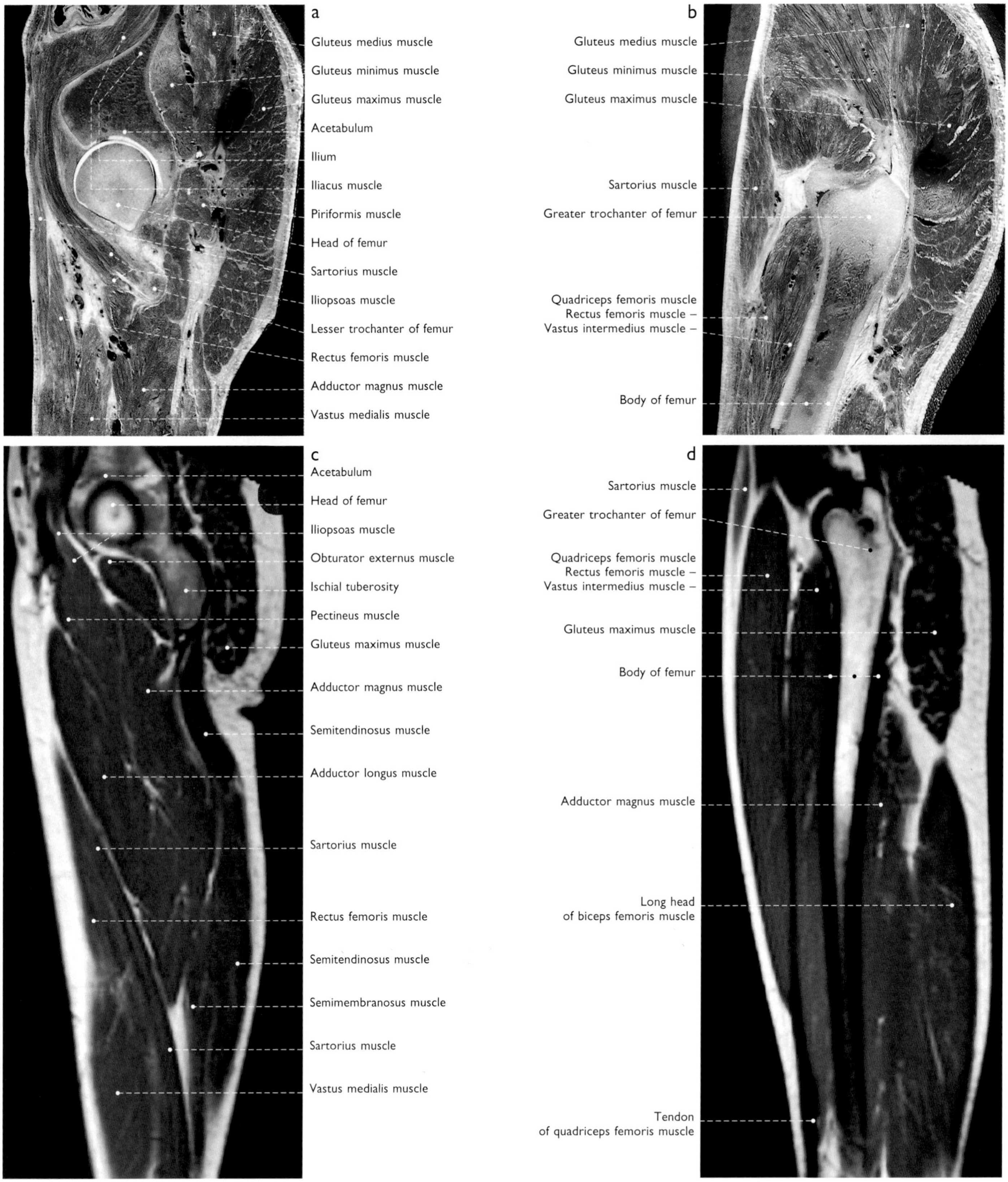
a
Gluteus medius muscle
Gluteus minimus muscle
Gluteus maximus muscle
Acetabulum
Ilium
Iliacus muscle
Piriformis muscle
Head of femur
Sartorius muscle
Iliopsoas muscle
Lesser trochanter of femur
Rectus femoris muscle
Adductor magnus muscle
Vastus medialis muscle
b
Gluteus medius muscle
Gluteus minimus muscle
Gluteus maximus muscle
Sartorius muscle
Greater trochanter of femur
Quadriceps femoris muscle
Rectus femoris muscle –
Vastus intermedius muscle –
Body of femur
c
Acetabulum
Head of femur
Iliopsoas muscle
Obturator externus muscle
Ischial tuberosity
Pectineus muscle
Gluteus maximus muscle
Adductor magnus muscle
Semitendinosus muscle
Adductor longus muscle
Sartorius muscle
Rectus femoris muscle
Semitendinosus muscle
Semimembranosus muscle
Sartorius muscle
Vastus medialis muscle
d
Sartorius muscle
Greater trochanter of femur
Quadriceps femoris muscle
Rectus femoris muscle –
Vastus intermedius muscle –
Gluteus maximus muscle
Body of femur
Adductor magnus muscle
Long head
of biceps femoris muscle
Tendon
of quadriceps femoris muscle

274 Thigh (30%)

a–d Sagittal sections through the head of femur (a, c) and, more laterally, through the greater trochanter and the body of femur (b, d)

a, b Anatomical sections

c, d Magnetic resonance images (MRI, T_1-weighted)

a

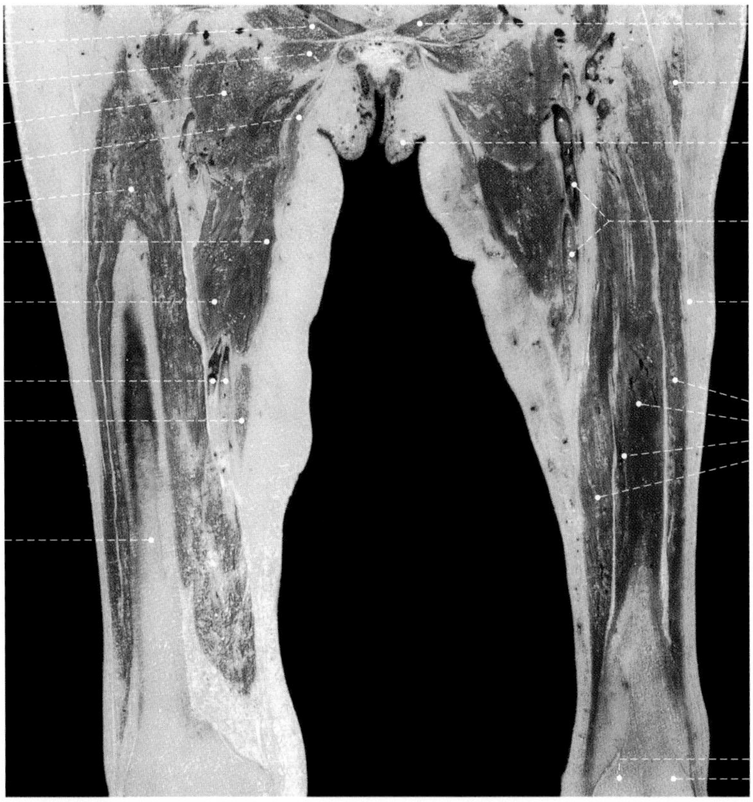
Obturator externus muscle
Pectineus muscle
Adductor brevis muscle
Gracilis muscle
Quadriceps femoris muscle
Adductor magnus muscle
Adductor longus muscle
Femoral artery and vein
Sartorius muscle
Body of femur
Pubis
Tensor fasciae latae muscle
Labium majus
Femoral artery and vein
Iliotibial tract
Quadriceps femoris muscle
– Vastus lateralis muscle
– Rectus femoris muscle
– Vastus intermedius muscle
– Vastus medialis muscle
Femur
– Medial condyle
– Lateral condyle

b

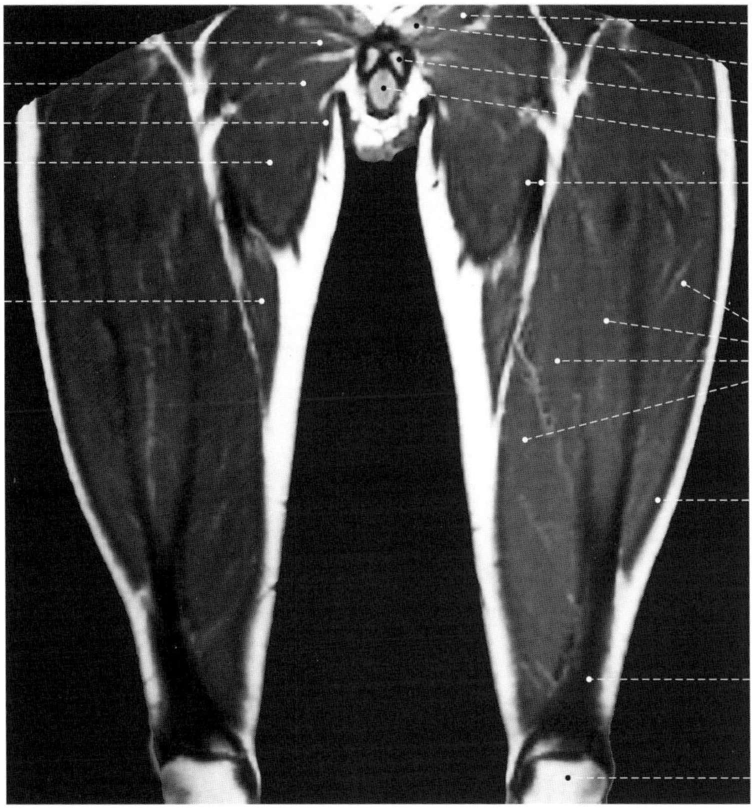
Pectineus muscle
Adductor brevis muscle
Gracilis muscle
Adductor longus muscle
Sartorius muscle
Obturator externus muscle
Pubis
Crus of penis
Bulb of penis
Femoral vein and artery
Quadriceps femoris muscle
– Vastus lateralis muscle
– Rectus femoris muscle
– Vastus intermedius muscle
– Vastus medialis muscle
Iliotibial tract
Tendon
of quadriceps femoris muscle
Patella

275 Thigh (20%)

a, b Coronal sections through the ventral parts of the thighs, ventral aspect

a Anatomical section of a female

b Magnetic resonance image (MRI, T_1-weighted) of a male

a

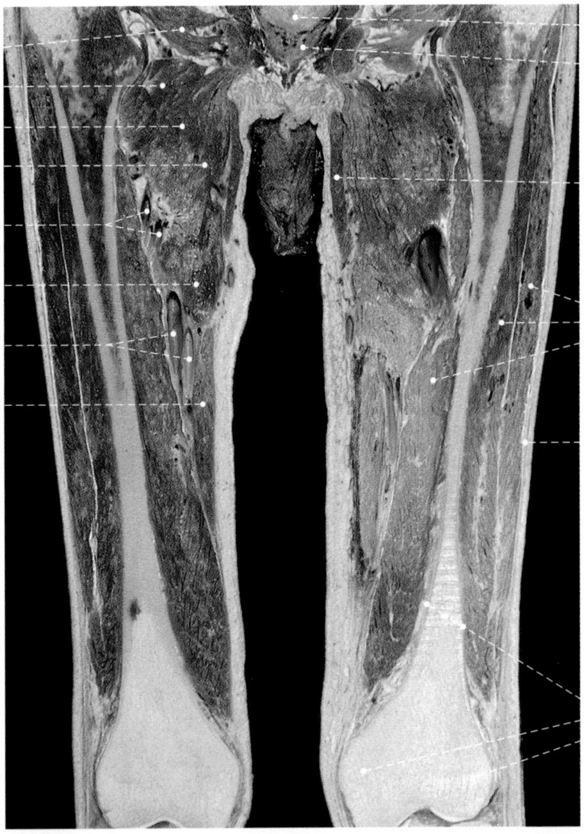
Obturator externus muscle
Pectineus muscle
Adductor brevis muscle
Adductor longus muscle
Deep artery and vein of thigh
Adductor magnus muscle
Femoral artery and vein
Sartorius muscle
Prostate
Seminal gland
Gracilis muscle
Quadriceps femoris muscle
– Vastus lateralis muscle
– Vastus intermedius muscle
– Vastus medialis muscle
Iliotibial tract
Femur
– Body of femur
– Medial condyle
– Lateral condyle

b

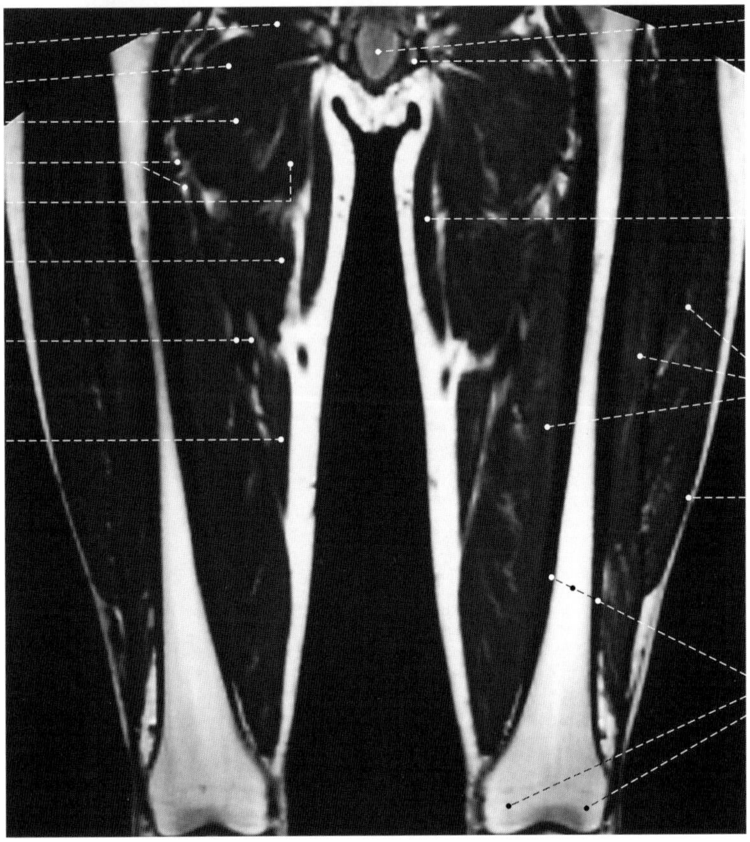
Obturator externus muscle
Pectineus muscle
Adductor brevis muscle
Deep artery and vein of thigh
Adductor longus muscle
Adductor magnus muscle
Femoral artery and vein
Sartorius muscle
Bulb of penis
Crus of penis
Gracilis muscle
Quadriceps femoris muscle
– Vastus lateralis muscle
– Vastus intermedius muscle
– Vastus medialis muscle
Iliotibial tract
Femur
– Body of femur
– Medial condyle
– Lateral condyle

276 Thigh (20%)

a, b Coronal sections through the middle parts of the thighs of a male, ventral aspect
a Anatomical section
b Magnetic resonance image (MRI, T_1-weighted)

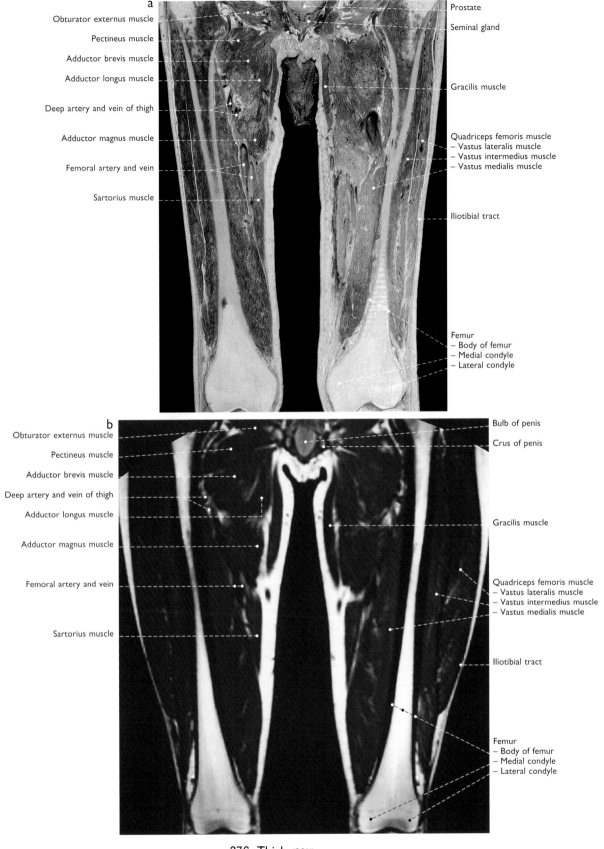

a

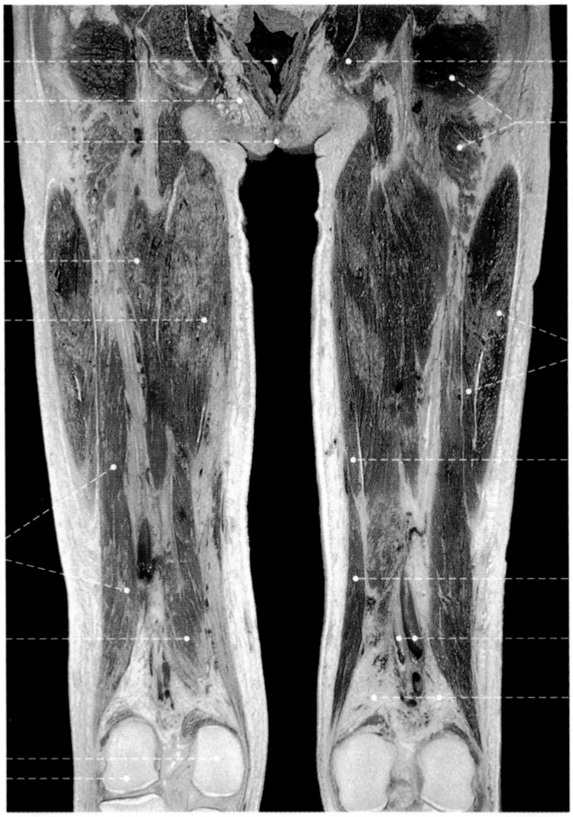
Rectum
Ischio-anal fossa
Anus
Semitendinosus muscle
Adductor magnus muscle
Biceps femoris muscle
Long head –
Short head –
Semimembranosus muscle
Femur
Medial condyle –
Lateral condyle –
Ischium
Gluteus maximus muscle
Quadriceps femoris muscle
– Vastus lateralis muscle
– Vastus intermedius muscle
Gracilis muscle
Sartorius muscle
Popliteal artery and vein
Popliteal fossa

b

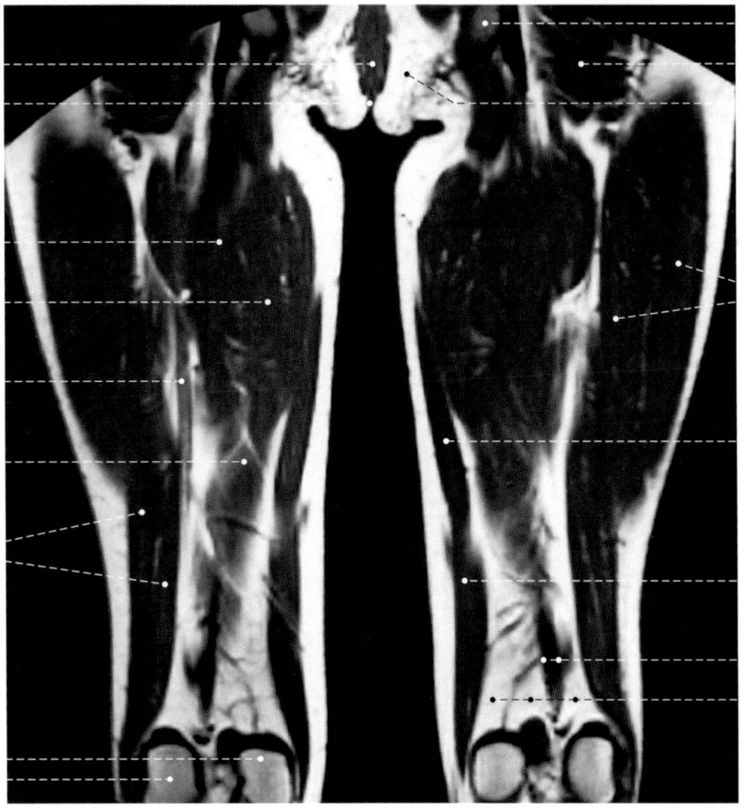
Rectum
Anus
Semitendinosus muscle
Adductor magnus muscle
Sciatic nerve
Semimembranosus muscle
Biceps femoris muscle
Long head –
Short head –
Femur
Medial condyle –
Lateral condyle –
Ischium
Gluteus maximus muscle
Ischio-anal fossa
Quadriceps femoris muscle
– Vastus lateralis muscle
– Vastus intermedius muscle
Gracilis muscle
Sartorius muscle
Popliteal artery and vein
Popliteal fossa

277 Thigh (20%)

a, b Coronal sections through the dorsal parts of the thighs of a male, ventral aspect

a Anatomical section

b Magnetic resonance image (MRI, T_1-weighted)

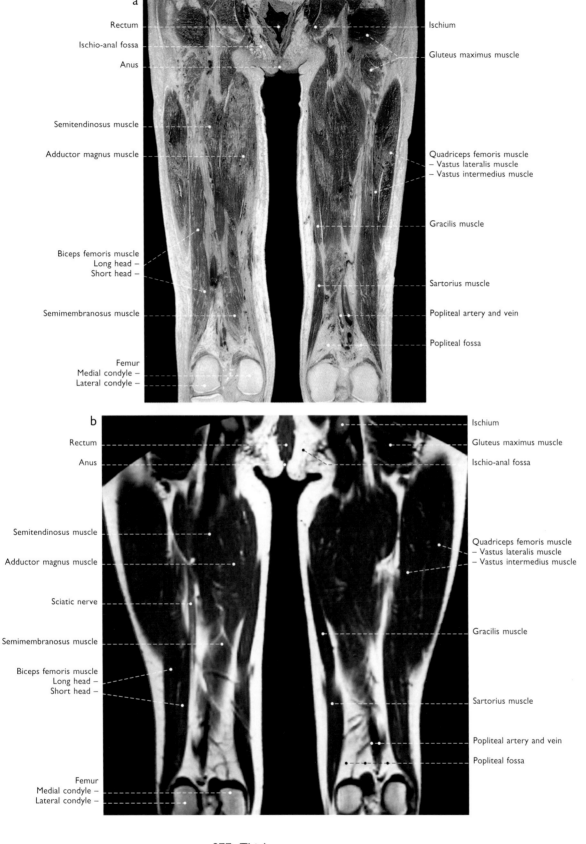

a

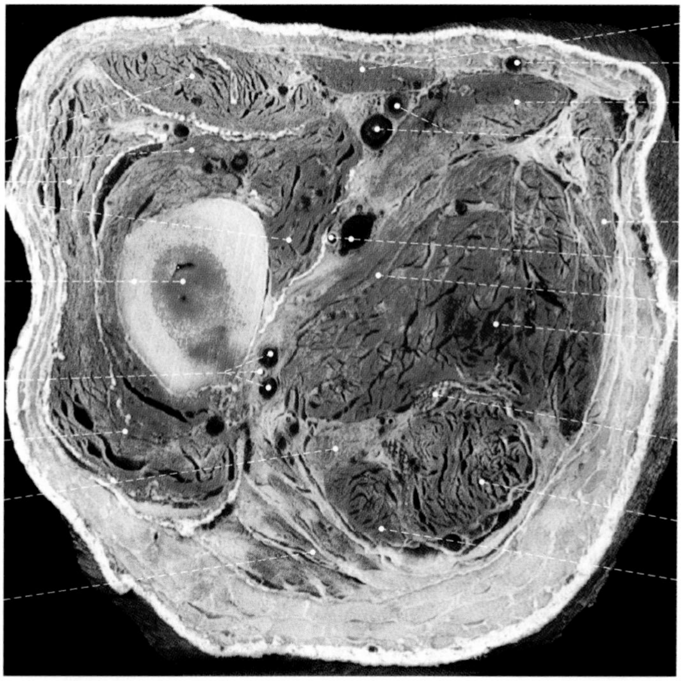
Sartorius muscle
Great saphenous vein
Adductor longus muscle
Femoral artery and vein
Gracilis muscle
Deep artery and vein of thigh
Adductor brevis muscle
Adductor magnus muscle
Tendon of semimembranosus muscle
Semitendinosus muscle
Long head of biceps femoris muscle
Quadriceps femoris muscle
Rectus femoris muscle –
Vastus intermedius muscle –
Vastus lateralis muscle –
Vastus medialis muscle –
Femur
Perforating artery and veins (of deep artery and vein of thigh)
Vastus lateralis muscle
Sciatic nerve
Gluteus maximus muscle

b

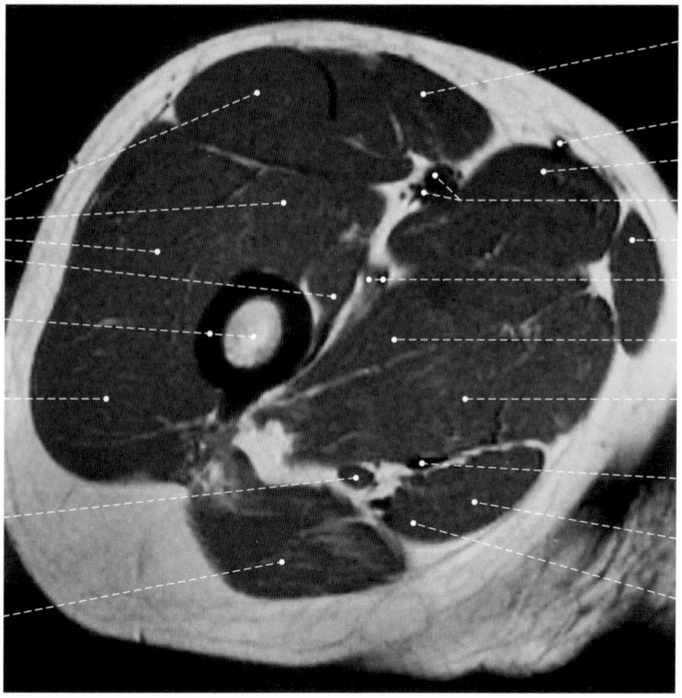
Sartorius muscle
Great saphenous vein
Adductor longus muscle
Femoral artery and vein
Gracilis muscle
Deep artery and vein of thigh
Adductor brevis muscle
Adductor magnus muscle
Tendon of semimembranosus muscle
Semitendinosus muscle
Long head of biceps femoris muscle
Quadriceps femoris muscle
Rectus femoris muscle –
Vastus intermedius muscle –
Vastus lateralis muscle –
Vastus medialis muscle –
Femur
Vastus lateralis muscle
Sciatic nerve
Gluteus maximus muscle

278 Right thigh (50%)

Axial (transverse) sections through the proximal thigh at the transition from the gluteal to the femoral region, inferior (distal) aspect

a Anatomical section

b Magnetic resonance image (MRI, T_1-weighted)

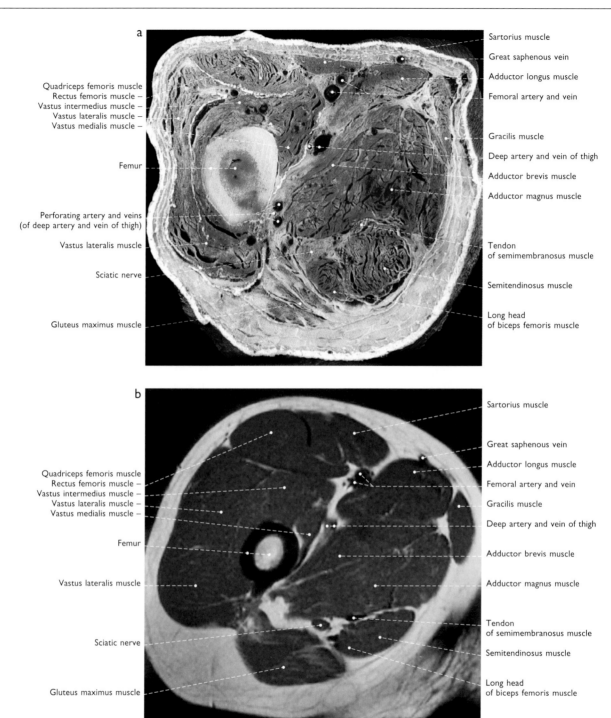

a

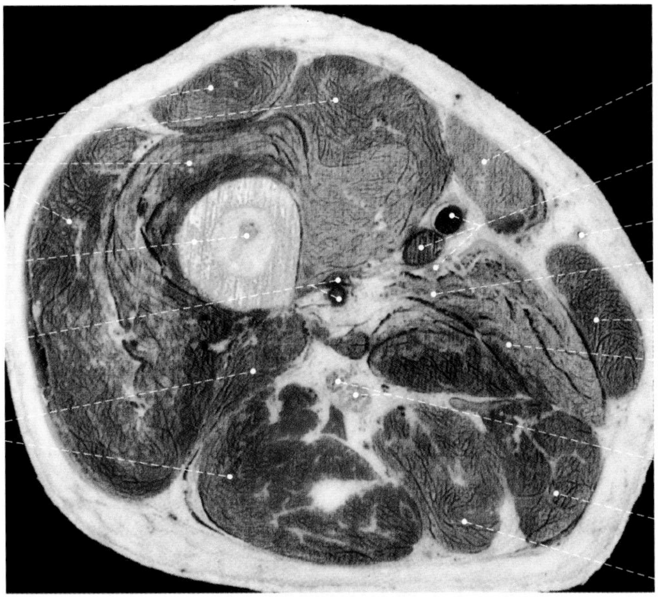
Quadriceps femoris muscle
Rectus femoris muscle –
Vastus medialis muscle –
Vastus intermedius muscle –
Vastus lateralis muscle –
Femur
Perforating vein and artery (of deep vein and artery of thigh)
Biceps femoris muscle
Short head –
Long head –
Sartorius muscle
Femoral artery and vein, Saphenous nerve
Great (= long) saphenous vein
Adductor longus muscle
Gracilis muscle
Adductor magnus muscle
Common fibular (= peroneal) nerve, Tibial nerve
Semimembranosus muscle
Semitendinosus muscle

b

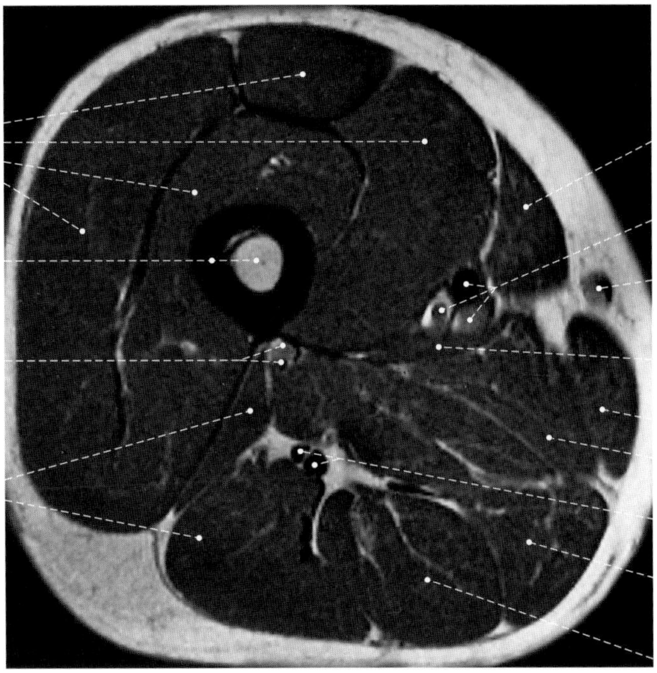
Quadriceps femoris muscle
Rectus femoris muscle –
Vastus medialis muscle –
Vastus intermedius muscle –
Vastus lateralis muscle –
Femur
Perforating vein and artery (of deep vein and artery of thigh)
Biceps femoris muscle
Short head –
Long head –
Sartorius muscle
Femoral artery and vein, Saphenous nerve
Great (= long) saphenous vein
Adductor longus muscle
Gracilis muscle
Adductor magnus muscle
Common fibular (= peroneal) nerve, Tibial nerve
Semimembranosus muscle
Semitendinosus muscle

279 Right thigh (60%)

Axial (transverse) sections through the proximal third of the thigh, inferior (distal) aspect

a Anatomical section

b Magnetic resonance image (MRI, T_1-weighted)

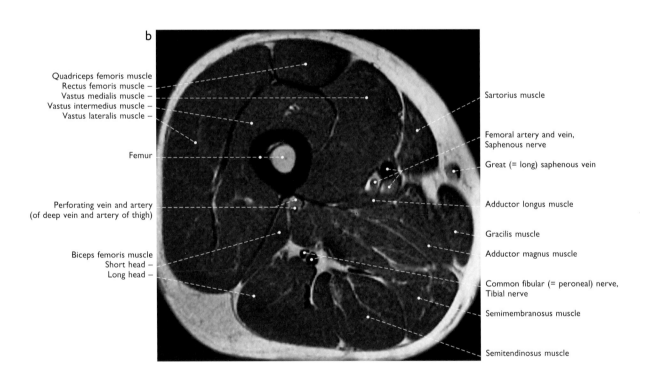

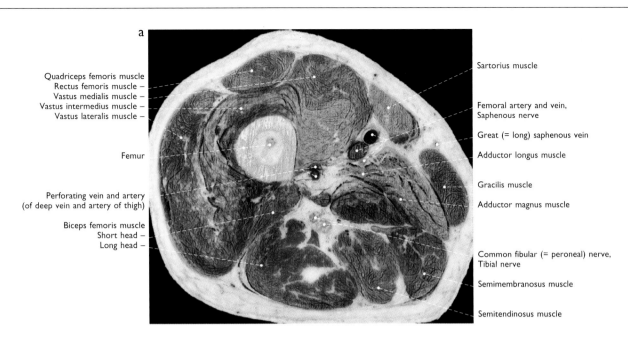

a

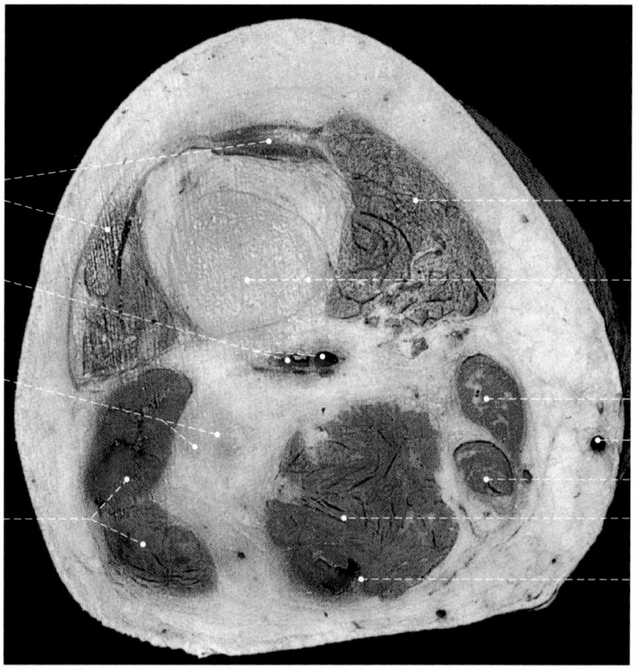
Quadriceps femoris muscle
Tendons
of rectus femoris and
vastus intermedius muscles –
Vastus lateralis muscle –
Popliteal artery and vein
Tibial nerve,
Common fibular (= peroneal) nerve
Biceps femoris muscle
Quadriceps femoris muscle
– Vastus medialis muscle
Femur
Sartorius muscle
Great (= long) saphenous vein
Gracilis muscle
Semimembranosus muscle
Tendon of semitendinosus muscle

b

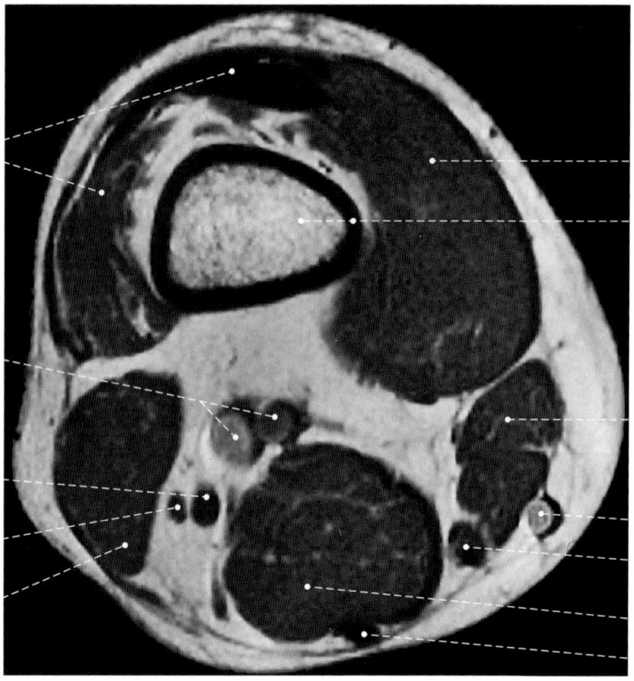
Quadriceps femoris muscle
Tendons
of rectus femoris and
vastus intermedius muscles –
Vastus lateralis muscle –
Popliteal artery and vein
Tibial nerve
Common fibular (= peroneal) nerve
Biceps femoris muscle
Quadriceps femoris muscle
– Vastus medialis muscle
Femur
Sartorius muscle
Great (= long) saphenous vein
Tendon of gracilis muscle
Semimembranosus muscle
Tendon of semitendinosus muscle

280 Right thigh (60%)

Axial (transverse) sections through the distal third of the thigh, inferior (distal) aspect

a Anatomical section

b Magnetic resonance image (MRI, T_1-weighted)

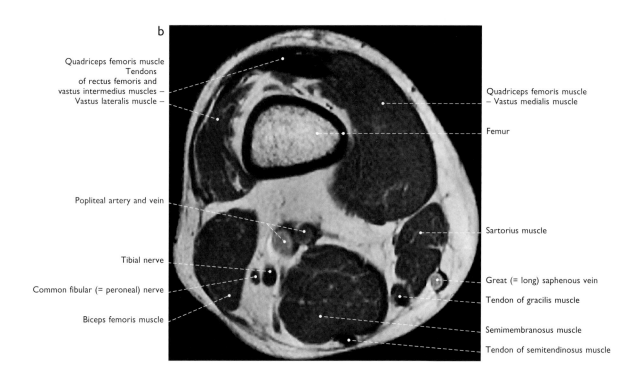

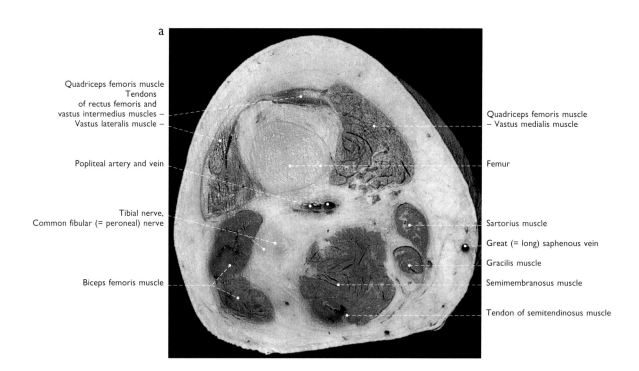

a

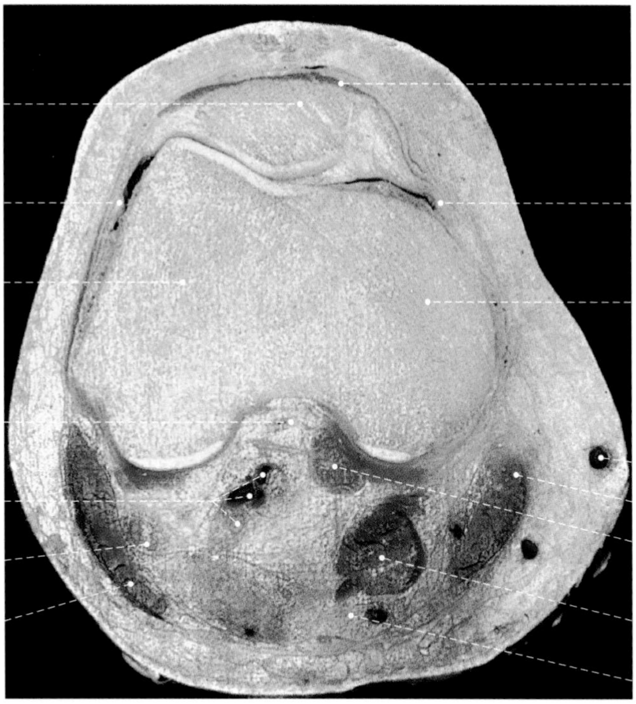
Patella
Lateral patellar retinaculum
Lateral condyle of femur
Anterior cruciate ligament
Popliteal artery and vein, Tibial nerve
Common fibular (= peroneal) nerve
Biceps femoris muscle
Patellar ligament
Medial patellar retinaculum
Medial condyle of femur
Great (= long) saphenous vein
Sartorius muscle
Tendon of medial head of gastrocnemius muscle
Semimembranosus muscle
Tendon of semitendinosus muscle

b

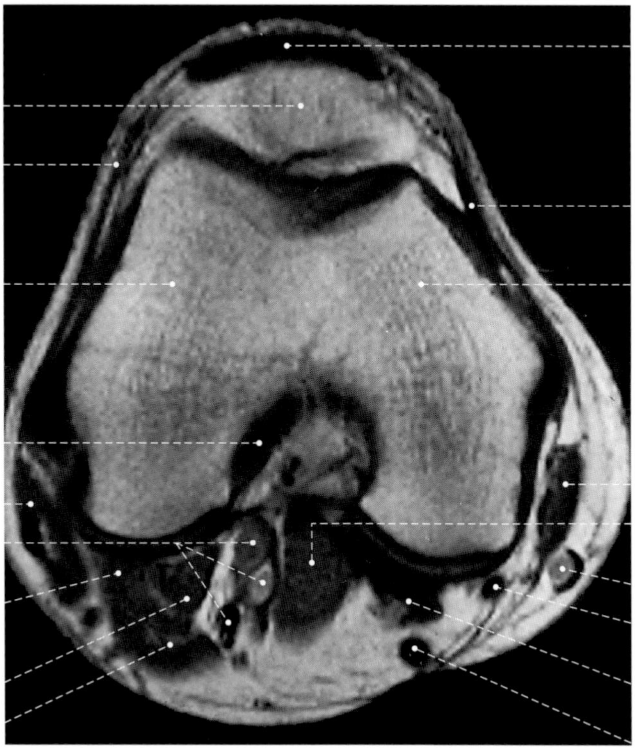
Patella
Lateral patellar retinaculum
Lateral condyle of femur
Anterior cruciate ligament
Biceps femoris muscle
Popliteal artery and vein, Tibial nerve
Common fibular (= peroneal) nerve
Popliteus muscle
Lateral head of gastrocnemius muscle
Patellar ligament
Medial patellar retinaculum
Medial condyle of femur
Sartorius muscle
Medial head of gastrocnemius muscle
Great (= long) saphenous vein
Tendon of gracilis muscle
Semimembranosus muscle
Tendon of semitendinosus muscle

281 Right thigh (60%)

Axial (transverse) sections through the proximal parts of the knee joint, inferior (distal) aspect

a Anatomical section

b Magnetic resonance image (MRI, T_1-weighted)

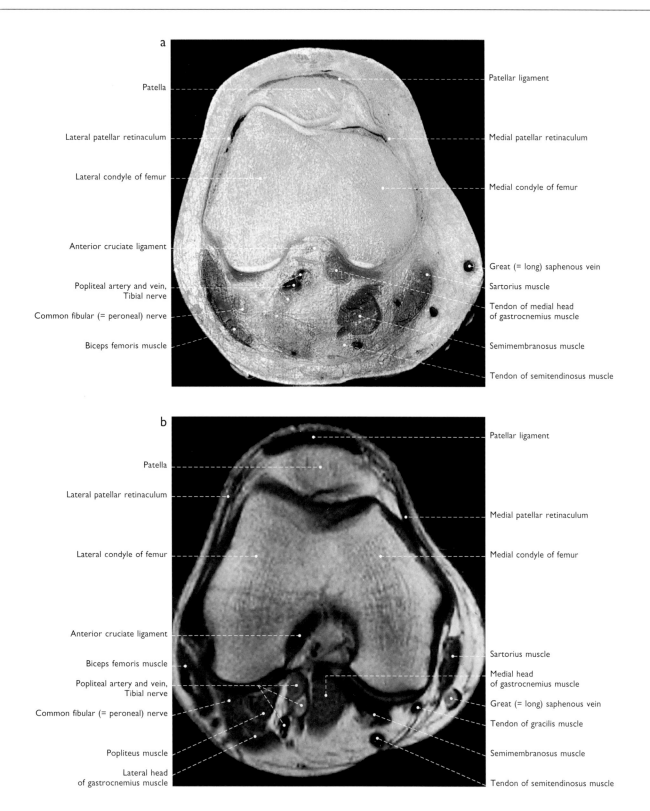

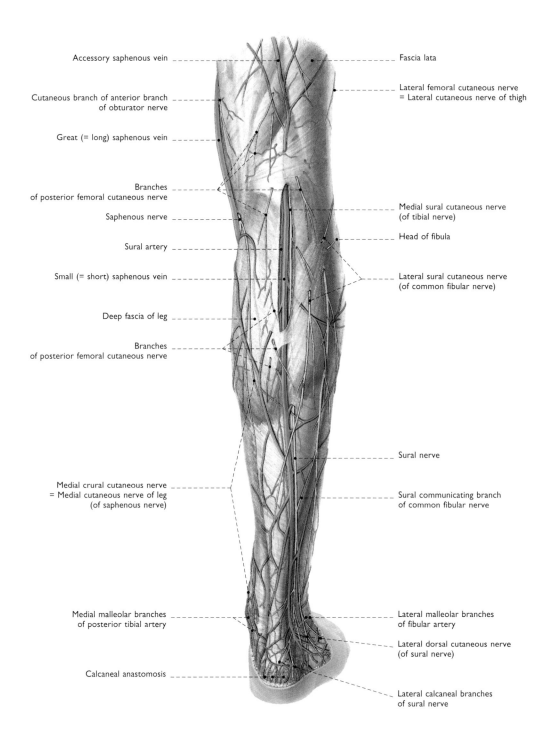

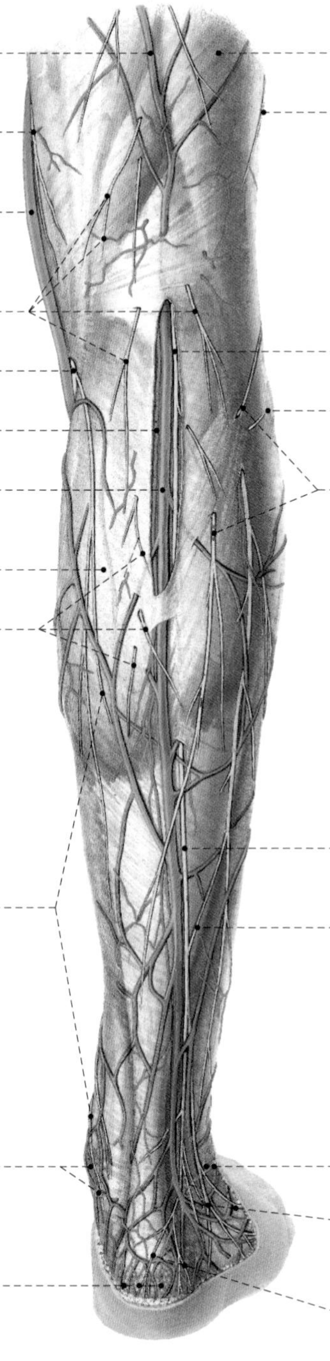
Accessory saphenous vein
Cutaneous branch of anterior branch of obturator nerve
Great (= long) saphenous vein
Branches of posterior femoral cutaneous nerve
Saphenous nerve
Sural artery
Small (= short) saphenous vein
Deep fascia of leg
Branches of posterior femoral cutaneous nerve
Medial crural cutaneous nerve = Medial cutaneous nerve of leg (of saphenous nerve)
Medial malleolar branches of posterior tibial artery
Calcaneal anastomosis
Fascia lata
Lateral femoral cutaneous nerve = Lateral cutaneous nerve of thigh
Medial sural cutaneous nerve (of tibial nerve)
Head of fibula
Lateral sural cutaneous nerve (of common fibular nerve)
Sural nerve
Sural communicating branch of common fibular nerve
Lateral malleolar branches of fibular artery
Lateral dorsal cutaneous nerve (of sural nerve)
Lateral calcaneal branches of sural nerve

282 Subcutaneous blood vessels and nerves of the popliteal fossa and the leg of the right side (30%)

Dorsal aspect

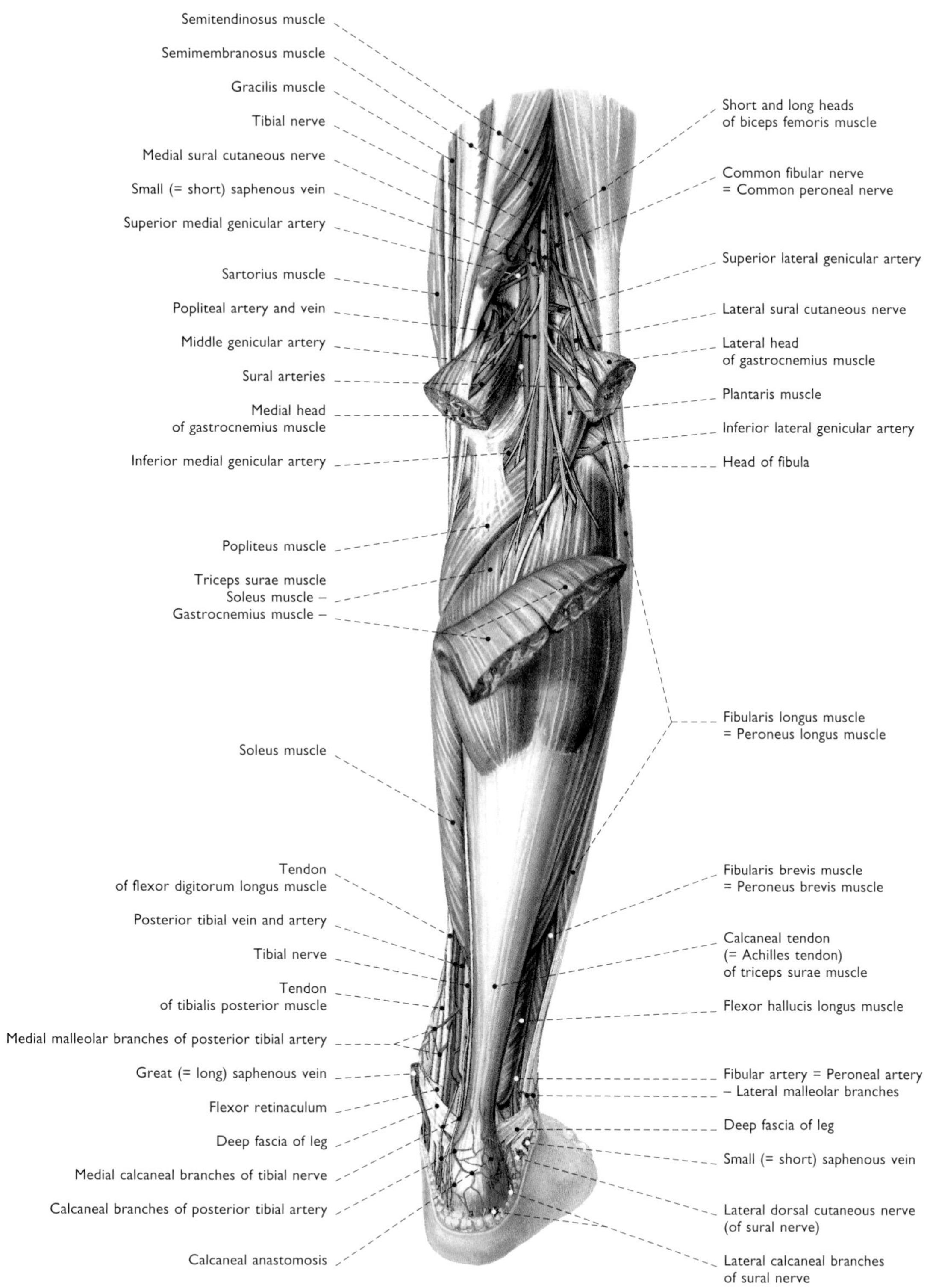
Semitendinosus muscle
Semimembranosus muscle
Gracilis muscle
Tibial nerve
Medial sural cutaneous nerve
Small (= short) saphenous vein
Superior medial genicular artery
Sartorius muscle
Popliteal artery and vein
Middle genicular artery
Sural arteries
Medial head
of gastrocnemius muscle
Inferior medial genicular artery
Popliteus muscle
Triceps surae muscle
Soleus muscle –
Gastrocnemius muscle –
Soleus muscle
Tendon
of flexor digitorum longus muscle
Posterior tibial vein and artery
Tibial nerve
Tendon
of tibialis posterior muscle
Medial malleolar branches of posterior tibial artery
Great (= long) saphenous vein
Flexor retinaculum
Deep fascia of leg
Medial calcaneal branches of tibial nerve
Calcaneal branches of posterior tibial artery
Calcaneal anastomosis
Short and long heads
of biceps femoris muscle
Common fibular nerve
= Common peroneal nerve
Superior lateral genicular artery
Lateral sural cutaneous nerve
Lateral head
of gastrocnemius muscle
Plantaris muscle
Inferior lateral genicular artery
Head of fibula
Fibularis longus muscle
= Peroneus longus muscle
Fibularis brevis muscle
= Peroneus brevis muscle
Calcaneal tendon
(= Achilles tendon)
of triceps surae muscle
Flexor hallucis longus muscle
Fibular artery = Peroneal artery
– Lateral malleolar branches
Deep fascia of leg
Small (= short) saphenous vein
Lateral dorsal cutaneous nerve
(of sural nerve)
Lateral calcaneal branches
of sural nerve

283 Blood vessels and nerves of the popliteal fossa and the leg of the right side (30%)

The gastrocnemius muscle was divided. Dorsal aspect

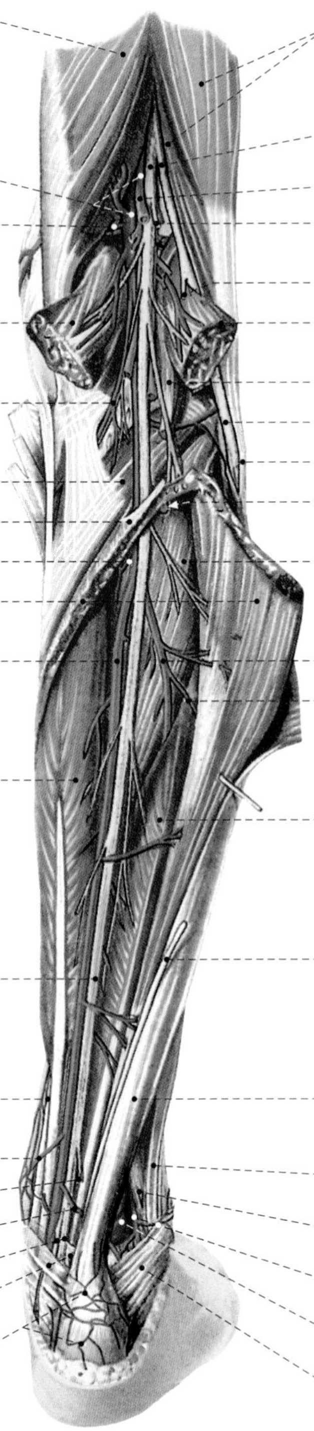
Semimembranosus muscle
Popliteal vein and artery
Superior medial genicular artery
Medial head of gastrocnemius muscle
Inferior medial genicular artery
Popliteus muscle
Tendinous arch of soleus muscle
Tibial nutrient artery
Soleus muscle
Posterior tibial artery
Flexor digitorum longus muscle
Tibial nerve
Tendon of tibialis posterior muscle
Medial malleolar branch of posterior tibial artery
Medial calcaneal branches of tibial nerve
Communicating branch of fibular artery
Medial and lateral plantar nerves
Deep fascia of leg, Flexor retinaculum
Calcaneal anastomosis
Long and short heads of biceps femoris muscle
Tibial nerve, Common fibular nerve
Small (= short) saphenous vein
Medial sural cutaneous nerve
Lateral sural cutaneous nerve
Lateral head of gastrocnemius muscle
Plantaris muscle
Common fibular (= peroneal) nerve
Head of fibula
Anterior tibial artery
Tibialis posterior muscle
Fibular artery = Peroneal artery
Fibular nutrient artery
Flexor hallucis longus muscle
Tendon of plantaris muscle
Calcaneal tendon (= Achilles tendon) of triceps surae muscle
Tendon of fibularis longus muscle
Tendon of fibularis brevis muscle
Lateral malleolar branches of fibular (= peroneal) artery
Flexor hallucis longus muscle
Superior fibular (= peroneal) retinaculum

284 Blood vessels and nerves of the popliteal fossa and the leg of the right side (30%)

The gastrocnemius and soleus muscles were divided, the deep veins removed. Dorsal aspect

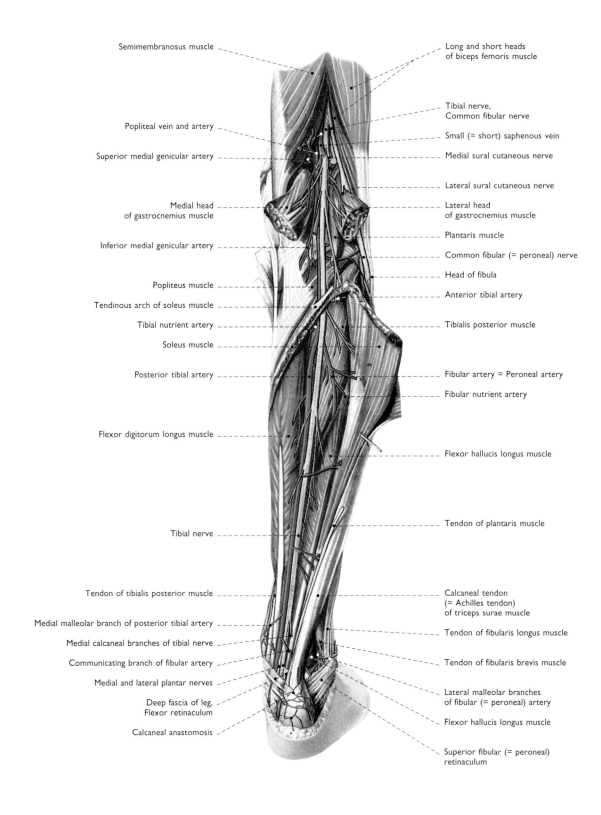

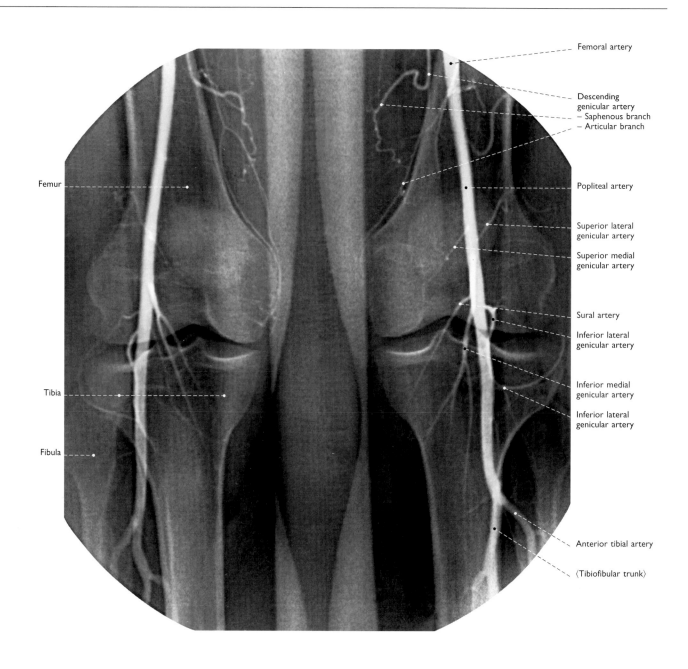

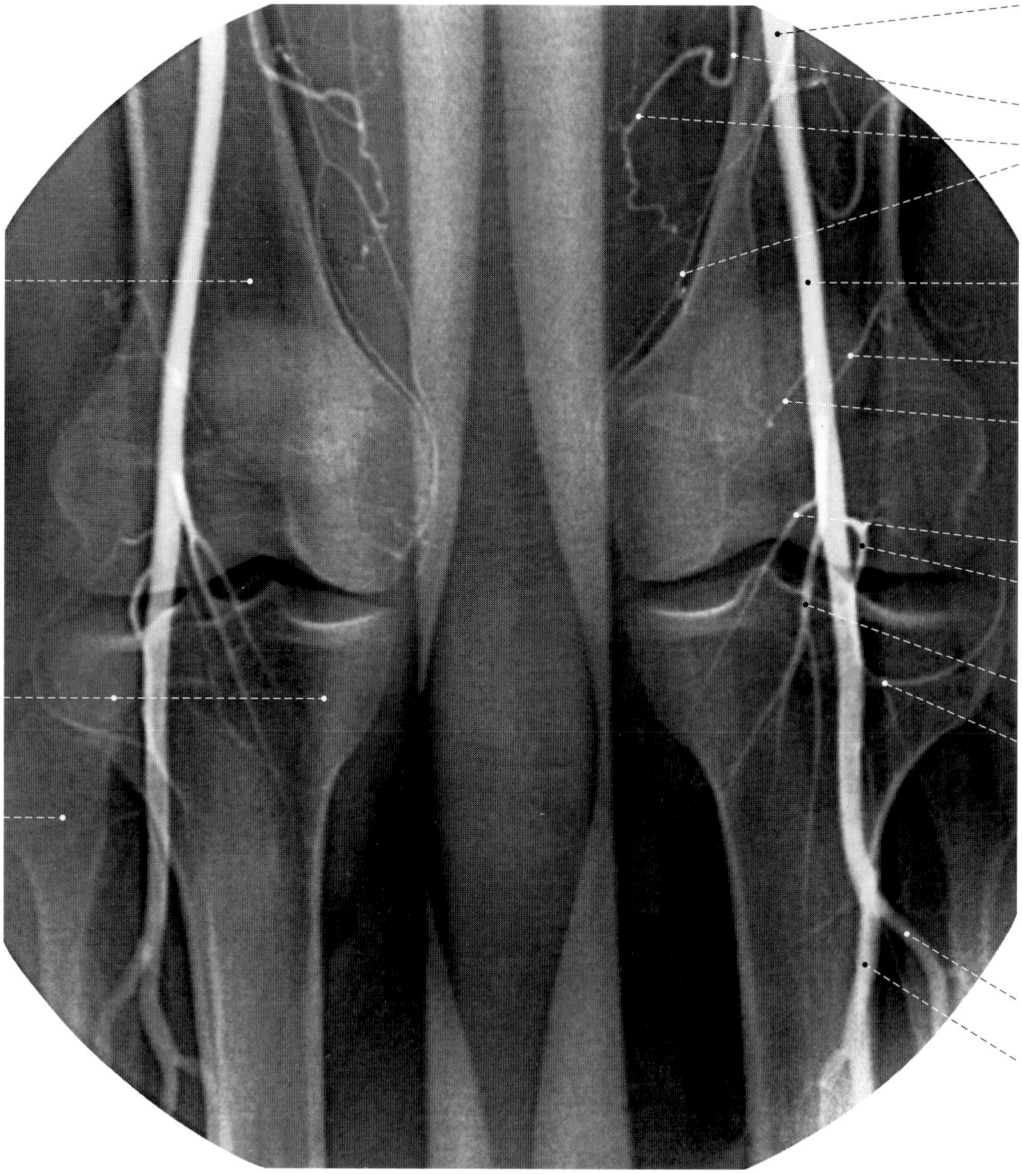
Femoral artery
Descending genicular artery
– Saphenous branch
– Articular branch
Femur
Popliteal artery
Superior lateral genicular artery
Superior medial genicular artery
Sural artery
Inferior lateral genicular artery
Tibia
Inferior medial genicular artery
Inferior lateral genicular artery
Fibula
Anterior tibial artery
⟨Tibiofibular trunk⟩

285 Arteries of the lower limb (60%)

Anteroposterior arteriogram of the femoral, popliteal, and tibial arteries

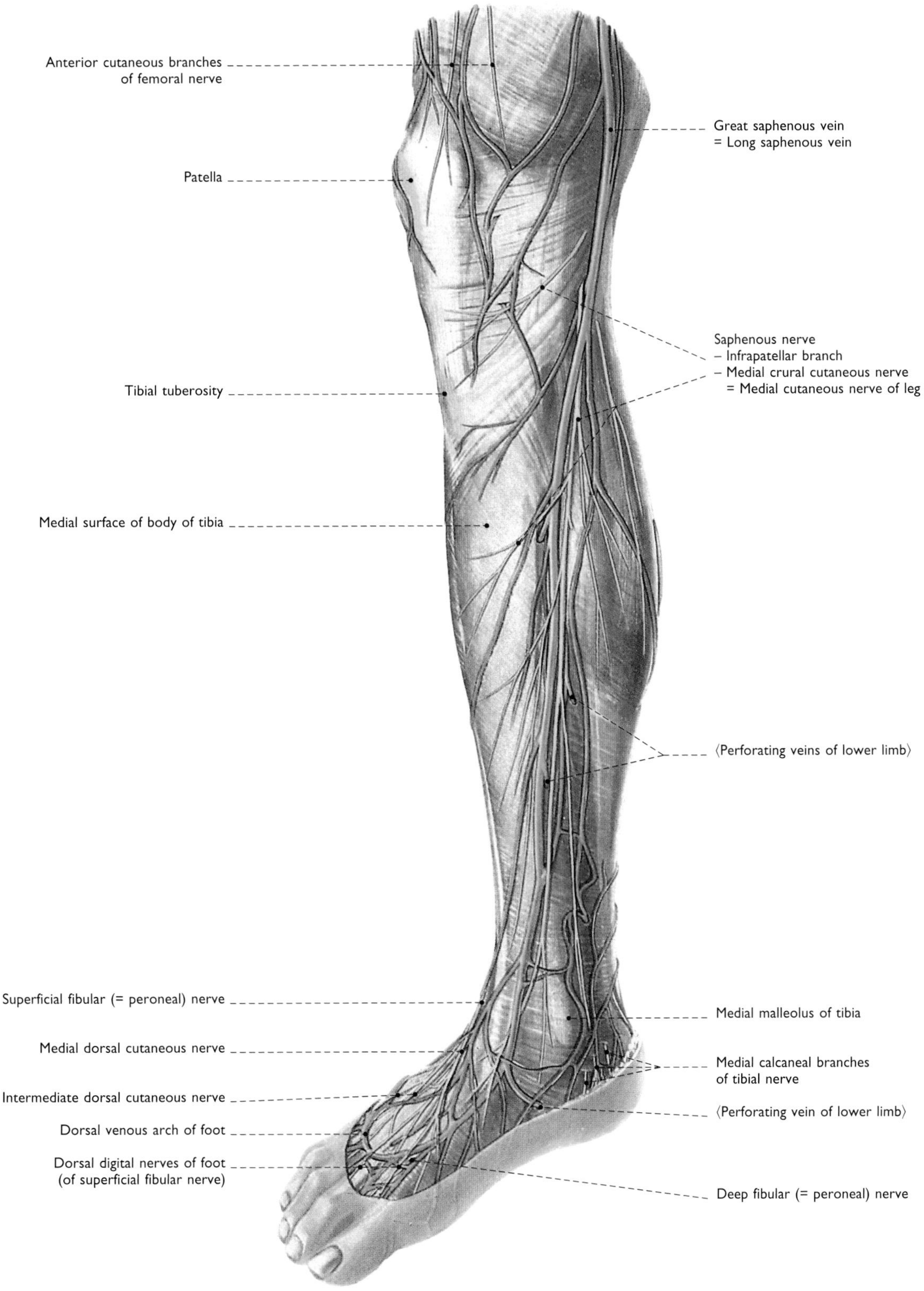
Anterior cutaneous branches of femoral nerve
Patella
Tibial tuberosity
Medial surface of body of tibia
Superficial fibular (= peroneal) nerve
Medial dorsal cutaneous nerve
Intermediate dorsal cutaneous nerve
Dorsal venous arch of foot
Dorsal digital nerves of foot (of superficial fibular nerve)
Great saphenous vein = Long saphenous vein
Saphenous nerve
– Infrapatellar branch
– Medial crural cutaneous nerve = Medial cutaneous nerve of leg
⟨Perforating veins of lower limb⟩
Medial malleolus of tibia
Medial calcaneal branches of tibial nerve
⟨Perforating vein of lower limb⟩
Deep fibular (= peroneal) nerve

286 Subcutaneous veins and nerves of the right leg and foot (30%)

Ventromedial aspect

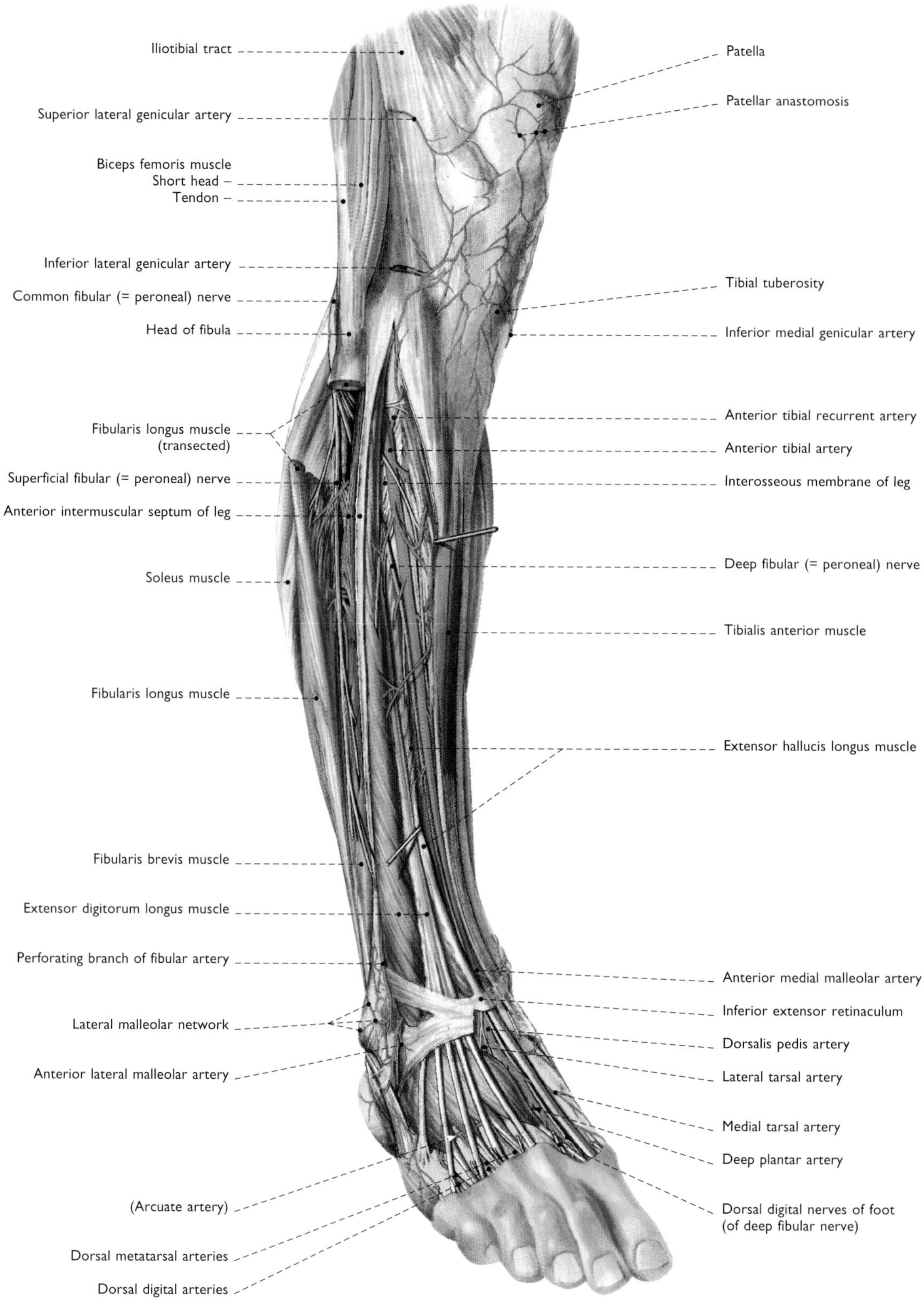
Iliotibial tract
Superior lateral genicular artery
Biceps femoris muscle
Short head
Tendon
Inferior lateral genicular artery
Common fibular (= peroneal) nerve
Head of fibula
Fibularis longus muscle (transected)
Superficial fibular (= peroneal) nerve
Anterior intermuscular septum of leg
Soleus muscle
Fibularis longus muscle
Fibularis brevis muscle
Extensor digitorum longus muscle
Perforating branch of fibular artery
Lateral malleolar network
Anterior lateral malleolar artery
(Arcuate artery)
Dorsal metatarsal arteries
Dorsal digital arteries
Patella
Patellar anastomosis
Tibial tuberosity
Inferior medial genicular artery
Anterior tibial recurrent artery
Anterior tibial artery
Interosseous membrane of leg
Deep fibular (= peroneal) nerve
Tibialis anterior muscle
Extensor hallucis longus muscle
Anterior medial malleolar artery
Inferior extensor retinaculum
Dorsalis pedis artery
Lateral tarsal artery
Medial tarsal artery
Deep plantar artery
Dorsal digital nerves of foot (of deep fibular nerve)

287 Arteries and nerves of the right leg and foot (30%)

The deep veins were removed. Ventrolateral aspect

a

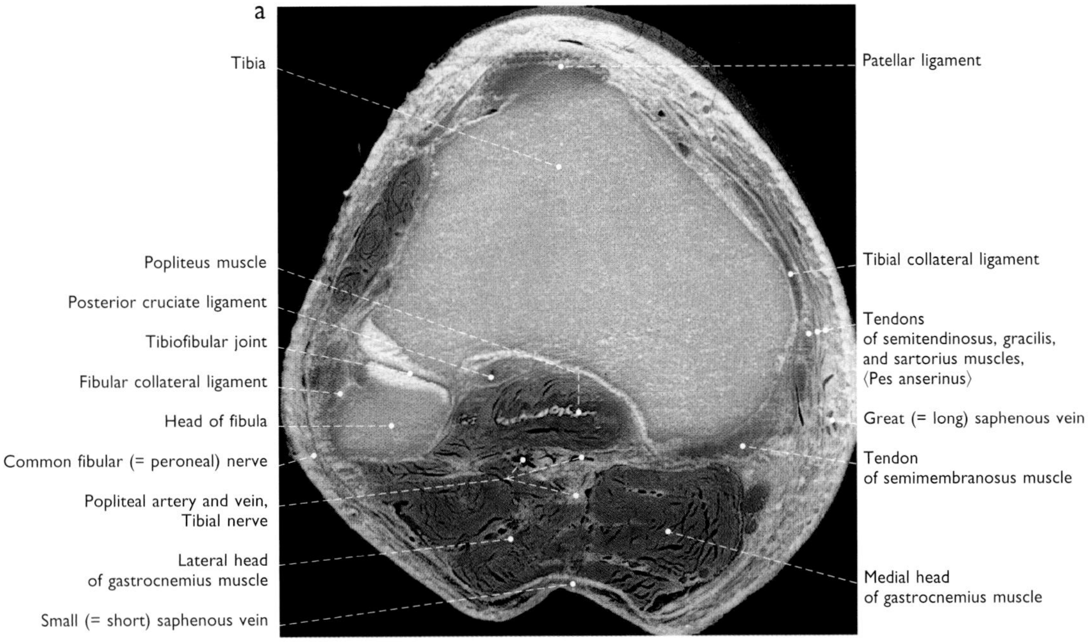
Tibia
Popliteus muscle
Posterior cruciate ligament
Tibiofibular joint
Fibular collateral ligament
Head of fibula
Common fibular (= peroneal) nerve
Popliteal artery and vein, Tibial nerve
Lateral head of gastrocnemius muscle
Small (= short) saphenous vein
Patellar ligament
Tibial collateral ligament
Tendons of semitendinosus, gracilis, and sartorius muscles, ⟨Pes anserinus⟩
Great (= long) saphenous vein
Tendon of semimembranosus muscle
Medial head of gastrocnemius muscle

b

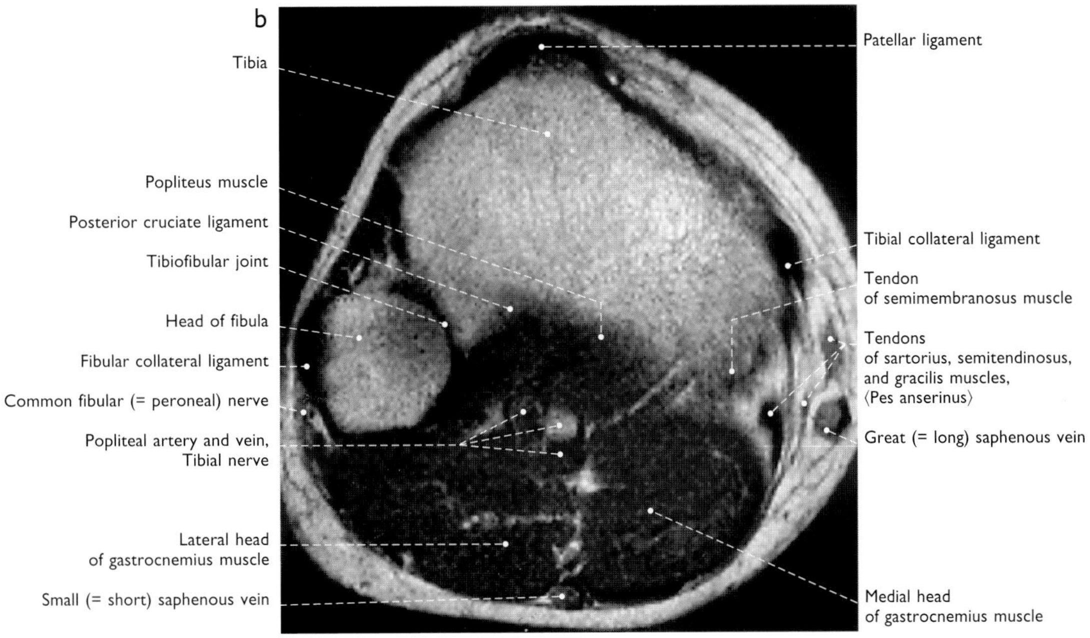
Tibia
Popliteus muscle
Posterior cruciate ligament
Tibiofibular joint
Head of fibula
Fibular collateral ligament
Common fibular (= peroneal) nerve
Popliteal artery and vein, Tibial nerve
Lateral head of gastrocnemius muscle
Small (= short) saphenous vein
Patellar ligament
Tibial collateral ligament
Tendon of semimembranosus muscle
Tendons of sartorius, semitendinosus, and gracilis muscles, ⟨Pes anserinus⟩
Great (= long) saphenous vein
Medial head of gastrocnemius muscle

288 Right leg (70%)

Axial (transverse) sections through the proximal leg at the level of the superior tibiofibular joint, inferior (distal) aspect

a Anatomical section

b Magnetic resonance image (MRI, T_1-weighted)

a

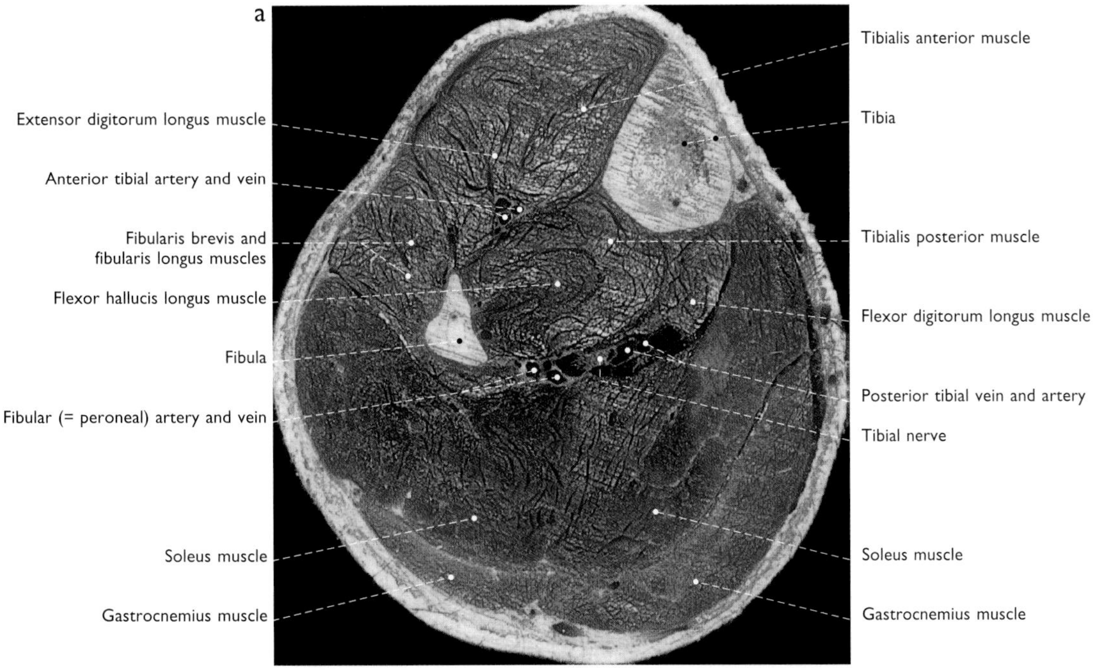
Extensor digitorum longus muscle
Anterior tibial artery and vein
Fibularis brevis and fibularis longus muscles
Flexor hallucis longus muscle
Fibula
Fibular (= peroneal) artery and vein
Soleus muscle
Gastrocnemius muscle
Tibialis anterior muscle
Tibia
Tibialis posterior muscle
Flexor digitorum longus muscle
Posterior tibial vein and artery
Tibial nerve
Soleus muscle
Gastrocnemius muscle

b

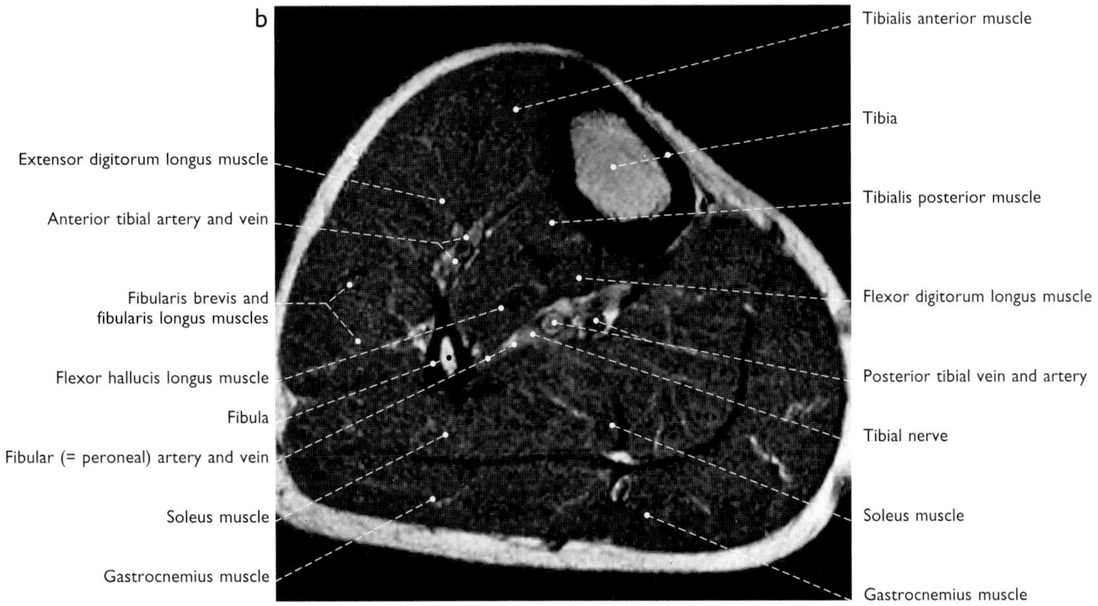
Extensor digitorum longus muscle
Anterior tibial artery and vein
Fibularis brevis and fibularis longus muscles
Flexor hallucis longus muscle
Fibula
Fibular (= peroneal) artery and vein
Soleus muscle
Gastrocnemius muscle
Tibialis anterior muscle
Tibia
Tibialis posterior muscle
Flexor digitorum longus muscle
Posterior tibial vein and artery
Tibial nerve
Soleus muscle
Gastrocnemius muscle

289 Right leg (70%)

Axial (transverse) sections through the proximal third of the leg, inferior (distal) aspect

a Anatomical section

b Magnetic resonance image (MRI, T_1-weighted)

a

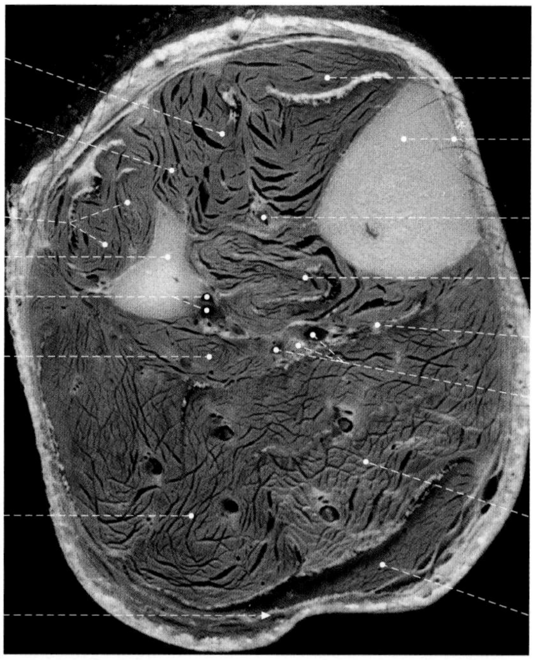
Extensor hallucis longus muscle
Extensor digitorum longus muscle
Fibularis brevis and fibularis longus muscles
Fibula
Fibular (= peroneal) artery and vein
Flexor hallucis longus muscle
Soleus muscle
Small (= short) saphenous vein
Tibialis anterior muscle
Tibia
Anterior tibial artery and vein,
Deep fibular (= peroneal) nerve
Tibialis posterior muscle
Flexor digitorum longus muscle
Posterior tibial artery and vein,
Tibial nerve
Soleus muscle
Gastrocnemius muscle

b

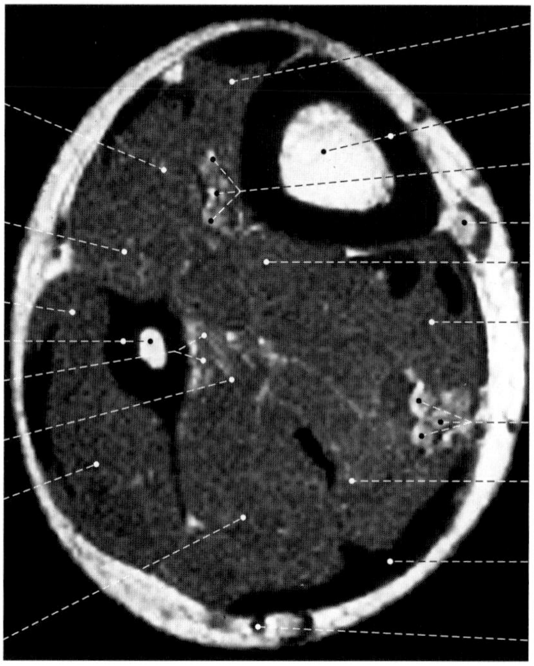
Extensor hallucis longus muscle
Extensor digitorum longus muscle
Fibularis brevis muscle
Fibula
Fibular (= peroneal) artery and vein
Flexor hallucis longus muscle
Fibularis longus muscle
Soleus muscle
Tibialis anterior muscle
Tibia
Anterior tibial artery and vein,
Deep fibular (= peroneal) nerve
Great (= long) saphenous vein
Tibialis posterior muscle
Flexor digitorum longus muscle
Posterior tibial artery and vein,
Tibial nerve
Soleus muscle
Gastrocnemius muscle
Small (= short) saphenous vein

290 Right leg (75%)

Axial (transverse) sections through the middle third of the leg, inferior (distal) aspect

a Anatomical section

b Magnetic resonance image (MRI, T_1-weighted)

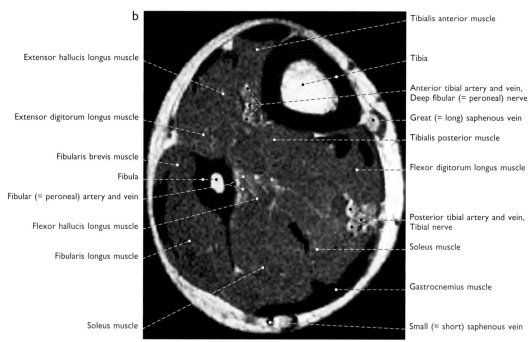

a

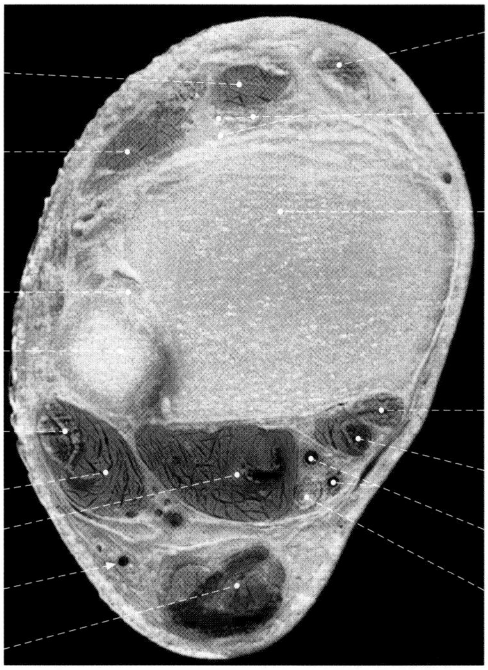
Extensor hallucis longus muscle
Extensor digitorum longus muscle
Tibiofibular syndesmosis
Fibula
Tendon of fibularis longus muscle
Fibularis brevis muscle
Flexor hallucis longus muscle
Small (= short) saphenous vein
Calcaneal tendon (= Achilles tendon)
Tendon of tibialis anterior muscle
Anterior tibial artery and vein, Deep fibular (= peroneal) nerve
Tibia
Tendon of tibialis posterior muscle
Tendon of flexor digitorum longus muscle
Posterior tibial artery and vein
Tibial nerve

b

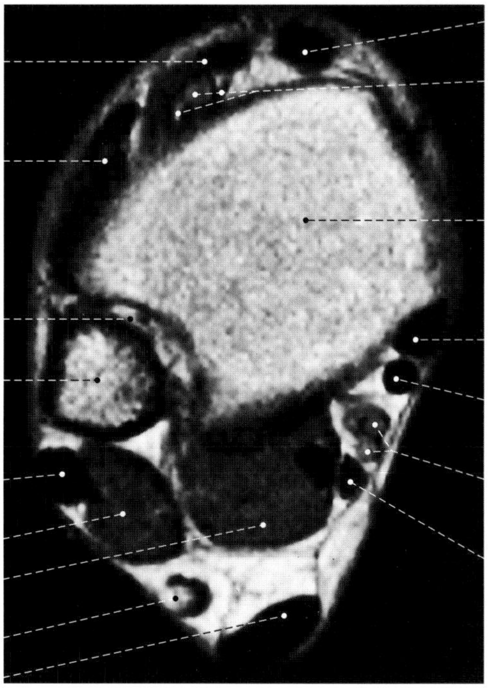
Extensor hallucis longus muscle
Extensor digitorum longus muscle
Tibiofibular syndesmosis
Fibula
Tendon of fibularis longus muscle
Fibularis brevis muscle
Flexor hallucis longus muscle
Small (= short) saphenous vein
Calcaneal tendon (= Achilles tendon)
Tendon of tibialis anterior muscle
Anterior tibial artery and vein, Deep fibular (= peroneal) nerve
Tibia
Tendon of tibialis posterior muscle
Tendon of flexor digitorum longus muscle
Posterior tibial artery and vein
Tibial nerve

291 Right leg (75%)

Axial (transverse) sections through the distal leg at the level of the inferior tibiofibular joint (= tibiofibular syndesmosis), inferior (distal) aspect

a Anatomical section

b Magnetic resonance image (MRI, T_1-weighted)

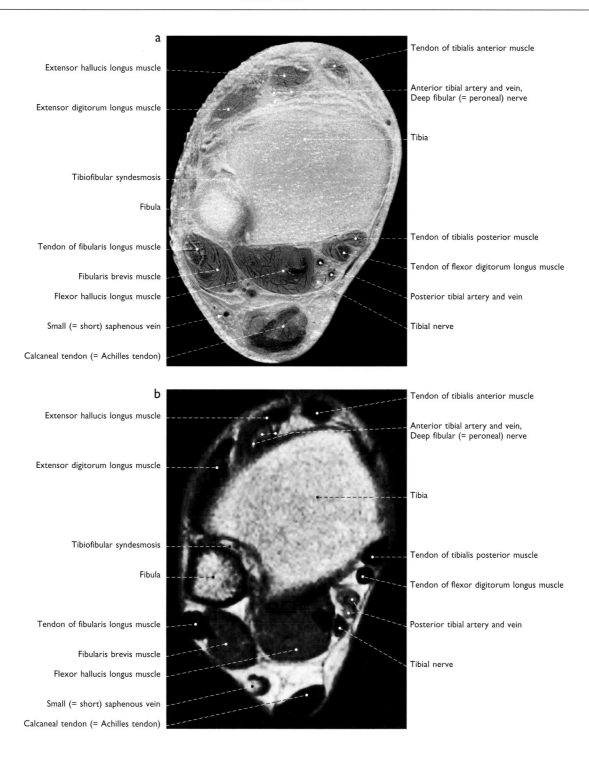

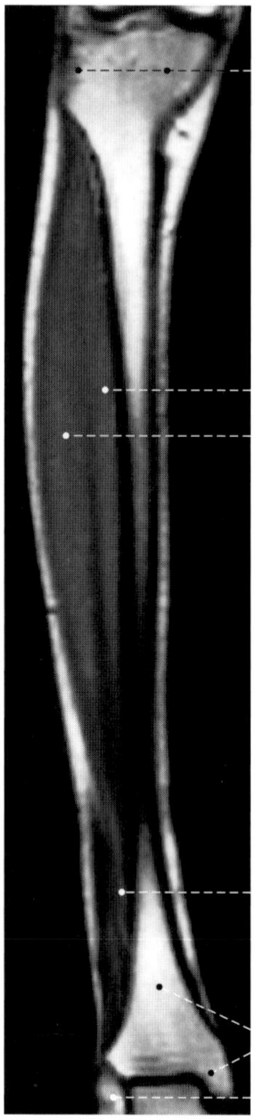
a
Lateral and medial condyles of tibia
Tibialis anterior muscle
Extensor digitorum longus muscle
Extensor hallucis longus muscle
Tibia
– Body of tibia
– Medial malleolus
Lateral malleolus of fibula

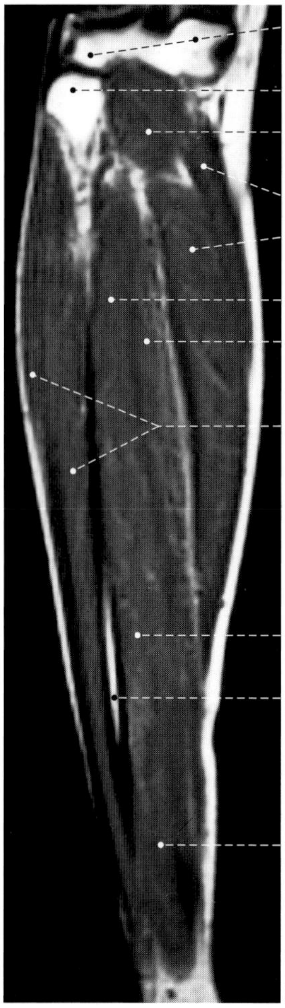
b
Lateral and medial condyles of tibia
Head of fibula
Popliteus muscle
Triceps surae muscle
– Medial head of gastrocnemius muscle
– Soleus muscle
Tibialis posterior muscle
Flexor digitorum longus muscle
Fibularis longus and fibularis brevis muscles
Flexor hallucis longus muscle
Fibula
Flexor hallucis longus muscle

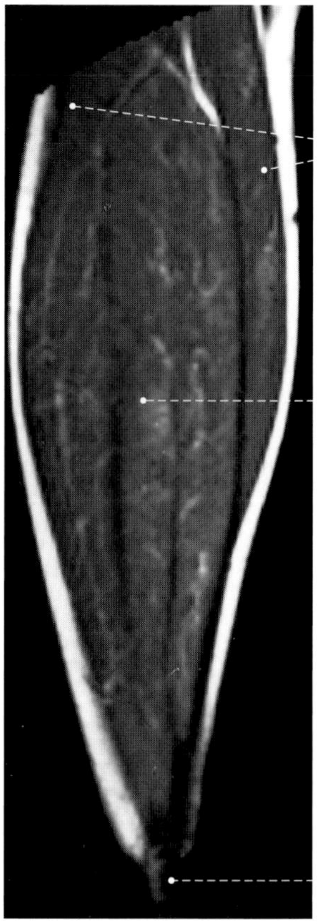
c
Gastrocnemius muscle
– Lateral head
– Medial head
Soleus muscle
Calcaneal tendon (= Achilles tendon) of triceps surae muscle

292 Right leg (30%)

a–c Coronal magnetic resonance images (MRI, T_1-weighted) through the
- a ventral part
- b middle part
- c dorsal part

of the leg, ventral aspect

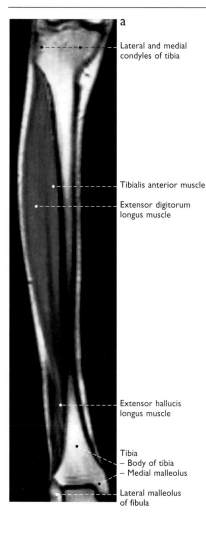

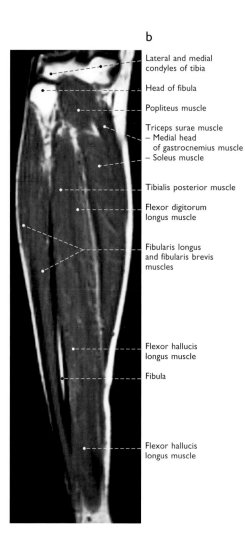

a

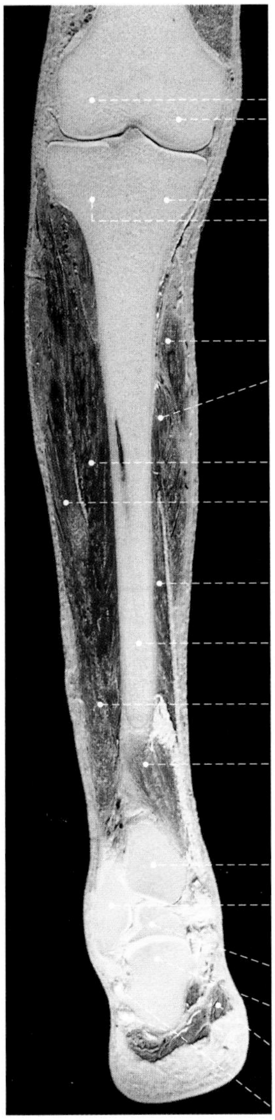
Femur
– Lateral condyle
– Medial condyle
Tibia
– Medial condyle
– Lateral condyle
Triceps surae muscle
– Medial head
of gastrocnemius m.
– Soleus muscle
Tibialis anterior muscle
Extensor digitorum
longus muscle
Flexor digitorum
longus muscle
Body of tibia
Extensor hallucis
longus muscle
Flexor hallucis
longus muscle
Tibia
Lateral malleolus
of fibula
Talus
Calcaneus
Abductor hallucis
muscle
Tendons
of fibularis brevis
and fibularis longus
muscles

b

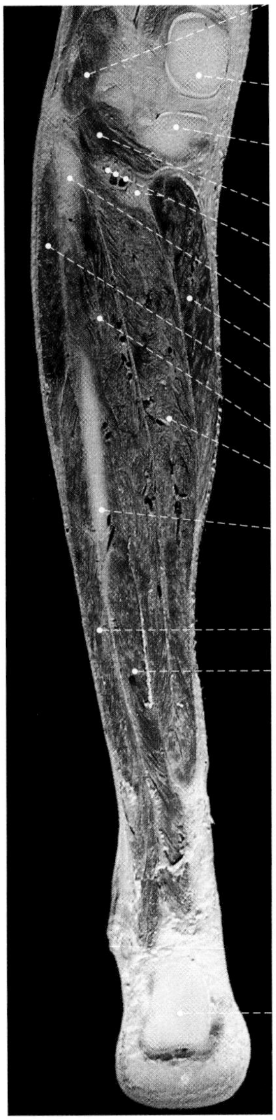
Lateral head
of gastrocnemius muscle
Medial condyle
of femur
Medial condyle
of tibia
Popliteus muscle
Posterior tibial a. and vv.,
Tibial nerve
Head of fibula
Soleus muscle
Fibularis longus m.
Tibialis posterior m.
Flexor digitorum
longus muscle
Body of fibula
Fibularis brevis muscle
Flexor hallucis longus
muscle
Calcaneus

c

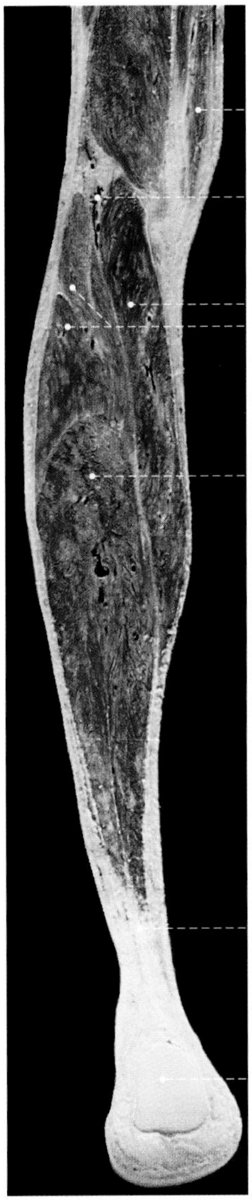
Sartorius muscle
Small (= short) saphenous vein
Gastrocnemius muscle
– Medial head
– Lateral head
Soleus muscle
Calcaneal tendon
(= Achilles tendon)
of triceps surae muscle
Calcaneus

293 Right leg (30%)

a–c Coronal anatomical sections through the
- a ventral part
- b middle part
- c dorsal part

of the leg, ventral aspect

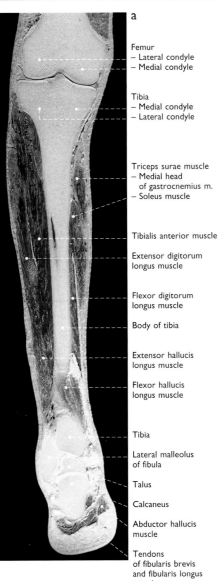

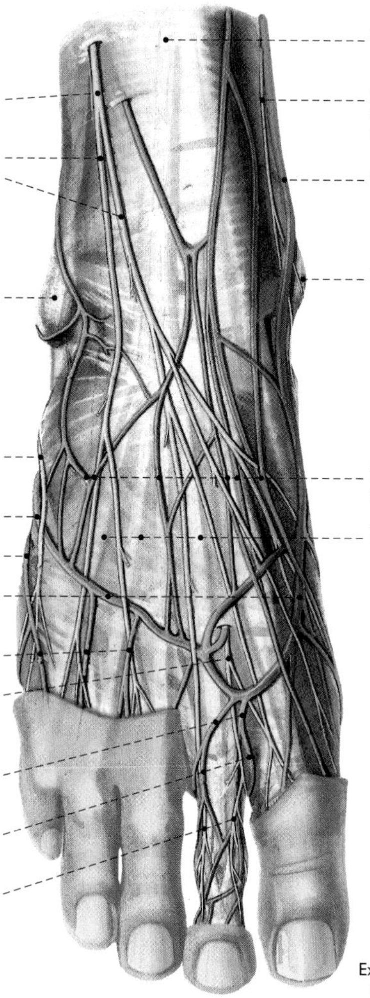
a
Deep fascia of leg
Superficial fibular nerve
Intermediate dorsal cutaneous nerve
Medial dorsal cutaneous nerve
Medial crural cutaneous nerve = Medial cutaneous nerve of leg (of saphenous nerve)
Great (= long) saphenous vein
Lateral malleolus of fibula
Medial malleolus of tibia
Lateral dorsal cutaneous nerve (of sural nerve)
Dorsal venous network of foot
Small (= short) saphenous vein
Dorsal fascia of foot
Lateral marginal vein
Dorsal venous arch of foot
Dorsal metatarsal veins
Deep fibular nerve
Intercapitular veins
Dorsal digital veins
Dorsal digital nerves of foot (of superficial and deep fibular nerves)

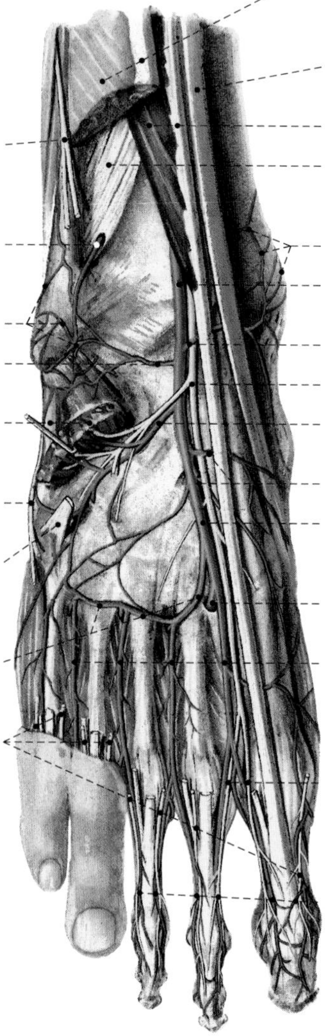
b
Extensor digitorum longus muscle (transected)
Tendon of tibialis anterior muscle
Superficial fibular nerve
Extensor hallucis longus muscle
Interosseous membrane of leg
Perforating branch of fibular artery
Medial malleolar network
Anterior tibial artery
Lateral malleolar network
Anterior medial malleolar artery
Anterior lateral malleolar artery
Deep fibular nerve
Extensor digitorum brevis and extensor hallucis brevis mm. (transected)
Lateral tarsal artery
Medial tarsal arteries
Lateral dorsal cutaneous nerve (of sural nerve)
Dorsalis pedis artery = Dorsal artery of foot
Tendon of fibularis tertius muscle
Deep plantar artery
(Arcuate artery)
Dorsal metatarsal arteries
Dorsal digital nerves of foot (of superficial fibular nerve)
Dorsal digital nerves of foot (of deep fibular nerve)
Dorsal digital arteries

294 Blood vessels and nerves of the dorsum of the right foot (50%)

Ventral aspect

a Subcutaneous veins and nerves

b Arteries and nerves after removal of the dorsal fascia of foot

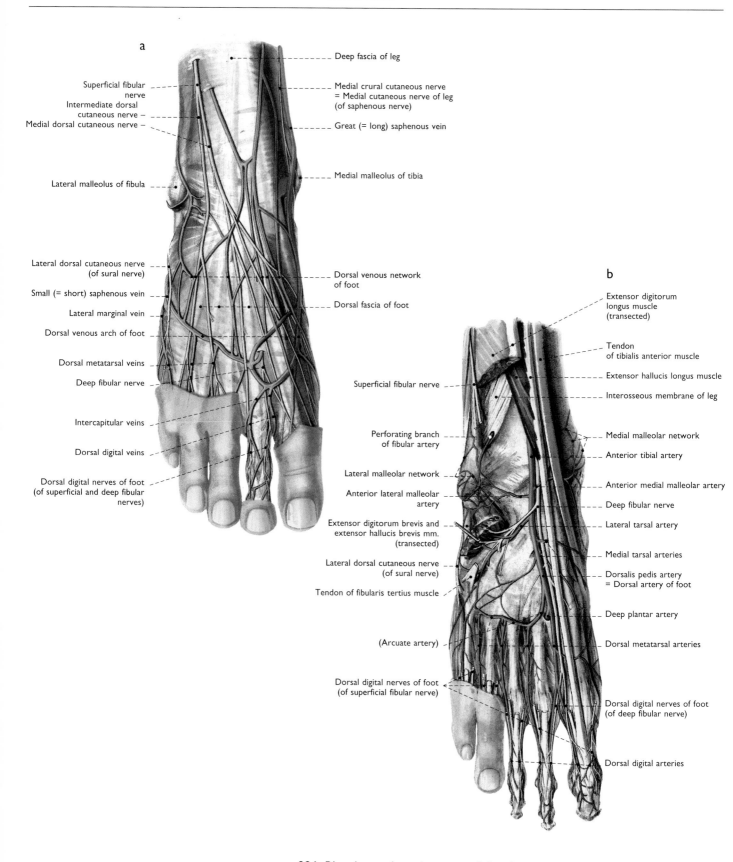

a

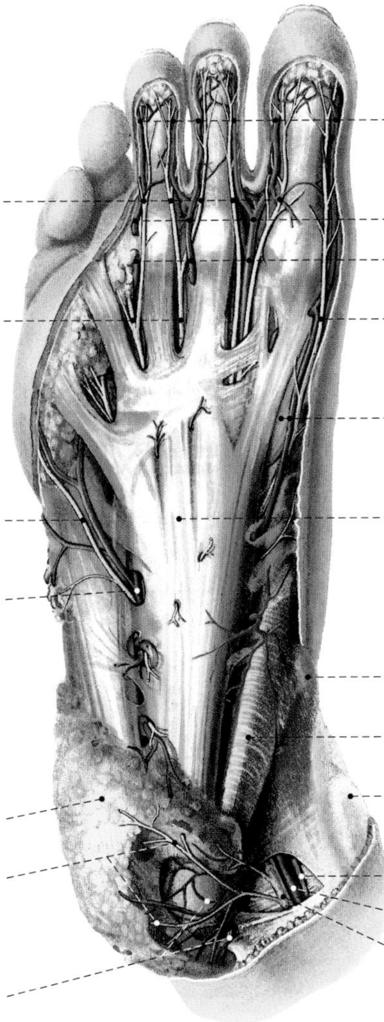
Proper plantar digital arteries
Proper plantar digital nerves
Common plantar digital arteries
Plantar metatarsal arteries
Common plantar digital nerves
⟨Medial plantar nerve of great toe⟩
Flexor hallucis brevis muscle, Superficial branch of medial plantar artery
Superficial branch of lateral plantar nerve
Plantar aponeurosis
Lateral plantar artery
Tuberosity of navicular
Abductor hallucis muscle
Medial malleolus of tibia
⟨Calcaneal fat body⟩
Medial calcaneal branches of tibial nerve
Medial plantar nerve
Posterior tibial artery
Lateral plantar nerve
Calcaneal anastomosis

b

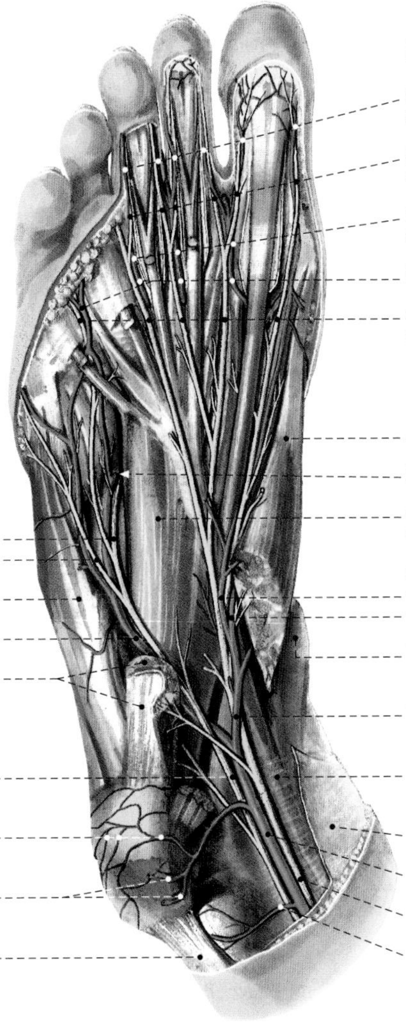
Proper plantar digital arteries
Proper plantar digital nerves
Common plantar digital arteries
Plantar metatarsal arteries
Common plantar digital nerves
Abductor hallucis muscle
Deep plantar arch
Quadratus plantae muscle = Flexor accessorius muscle
Lateral plantar nerve
Deep branch –
Superficial branch –
Medial plantar artery
– Superficial branch
– Deep branch
Abductor digiti minimi muscle
Lateral plantar artery
Tuberosity of navicular
Flexor digitorum brevis muscle (cut surface), Plantar aponeurosis
Medial plantar artery
Lateral plantar nerve
Flexor retinaculum
Calcaneal anastomosis
Deep fascia of leg
Posterior tibial artery
Calcaneal branches of posterior tibial artery
Medial plantar nerve
Calcaneal tendon (= Achilles tendon) of triceps surae muscle
Communicating branch of fibular artery

295 Arteries and nerves of the sole of the right foot (50%)

Plantar aspect

a Superficial layer

b The abductor hallucis muscle and the short flexor muscle of toes were partially removed.

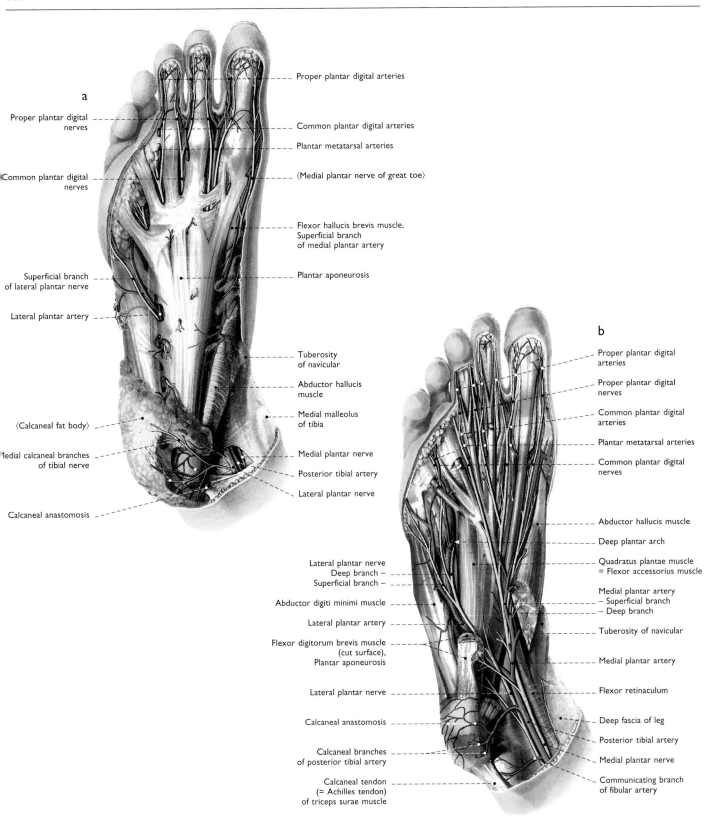

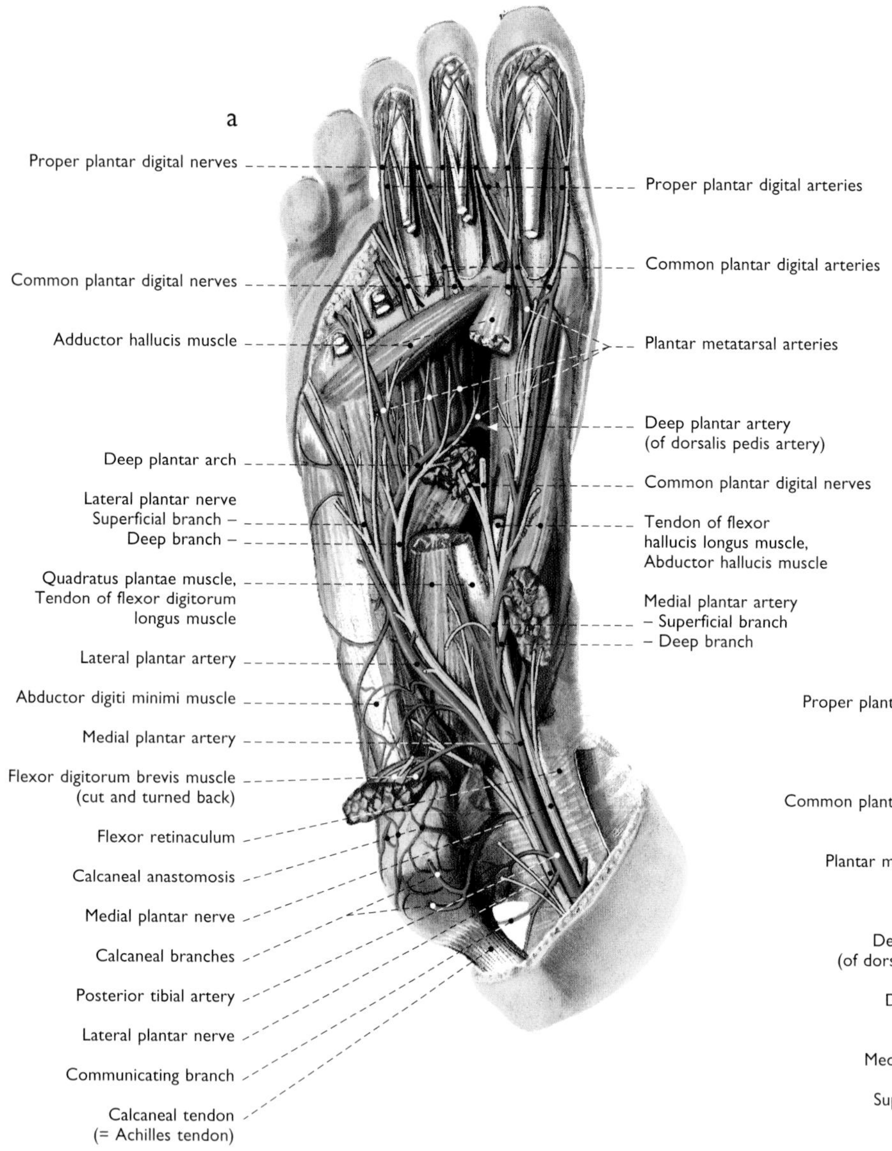
a
Proper plantar digital nerves
Common plantar digital nerves
Adductor hallucis muscle
Deep plantar arch
Lateral plantar nerve
Superficial branch –
Deep branch –
Quadratus plantae muscle,
Tendon of flexor digitorum
longus muscle
Lateral plantar artery
Abductor digiti minimi muscle
Medial plantar artery
Flexor digitorum brevis muscle
(cut and turned back)
Flexor retinaculum
Calcaneal anastomosis
Medial plantar nerve
Calcaneal branches
Posterior tibial artery
Lateral plantar nerve
Communicating branch
Calcaneal tendon
(= Achilles tendon)
Proper plantar digital arteries
Common plantar digital arteries
Plantar metatarsal arteries
Deep plantar artery
(of dorsalis pedis artery)
Common plantar digital nerves
Tendon of flexor
hallucis longus muscle,
Abductor hallucis muscle
Medial plantar artery
– Superficial branch
– Deep branch

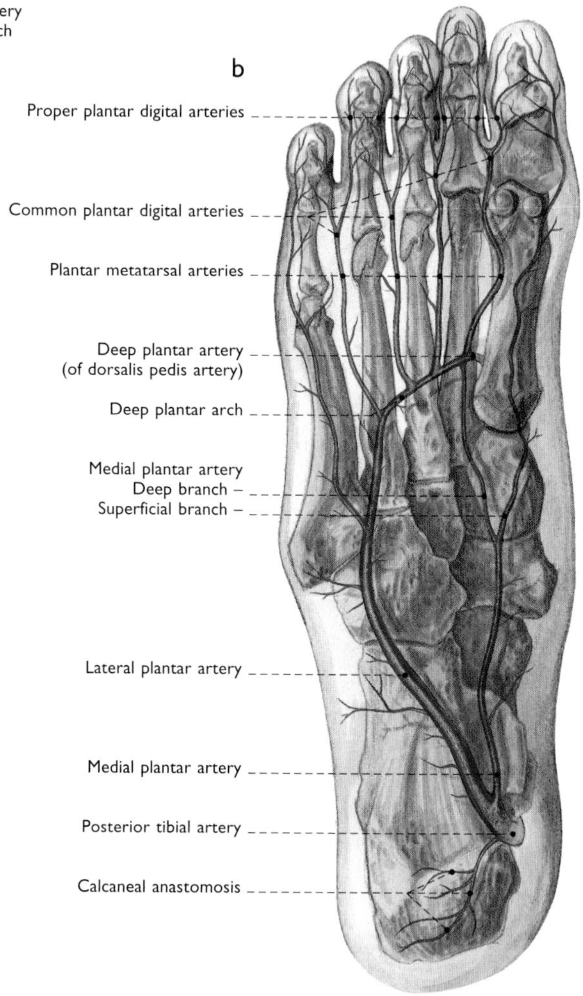
b
Proper plantar digital arteries
Common plantar digital arteries
Plantar metatarsal arteries
Deep plantar artery
(of dorsalis pedis artery)
Deep plantar arch
Medial plantar artery
Deep branch –
Superficial branch –
Lateral plantar artery
Medial plantar artery
Posterior tibial artery
Calcaneal anastomosis

296 Arteries and nerves of the sole of the right foot (50%)

Plantar aspect

a The oblique head of the abductor hallucis muscle and the short flexor muscle of toes were partially removed.

b Arteries of the sole of the right foot, schematic representation

a

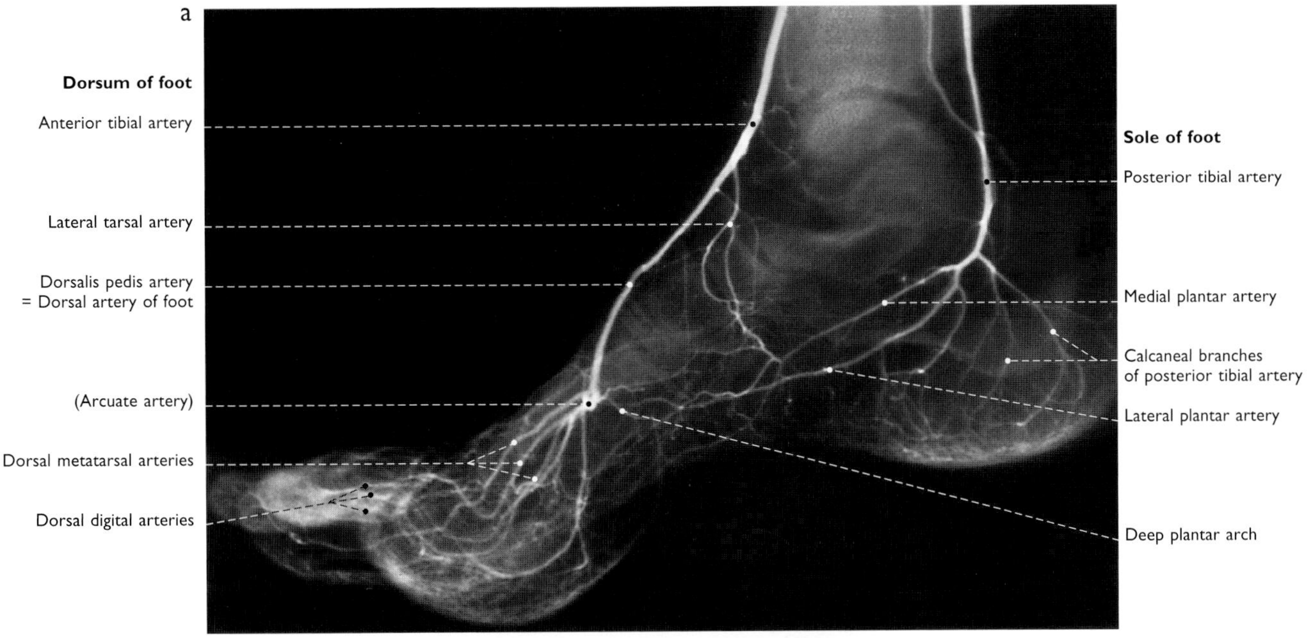
Dorsum of foot
Anterior tibial artery
Lateral tarsal artery
Dorsalis pedis artery
= Dorsal artery of foot
(Arcuate artery)
Dorsal metatarsal arteries
Dorsal digital arteries
Sole of foot
Posterior tibial artery
Medial plantar artery
Calcaneal branches
of posterior tibial artery
Lateral plantar artery
Deep plantar arch

b

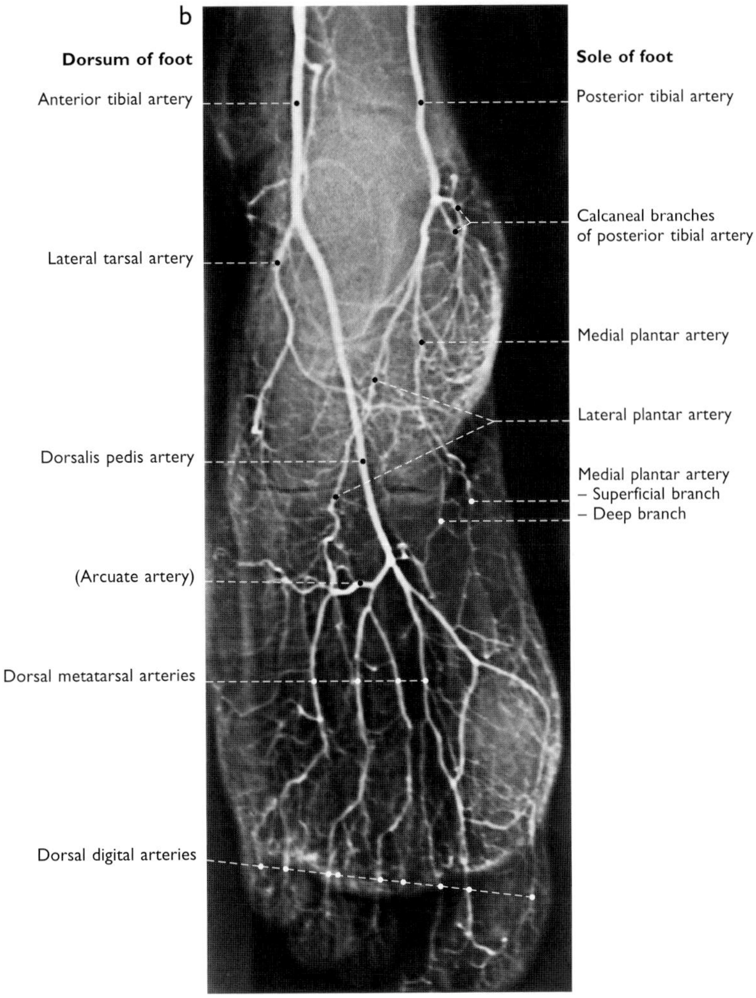
Dorsum of foot
Anterior tibial artery
Lateral tarsal artery
Dorsalis pedis artery
(Arcuate artery)
Dorsal metatarsal arteries
Dorsal digital arteries
Sole of foot
Posterior tibial artery
Calcaneal branches
of posterior tibial artery
Medial plantar artery
Lateral plantar artery
Medial plantar artery
– Superficial branch
– Deep branch

297 Arteries of the right foot (45%)

a Lateromedial arteriogram
b Dorsoplantar (anteroposterior) arteriogram of the arteries of the right foot

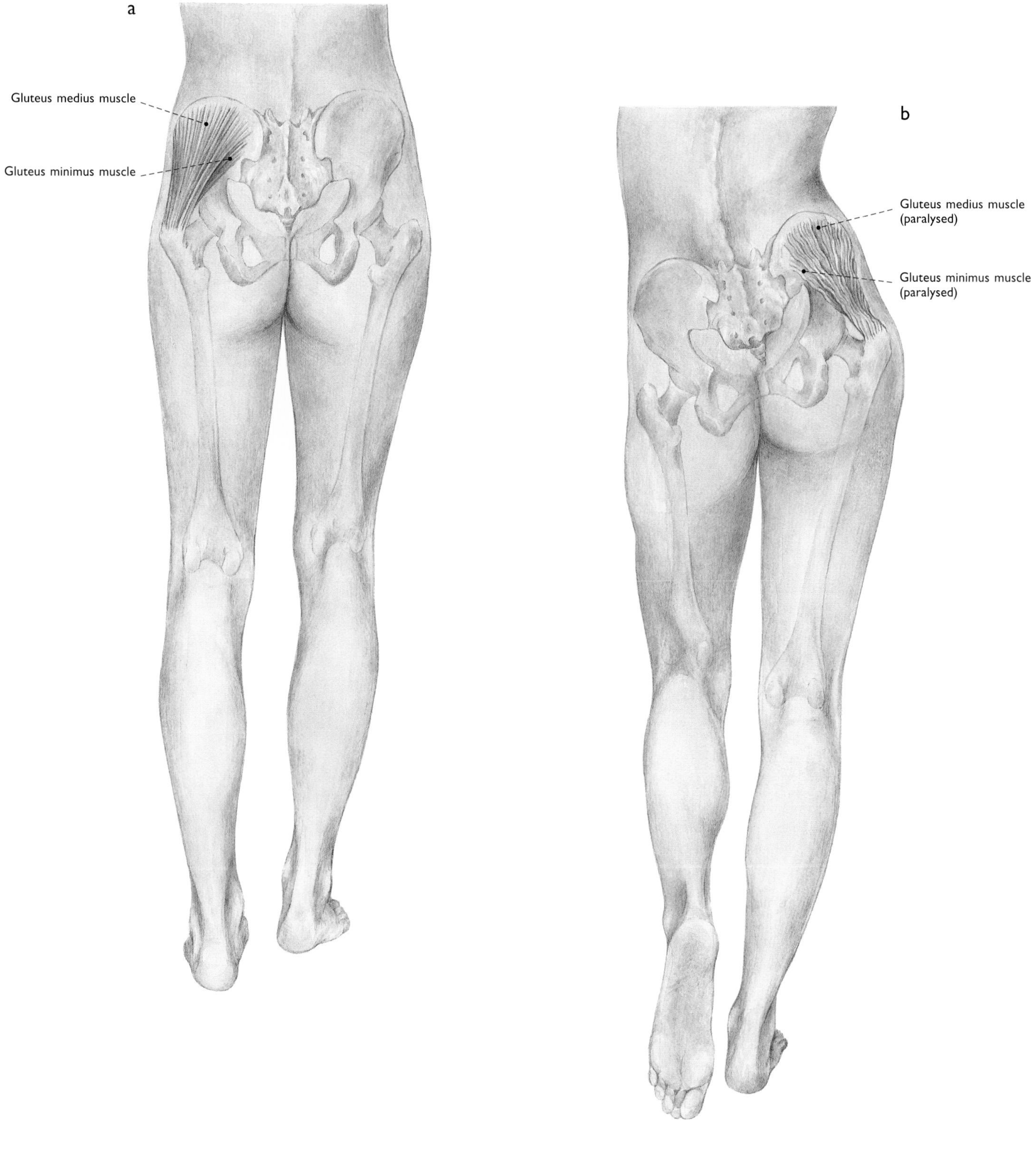
a
Gluteus medius muscle
Gluteus minimus muscle
b
Gluteus medius muscle
(paralysed)
Gluteus minimus muscle
(paralysed)

298 Paralysis of nerves of the lower limb (20%)

Dorsal aspect

a Normal function of the left lower limb in walking

b Palsy of the right **superior gluteal nerve** and following defects of the abductors of the right hip joint (gluteus medius and minimus muscles). When walking, the pelvis tilts downwards on the contralateral, unsupported side (positive 'TRENDELENBURG's sign').

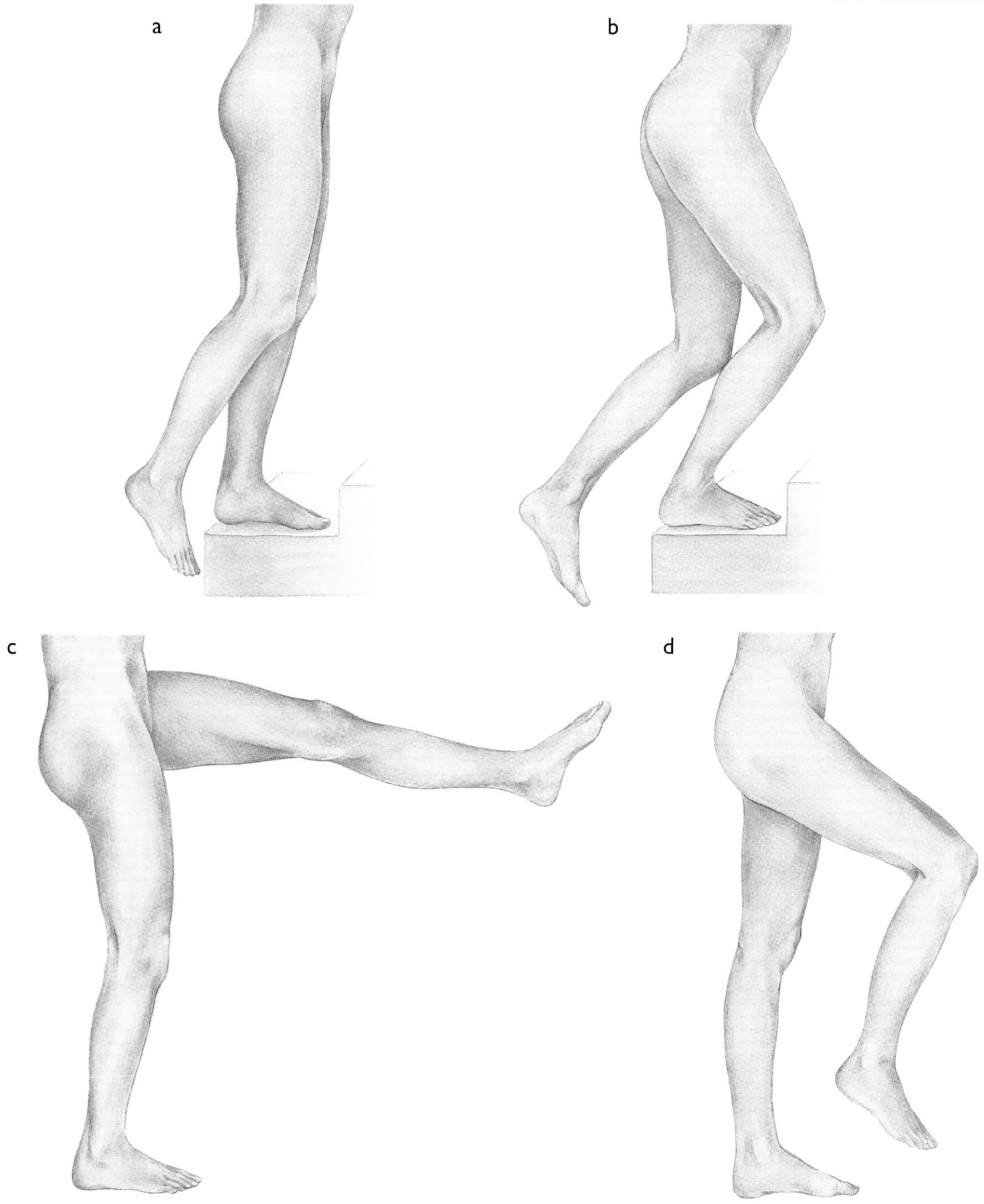

299 Paralysis of nerves of the lower limb (10%)

Right lateral aspect

a Normal function of the left lower limb in going upstairs

b Palsy of the right **inferior gluteal nerve** and following defect of the gluteus maximus muscle of the right side. As a result difficulties develop in going upstairs, especially in lifting the body upon the standing leg.

c Normal function of the left lower limb in regard to full flexion of the hip joint and to full extension of the knee joint

d Palsy of the right **femoral nerve** and resulting defects of the iliopsoas, sartorius, and quadriceps femoris muscles. The skin area marked by blue color indicates the autonomous area of the femoral nerve.

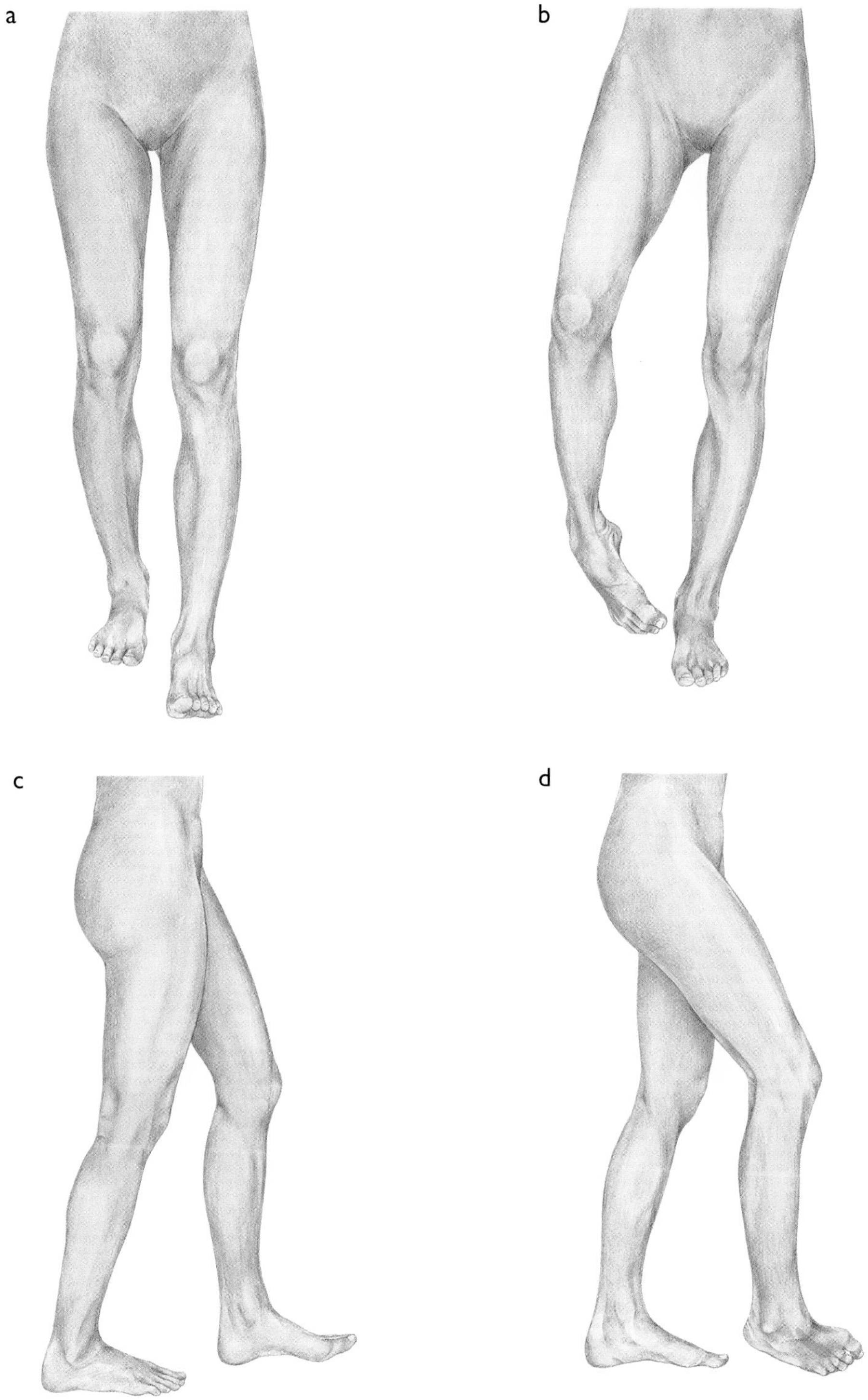

300 Paralysis of nerves of the lower limb (10%)

a, c Normal function of the left lower limb in walking

b, d Palsy of the right **common fibular nerve** and resulting defects of the lateral (= fibular or peroneal) and the anterior (= extensor) muscle groups of the right leg ('foot drop', 'steppage gait'). The skin region marked by blue color indicates the autonomous area of the common fibular nerve which is identical with the autonomous area of the superficial fibular nerve.

a, b Ventral aspect

c, d Right lateral aspect

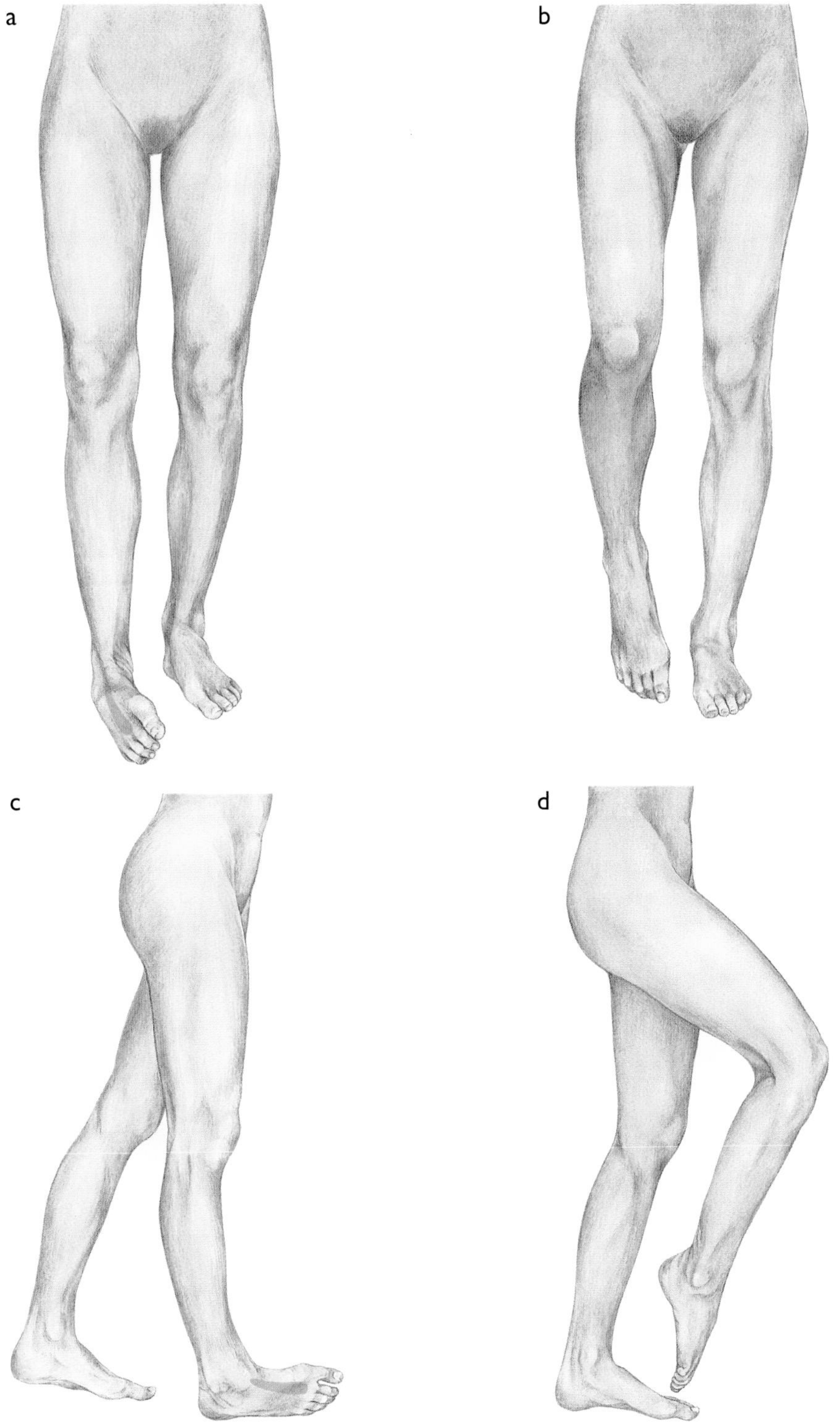

301 Paralysis of nerves of the lower limb (10%)

a, c Palsy of the right **superficial fibular nerve** and non-functioning of the lateral (= fibular or peroneal) muscle group of the right leg. The skin region marked by blue color indicates the autonomous area of the superficial fibular nerve.
b, d Palsy of the right **deep fibular nerve** and non-functioning of the anterior (= extensor) muscle group of the right leg ('foot drop', 'steppage gait')
a, b Ventral aspect
c, d Right lateral aspect

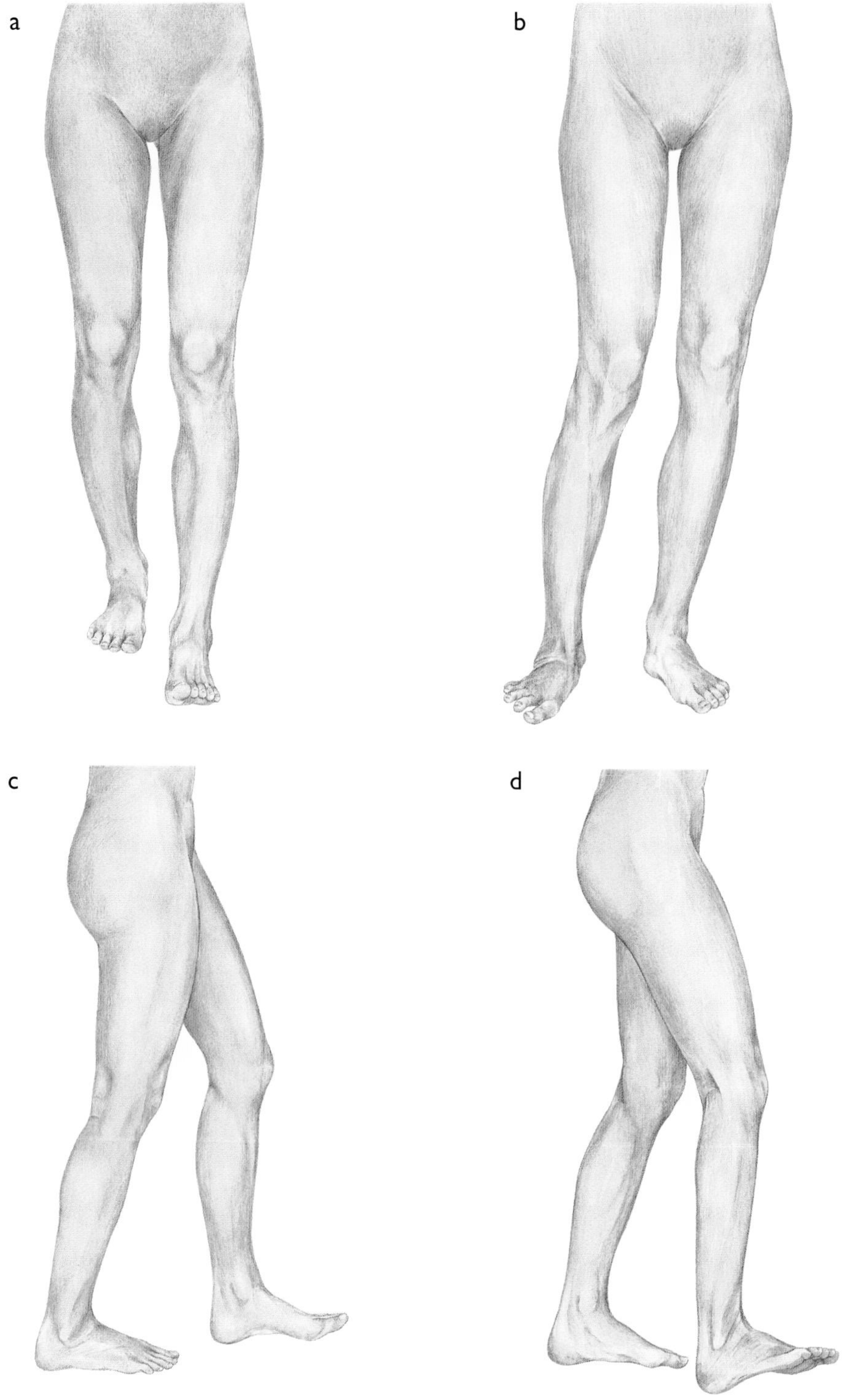

302 Paralysis of nerves of the lower limb (10%)

a, c Normal function of the left lower limb in walking

b, d Palsy of the right **tibial nerve** and resulting defects of the muscles of the superficial and deep posterior (= superficial and deep flexor) muscle groups of the right leg. The muscles of the calf are atrophied. When walking, it is impossible to produce plantarflexion and to push off with the foot. The skin area marked by blue color indicates the autonomous area of the tibial nerve.

a, b Ventral aspect

c, d Right lateral aspect

Indexes of Eponyms

Alphabetical Index of Common Used Eponyms

Eponyms are terms containing proper names of persons who usually described the concerned structures first. Eponyms are frequently utilized in clinical linguistic usage and commonly preferred to the anatomical terms. For this reason the proper names which are contained in commonly used eponyms are placed in brackets following the anatomical terms in the lettering text of the present atlas. In the subsequent table the eponyms and the corresponding anatomical terms are specified, additionally some biographical data of the persons named in the eponyms are given. Only those eponyms are considered that are cited with high frequency in the literature.

English Eponym	**Anatomical Term**	**Name and Related Data**
Achilles tendon	Calcaneal tendon	Named after Achilles (Greek legendary man, hero in Homer´s Ilias). He was killed by Paris at the heel which was the only vulnarable spot of his body.
Adam´s apple	Laryngeal prominence of thyroid cartilage	Named after Adam (biblically Adam = first man of the Old Testament who got a fright upon God´s call so that the fruit from the prohibited tree stuck in his throat; in Arabic language, adam = vir = man)
ALCOCK´s canal	Pudendal canal	ALCOCK, Benjamin, 1801– ? , Professor of Anatomy, Physiology, and Pathology in Dublin, later Professor of Anatomy in Cork/Ireland, he emigrated to America in 1855
Ammon´s horn	Hippocampus proper	Named after Ammon (Egyptian sun-god who was often adored in the guise of the head of a ram resembling the shape of both proper hippocampi with diencephalon and brainstem)
ARANTIUS, Duct of	Ductus venosus	ARANTIUS (ARANZIO), Giulio Cesare, 1530–1589, Professor of Medicine, Surgery, and Anatomy in Bologna, pupil of Vesalius, Physician to Pope Gregory XIII
ARANTIUS, Ligament of	Ligamentum venosum	ARANTIUS, Giulio Cesare, see before
ARANTIUS, Nodules of Bodies of ARANTIUS	Nodules of semilunar cusps	ARANTIUS, Giulio Cesare, see before
ARNOLD, Tract of	Frontopontine fibers	ARNOLD, Friedrich, 1803–1890, Professor of Anatomy in Zurich, Freiburg, Tübingen, and Heidelberg
ASCHOFF-TAWARA node, Node of TAWARA	Atrioventricular node	ASCHOFF, Karl Albert Ludwig, 1866–1942, Professor of Pathology in Marburg, Freiburg, and Berlin; TAWARA, Sunao, see there
BARTHOLIN´s duct	Major sublingual duct	BARTHOLIN, Caspar Secundus, 1655–1738, Professor of Philosophy, and then Professor of Medicine, Anatomy, and Physics in Copenhagen
BARTHOLIN´s gland	Greater vestibular gland	BARTHOLIN, Caspar Secundus, see before
BAUHIN´s valve	Ileal orifice	BAUHIN, Caspar, 1560–1624, Professor of Greek, Medicine, Anatomy, and Botany in Basle
BELL´s nerve	Long thoracic nerve	BELL, Sir Charles, 1774–1842, Professor of Anatomy and Surgery in London, later Professor of Surgery in Edinburgh
BERTIN´s columns	Renal columns	BERTIN, Exupère Joseph, 1712–1781, Anatomist in Paris
BICHAT´s fat pad	Buccal fat pad	BICHAT, Marie François Xavier, 1771–1802, Professor of Anatomy in Paris
BOCHDALEK´s triangle	Lumbocostal triangle	BOCHDALEK, Victor (junior), 1835–1868, Anatomist in Prague
BOTALLO´s duct	Ductus arteriosus	BOTALLO (BOTAL), Leonardo, 1530– ?, Italian Anatomist and Military Surgeon in France, Physician to the Kings Charles IX and Henry III of France
BOTALLO´s ligament	Ligamentum arteriosum	BOTALLO, Leonardo, see before
BOYD´s veins	Perforating veins (below knee joint)	BOYD, Alexander Michael, 1905–1973, Anatomist and Professor of Surgery (mainly Vascular Surgery) in Manchester
BROCA´s diagonal band	Diagonal band	BROCA, Pierre Paul, 1824–1880, Anatomist and Anthropologist, Professor of Clinical Surgery and Director of the Anthropological Laboratories in Paris
BUCK´s fascia	(Deep) fascia of penis	BUCK, Gurdon, 1807–1877, Surgeon in New York
BURDACH´s tract	Cuneate fasciculus	BURDACH, Karl Friedrich, 1776–1847, Professor of Anatomy and Physiology in Dorpat and Königsberg
CARABELLI formation, Cusp of CARABELLI	Anomalous tubercle of tooth	CARABELLI, Gregor, Edler von Lunkaszprie, 1787–1842, Professor of Dental Surgery in Vienna
CHASSAIGNAC´s tubercle	Carotid tubercle	CHASSAIGNAC, Charles Marie Edouard, 1805–1879, Professor of Anatomy and Surgery in Paris
CHOPART´s line	(Line of amputation through the transverse tarsal joint)	CHOPART, François, 1743–1795, Professor of Surgery in Paris
CLOQUET´s gland, CLOQUET´s node, ROSENMÜLLER-CLOQUET lymph node	Proximal deep inguinal lymph node	CLOQUET, Baron de, Jules Germain, 1790–1883, Professor of Pathology and Surgery in Paris, Surgeon to Napoléon III; ROSENMÜLLER, Johann Christian, see there
CLOQUET´s septum	Femoral septum	CLOQUET, Baron de, Jules Germain, see before

English Eponym	Anatomical Term	Name and Related Data
COCKETT´s veins	Perforating veins (at distal leg)	COCKETT, Frank Bernard, born 1916, Surgeon (mainly Vascular Surgeon) in London
COLLES´ ligament	Reflected inguinal ligament	COLLES, Abraham, 1773–1843, Professor of Anatomy and Surgery in Dublin
COOPER´s fascia	Cremasteric fascia	COOPER, Sir Astley Paston, 1768–1841, Professor of Anatomy and Surgery in London, eminent Surgeon and Physician to the Kings George IV and William IV and to Queen Victoria of England
COOPER´s ligament (groin)	Pectineal inguinal ligament	COOPER, Sir Astley Paston, see before
COOPER´s ligaments (breast)	Suspensory ligaments of breast	COOPER, Sir Astley Paston, see before
CORTI´s ganglion, Ganglion of CORTI	Cochlear ganglion	CORTI, Marchese de, Alfonso, 1822–1888, native Italian, Anatomist in Vienna, Würzburg, Utrecht, and Turin
CORTI´s organ, Organ of CORTI	Spiral organ	CORTI, Marchese de, Alfonso, see before
COWPER´s gland	Bulbo-urethral gland	COWPER, William, 1666–1709, Professor of Anatomy and Surgery in London
DARWIN´s tubercle	Auricular tubercle	DARWIN, Charles Robert, 1809–1882, English Naturalist, founder of the Theory of Evolution
DODD´s veins	Perforating veins (at the level of adductor canal)	DODD, Harold, 1899–1987, Surgeon in Liverpool and London
DOUGLAS, Fold of	Recto-uterine fold	DOUGLAS, James, 1675–1742, native Scotsman, Anatomist and Gynecologist in London
DOUGLAS, Line of, Arcuate line of DOUGLAS, Arch of DOUGLAS	Arcuate line of rectus sheath	DOUGLAS, James, see before
DOUGLAS, Pouch of	Recto-uterine pouch	DOUGLAS, James, see before
ERB´s point	Punctum nervosum	ERB, Wilhelm Heinrich, 1840–1921, Professor of Medicine and Neurology in Leipzig and Heidelberg
EUSTACHIAN tube	Pharyngotympanic tube	EUSTACHI (EUSTACHIO), Bartolomeo, about 1515–1574, Professor of Anatomy in Rome, Papal Physician
EUSTACHIAN valve	Valve of inferior vena cava	EUSTACHI, Bartolomeo, see before
FALLOPIAN canal	Facial canal	FALLOPIO (FALLOPIA, FALLOPPIUS), Gabriele, 1523–1563, Professor of Anatomy, Surgery, and Botany in Padua, pupil of Vesalius
FALLOPIAN tube	Uterine tube	FALLOPIO, Gabriele, see before
FLACK´s node, Node of KEITH-FLACK	Sinu-atrial node	FLACK, Martin William, 1882–1931, Physiologist in London; KEITH, Sir Arthur, see there
FLECHSIG´s tract	Posterior (= dorsal) spinocerebellar tract	FLECHSIG, Paul Emil, 1847–1929, Professor of Psychiatry in Leipzig
FOLLIAN process	Anterior process of malleus	FOLLI (FOLIUS), Cecilio, 1615–1660, Professor of Anatomy in Venice
FONTANA, Spaces of	Spaces of iridocorneal angle	FONTANA, Abbada Felice, 1720–1805, Professor of Philosophy in Pisa and Professor of Anatomy in Florence, founder of the Museum of Natural History in Florence
FRANKENHÄUSER´s ganglion	Uterovaginal plexus	FRANKENHÄUSER, Ferdinand, 1832–1894, Professor of Gynecology in Jena and Zurich
GALEN´s vein, Vein of GALEN	Great cerebral vein	GALEN (GALENOS), Claudius (Clarissimus), about 130 – about 200, important Greek Physician of the classical antiquity, his influence persisting for 15 centuries until the Renaissance; Physician to the Roman Emperors Marcus Aurelius, Commodus, and Septimus Severus
GASSERIAN ganglion	Trigeminal ganglion	GASSER, Johann Lorenz (Laurentius), about 1723 – about 1765, Professor of Anatomy in Vienna
GEROTA´s fascia, GEROTA´s capsule	Renal fascia	GEROTA, Dumitru, 1867–1939, Professor of Surgery and Experimental Surgery in Bucharest
GIACOMINI, Band of, Limbus of GIACOMINI	(Ventral continuation of the dentate gyrus on to the surface of uncus)	GIACOMINI, Carlo, 1840–1898, Professor of Anatomy in Turin

English Eponym	Anatomical Term	Name and Related Data
GIMBERNAT´s ligament	Lacunar inguinal ligament	GIMBERNAT, Don de, Manuel Louise Antonio, 1734-1816, Professor of Anatomy in Barcelona and Professor of Surgery in Madrid, Surgeon to King Charles III of Spain
GLASERIAN fissure	Petrotympanic fissure	GLASER, Johann Heinrich, 1629–1675, Professor of Greek, Anatomy, and Botany in Basle
GLISSON´s capsule, Capsule of GLISSON	Fibrous capsule and perivascular fibrous capsule of liver	GLISSON, Francis, 1597–1677, Professor of Anatomy in Cambridge and Physician in London
GOLL´s tract	Gracile fasciculus	GOLL, Friedrich, 1829–1903, Neurologist and Professor of Anatomy and Pharmacology in Zurich
GOWERS´ tract	Anterior (= ventral) spinocerebellar tract	GOWERS, Sir William Richard, 1845–1915, Neurologist and Professor of Clinical Medicine in London
GRAAFIAN follicles	Vesicular ovarian follicles	GRAAF, de, Regnier, 1641–1673, Anatomist and Physician in Leyden, Delft, and Paris
GRATIOLET´s radiation	Optic radiation	GRATIOLET, Louis Pierre, 1815–1865, Anatomist and Professor of Zoology in Paris
GUDDEN´s tract	Mammillotegmental fasciculus	GUDDEN, von, Johann Bernhard Aloys, 1824–1886, Professor of Psychiatry in Zurich and Munich, psychiatric surveyor of King Louis II of Bavaria, was drowned with King Louis II in Lake Starnberg
Loge de GUYON	Ulnar canal	GUYON, Jean Casimir Félix, 1831–1920, Professor of Surgery and Pathology in Paris
HALLER´s arches	Lateral and medial arcuate ligaments of diaphragm	HALLER, von, Albrecht, 1708–1777, native Swiss and known poet ('The Alpes', 1729), Professor of Anatomy, Physiology, Surgery, and Botany in Göttingen
HALLER´s artery	Dorsal pancreatic artery	HALLER, von, Albrecht, see before
HALLER´s tripus	Celiac trunk	HALLER, von, Albrecht, see before
HASNER´s valve	Lacrimal fold	HASNER, Joseph, Ritter von Artha, 1819–1892, Anatomist and Professor of Ophthalmology in Prague
HEAD´s zones	(Zones of hyperalgesia of inner organs at the body surface)	HEAD, Sir Henry, 1861–1940, Neurologist in London
HEISTER´s valve	Spiral fold of cystic duct	HEISTER, Lorenz (Laurentius), 1683–1758, Professor of Anatomy, Surgery, and Botany in Altdorf near Nuremberg and later in Helmstedt
HEROPHILUS, Torcular of	Confluence of sinuses	HEROPHILUS (HEROPHILOS), 335–280 B.C., Greek Physician in Alexandria under the government of Ptolemaeus I Soter
HESCHL´s transverse convolutions	Transverse temporal gyri	HESCHL, Richard, 1824–1881, Professor of Anatomy in Olmütz, then Professor of Pathology in Krakau and of Clinical Medicine in Graz and Vienna
HESSELBACH´s fascia	Cribriform fascia	HESSELBACH, Franz Kaspar, 1759–1816, Anatomist and Professor of Surgery in Würzburg
HESSELBACH´s ligament	Interfoveolar ligament	HESSELBACH, Franz Kaspar, see before
HESSELBACHS's triangle	Inguinal triangle	HESSELBACH, Franz Kaspar, see before
HIGHMORE, Body of, Corpus of HIGHMORE	Mediastinum of testis	HIGHMORE, Nathaniel, 1613–1685, Physician in Sherborne, Dorsetshire/England
HIGHMORE´s cavity, Antrum of HIGHMORE	Maxillary sinus	HIGHMORE, Nathaniel, see before
HIS, Angle of	Cardial notch	HIS, Wilhelm (senior), 1831–1904, Professor of Anatomy and Physiology in Basle and Leipzig
HIS, Bundle of	Atrioventricular bundle	HIS, Wilhelm (junior), 1863–1934, Professor of Anatomy and Medicine in Leipzig, Basle, Göttingen, and Berlin
HOLZKNECHT´s space	Retrocardial space	HOLZKNECHT, Guido, 1872–1931, Radiologist in Vienna
HORNER´s muscle	Deep part of palpebral part of orbicularis oculi muscle	HORNER, William Edmonds, 1793–1853, Professor of Anatomy in Philadelphia
HOUSTON´s valve, HOUSTON-KOHLRAUSCH fold	(Middle) transverse fold of rectum	HOUSTON, John, 1802–1845, Surgeon in Dublin; KOHLRAUSCH, Otto Ludwig Bernhard, see there

English Eponym	Anatomical Term	Name and Related Data
HUNTER´s canal	Adductor canal	HUNTER, John, 1728–1793, native Scotsman, Professor of Surgery in London, Surgeon to King George III of England
JACOBSON´s nerve	Tympanic nerve	JACOBSON, Ludwig Levin, 1783–1843, native Dane, Anatomist in Copenhagen, for a period Military Physician in the French Army
JACOBSON´s plexus	Tympanic plexus	JACOBSON, Ludwig Levin, see before
KEITH-FLACK, Node of, FLACK´s node	Sinu-atrial node	KEITH, Sir Arthur, 1866–1955, Professor of Anatomy in London, later Rector of the Aberdeen University; FLACK, Martin William, see there
KERCKRING´s valves	Circular folds of small intestine	KERCKRING, Theodor, 1640–1693, native German, Anatomist and Physician in Amsterdam, later in Hamburg
KIESSELBACH, Area of	(Area rich in blood vessels at the anterior nasal septum, frequent source of nosebleed)	KIESSELBACH, Wilhelm, 1839–1902, Professor of Otorhinolaryngology in Erlangen
KOHLRAUSCH´s fold, HOUSTON-KOHLRAUSCH fold	(Middle) transverse fold of rectum	KOHLRAUSCH, Otto Ludwig Bernhard, 1811–1854, Physician in Hannover; HOUSTON, John, see there
KRISTELLER´s plug	(Mucous plug in the cervical canal)	KRISTELLER, Samuel, 1820–1900, Gynecologist in Berlin
LAIMER´s triangle	(Weak triangle at the transition of pharynx to esophagus)	LAIMER, Eduard, about 1860– ?, Anatomist in Graz
LANGER´s lines	Tension lines, Cleavage lines	LANGER, Karl, Ritter von Edenberg, 1819–1887, Professor of Zoology in Budapest, later Professor of Anatomy in Vienna
LANGERHANS, Islets of	Pancreatic islets	LANGERHANS, Paul, 1847–1888, Anatomist and Professor of Pathological Anatomy in Freiburg, later Physician at Madeira
LARREY´s fissure	Sternocostal triangle	LARREY, Baron de, Dominique Jean, 1766–1842, Surgeon in Paris, famous Military Physician and Physician to Napoléon I
LISFRANC´s line	(Line of amputation through the tarsometatarsal joints)	LISFRANC de ST. MARTIN, Jacques, 1790–1847, Military Surgeon, later Professor of Surgery in Paris
LISTER´s tubercle	Dorsal tubercle of radius	LISTER, Lord Joseph, 1827–1912, Professor of Surgery in Glasgow, Edinburgh, and London, Surgeon to King Edward VII of England
LITTRÉ, Glands of	Urethral glands of male urethra	LITTRÉ, Alexis, 1658–1726, Anatomist and Surgeon in Paris
LOUIS, Angle of, Angle of LUDOVICUS	Sternal angle	LOUIS (LUDOVICUS), Pierre Charles Alexandre, 1787–1872, Pathologist and Pulmonologist in Paris
LUSCHKA, Foramen of	Lateral aperture of fourth ventricle	LUSCHKA, von, Hubert, 1820–1875, Professor of Anatomy in Tübingen
LUYS, Nucleus of, Corpus LUYSI	Subthalamic nucleus	LUYS, Jules Bernard, 1828–1897, Professor of Neurology in Paris
MAGENDIE, Foramen of	Median aperture of fourth ventricle	MAGENDIE, François, 1783–1855, Professor of Physiology and Pathology in Paris
MARSHALL´s vein	Oblique vein of left atrium of heart	MARSHALL, John, 1818–1891, Professor of Physiology, Anatomy, and Surgery in London
MECKEL´s cave	Trigeminal cave	MECKEL, Johann Friedrich (senior), 1714–1774, Professor of Anatomy, Botany, and Gynecology in Berlin
MEIBOMIAN glands	Tarsal glands	MEIBOM (MEIBOMIUS), Heinrich, 1638–1700, Professor of Medicine, History, and Poetry in Helmstedt
MÉNARD-SHENTON line, SHENTON´s line	(Radiological line of orientation at the infantile pelvic girdle and femur)	MÉNARD, Maxime, 1872–1929, Forensic Physician in Paris; SHENTON, Edward Warren Hine, see there
MOHRENHEIM´s fossa	Clavipectoral triangle, Deltopectoral triangle	MOHRENHEIM, Freiherr von, Joseph Jakob, 1759–1799, Surgeon, Obstetrician, and Ophthalmologist in Vienna, later Professor of Surgery and Obstetrics in St. Petersburg
MOLL´s glands	Ciliary glands	MOLL, Jakob Anton, 1832–1914, Ophthalmologist in Utrecht and Den Haag
MONRO, Foramen of	Interventricular foramen	MONRO, Alexander (junior), 1733–1817, Professor of Anatomy in Edinburgh
MORGAGNI, Columns of	Anal columns	MORGAGNI, Giovanni Battista, 1682–1771, Professor of Anatomy in Padua, pupil of Valsalva, founder of morbid anatomy
MORGAGNI, Ventricle of	Laryngeal ventricle	MORGAGNI, Giovanni Battista, see before

English Eponym	Anatomical Term	Name and Related Data
MORISON´s pouch	Hepatorenal recess of subhepatic space	MORISON, James Rutherford, 1853–1939, Surgeon in England
MÜLLER´s muscle	Superior tarsal muscle	MÜLLER, Heinrich, 1820–1864, Professor of Anatomy in Würzburg
PACCHIONIAN granulations	Arachnoid granulations	PACCHIONI, Antonio, 1665–1726, Physician in Tivoli and Professor of Anatomy in Rome
PECQUET, Cistern of	Cisterna chyli, Chyle cistern	PECQUET, Jean, 1622–1674, Physician in Fouquet, Montpellier, and Paris
PETIT, Triangle of	Inferior lumbar triangle	PETIT, Jean Louis, 1664–1750, Anatomist and Professor of Surgery in Paris
POUPART´s ligament	Inguinal ligament	POUPART, François, 1616–1708, Naturalist, Anatomist, and Surgeon in Reims and Paris
PURKINJE fibers	Subendocardial branches of atrioventricular bundle	PURKYNĚ (PURKINJE), Johannes (Jan) Evangelista, 1787–1869, Professor of Physiology in Breslau, later in Prague
REISSNER´s membrane	Vestibular surface of cochlear duct	REISSNER, Ernst, 1824–1878, Professor of Anatomy in Dorpat, later in Breslau
RETZIUS´ space, Cave of RETZIUS	Retropubic space	RETZIUS, Anders Adolf, 1796–1860, Anthropologist and Professor of Anatomy and Physiology in Stockholm
RIOLAN, Arcade of	(Anastomosis between middle and left colic arteries and veins)	RIOLAN, Jean (junior), 1577–1657, Professor of Anatomy, Botany, and Pharmacology in Paris, Physician to the Kings Henry IV and Louis XIII of France
ROLANDO, Fissure of, Sulcus of ROLANDO	Central sulcus of cerebrum	ROLANDO, Luigi, 1773–1831, Professor of Medicine in Sassari/Sardinia, later Professor of Anatomy in Turin, Physician to Victor Emanuel of Sardinia
ROSENMÜLLER, Fossa of	Pharyngeal recess	ROSENMÜLLER, Johann Christian, 1771–1820, Professor of Anatomy and Surgery in Leipzig
ROSENMÜLLER´s gland, ROSENMÜLLER´s node, ROSENMÜLLER-CLOQUET lymph node	Proximal deep inguinal lymph node	ROSENMÜLLER, Johann Christian, see before; CLOQUET, Baron de, Jules Germain, see there
SANTORINI´s cartilage	Corniculate cartilage	SANTORINI, Giovanni Domenico (Giandomenico), 1681–1737, Professor of Anatomy and Medicine in Venice
SANTORINI´s duct	Accessory pancreatic duct	SANTORINI, Giovanni Domenico, see before
SCARPA´s ganglion	Vestibular ganglion	SCARPA, Antonio, 1747–1832, Professor of Surgery in Modena and Professor of Anatomy in Pavia, Surgeon to Napoléon I
SCARPA´s nerve	Nasopalatine nerve	SCARPA, Antonio, see before
SCARPA´s triangle	Femoral triangle	SCARPA, Antonio, see before
SCHLEMM, Canal of	Scleral venous sinus	SCHLEMM, Friedrich, 1795–1858, Professor of Anatomy in Berlin
SCHULTZE´s comma tract	Interfascicular fasciculus	SCHULTZE, Maximilian Johann Sigismund, 1825–1874, Professor of Anatomy in Halle, later in Bonn
SHENTON´s line, MÉNARD-SHENTON line	(Radiological line of orientation at the infantile pelvic girdle and femur)	SHENTON, Edward Warren Hine, 1872–1955, Radiologist in London; MÉNARD, Maxime, see there
SHRAPNELL´s membrane	Pars flaccida of tympanic membrane	SHRAPNELL, Henry Jones, 1761–1834, English Military Surgeon, later Anatomist and Surgeon in London
SPIEGEL´s line, SPIGHEL´s line	Semilunar line, Linea semilunaris	SPIEGEL (SPIGHEL, van den, SPIEGHEL, SPIGELIUS), Adriaan, 1578–1625, native Fleming, Professor of Anatomy in Venice, later in Padua
SPIEGELIAN lobe	Caudate lobe of liver	SPIEGEL, Adriaan, see before
STENSEN´s canal, STENON´s canal	Incisive canal	STENSEN (STENO, STENONIUS), Niels, 1638–1686, Geologist and Professor of Anatomy in Copenhagen, pupil of Bartholin and Sylvius, later Theologian and catholic Bishop
STENSEN´s duct, STENON´s duct	Parotid duct	STENSEN, Niels, see before
STILLING´s decussation	(Scissor-like decussation of cerebellorubral fibers in the midbrain)	STILLING, Benedikt, 1810–1879, Anatomist and Surgeon in Kassel and Vienna
SYLVIAN aqueduct, Aqueduct of SYLVIUS	Aqueduct of midbrain, Cerebral aqueduct	SYLVIUS, Franciscus (originally De La BOË, François), 1614–1672, Physician in Amsterdam and Professor of Practical Medicine in Leyden
SYLVIAN fissure, SYLVIAN sulcus	Lateral sulcus of cerebrum	SYLVIUS, Franciscus, see before

English Eponym	Anatomical Term	Name and Related Data
TAWARA, Node of, ASCHOFF-TAWARA node	Atrioventricular node	TAWARA, Sunao, 1873–1952, Professor of Pathology in Fukuoka/Japan, before assistant of Aschoff in Marburg; ASCHOFF, Karl Albert Ludwig, see there
TENON´s capsule	Fascial sheath of eyeball	TENON, Jacques René, 1724–1816, Surgeon, Ophthalmologist, and Professor of Pathology in Paris
THEBESIAN valve	Valve of coronary sinus	THEBESIUS, Adam Christian, 1686–1732, native Silesian, Anatomist and Pathologist in Leyden, later Physician in Hirschberg/Silesia
TRENDELENBURG´s sign	(Dipping gait in case of defects of the hip abductors)	TRENDELENBURG, Wilhelm, 1844–1924, Professor of Surgery in Rostock, Bonn, and later in Leipzig
VALSALVA, Sinus of	Aortic sinus	VALSALVA, Antonio Maria, 1666–1723, Professor of Anatomy in Bologna, teacher of Morgagni
VATER´s papilla, Tubercle of VATER	Major duodenal papilla	VATER, Abraham, 1684–1751, Professor of Anatomy and Botany in Wittenberg, later Professor of Pathology and Therapeutics at the same University
VICQ D´AZYR´s bundle	Mammillothalamic fasciculus	VICQ D´AZYR, Félix, 1748–1794, Anatomist and Physician in Paris, Physician to Queen Marie-Antoinette of France
VIDIAN artery	Artery of pterygoid canal	VIDIUS, Vidus (originally GUIDI, Guido), 1500 – about 1567, native Italian, Professor of Medicine in Paris, later Professor of Philosophy and Medicine in Pisa, Physician to King Francis I of France, teacher of Vesalius
VIDIAN canal	Pterygoid canal	VIDIUS, Vidus, see before
VIDIAN nerve	Nerve of pterygoid canal	VIDIUS, Vidus, see before
WALDEYER´s ring	Pharyngeal lymphoid ring	WALDEYER-HARTZ, von, Heinrich Wilhelm Gottfried, 1836–1921, Professor of Pathological Anatomy in Breslau, later Professor of Anatomy in Strasbourg and Berlin
WARD´s triangle	(Triangle deficient in spongy bone in the neck of femur)	WARD, Frederick Oldfried, 1818–1877, Physician in London
WHARTON´s duct	Submandibular duct	WHARTON, Thomas, about 1616–1673, Physician in London
WILLIS, Circle of	Cerebral arterial circle	WILLIS, Thomas, 1621–1675, Professor of Natural Philosophy in Oxford and Physician in London, Physician to King James II of England
WINSLOW, Foramen of	Omental foramen, Epiploic foramen	WINSLOW, Jacob Benignus, 1669–1760, native Dane, Professor of Anatomy, Medicine, and Surgery in Paris
WIRSUNG, Duct of	Pancreatic duct	WIRSUNG, Johann Georg, 1600–1643, native German, Professor of Anatomy in Padua
WRISBERG, Ligament of	Posterior meniscofemoral ligament	WRISBERG, Heinrich August, 1739–1808, Professor of Anatomy in Göttingen
ZEISIAN glands, Glands of ZEIS	Sebaceous glands of eyelid	ZEIS, Eduard, 1807–1868, Physician in Dresden and Professor of Surgery in Marburg
ZENKER´s diverticulum	(Pulsion diverticulum at the transition of pharynx to esophagus)	ZENKER, von, Friedrich Albert, 1825–1898, Professor of Pathology in Dresden and Erlangen
ZINN, Anulus of	Common tendinous ring of extra-ocular muscles	ZINN, Johann Gottfried, 1727–1759, Professor of Anatomy and Medicine as well as Director of the Botanical Gardens in Göttingen
ZINN, Zonule of	Ciliary zonule	ZINN, Johann Gottfried, see before

Alphabetical Index of Anatomical Terms with Corresponding Eponyms

Anatomical Terms	Common English Eponyms
Accessory pancreatic duct	SANTORINI´s duct
Adductor canal	HUNTER´s canal
Anal columns	Columns of MORGAGNI
Anomalous tubercle of tooth	CARABELLI formation, Cusp of CARABELLI
Anterior process of malleus	FOLLIAN process
Anterior spinocerebellar tract	GOWERS´ tract
Aortic sinus	Sinus of VALSALVA
Aqueduct of midbrain	SYLVIAN aqueduct, Aqueduct of SYLVIUS
Arachnoid granulations	PACCHIONIAN granulations
Arcuate line of rectus sheath	Arcuate line of DOUGLAS, Arch of DOUGLAS, Line of DOUGLAS
Artery of pterygoid canal	VIDIAN artery
Atrioventricular bundle	Bundle of HIS
Atrioventricular node	ASCHOFF-TAWARA node
Auricular tubercle	DARWIN´s tubercle
Buccal fat pad	BICHAT´s fat pad
Bulbo-urethral gland	COWPER´s gland
Calcaneal tendon	Achilles tendon
Cardial notch	Angle of HIS
Carotid tubercle	CHASSAIGNAC´s tubercle
Caudate lobe of liver	SPIEGELIAN lobe
Celiac trunk	HALLER´s tripus
Central sulcus of cerebrum	Fissure of ROLANDO, Sulcus of ROLANDO
Cerebral aqueduct	SYLVIAN aqueduct, Aqueduct of SYLVIUS
Cerebral arterial circle	Circle of WILLIS
Chyle cistern	Cistern of PECQUET
Ciliary glands	MOLL´s glands
Ciliary zonule	Zonule of ZINN
Circular folds of small intestine	KERCKRING´s valves
Cisterna chyli	Cistern of PECQUET
Clavipectoral triangle	MOHRENHEIM´s fossa
Cleavage lines	LANGER´s lines
Cochlear ganglion	CORTI´s ganglion, Ganglion of CORTI
Common tendinous ring of extra-ocular muscles	Anulus of ZINN
Confluence of sinuses	Torcular of HEROPHILUS
Corniculate cartilage	SANTORINI´s cartilage
Cremasteric fascia	COOPER´s fascia
Cribriform fascia	HESSELBACH´s fascia
Cuneate fasciculus	BURDACH´s tract

Anatomical Terms	Common English Eponyms
Deep fascia of penis	BUCK´s fascia
Deep part of palpebral part of orbicularis oculi muscle	HORNER´s muscle
Deltopectoral triangle	MOHRENHEIM´s fossa
Diagonal band	BROCA´s diagonal band
Dorsal pancreatic artery	HALLER´s artery
Dorsal spinocerebellar tract	FLECHSIG´s tract
Dorsal tubercle of radius	LISTER´s tubercle
Ductus arteriosus	BOTALLO´s duct
Ductus venosus	Duct of ARANTIUS
Epiploic foramen	Foramen of WINSLOW
Facial canal	FALLOPIAN canal
Fascia of penis	BUCK´s fascia
Fascial sheath of eyeball	TENON´s capsule
Femoral septum	CLOQUET´s septum
Femoral triangle	SCARPA´s triangle
Fibrous capsule and perivascular fibrous capsule of liver	GLISSON´s capsule, Capsule of GLISSON
Frontopontine fibers	Tract of ARNOLD
Gracile fasciculus	GOLL´s tract
Great cerebral vein	GALEN´s vein, Vein of GALEN
Greater vestibular gland	BARTHOLIN´s gland
Hepatorenal recess of subhepatic space	MORISON´s pouch
Hippocampus proper	Ammon´s horn
Ileal orifice	BAUHIN´s valve
Incisive canal	STENSEN´s canal
Inferior lumbar triangle	Triangle of PETIT
Inguinal ligament	POUPART´s ligament
Inguinal triangle	HESSELBACH´s triangle
Interfascicular fasciculus	SCHULTZE´s comma tract
Interfoveolar ligament	HESSELBACH´s ligament
Interventricular foramen	Foramen of MONRO
Lacrimal fold	HASNER´s valve
Lacunar inguinal ligament	GIMBERNAT´s ligament
Laryngeal prominence of thyroid cartilage	Adam´s apple
Laryngeal ventricle	Ventricle of MORGAGNI
Lateral and medial arcuate ligaments of diaphragm	HALLER´s arches
Lateral aperture of fourth ventricle	Foramen of LUSCHKA
Lateral sulcus of cerebrum	SYLVIAN fissure, SYLVIAN sulcus
Ligamentum arteriosum	BOTALLO´s ligament
Ligamentum venosum	Ligament of ARANTIUS

Anatomical Terms	Common English Eponyms
Linea semilunaris	SPIEGEL´s line, SPIGHEL´s line
Long thoracic nerve	BELL´s nerve
Lumbocostal triangle	BOCHDALEK´s triangle
Major duodenal papilla	VATER´s papilla, Tubercle of VATER
Major sublingual duct	BARTHOLIN´s duct
Mammillotegmental fasciculus	GUDDEN´s tract
Mammillothalamic fasciculus	VICQ D´AZYR´s bundle
Maxillary sinus	HIGHMORE´s cavity, Antrum of HIGHMORE
Median aperture of fourth ventricle	Foramen of MAGENDIE
Mediastinum of testis	Body of HIGHMORE, Corpus of HIGHMORE
Middle transverse fold of rectum	HOUSTON´s valve, KOHLRAUSCH´s fold, HOUSTON-KOHLRAUSCH fold
Nasopalatine nerve	SCARPA´s nerve
Nerve of pterygoid canal	VIDIAN nerve
Nodules of semilunar cusps	Nodules of ARANTIUS
Oblique vein of left atrium of heart	MARSHALL´s vein
Omental foramen	Foramen of WINSLOW
Optic radiation	GRATIOLET´s radiation
Pancreatic duct	Duct of WIRSUNG
Pancreatic islets	Islets of LANGERHANS
Parotid duct	STENSEN´s duct
Pars flaccida of tympanic membrane	SHRAPNELL´s membrane
Pectineal inguinal ligament	COOPER´s ligament (groin)
Perforating veins of lower limb	BOYD´s, COCKETT´s, and DODD´s veins
Petrotympanic fissure	GLASERIAN fissure
Pharyngeal lymphoid ring	WALDEYER´s ring
Pharyngeal recess	Fossa of ROSENMÜLLER
Pharyngotympanic tube	EUSTACHIAN tube
Posterior meniscofemoral ligament	Ligament of WRISBERG
Posterior spinocerebellar tract	FLECHSIG´s tract
Proximal deep inguinal lymph node	CLOQUET´s gland, CLOQUET´s node, ROSENMÜLLER´s gland, ROSENMÜLLER´s node, ROSENMÜLLER-CLOQUET lymph node
Pterygoid canal	VIDIAN canal
Pudendal canal	ALCOCK´s canal
Punctum nervosum	ERB´s point
Recto-uterine fold	Fold of DOUGLAS
Recto-uterine pouch	Pouch of DOUGLAS

Anatomical Terms	Common English Eponyms
Reflected inguinal ligament	COLLES´ ligament
Renal columns	BERTIN´s columns
Renal fascia	GEROTA´s capsule, GEROTA´s fascia
Retrocardial space	HOLZKNECHT´s space
Retropubic space	RETZIUS´ space, Cave of RETZIUS
Scleral venous sinus	Canal of SCHLEMM
Sebaceous glands of eyelid	ZEISIAN glands, Glands of ZEIS
Semilunar line	SPIEGEL´s line, SPIGHEL´s line
Sinu-atrial node	Node of KEITH-FLACK
Spaces of iridocorneal angle	Spaces of FONTANA
Spiral fold of cystic duct	HEISTER´s valve
Spiral organ	CORTI´s organ, Organ of CORTI
Sternal angle	Angle of LOUIS
Sternocostal triangle	LARREY´s fissure
Subendocardial branches of atrioventricular bundle	PURKINJE fibers
Submandibular duct	WHARTON´s duct
Subthalamic nucleus	Nucleus of LUYS, Corpus LUYSI
Superior tarsal muscle	MÜLLER´s muscle
Suspensory ligaments of breast	COOPER´s ligaments (breast)
Tarsal glands	MEIBOMIAN glands
Tension lines	LANGER´s lines
Transverse fold of rectum (middle of three)	HOUSTON´s valve, KOHLRAUSCH´s fold, HOUSTON-KOHLRAUSCH fold
Transverse temporal gyri	HESCHL´s transverse convolutions
Trigeminal cave	MECKEL´s cave
Trigeminal ganglion	GASSERIAN ganglion
Tympanic nerve	JACOBSON´s nerve
Tympanic plexus	JACOBSON´s plexus
Ulnar canal	Loge de GUYON
Urethral glands of male urethra	Glands of LITTRÉ
Uterine tube	FALLOPIAN tube
Uterovaginal plexus	FRANKENHÄUSER´s ganglion
Valve of coronary sinus	THEBESIAN valve
Valve of inferior vena cava	EUSTACHIAN valve
Ventral spinocerebellar tract	GOWERS´ tract
Vesicular ovarian follicles	GRAAFIAN follicles
Vestibular ganglion	SCARPA´s ganglion
Vestibular surface of cochlear duct	REISSNER´s membrane

Subject Index

Volume numbering is given in bold print, followed by page numbers.
Adjectives generally precede nouns (as in the index of the Terminologia Anatomica).
Brackets in the text of illustrations were omitted in the subject index.

A

B

C

D

E

F

G

H

J

M

P

S

T

U

V

W

X

Y

Z